ESSENTIALS OF MEDICAL LABORATORY PRACTICE

ESSENTIALS OF MEDICAL LABORATORY PRACTICE

Constance L. Lieseke, CMA (AAMA), PBT, MLT(ASCP)
Medical Assisting Faculty and Program Coordinator
Business and Technology Division
Olympic College
Bremerton, Washington

Elizabeth A. Zeibig, PhD, MLS(ASCP)
Associate Dean for Graduate Education
Doisy College of Health Sciences
Associate Professor
Department of Clinical Laboratory Science
Saint Louis University
St. Louis, Missouri

F.A. Davis Company • Philadelphia

F.A. Davis Company
1915 Arch Street
Philadelphia, PA 19103
www.fadavis.com

Printed in the United States of America

Last digit indicates print number: 10 9 8 7 6 5 4 3 2 1

Senior Acquisitions Editor: Andy McPhee
Manager of Content Development: George W. Lang
Developmental Editor: Karen Lynn Carter
Design and Illustration Manager: Carolyn O'Brien

As new scientific information becomes available through basic and clinical research, recommended treatments and drug therapies undergo changes. The author(s) and publisher have done everything possible to make this book accurate, up to date, and in accord with accepted standards at the time of publication. The author(s), editors, and publisher are not responsible for errors or omissions or for consequences from application of the book, and make no warranty, expressed or implied, in regard to the contents of the book. Any practice described in this book should be applied by the reader in accordance with professional standards of care used in regard to the unique circumstances that may apply in each situation. The reader is advised always to check product information (package inserts) for changes and new information regarding dose and contraindications before administering any drug. Caution is especially urged when using new or infrequently ordered drugs.

Library of Congress Cataloging-in-Publication Data

Lieseke, Constance L.
    Essentials of medical laboratory practice / Constance L. Lieseke, Elizabeth A. Zeibig.
        p. ; cm.
    Includes bibliographical references.
    ISBN 978-0-8036-1899-2
    I. Zeibig, Elizabeth A. II. Title.
    [DNLM: 1. Laboratory Techniques and Procedures. 2. Laboratories--organization & administration. 3. Laboratory Personnel--standards. QY 25]
    610.78--dc23
                            2011047184

Authorization to photocopy items for internal or personal use, or the internal or personal use of specific clients, is granted by F.A. Davis Company for users registered with the Copyright Clearance Center (CCC) Transactional Reporting Service, provided that the fee of $.25 per copy is paid directly to CCC, 222 Rosewood Drive, Danvers, MA 01923. For those organizations that have been granted a photocopy license by CCC, a separate system of payment has been arranged. The fee code for users of the Transactional Reporting Service is: 978-0-8036-1899-2/12 0 + $.25.

I could not have completed this immense task without the love and support of my family. This book is dedicated to:

Dan, my best friend and the love of my life.

Caty and Clint, who give my life meaning and inspire me to do my best.

My mother, LaVonne, who taught me about hard work and determination.

CLL

This book is dedicated to:

My coauthor, Constance Lieseke, who took on more than she initially bargained for and who worked tirelessly to bring the book to fruition. I am proud to have been part of this project with her.

My mother, Shirley Gockel, for her unending support and love.

My boyfriend Robert (Bob) A. Blessing for being my source of strength, support, and love and for helping me get my life organized and in order—You are truly my "blessing."

AZ

The clinical laboratory plays an important role in patient care by providing timely, accurate, reliable test results to health-care team members. The results provided by the clinical laboratory are used by appropriate team members to make important diagnosis, treatment, and monitoring decisions. With recent advances in technology, some laboratory tests may now be performed by appropriately trained individuals in alternative settings, such as in physician offices. Medical assistants and phlebotomists may be called upon to perform this testing. It is thus imperative that individuals who collect or oversee collection of samples for laboratory testing, perform laboratory tests, or interpret laboratory test results be educated in this important area of medicine.

The purpose of this text is to introduce the reader to the clinical laboratory. The text is organized into six sections. Each of these sections is presented as a complete package. Section I covers the structure and organization of the clinical laboratory and important considerations, including regulations, safety, quality, legal and ethical issues, and laboratory equipment. Section II introduces the importance of techniques associated with proper specimen collection and handling. The remaining sections are dedicated to specific laboratory tests organized by general type: hematology, chemistry, urinalysis, and immunology.

Each section opens with *On the Horizon,* an overview of the chapters in that section. *On the Horizon* consists of a content overview, and a description of the relevance of the content to medical assistants and other health-care professionals. A patient scenario called *Case in Point* follows, and then a series of questions about upcoming content, called *Questions for Consideration.* Completing this section are brief narratives that summarize each chapter in the section.

Chapters begin with a Chapter Outline for easy reference. Learning Outcomes appear next. These serve as a helpful resource to guide readers as they study chapter content. A list of References to the Commission on Accreditation of Allied Health Education Programs (CAAHEP) and the Accrediting Bureau of Health Education Schools (ABHES) standards appear after the Learning Outcomes. Key Terms then follow organized in alphabetical order. Each key term is bolded and defined, as appropriate, where the term first appears in the text.

Test Your Knowledge sections offer self-assessment questions coded to the appropriate learning outcomes and are strategically placed throughout the chapter. Tables, figures, and procedures coded to CAAHEP and ABHES standards complement the organized, logically presented chapter content. Following a chapter summary readers have an opportunity to review content through a series of questions and a chapter case study, a component called *Time to Review.* A list of resources and suggested readings is included at the end of each chapter.

The feature *What Does It All Mean?* is located at the end of each section and reiterates the purpose of the section and its importance to medical assistants and other health-care professionals. The case study introduced in *On the Horizon* is revisited here and discussed. This discussion does not include the answers to questions posed for consideration. The answers to those questions may be found in the Instructor's Guide.

An interactive CD-ROM is packaged with this text, allowing students an opportunity to apply their knowledge in a variety of situations. There are a total of 29 exercises available in the following formats: Don't Tip the Scale, Drag and Drop, Multiple Choice, Picture It, and Quiz Show.

Students will find an additional 12 interactive activities on the F.A. Davis website at http://www.davisplus.fadavis.com/ keyword Lieseke. Instructors will find an electronic test bank, chapter-by-chapter PowerPoints, and numerous other instructional resources on DavisPlus.

In addition to the core chapter content, a comprehensive list of abbreviations is included at the beginning of the book for quick reference. A list of all CAAHEP and ABHES competencies covered in each chapter also appears in the front of the book, to quickly access information about specific procedures. A list of reference ranges for common laboratory tests are included in the appendices and a complete glossary of key terms follows.

We've made every effort to create an accurate, reader-friendly, informative text that contains practical information about the clinical laboratory and the medical assistant's role in it. We hope you find this book to be a rich and rewarding resource for your studies.

— *Constance A. Lieseke*
Elizabeth A. Zeibig

Nikki A. Marhefka, EdM, MT(ASCP), CMA (AAMA)
Medical Assistant Program Director
Central Penn College
Summerdale, Pennsylvania

Nancy M. Jones-Bermea, BS (Education), BA (Education), BS (Business Administration)
Professor, Business and Technology Division
Olympic College
Bremerton, Washington

Roxanne Alter, MS, MT(ASCP)
Assistant Professor
Clinical Laboratory Science Program
University Nebraska Medical Center
School of Allied Health Professions
Omaha, Nebraska

Lou M. Brown, MT(ASCP), CMA (AAMA)
Program Director
Medical Assisting and Phlebotomy
Wayne Community College
Goldsboro, North Carolina

Catherine Chevalier, CMA (AAMA), CPT, AS
Externship Coordinator and Assistant Professor
Medical Assisting
Hesser College
Manchester, New Hampshire

Susan Conforti, EdD, MT(ASCP)SBB
Assistant Professor
Medical Laboratory Technology Program
Farmingdale State College
School of Health Sciences
Farmingdale, New York

Andrea Renea Craven, MLT, RMA, BCLS
Instructor
Medical Assisting
Richmond Community College
Hamlet, North Carolina

Anne Davis-Johnson CMA (AAMA)
Medical Assisting Instructor
Health Sciences
Central Carolina Community College
Lillington, North Carolina

Deborah R. Flowers, MS
Instructor
Medical Assisting
Guilford Technical Community College
Jamestown, North Carolina

Mary Gjernes, MLT(ASCP), CLT, CMA (AAMA)
Director
Medical Assisting Program
Presentation College
Allied Health Department
Aberdeen, South Dakota

Cheri Goretti, MA, MT(ASCP), CMA (AAMA)
Associate Professor and Coordinator
Medical Assisting and Allied Health Programs
Quinebaug Valley Community College
Danielson, Connecticut

Debbie Heinritz, MT(ASCP), CLS(NCA)
Instructor
Clinical Laboratory Technician Program
Northeast Wisconsin Technical College
Health Sciences Department
Green Bay, Wisconsin

Lynne Hendrick, CMA (AAMA)
Instructor and Chair
Medical Assistant Program
Globe University Minnesota School of Business
Elk River, Minnesota

Hiba M. Ismail, MLS(ASCP)
Instructor
Health and Human Services
Youngstown State University
Youngstown, Ohio

Sharon M. King, RT(CSMLS), BS, MEd, H(ASCP)
Instructor
Allied Health
Massasoit Community College
Canton, Massachusetts

Michelle Mantooth, MSc, MLS(ASCP), CG (ASCP)
Faculty
Allied Health
Trident Technical College
Charleston, South Carolina

Patrice Nadeau, MS MT(ASCP)
Program Director, Medical Assistant
Health and Human Services
Dakota County Technical College
Rosemount, Minnesota

Joyce B. Thomas, CMA (AAMA)
Instructor
Medical Assisting
Central Carolina Community College
Pittsboro, North Carolina

Lynette M. Veach, CMA, MLT(ASCP)
Former adjunct faculty member
Medical Assisting Technology
Columbus State Community College
Columbus, Ohio

Jo Ann Wilson, PhD
Professor, Director of Professional Programs
Biological Sciences
Florida Gulf Coast University
Fort Myers, Florida

Stacey F. Wilson, MT/PT(ASCP), CMA (AAMA), MHA
Program Chair
Medical Assisting
Cabarrus College of Health Sciences
Concord, North Carolina

Carole A. Zeglin, MS, BS, MT, RMA
Asst. Professor/Director Medical Assisting/
    Phlebotomy Programs
Health Professions
Westmoreland County Community College
Youngwood, Pennsylvania

Dianna Zometsky, CMA (AAMA), CMM
Medical Assisting Instructor
Health Science
Lorenzo Walker Institute of Technology
Naples, Florida

Acknowledgments

We would like to express our gratitude to the colleagues, friends, and family members who have provided resources, technical advice, and support throughout this endeavor. We would like to offer a special thank you to:

- Nancy M. Jones-Bermea, for her photography skills and patience while shooting the majority of the photos in the textbook.

- Caitlin Lieseke, who contributed to the ancillary development for this book.

- Clinton Lieseke, who created the PowerPoint slides for the instructor resources.

In addition, we would like to acknowledge these professionals from F.A. Davis:

- Christa Fratantoro, Senior Acquisitions Editor, for introducing Beth to Andy McPhee.

- Andy McPhee, Senior Acquisitions Editor, who enticed Beth to start this project, then continued to provide support and guidance to both of us as we completed the task.

- Karen Lynn Carter, Developmental Editor, whose patience and guidance was essential to our work.

- Yvonne N. Gillam, Developmental Editor, whose detailed instructions provided structure as needed.

- Stephanie Rukowicz, Associate Developmental Editor, for her patience with our questions and her assistance with the ancillaries for the text.

- Jennifer Pine, Senior Developmental Editor, for all her help and enthusiasm at Book Camp.

- The rest of the members of our F. A. Davis team.

List of Procedures

Ab: Antibody

ABGs: Arterial blood gases

ABN: Advanced Beneficiary Notice of Noncoverage

ABO: Blood Group

ACTH: Adrenocorticotropic hormone

ADA: American Diabetes Association

ADH: Antidiuretic hormone

Ag: Antigen

AIDS: Acquired immune deficiency syndrome

ALP: Alkaline phosphatase

ALT: Alanine aminotransferase

AMT: American Medical Technologists

ANA: Antinuclear antibody

aPTT: Activated partial thromboplastin time (PTT)

ASAP: As soon as possible

ASCP: American Society for Clinical Pathology

ASO: Antistreptolysin O

AST: Aspartate aminotransferase

BBPs: Bloodborne pathogens

bid: Two times daily

BMI: Body mass index

BMP: Basic metabolic panel

BNP: Brain natriuretic peptide

BSI: Body substance isolation

BT: Bleeding time

BUN: Blood urea nitrogen

Bx: Biopsy

C&S: Culture and sensitivity

Ca: Calcium

CAP: College of American Pathologists

CBC: Complete blood count

CDC: Centers for Disease Control and Prevention

CEA: Carcinoembryonic antigen

CK: Creatine kinase

CK-BB, -MB, -MM: Creatine kinase isoenzymes

Cl: Chloride

CLIA '88: Clinical Laboratory Improvement Amendment of 1988

CLSI: Clinical and Laboratory Standards Institute

CMP: Comprehensive Metabolic Panel

CMS: Centers for Medicare & Medicaid Services

CMV: Cytomegalovirus

CO$_2$: Carbon dioxide

COC: Chain of custody

COLA: Commission on Laboratory Assessment

COPD: Chronic obstructive pulmonary disease

CPT: Current procedural terminology

CRP: C-reactive protein

CSF: Cerebrospinal fluid

DIC: Disseminated intravascular coagulation

Diff: White blood cell differential

DOB: Date of birth

DVT: Deep vein thrombosis

Dx: Diagnosis

EBV: Epstein-Barr virus

ECG/EKG: Electrocardiogram

EDTA: Ethylenediaminetetraacetic acid

EIA: Enzyme immunoassay

ESR: Erythrocyte sedimentation rate

FBS: Fasting blood sugar

FDA: Food and Drug Administration

FDPs: Fibrin degradation products

FOBT: Fecal occult blood testing

FPG: Fasting plasma glucose

FSH: Follicle-stimulating hormone

FTA-ABS: Fluorescent treponemal antibody-absorbed

FUO: Fever of unknown origin

G/gm/g: Gram

GGT: Gamma glutamyl transferase

GH: Growth hormone

GTT: Glucose tolerance test

HAI: Health-care acquired infection

H. pylori: Helicobacter pylori

H&H: Hemoglobin and hematocrit

HAV: Hepatitis A virus

HBIg: Hepatitis B immune globulin

HB$_s$Ag: Hepatitis B surface antigen

HBV: Hepatitis B virus

HCG: Human chorionic gonadotropin

HCl: Hydrochloric acid

HCO$_3$⁻: Bicarbonate

Hct: Hematocrit

HCV: Hepatitis C virus

HDL: High-density lipoprotein

HDN: Hemolytic disease of the newborn

Hgb: Hemoglobin

HgbA1c; HbA1c: Hemoglobin A1c

HHS: United States Department of Health and Human Services

HIPAA: Health Information Portability and Accountability Act

HIV: Human immunodeficiency virus

HLA: Human leukocyte antigen

ICD-9: International Classification of Procedures, 9th edition

IFG: Impaired fasting glucose

iFOB: Immunoassay fecal occult blood

Ig: Immunoglobulin

IGT: Impaired glucose tolerance

IM: Infectious mononucleosis

INR: International normalized ratio

K: Potassium

KOH: Potassium hydroxide

LD: Lactate dehydrogenase

LDL: Low-density lipoprotein

LH: Luteinizing hormone

Li: Lithium

LPN: Licensed practical nurse

Lytes: Electrolytes

MCH: Mean corpuscular hemoglobin

MCHC: Mean corpuscular hemoglobin concentration

MCV: Mean corpuscular volume

MIC: Minimum inhibitory concentration

mg: Milligram

Mg: Magnesium

MI: Myocardial infarction

mL: Milliliter

MRSA: Methicillin-resistant *Staphylococcus aureus*

MSDS: Material safety data sheets

MSH: Melanocyte-stimulating hormone

Na: Sodium

NFPA: National Fire Protection Association

NIH: National Institutes of Health

NP: Nasopharyngeal

NPO: Nothing by mouth

O&P: Ova and parasites

O$_2$: Oxygen

OGTT: Oral glucose tolerance test

OPIM: Other potentially infectious materials

OSHA: Occupational Safety and Health Administration

P: Phosphorus

Pap: Papanicolaou test and stain for detection of cervical cancer

PAP: Prostatic acid phosphatase

PEP: Postexposure prophylaxis

PHI: Protected health information

PKU: Phenylketonuria

Plt: Platelet

POCT: Point-of-care testing

POL: Physician office laboratory

Pp: Postprandial (after eating)

PPE: Personal protective equipment

PPM: Provider-performed microscopy

PPMP: Provider-performed microscopy procedures

Prl: Prolactin

PSA: Prostate-specific antigen

PST: Plasma separator tube

PT: Protime or Prothrombin time

PTH: Parathyroid hormone

QA: Quality assurance

QC: Quality control

qh: Every hour

qid: Four times a day

QNS: Quantity not sufficient

RA: Rheumatoid arthritis

RACE: Rescue, Alarm, Contain, Extinguish

RBC: Red blood cell

Retic: Reticulocyte count

RF: Rheumatoid factor

Rh: Rh (Rhesus) factor present on red blood cells

RIA: Radioimmunoassay

RN: Registered nurse

RPM: Rotations or Revolutions per minute

RPR: Rapid plasma regain

RSV: Respiratory syncytial virus

Sed Rate: Erythrocyte sedimentation rate

SG: Specific gravity

SST: Serum separator tube

STAT: Urgent or immediately

STD: Sexually transmitted disease

T&C: Type and crossmatch

T3: Triiodothyronine

T4: Thyroxine

TAT: Turnaround time

TB: Tuberculosis

TC: Throat culture

TSH: Thyroid-stimulating hormone

VDRL: Venereal Disease Research Laboratory

VLDL: Very Low-density lipoprotein

WBC: White blood cell

WHO: World Health Organization

Contents in Brief

Contents

On the Horizon

Laboratory testing is an essential component of effective patient care. The results obtained from laboratory testing provide valuable information that assists physicians and other primary health providers with the diagnosis and monitoring of disease.

Relevance for the Medical Assistant (Health-Care Provider)

Medical assistants and other health-care support personnel are frequently involved in the collection of samples for laboratory testing. In many settings, these individuals perform select laboratory tests that are typically considered basic and uncomplicated. Laboratorians who have completed extensive education and training are able to perform complex laboratory testing. Medical assistants and other health-care support personnel may be responsible for the collection of samples and, in many cases, performance of the tasks associated with the processing and transport of samples to the laboratory for complex testing. On occasion, these individuals may have the opportunity to examine laboratory test results as part of their encounters with patients.

Case in Point

It is the first week of your student practicum at Maple Grove Clinic. You have been assigned to work for Dr. Pueblo under the direction of your clinical instructor, Doris. The second patient of the day is Mr. Hershey. You observe Doris interact with Mr. Hershey and perform the preliminary appropriate tasks associated with Mr. Hershey's appointment. After examining the patient, Dr. Pueblo emerges and informs Doris that he will be ordering laboratory tests. Doris takes this opportunity to introduce you to the laboratory.

Questions for Consideration:

- Compare and contrast the three phases of laboratory testing: preanalytical, analytical, and postanalytical.
- Government regulations allow medical assistants and other health-care support staff to perform what category of laboratory tests?
- What is the purpose of practicing universal precautions when dealing with laboratory specimens?
- True or False. Laboratory test results can be reported only if the quality control samples are tested and found to be in range.
- What is the name of the federal act that regulates laboratory-testing personnel?

Section I
Overview of the Laboratory

Chapter 1: The Clinical Laboratory provides the reader with basic definitions of terms such as *laboratory test* and *normal range*; identification of the areas of a typical laboratory; and an introduction to preanalytical, analytical, and postanalytical testing. A discussion of the importance of the laboratory and role of the medical assistant and other health-care support personnel as they relate to laboratory testing is presented. The difference between the regulations governing clinical laboratories and laboratories housed in a physician office is introduced in terms of the testing that can be performed in each setting.

Chapter 2: Regulations Governing Laboratory Personnel identifies the individuals who perform testing in clinical laboratories, including the Medical Laboratory Technician (MLT) and the Medical Laboratory Scientist (MLS), along with the range of tasks that each level of practitioner can perform. A detailed description and justification for the role that medical assistants and other health-care support personnel may assume in the laboratory under federal regulations, specifically in a physician office setting, is presented.

Chapter 3: Laboratory Safety and Preventing the Spread of Disease covers associated key concepts and documentation procedures, including those for Material Safety Data Sheets (MSDS); the handling of fire and chemical spills; and biological and electrical considerations. Personal protective equipment (PPE) and hand-washing concepts are addressed. This chapter contains sections dedicated to blood-borne pathogen standards, universal precautions, handling of needles and sharps, and preventing the spread of disease.

Chapter 4: Assuring Quality covers the essential aspects and importance of quality assurance and quality control. The performance and documentation of quality control procedures, as well as the recognition and resolution of quality control results that are not in range, are detailed. The concepts, considerations, and reasoning behind proficiency/competency testing are explored.

Chapter 5: Legal and Ethical Issues explores a number of legal and ethical issues associated with laboratory testing. Topics include the Clinical Laboratory Improvement Act of 1988 (CLIA '88), fraud and abuse, informed consent, "the right to know," and the Health Insurance Portability and Accountability Act (HIPAA).

Chapter 6: Laboratory Equipment introduces the reader to key pieces of equipment used in a typical physician office laboratory, including centrifuges, microscopes, and point-of-care instruments. A brief overview of the principles behind these and other key hematology and chemistry analyzers are introduced and described.

Chapter 1

The Clinical Laboratory

Constance L. Lieseke, CMA (AAMA), MLT, PBT(ASCP)

CHAPTER OUTLINE

Learning Outcomes

After reading this chapter, the successful student will be able to:

1-1 Define the key terms for this chapter.

1-2 Describe the different types of laboratories presented in the text and the common tests available in each.

1-3 Identify the different departments in a hospital or reference laboratory and list some of the tests performed in these departments.

1-4 Provide several reasons that laboratory testing might be performed.

1-5 Explain the roles a medical assistant might play in a laboratory setting.

1-6 List and justify the various pieces of information that must be included on a laboratory requisition.

1-7 Explain the concept of Advance Beneficiary Notice of Noncoverage (ABN) and how it affects laboratory reimbursement.

1-8 Explain the purpose of a laboratory directory, as well as how a laboratory directory may be used when preparing to collect a specimen.

1-9 Compare and contrast the function of a laboratory requisition and a laboratory report.

1-10 Identify the different phases of laboratory testing, and explain the flow of the laboratory testing process.

1-11 Provide examples of preanalytical, analytical, and postanalytical procedures and how they affect the quality of laboratory testing.

CAAHEP/ABHES STANDARDS

 CAAHEP 2008 Standards

II.A.2: Distinguish between normal and abnormal test results

 ABHES Standards

- None

KEY TERMS

Advance Beneficiary Notice of Noncoverage (ABN)	ICD-9 code	Point-of-care testing (POCT)
Ambulatory	Laboratory	Profiles
Asymptomatic	Laboratory directory	Quality control (QC)
CLIA-waived	Laboratory report	Reference laboratories
Complexity	Laboratory requisition	Reference ranges
CPT code	Normal ranges	Serum
Efficacy	Panels	Specimens
Hospital laboratories	Physician office laboratories (POLs)	STAT
	Plasma	

The clinical laboratory plays a vital role in patient care. Diagnostic puzzles are solved each day by using results obtained from testing procedures performed on blood, tissue, and other body fluids. Quality patient care depends on excellent laboratory practices, so it is important to build a solid understanding of the structure and function of the clinical laboratory before performing testing procedures. This chapter explains the reasons that laboratory testing may be ordered and identifies the types of laboratories where testing is performed. The role of the medical assistant in the clinical laboratory as well as the roles played by other laboratory personnel are also introduced. To expand understanding of how the clinical laboratory operates, the flow of information in the laboratory setting is also explained.

THE CLINICAL LABORATORY

A clinical **laboratory** is any place where **specimens** from the human body may be collected, processed, examined, or analyzed. With this broad definition in mind, then, a laboratory might be someone's home, a long-term care facility, the office of a health-care provider, a free clinic, a hospital, a small facility used strictly for specimen collection and processing, or a large and complex reference laboratory. As of January 2010, the Centers for Medicare & Medicaid Services identified more than 216,000 clinical laboratories in the United States.[1] To simplify our discussion of the various types of laboratories, we will classify them into three basic groups as described below (Table 1-1).

Physician Office Laboratories

Physician office laboratories (POLs) are clinical laboratories within physician offices where laboratory testing is carried out on specimens obtained from the practices' own patients. More than half of all the laboratories in the United States are POLs. This type of laboratory can be advantageous because the results for tests performed on site are available quickly and patient treatment can begin immediately if necessary. Testing and specimen collection in these office laboratories may be accomplished by various members of the health-care team, such as medical assistants,

[1]Data From CLIA Update—January 2010
Division of Laboratory Services
Centers for Medicare & Medicaid Services
Laboratories by Type of Facility
https://www.cms.gov/CLIA/downloads/factype.pdf

TABLE 1-1	
Types of Laboratories and Sample of Testing Performed	
Type of Laboratory	**Testing Performed**
Physician office laboratory	CLIA-waived tests Moderate complexity testing (with appropriate training, staffing, and supervision) Microscopic examinations (performed by health-care provider or qualified staff)
Hospital laboratory	CLIA-waived tests CLIA moderate- and high-complexity tests (based on the needs of the patients served in the facility) Point-of-care testing Microscopic examinations
Reference laboratory	CLIA-waived tests Moderate- and high-complexity tests Microscopic examinations

clinical or medical laboratory technicians who have been trained in laboratory testing, or phlebotomists who are trained to draw blood and perform some simple laboratory procedures. These **ambulatory** (outpatient) laboratories generally perform low **complexity** tests that are designated as Clinical Laboratory Improvement Amendment–waived (**CLIA-waived**) tests by the U.S. Food and Drug Administration (FDA). CLIA-waived tests are laboratory examinations and procedures that use simple and accurate methods requiring very little interpretation to report correct results. These tests may include the following:

- Rapid microbiology testing for the presence of group A *Streptococcus* and influenza
- Urine analysis
- Pregnancy testing
- Tests such as those for mononucleosis, *Helicobacter pylori*, and HIV
- Coagulation testing to monitor patients who are taking anticoagulants
- Glucose levels and other tests used to monitor diabetic patients
- Fecal occult blood tests for the presence of blood in the stool
- Cholesterol testing

Physician office laboratories may also provide testing that is more complex if staff members are properly trained to perform such procedures. More details about the Clinical Laboratory Improvement Amendment and the classification of laboratory tests are provided in Chapter 2.

Hospital Laboratories

Hospital laboratories generally offer laboratory testing that meets the needs of their respective institution. For instance, if a hospital specializes in a certain type of surgical procedure or treatment, the hospital laboratory will offer extensive testing in that specialty area, in addition to the standard tests required to monitor the health of the other patients in the hospital. In most situations, hospital laboratories perform high volumes of routine test procedures. Hospital laboratories may also serve as a reference laboratory for the local community, especially for **STAT** testing needs. (STAT tests are those that require immediate results.) Tests performed at a hospital laboratory may include the following:

- Electrolytes
- Kidney function tests
- Liver function analysis
- Blood typing and crossmatches for transfusions
- Identification of microorganisms and antibiotic sensitivity testing
- Urine analysis
- Coagulation testing
- Cardiac enzyme assays
- Complete blood counts (CBCs) and other hematology testing

Hospital laboratories may also offer another method for testing samples, called **point-of-care testing (POCT)**. Point-of-care tests are actually performed at the patient's bedside rather than in the laboratory, using a portable instrument that gives immediate results. These tests may be performed by laboratory personnel or in some situations by other hospital employees who have been trained to perform the testing.

Reference Laboratories

Reference laboratories perform more tests annually than either POLs or the hospital laboratories, processing perhaps thousands of specimens per day. These tests include those that are performed at hospital laboratories, but reference laboratories may offer specialized testing that is not performed at either hospital laboratories or POLs. Specimens may be sent to a reference laboratory from all over the country.

LABORATORY DEPARTMENTS

Testing in hospital and reference laboratories is usually departmentalized for efficiency, as presented in Table 1-2. This allows all testing that uses similar instrumentation or methods to be performed in the same area of the laboratory. These departments may include the following:

- **Specimen Processing:** The area of the laboratory where all incoming specimens are sorted, accessioned into the computer system of the laboratory, and appropriately labeled for transport to their respective departments for testing. The specimen processing department may also prepare specimens for transport to reference laboratories.

- **Hematology:** Whole blood testing, which focuses on the formed elements (the blood cells) in the blood. Coagulation testing is also performed in this department.

- **Clinical Chemistry:** Testing performed on **plasma** or **serum** (the liquid portion of the blood) and includes analysis of the substances dissolved in the bloodstream. Most testing is automated, and many of the tests are performed as panels or groups of tests.

- **Serology/Immunohematology:** Testing that focuses primarily on the presence of antigens or antibodies on cells or in the liquid portion of the blood. Blood typing and antibody screens and crossmatches for transfusions may also be performed in this department.

TABLE 1-2

Summary of Laboratory Departments, Common Tests Performed, and Specimen Types

Laboratory Department	Common Tests Performed	Specimen Types
Specimen Processing	Incoming specimens sorted Specimens accessioned into computer system Specimens labeled and prepared for testing in separate department	All types
Hematology	Complete blood count Hemoglobin and hematocrit measurements Coagulation studies Erythrocyte sedimentation rate Differential white blood cell count Platelet counts	Whole blood
Clinical Chemistry	Electrolytes Glucose Blood urea nitrogen Creatinine Thyroid testing Cardiac enzyme testing Comprehensive metabolic panel Cholesterol/lipid testing Many automated chemistry tests and panels	Serum, plasma, urine, cerebrospinal fluid, amniotic fluid
Serology and Immunohematology	Various tests looking for antigens and/or antibodies such as: RPR Mononucleosis testing HIV tests Chlamydia testing Antistreptolysin O test Pregnancy testing C-reactive protein ABO/Rh blood typing Antibody screens and crossmatches for transfusions Newborn testing Prenatal testing	Serum, plasma, whole blood

TABLE 1-2–cont'd		
Summary of Laboratory Departments, Common Tests Performed, and Specimen Types		
Laboratory Department	**Common Tests Performed**	**Specimen Types**
Urinalysis	Physical appearance of urine Urine chemical analysis Microscopic urine analysis	Urine
Microbiology/Parasitology	Identification of pathogenic microorganisms Streptococcal screens Antibiotic sensitivity testing	Blood, urine, wound specimens, tissue, stool, cerebrospinal fluid, sputum, urethral and vaginal discharge, nails, skin scrapings
Cytology	Examination of various specimens for abnormal cells Chromosomal studies Pap smears	Urine, skin, tissue specimens, sputum
Coagulation	Testing for presence or absence of adequate clotting factors	Whole blood
Histology/Pathology	Examination for abnormal form and structure in tissues	Tissue/organs, biopsy specimens from various parts of the body, preserved and fresh specimens examined

- **Urinalysis:** The physical appearance of urine is assessed, and urine chemical and microscopic analysis is performed.
- **Microbiology/Parasitology:** Identification of pathogenic microorganisms and antibiotic sensitivity testing.
- **Cytology:** Examination of various specimens for abnormal cells, chromosomal studies, Pap smears.
- **Coagulation:** Specimens testing for the presence of various clotting factors.
- **Histology/Pathology:** Tissue samples examined for abnormal function and form.

> **Test Your Knowledge 1-2**
>
> Which laboratory department would perform a test to see if someone had a pathogenic microorganism in a wound?   (Outcome 1-3)

WHY IS LABORATORY TESTING PERFORMED?

Laboratory testing is critical for appropriate patient treatment. The results obtained from a blood test or evaluation of other types of specimens from the human body are essential for the health-care provider to gain information that is not available through the patient history or physical examination. Health-care providers generally order laboratory tests for at least one of these reasons:

1. *To assign a diagnosis.* Laboratory testing may be used to help with a differential diagnosis when the patient's symptoms are vague or similar to those of other disease states. Diagnostic testing can also confirm a clinical diagnosis (such as diabetes or a myocardial infarction) when that confirmation could lead to more effective treatment for the patient. Microbiological testing may also fall into this category, as the identification of the bacteria and/or virus involved in the infection will be essential to establish an appropriate plan of action.

2. *Prevention or early detection of disease through screening tests.* Many chronic health conditions are **asymptomatic** in the early disease stages. If these conditions are identified with routine screening tests (such as cholesterol measurements and routine prostate cancer screening) early in the disease process, treatment may be much more effective in keeping the patient healthy. These screening tests are being ordered with more frequency in the general population as more

information becomes available about the advantages of early diagnosis and treatment.

3. *Ongoing assessment of the patient's progress and treatment.* Once a diagnosis has been established and treatment has begun, it is very important that the patient is monitored closely. This often requires frequent blood tests to determine therapeutic drug levels, hepatic profiles when a particular medication may cause liver damage, or hemoglobin tests to see how effective the treatment might be for someone who is anemic. Patients may need to have their blood drawn daily, monthly, or quarterly. The frequency is dependent on the pathological condition. It may be necessary to use specimens other than blood to monitor the treatment for a patient. Sometimes repeat cultures are also necessary to verify the **efficacy** (effectiveness) of the antibiotic used to fight an infection.

Test Your Knowledge 1-3

When a pregnant young woman sees her nurse-midwife for a routine checkup, the practitioner requests a test to see if the patient is developing diabetes during the pregnancy. Why is the test being performed?
  a. To assign a diagnosis
  b. To screen for prevention or early disease detection
  c. To assess the ongoing status of treatment
  d. None of the above   (Outcome 1-4)

THE ROLE OF THE MEDICAL ASSISTANT IN THE CLINICAL LABORATORY

A medical assistant can contribute in the clinical laboratory in various ways. The comprehensive training received by medical assistants allows them to perform clinical duties with direct patient contact, as well as offering employment opportunities in an administrative capacity. A clinical medical assistant working in a physician office laboratory may be called on to perform phlebotomy or supervise urine drug screen collections for routine employment purposes, educate patients concerning collection protocols, collect and process microbiology specimens, and perform various test procedures. Medical assistants performing clinical duties may also be asked to prepare microscopic specimens for examination, and focus the microscope for providers to evaluate the specimen. In addition, the medical assistant with appropriate training may also perform microscopic examinations such as white blood cell differential counts and urine microscopy examinations.

A clinical medical assistant working in a hospital or reference laboratory may function as a phlebotomist or may work as a laboratory assistant. A laboratory assistant may be responsible for setting up microbiology cultures, answering phones and responding to requests for laboratory results, assisting with bone marrow aspiration or other collection procedures, processing specimens and delivering them to the various laboratory departments, performing CLIA-waived or moderate-complexity tests available in that laboratory setting, or assisting with preparation of tissue and cellular samples for examination. Medical assistants may also perform point-of care testing and assist with quality assurance in the laboratory.

An administrative medical assistant in a laboratory setting might help with inventory and ordering of supplies, data input, answering telephone calls, scheduling, billing and coding, production and transmission of laboratory reports, creation of other laboratory forms, and various nonclinical patient interactions. These duties are necessary in every laboratory, regardless of size or location.

Test Your Knowledge 1-4

True or False: A medical assistant can work only in an administrative capacity in a hospital or reference laboratory.   (Outcome 1-4)

Test Your Knowledge 1-5

Are medical assistants able to perform laboratory testing?   (Outcome 1-5)

INFORMATION FLOW IN THE CLINICAL LABORATORY

In addition to understanding the organization of the clinical laboratory setting and identifying the reason laboratory testing might be performed, it is important to know how information is exchanged within the laboratory. To ensure that laboratory test results are as meaningful as possible to the health-care provider, all those involved with specimen collection, processing, and testing must use the required paperwork and database correctly. This information exchange will involve a **laboratory requisition,** a **laboratory directory,** a computer database, and a **laboratory report.**

Laboratory Requisitions

A laboratory requisition (Fig. 1-1) is the form used by a physician (or other qualified health-care professional) to

CB LABORATORY

Patient (Last, First, MI)		774911
Sex ☐ Male ☐ Female	Date of Birth (required)	
Patient Number	Room #	774911
Guarantor Required if insurance or patient billing	Day Phone	774911
Address	PM Phone	
City State	Zip	774911

CLIENT ACCOUNT NO. 790338
Shore Physicians
13 Waterview Dr.
Seattle, WA 98103
☐ CALL RESULTS TO: 425-377-8571
☐ FAX RESULTS TO: 425-792-1608

INSURANCE INFO (PLEASE ATTACH COPY OF CARD, W/GROUP # & ADDRESS)   774911

ORDERING PRACTITIONER - FULL NAME(S) REQUIRED
DRS NAME (Last, First, MI): _____
ADDL. COPY TO: _____
ADDRESS: _____

PATIENT RELATIONSHIP TO SUBSCRIBER: ☐ SPOUSE ☐ CHILD ☐ OTHER   774911

PHONE: _____ FAX: _____

ADDITIONAL TESTS/COMMENTS - DIAGNOSIS CODES REQUIRED FOR EACH TEST ORDERED

Collection Code: B = LIGHT BLUE   FS = FROZEN SERUM   L = LAVENDER   R = RED TOP (PLAIN)
S = SERUM (GOLD TOP OR TIGER TOP)   U = URINE

TESTS HIGHLIGHTED IN RED OR MARKED WITH A Δ MAY REQUIRE A SIGNED ADVANCE BENEFICIARY NOTICE (ABN), IF BILLING MEDICARE. ADDITIONAL LCD TESTS NOT LISTED MAY REQUIRE AN ABN.

Specimen Information

■ STAT   ☐ Phone ( ) _____ or ☐ Fax ( ) _____ | Collected by | Date Drawn / / | Time Drawn A.M. P.M. | ☐ Fasting ☐ Random | 24 Hour Urine Volume _____

CPT	✓	Tests or Panels	ICD9-CM	CPT	✓	Tests or Panels (cont'd)	ICD9-CM	CPT	Single Tests (cont'd)	ICD9-CM	CPT	✓	Single Tests (cont'd)	ICD9-CM
		Panel or Single tests may be selected				Panel or Single tests may be selected		82378	CEA	S	84702		Beta HCG Quant	S
80051		Electrolytes Panel	S	80069		Renal Function Panel	S	82550	CK (CPK)	S	84146		Prolactin	S
84295		Sodium	S								84153		PSA	S
84132		Potassium	S					80162	Digoxin ★	R	G0103		PSA Screen	S
82435		Chloride	S	84100		Phosphorus	S	80101	Drug, Screen, Urine	U	85610		PT with INR ★	B
82374		Carbon Dioxide	S	80061		Lipid Profile	S	x7					Is pt. taking Coumadin? ☐ Y ☐ N ★	
80048		Basic Metabolic Panel	S	82465		Cholesterol	S	82728	Ferritin	S	85730		PTT ★	B
80051		Na, K, CL, CO2	S	84478		Triglycerides	S	82746	Folate	FS			Is pt. taking Heparin? ☐ Y ☐ N ★	
84520		BUN	S	83718		HDL Cholesterol	S	83001	FSH	FS	85044		Retic Count	L
82310		Calcium	S	80074		Acute Hepatitis Panel	S	82977	Gamma GT	S	86592		RPR	S
82465		Creatinine	S	86709		Hepatitis A Antobidy IGM	S	83036	Hgb A1C (Glycohemo)	L	86762		Rubella Ab	S
82947		Glucose	S	86705		Hepatitis B Core Antibody IGM	S	85014	Hematocrit	L	85651		Sed Rate	L
80053		Comprehensive Metabolic Panel	S					85018	Hemoglobin	L	84480		T3 Total	S
				87340		Hepatitis B Surface Antigen	S	86701	HIV 1 Ab w/Western Blot confirmation	S	84479		T3 Uptake	S
80048		Basic Metabolic Panel	S								84439		T4 Free	S
82040		Albumin	S	86803		Hepatitis C Antibody	S	83540	Iron	S	84436		T4 Total	S
84075		Alkaline Phos.	S					83550	Iron Binding (TIBC)	S	84403		Testosterone Total	S
82247		Bilirubin, Total	S					83615	LD (LDH)	S	80198		Theophylline ★	R
84450		SGOT/AST	S								84443		TSH	S
84460		SGPT/ALT	S	CPT	✓	Single Tests	ICD9-CM	83002	LH Luteinizing Hormone	FS	81001		Urinalysis w/Micro, auto if indicated	U
84155		Total Protein	S	86900		ABO Blood Group	L, R	80178	Lithium	R				
80076		Hepatic Function (Liver) Panel	S	86901		RH (D) Type	L, R	83735	Magnesium	S	82575		Urine Creatinine Clearance 24 hr	U/S
				86850		Antibody Screen	L, R	86308	Mono	S	84156		Urine Total Protein 24 hr	U
82040		Albumin	S					80184	Phenobarbital ★	R	84540		Urine Urea Nitrogen 24 hr	U
82247		Bilirubin, Total	S	82150		Amylase	S	80185	Phenytoin/Dilantin ★	R	CPT	✓	Microbiology	ICD9-CM
82248		Bilirubin, Direct	S	86038		Antinuclear Antibody	S	85049	Platelet Count Auto	L			Aerobic Culture Source _____	
84450		AST/SGOT	S	82607		B-12 Vitamin	FS	84703	Pregnancy, Qual. Serum	S				
84460		ALT/SGPT	S	86141		hs-CRP	S	81025	Pregnancy, Qual. Urine	U			Anaerobic Culture Source _____	
84075		Alkaline Phos.	S	80156		Carbamazepine/Tegretol ★	R		★ REQUIRED LAST CODE					
84155		Total Protein	S	85025		CBC w/auto diff	L		DATE _____ A.M.				Other Source _____	
				85007		Manual Diff.	L		TIME _____ P.M.					

Other Tests

Only tests or Medicare Approved Panels that are medically necessary for the diagnosis or treatment of a Medicare or Medicaid patient will be reimbursed. Screening tests will not be reimbursed and should not be submitted for payment. The OIG states that a physician who orders medically unnecessary tests for which Medicare or Medicaid reimbursement is claimed may be subject to civil penalties under the False Claims Act.

Figure 1-1 Sample laboratory requisition. Current Procedural Terminology © 2011 American Medical Association, All Rights Reserved.

document the tests that are to be performed for a patient. The form is filled out by the health-care provider who orders the test or by the provider's office staff. This requisition must be complete with various data linking the patient to the tests ordered, and must provide billing information for that patient. The laboratory staff will use this requisition to enter the orders into their database for the patient, and the form is often used for reimbursement procedures as well. Although all laboratories may use unique formats, standardized information should be present on all requisitions for testing and reimbursement purposes:

- Patient demographic information, including name, address, phone number, and birth date.
- Patient gender.
- Complete patient insurance and billing information.
- Date and time of collection, and identification of the person who performed the collection.
- Documentation of how the results are to be relayed to the health-care provider who ordered the tests, and documentation of any other practitioner who is to receive a copy of the results.
- Appropriate diagnostic information in the form of an **ICD-9 code** to allow for reimbursement for the test ordered. An ICD-9 code is the numeric indicator for the diagnosis or symptom associated with the laboratory test ordered.
- Test selection, clearly marked with a check, circle, or X in the appropriate area on the requisition. Tests may also be written in if they are not preprinted on the requisition used.
- Any additional comments that may assist with the ordering or interpretation of the test.

Test Your Knowledge 1-6

Why is it important to have the name of the ordering physician/practitioner on a requisition when ordering laboratory testing?   (Outcome 1-6)

Laboratory tests may be ordered as **panels** or **profiles,** which consist of a group of tests that are designed to indicate a problem with a specific organ system or disease process. Tests may also be ordered individually, or the requisition may contain orders for a combination of both. Often the requisitions are organized according to the general types of tests, such as hematology, serology, or chemistry. On the requisition, each test will have a five-digit procedure code (known as a **CPT code),** which is necessary for reimbursement purposes. There may also be a code or symbol included on the requisition, indicating the type of tube or specimen container that is necessary for that specific test. This information is valuable as a quick reference for the phlebotomist when collecting the specimen.

Most requisitions also include some sort of label that can be peeled off and applied to the specimen container. This label may have numbers, bar-code symbols, or both. These labels link the patient information provided on the requisition with that specific sample once it has been entered into the database for the laboratory.

Advance Beneficiary Notice of Noncoverage

An **Advance Beneficiary Notice of Noncoverage (ABN)** is a document that may be necessary to receive

---

Procedure 1-1: Completing a Laboratory Requisition

TASK

Correctly fill out a laboratory requisition, including all necessary information for reimbursement. Include an ABN if necessary.

CAAHEP/ABHES Standards

None

CONDITIONS

- Laboratory requisition
- Patient demographic information
- Patient insurance information
- Laboratory order from qualified health-care professional
- ICD-9 code for diagnosis or symptoms
- Advance Beneficiary Notice of Noncoverage

Procedure	Rationale
1. Greet and identify patient using at least two unique identifiers.	All patients must be identified properly before collecting samples or performing laboratory testing.
2. Verify test ordered.	All laboratory test orders should be verified by checking the chart and/or requisition more than once.
3. Fill in the requisition with the patient's demographic information by printing it clearly, or by using a data entry program if available at your location.	The patient's demographic information (including age and gender) is used for reimbursement as well as establishing reference ranges for the tests ordered.
4. Ask patient for an insurance card if he or she is insured.	The insurance card should be used for the information added to the requisition; do not rely on information that the patient provides from memory.
5. Copy both sides of the insurance card, and add the information to the requisition in the appropriate site.	Be sure to include the insurance identification number as well as the group number for appropriate reimbursement. The back of the card is important to copy, as it provides the insurance company's contact information in case of claim questions.
6. Establish the relationship of the patient to the insured. Document that on the requisition.	Sometimes the patient is not listed on the insurance card; it may be a spouse or a child or other dependent.
7. If the patient has a medication level ordered (such as digoxin), ask when the patient took the last dose. Use the laboratory directory if necessary to verify whether it is the correct time to draw the specimen. Note the time of the last dose on the requisition.	Some medication levels are clinically significant only when drawn at a specific interval after the last dose.
8. If the patient has Medicare Part B as his or her primary insurance coverage, verify whether an Advance Beneficiary Notice of Noncoverage is necessary. This must be completed and signed before the specimen collection begins.	The laboratory may have a database established in which the employee can type in the name of the test ordered and the diagnosis code provided, and the software will be able to determine whether an ABN is necessary. If there is no automated system in place, the employee may need to use an alternative reference. Many laboratories provide their clients with a book of covered diagnosis codes for the tests with limited coverage.
9. Clarify which physician ordered the test and document that on the requisition. If additional copies are to be sent to other health-care providers, add this information to the requisition as well.	Many times the requisitions will be preprinted with the name of the physician office or practice group. It is still necessary to document which physician within the practice actually ordered the laboratory test to be performed.
10. Document whether the test was ordered as STAT or routine.	If the test was ordered as STAT, it needs to be drawn and processed immediately. It may be necessary to contact a laboratory courier to pick up the sample immediately, or to notify the technician that there is a STAT order.

Continued

Procedure 1-1: Completing a Laboratory Requisition—cont'd

Procedure	Rationale
11. Check the requisition for an ICD-9 code for each test to be performed. If a code is not present, contact the health-care provider or check the chart to obtain a code.	An ICD-9 code is necessary for every test for successful reimbursement.
12. Have the patient wait in a comfortable environment until the sample can be collected. Place the requisition in an appropriate location to alert other staff members that a specimen collection is waiting.	Sometimes the employee who fills out the requisition is not the same person who will collect the sample.

reimbursement for laboratory services. It is specifically used for patients who have Medicare Part B as their primary insurance coverage. The purpose of an ABN is to inform Medicare-covered patients that payment may be denied for a specific laboratory test and that the patient will be billed for the full cost of that test if he or she chooses to have it performed. The ABN allows the patients to make an informed decision about whether they wish to have the tests performed, with the realization that they may be responsible for the total cost.

The ABN must be verbally reviewed with the patient, and any questions about potential reimbursement must be answered before it is signed, whether or not the patient wishes to have the laboratory work performed. This process must occur before the specimen is collected from the patient. The person collecting the specimen must ensure that the test ordered has been identified on the ABN form and that there is documentation of the anticipated reason for noncoverage. Figure 1-1 shows an example of an ABN. The employee filling out the form also must provide an estimated cost in writing so that the patient knows what the financial responsibility may be if he or she decides to have the laboratory test performed. The patient's decision about having the test performed must be documented on the form, along with the patient's signature and that day's date. The patient must receive a copy of the form after it is signed, and a copy must also be kept on file with the laboratory.

Medicare coverage for laboratory tests may be denied for various reasons, including frequency of testing, the diagnosis provided by the health-care provider for a specific test, or because the test ordered is considered experimental. Whenever a patient with Medicare coverage has

a specimen collected, the laboratory employee responsible for the specimen collection must verify whether the test ordered will be covered by Medicare for the reason that the test is ordered. The regulations affecting coverage are different for geographical regions across the country, and change frequently. Most laboratories now have a way to verify coverage by using a computer database, but it can be difficult to keep abreast of changes. It is unlawful to have every Medicare patient fill out an ABN "just in case"; it is the responsibility of those collecting the specimen to make their best effort to verify coverage before an ABN is signed.

The format for this Advance Beneficiary Notice of Noncoverage document is defined by the Centers for Medicare & Medicaid Services (CMS), and is updated periodically (CMS document number CMS-R-131). Medicare bases its decision for coverage on "medical necessity" rules, which define those tests that the agency deems medically necessary for specific health conditions, and how frequently these tests should be performed. It is important to remember that just because Medicare has limited coverage on specific tests, the patient should never be told that the health-care provider gave a "bad code" or that the test was ordered for the "wrong reason."

Test Your Knowledge 1-7
What is the purpose of an ABN?   (Outcome 1-7)

Laboratory Directory

As discussed, laboratory requisitions often provide information about what type of tube to use for a blood draw for a specific test by using a code or symbol, but

CB LABORATORY 2692 Millenium Rd. • Seattle, WA 98103   **ADVANCE BENEFICIARY NOTICE (ABN)**
425-353-8778

Patient's Name: _____John Smith_____   Identification Number: ___23995500___

ADVANCE BENEFICIARY NOTICE OF NONCOVERAGE (ABN)

NOTE: If Medicare doesn't pay for the Laboratory Test(s) Below you may have to pay.

Medicare does not pay for everything, even some care that you or your health-care provider have good reason to think you need. We expect Medicare may not pay for the Laboratory Test(s) below.

Laboratory Test(s):	Reason Medicare May Not Pay:	Estimated Cost:
PROSTATIC SPECIFIC AG	Denied as too frequent	$50.10
TSH	Denied for your condition	$41.34

WHAT YOU NEED TO DO NOW:
- Read this notice, so you can make an informed decision about your care.
- Ask us any questions that you may have after you finish reading.
- Choose an option below about whether to receive the Laboratory Test(s) listed above.
   Note: If you choose Option 1 or 2, we may help you use any other insurance that you may have, but Medicare cannot require us to do this.

OPTIONS:	Check only one box. We cannot choose a box for you.

☐ **OPTION 1.** I want the Laboratory Test(s) listed above. You may ask to be paid now, but I also want Medicare billed for an official decision on payment, which is sent to me on a Medicare Summary Notice (MSN). I understand that if Medicare doesn't pay, I am responsible for payment, but **I can appeal to Medicare** by following the directions on the MSN. If Medicare does pay, you will refund any payments I made to you, less co-pays or deductibles.

☐ **OPTION 2.** I want the Laboratory Test(s) listed above, but do not bill Medicare. You may ask to be paid now as I am responsible for payment. **I cannot appeal if Medicare is not billed.**

☐ **OPTION 3.** I do not want the Laboratory Test(s) listed above. I understand with this choice I am not responsible for payment, and **I cannot appeal to see if Medicare would pay**.

Additional Information:

This notice gives our opinion, not an official Medicare decision. If you have any other questions on this notice or Medicare Billing, call **1-800-MEDICARE** (1-800-633-4227/**TTY:** 1-877-486-2048).
Signing below means you have received and understand this notice. You also receive a copy.

Signature:	Date:

According to the Paperwork Reduction Act of 1995, no persons are required to respond to a collection of information unless it displays a valid OMB control number. The valid OMB control number for this information collection is 0938-0566. The time required to complete this information collection is estimated to average 7 minutes per response, including the time to review instructions, search existing data resources, gather the data needed, and complete and review the information collection. If you have comments concerning the accuracy of the time estimate or suggestions for improving this form, please write to: CMS, 7500 Security Boulevard, Attn: PRA reports Clearance Officer, Baltimore, Maryland 21244-1850.

Form CMS-R-131 (03/08)   Form Approved OMB No. 0938-0566

HNL-18 (03/09)   WHITE: LAB COPY   CANARY: PATIENT COPY   **ADVANCE BENEFICIARY NOTICE (ABN)**

Figure 1-2 Example of an Advance Beneficiary Notice of Noncoverage (ABN).

the information provided on the requisition is limited at best. The requisition does not include information about how to process and store the specimen, or what the minimum volume may be for the test ordered. It also does not include information about how often the laboratory performs that specific analysis if the physician needs to know this information. This additional information about specimen collection and handling may be found in a laboratory directory (Fig. 1-3).

POINT OF INTEREST 1-1
Advance beneficiary notice of noncoverage

If a laboratory accepts Medicare assignment, it is not legal to bill Medicare beneficiaries for laboratory tests that are covered by Medicare Part B. However, Medicare does not cover all laboratory tests, so there are many situations in which the health-care providers may order tests that are not covered by Medicare but that provide valuable information for patient treatment. The only way that the laboratory can be reimbursed for these tests is to have the patient complete a valid Advance Beneficiary Notice of Noncoverage, also known as an ABN. This form must be completed and signed prior to the specimen collection. The ABN form informs the Medicare beneficiary of the test that has been ordered, and specifies the reason that Medicare may not pay for the tests, as well as providing the estimated cost for the test. The ABN is necessary in these situations:

- When the test ordered is not medically necessary in Medicare's opinion for the ICD-9 code (diagnosis) that is provided. This situation is also present if there is no ICD-9 code given for the test ordered.
- Many screening tests are not covered by Medicare; these are often not covered if there is no evidence of disease.
- Tests that are ordered more frequently than what is recommended by Medicare.
- Any test that is still considered to be investigational or experimental in nature. These tests have not yet been approved by the FDA.

Often those who work with Medicare patients will use the term *limited coverage* to refer to the rules that govern laboratory reimbursement. This means that Medicare will pay for laboratory tests only when they meet certain criteria. These may be national coverage decisions or local coverage decisions. Nationally, there are several tests established that have limited coverage (based on the ICD-9 codes, frequency of testing, or the investigational status) and regional restrictions may add to the list that is established on a national basis.

By signing the ABN, the Medicare patient is giving the laboratory permission to bill him or her directly for the test to be performed. If the employee who draws the blood does not get an ABN signed when appropriate, the laboratory will be performing the test for free, as it cannot have the ABN signed after the process is completed. If the specimen was collected by an employee at a physician office and transported to the laboratory for testing, the physician office will often receive a bill for the service from the laboratory, because that laboratory cannot be reimbursed in any other way.

It is illegal to have every Medicare patient fill out an ABN; these forms are to be used only when necessary for noncovered tests. In addition, the laboratory must retain a copy of the ABN and the patient must also be given a copy. Advanced Beneficiary Notices of Noncoverage are also used for other medical services; it is necessary to have a specific one for each type of noncovered service.

Commonly, a laboratory directory is a computer database of specific information about tests that are performed by that laboratory. The directory may also be provided in a book format, which can be consulted by facilities that do not have Internet access. The laboratory directory (also known as a directory of services) provides the following types of information:

- The internal test number used to enter the test order into the database
- CPT five-digit code used for reimbursement for that test
- Related information if there is more than one place within the directory where the test is addressed
- Acronyms or abbreviations that may be listed on the requisition for that test, or perhaps used to order the test in the computer system for that laboratory
- The type of specimen required, and in some cases the type or color of tubes to use for the blood draw or identification of the additives that must be present in the tubes
- The requested specimen volume and the minimum acceptable specimen volume
- Collection notes and/or specific requirements necessary for some tests
- Storage instructions for the specimen after collection and during transportation (room temperature, frozen, refrigerated, etc.)
- **Reference ranges** (also known as **normal ranges**) for the test ordered
- Clinical significance and interpretation of the test results
- Testing intervals/frequency and testing locations

Once the specimen requirements have been established, the collection process can continue. The employee who is performing the collection must document two unique

CB LABORATORY

2692 Millenium Rd - Seattle, WA 98103
425-353-8778

GLYCOHEMOGLOBIN	
Order Test GLYCO GLYCO Represents average glucose concentration over a 6–8 week period.	
Synonyms	HbA1C; Hemoglobin A1C
Specimen Required	
Container Type	Lavender top tube (EDTA)
Specimen Type	Whole blood
Minimum Volume	1 mL
Specimen Processing	Store and transport refrigerated.
Stability	**Room Temp** 24 hours **Refrigerated** 7 days **Frozen** ($-20°C$) 2 weeks
Alternate Specimens	Sodium flouride/potassium oxalate whole blood (grey top tube).
Department	Immunochemistry
CPT Codes	83036
Test Schedule	Sun-Fri nights
Turnaround Time	24–48 hours
Method	HPLC
Test Includes	
HbA1c, %	
Reference Ranges	

HbA1c 4.0–6.0 Non-diabetic %
  The American Diabetes Association
  considers a result of less than 7% to be
  the goal of diabetic therapy.	

Figure 1-3 Sample of information found in a laboratory directory.

Procedure 1-2: Use a Laboratory Directory

TASK

Use a laboratory directory to clarify the collection requirements and processing procedures for a laboratory order.

CAAHEP/ABHES Standards

None

CONDITIONS

- Laboratory requisition
- Laboratory order from qualified health-care professional
- Laboratory directory book or database including laboratory service information

Continued

Procedure 1-2: Use a Laboratory Directory—cont'd

Procedure	Rationale
1. Obtain the laboratory requisition or the laboratory order from the health-care provider. Verify the test ordered, especially if it is a test that may be performed on more than one body fluid.	Some tests, such as creatinine or total protein, are commonly ordered on blood but may also be ordered using a urine specimen.
2. Look up the test alphabetically using the computer database or the laboratory directory reference book.	This can sometimes be difficult if the test is ordered under an acronym or abbreviation or if there are two names used for the test, such as Tegretol, which may also be known as carbamazepine. Many laboratory directories will include a cross-reference that may help the user to find the correct entry.
3. Identify the type of specimen to be collected.	The information may be very straightforward, specifying the color of tube to be used. (For example, lavender-top or green-top tube.) However, sometimes the specimen requirements are described as "heparinized plasma" or "EDTA plasma." The employee needs to know which type of tube to use for this type of specimen.
4. Verify any restrictions on specimen type, or notations of unacceptable specimens.	For instance, many tests cannot use hemolyzed samples, or sometimes samples that are over 2 hours old cannot be used.
5. Verify the acceptable minimum volume, if listed.	There may be a requested volume (e.g., 1 mL) as well as a minimum volume listed. The minimum volume may be important if drawing the specimen from a child or other patient with difficult-to-access veins.
6. Identify the specimen processing instructions.	Is the specimen supposed to be spun within a certain time after the blood draw? Is the plasma or serum to be frozen? The processing instructions are very important for the specimen to be acceptable when it arrives at the testing laboratory.
7. Identify the schedule for performance of the test ordered.	The reference laboratory may list the testing schedule so that the health-care provider will be aware of how long it will take before he or she can expect the results for the test.
8. Prepare the necessary supplies to perform the specimen collection.	If a specimen must be frozen immediately or kept at a certain temperature, it is necessary to have the supplies at hand immediately after the specimen is collected. These should be prepared before proceeding.

identifiers for the patient, the employee ID (or initials), the date of collection, and the time of collection on the requisition and on the tube or alternative collection container. This same employee may also be responsible for entering the patient information into the computer database, whereas in other laboratories the specimen and paperwork may be prepared for transport to another location where the information will be added to the database upon arrival.

Test Your Knowledge 1-8

Why would a medical assistant use a laboratory directory before performing a blood draw?   (Outcome 1-8)

Laboratory Reports

Once the specimen has been processed, delivered to the correct department, and tested within the laboratory, a laboratory report is generated to transmit the test results back to the health-care provider. An example of a laboratory report is presented in Figure 1-4. The laboratory report document will list the results for the tests performed, as well as the reference ranges (also known as normal ranges) that have been established by the laboratory for that test. Reference ranges are the results that are expected in the general healthy population 95% of the time for a particular laboratory test. A range is necessary (instead of a specific value) because of differences in the population due to age, race, and gender. Geographical locations may also affect the reference range, as will the testing methods used by that laboratory. A notation will be present on the laboratory report for all results that are outside the expected reference range for that patient, based on demographics, the testing method, and the test ordered. The gender and age of the patient may affect the reference ranges used for interpretation of the results, so it is critical that this information is provided whenever a sample is collected.

The laboratory report will also include the date and time of the specimen collection, the name and identification number for the patient, and the name and address of the laboratory where the test was performed. The specimen source is identified, as well as the date and time the report was generated.

◄ CB LABORATORY ►

Patient: Sally Seashore
DOB: 08/07/1957   Sex: Fe
ID# 774909

Date/Time: 7/20/2012 16:50
Report Status: Final

PROCEDURE	RESULT VALUES	ABN	REFERENCE RANGES	UNITS
Rapid strep screen				
Rapid strep screen	Positive			
Dipstick UA only				
Appearance-UA	Clear			
Color-UA	Yellow			
Glucose-UA	Neg			
Ketone-UA	Neg			
UA spec gravity	1.010		1.002 – 1.030	
Occult-blood-UA	Neg			
pH-UA	6.0		5 – 7.9	
Protein-UA	Neg			
Nitrite	Neg			
Leukocyte esterase	Neg			
Electrolytes				
Sodium	141		136 – 145	mEq/L
Potassium	4.8		3.5 – 5.0	mEq/L
Chloride	100		96 – 106	mEq/L
CO2	25		22 – 30	mEq/L
Hemoglobin + Hematocrit				
Hgb	10.9	L	12 – 16	g/dL
HCT	33	L	37 – 48	g/dL

Flags: H = High   L= Low   A = Abnormal   Crit = Critical

Tests performed at: CB Laboratory, 2692 Millenium Rd., Seattle, WA 98103

Figure 1-4 Sample laboratory report.

Procedure 1-3: Distinguish Between Normal and Abnormal Test Results

TASK

Use a laboratory report to identify normal and abnormal test results for a patient.

CAAHEP/ABHES Standards

 CAAHEP 2008 Standards

II.A.2: Distinguish between normal and abnormal test results

 ABHES Standards

None

Conditions

- Laboratory report
- Pen, pencil, or highlighter

Procedure	Rationale
1. Examine the laboratory report for all necessary information.	All laboratory reports must include the following: 1. The name of the patient 2. The patient ID 3. The gender and age of the patient 4. Laboratory results with documented reference ranges 5. The name of the ordering health-care provider 6. The date and time of specimen collection 7. The date and time that the specimen was tested 8. The name of the laboratory where the test was performed
2. Identify the column on the laboratory report where the reference ranges are noted for each of the test results.	This column is usually near the patient results, and the data are often listed as a range, except in the case of tests that provide a positive and negative test result, or in the case of microbiology testing, antibiotic sensitivity testing, or immunology testing.
3. Compare the patient results to the reference range column.	Remember that the reference ranges may take the age and gender of the patient into consideration; the ranges will not necessarily be the same for all patients tested.
4. Circle or highlight the results that are not within the reference ranges. Document High or Low next to the values in the provided area.	Highlighting or circling these results may bring them to the attention of the provider. When a laboratory report is printed in the office (rather than one used in the classroom) the High or Low results are noted on the laboratory report when it is printed. However, the office protocol may also include highlighting or circling the results when the report arrives in the office to make certain that they are not overlooked.

Laboratory reports may be hand-delivered to the ordering health-care provider by a medical assistant within an office or via a courier service from a reference laboratory. They may also be faxed, mailed, or in some cases transmitted via e-mail. In some situations, the laboratory reports may also be available online through a dedicated laboratory link so that the provider can view the results on site. These results must be reviewed as soon as possible so that appropriate action can be taken for those outside of the normal reference range. Laboratory reports are a legal document that becomes part of the patient's health record.

Test Your Knowledge 1-9

In which ways are laboratory requisitions and laboratory reports similar?   (Outcome 1-9)

THREE PHASES OF LABORATORY TESTING

As we begin to understand the way that a laboratory is organized and how information is transferred through the testing process, it is important to realize that there are three components, known in laboratory jargon as *phases,* associated with laboratory testing: preanalytical, analytical, and postanalytical. A description of each phase of testing is detailed below and summarized in Table 1-3.

- **Preanalytical Phase:** The preanalytical phase of laboratory testing refers to the situations and actions that take place prior to the collection, during the collection, and during the processing/storage/transportation of the specimen. Phlebotomists and medical assistants often participate in this phase of laboratory testing. The importance of this phase cannot be emphasized enough. Generally speaking, the majority of problems associated with laboratory tests result from inadequate or inappropriate specimen collection, processing, storage, and transportation (i.e., the preanalytical phase of testing).
- **Analytical Phase:** The analytical phase of laboratory testing refers to the performance of the tests that have been ordered. This phase also includes maintenance and calibration of laboratory equipment and instruments associated with the testing and performing

TABLE 1-3		
Identification of, Definition of, and the Personnel Responsible for the Three Phases of Laboratory Testing		
Phase	**Definition**	**Personnel Responsible**
Preanalytical	All procedures/processes that occur before the specimen is actually tested. Includes patient preparation, accurate paperwork and data entry, appropriate specimen collection, processing, storage and transportation.	Medical assistant, phlebotomist, CLT or MLT, other laboratory professionals involved in this process
Analytical	All procedures/processes involved in the testing of the specimen. This includes the way the testing instrument was prepared and maintained, how the testing supplies were stored, appropriate training of the personnel performing the test, and quality control to ensure that the testing methods are working properly.	Medical assistant, medical laboratory professional performing the test, supervisor responsible for training and overseeing the process, personnel performing maintenance on instruments
Postanalytical	All procedures/processes that affect how the test results are handled when the analysis has been completed. These may include review and analysis of the results by the person performing the test, appropriate follow-through on extremely high or low results, how the results are recorded (in a computer or on paper, etc.) phone calls, report printing, report sorting, appropriate fax procedures, charting procedures within an office, physician review procedures, contact with patient if necessary for follow-up.	Various laboratory professionals that perform the test, administrative laboratory support personnel that process the results, medical assistants or other physician office personnel who perform charting procedures, physicians and other health-care professionals who interact directly with the patients.

quality control (QC) measures, which are in place to validate the test reagents/kits, the testing process, and training of the laboratory personnel performing the test.

- **Postanalytical Phase:** The postanalytical phase of laboratory testing includes the processes associated with the recording and reporting of laboratory results, storage and/or disposal of specimens after testing, and provider and patient notification of test results. Even if the other two phases of testing occur without any exceptions, if this phase isn't handled appropriately, then the overall experience will not be a positive one, and may negatively affect patient treatment.

Test Your Knowledge 1-10

List the three phases of laboratory testing.

(Outcome 1-10)

Test Your Knowledge 1-11

If a specimen is collected into a tube with the wrong type of anticoagulant for the test ordered, which phase of laboratory testing has gone wrong?   (Outcome 1-11)

SUMMARY

Laboratory testing is vital to the diagnosis of patient disease and implementation of proper patient treatment, as it provides critical information that cannot be gathered with a physical examination alone. Testing may occur in physician office laboratories, in hospital laboratories, or in large reference laboratories. The larger laboratories may be organized by departments as needed for efficient specimen handling. Various personnel perform the testing procedures, and their education and titles will vary depending on their responsibilities and the type of testing performed in the respective laboratory. Medical assistants play an important role in the laboratory by providing direct patient interaction, specimen collection, and processing or performance of laboratory tests.

Laboratory information, such as that provided on a requisition, is vital for proper testing procedures, result interpretation, and reimbursement for services provided. The exchange of information begins with a requisition and may involve the use of a laboratory directory for specimen requirements and other specifics. The process ends with the laboratory reports that provide the ordering practitioner with the final test results and reference ranges. Reimbursement procedures may involve laboratory personnel, so it is important that these individuals understand the processes involved with the necessary documentation on a requisition and the use of an ABN.

There are three phases of laboratory testing, including the procedures surrounding specimen collection and handling, the actual testing process, and the manner in which the results are reported back to the physician. These are the preanalytical phase, the analytical phase, and the postanalytical phase. All three phases must be handled correctly for laboratory results to be as meaningful as possible as part of quality patient care.

TIME TO REVIEW

1. If a patient is asymptomatic, it means   Outcome 1-1
   that he or she:
   a. Demonstrates specific symptoms of a disease state
   b. Complains of multiple symptoms
   c. Does not exhibit symptoms
   d. Is not ill

2. True or False: A specimen may be   Outcome 1-1
   defined as a part of something that demonstrates the characteristics of the whole.

3. What do hospital and reference   Outcome 1-2
   laboratories have in common?

4. Is urine analyzed only in physician   Outcome 1-2
   office laboratories?

5. A medical assisting student needs to   Outcome 1-3
   have a blood test performed to see if she has antibodies to hepatitis B in her bloodstream. This test would most likely be performed in this laboratory department:
   a. Blood Banking
   b. Hematology
   c. Serology
   d. Microbiology

6. Which laboratory department is   Outcome 1-3
   responsible for accessioning specimens into the laboratory information system when they arrive at the laboratory?

7. Mr. Earl has a laboratory test performed   Outcome 1-4
   to see if the diet and exercise changes suggested by

his health-care provider have helped to lower his cholesterol levels. Which of these reasons explains why this test is being ordered?

a. Assignment of a diagnosis
b. Ongoing assessment of the patient's progress and treatment
c. Prevention or possible early detection through screening tests
d. None of the above

8. Which of these duties might a medical assistant perform in a laboratory setting? *Outcome 1-5*

a. Urine drug screen collections
b. Phlebotomy
c. Urinalysis testing
d. Preparation of microbiology specimens for testing and/or analysis
e. All of the above

9. True or False: A diagnosis code does not need to be included on a requisition at the time the laboratory test is ordered. *Outcome 1-6*

10. True or False: A requisition is used only for ordering the laboratory tests. *Outcome 1-6*

11. The abbreviation ABN stands for: *Outcome 1-7*

a. Advance Beneficiary Notice of Noncoverage
b. Advance Beneficiary Notification
c. Action Bulletin of Noncoverage
d. Advance Bulletin of Noncoverage

12. The laboratory directory will include *Outcome 1-8* _____ instructions for a specimen after collection and during transportation.

13. True or False: The terms *laboratory requisition* and *laboratory report* may be used interchangeably. *Outcome 1-9*

14. Which phases of laboratory testing might be affected by the actions of a medical assistant in his or her various laboratory roles? *Outcome 1-11*

Case Study 1-1: Potential for growth

Cindy Lee, a certified medical assistant (CMA) working in a gynecology office, leaves early one Friday before her office closes. When she returns on Monday morning, she finds a box containing agar plates for microbiology specimen growth on the counter in the laboratory area. Cindy notices that the box has KEEP REFRIGERATED printed on the outside, but it appears that the box has been left out all night, and the cold packs within the box are at room temperature.

- Should Cindy be concerned about this situation?
- Which phase of laboratory testing may be affected by this oversight?

RESOURCES AND SUGGESTED READINGS

American Society for Clinical Laboratory Science Consumer Lab Testing Information
http://www.ascls.org/labtesting/index.asp
Numerous questions and answers on general laboratory testing.
American Society for Clinical Laboratory Science Introduction to Laboratory Testing
http://www.ascls.org/labtesting/labintro.asp
Introduction to the three phases of laboratory testing; also basic terms referring to analytical aspects of quality control.
Centers for Medicare & Medicaid Services Overview of Beneficiary Notices Initiative
http://www.cms.hhs.gov/bni
Links to various ABN information, including the new and old forms in use and answers to various commonly asked questions.
Good Laboratory Practices for Waived Sites
http://www.cdc.gov/mmwr/preview/mmwrhtml/rr5413a1.html
An overview of some problems that have occurred in waived test sites and an introduction to the three phases of laboratory testing. Recommendations for good practices overall.
CLIA Update—January 2010. Division of Laboratory Services, Centers for Medicare & Medicaid Services; Laboratories by Type of Facility (Exempt/Nonexempt combined)
http://www.cms.gov/CLIA/downloads/factype.pdf
Lists the number of different types of laboratories registered with CMS as of January 2010.

Chapter 2

Regulations Governing Laboratory Personnel

Constance L. Lieseke, CMA (AAMA), MLT, PBT(ASCP)

CHAPTER OUTLINE

Learning Outcomes
After reading this chapter, the successful student will be able to:

2-1 Define the key terms.

2-2 List the laboratory professionals present in a typical hospital, reference, or physician office laboratory.

2-3 Describe the personnel structure of the laboratory settings presented in the text.

2-4 Explain how the duties of laboratory professionals may vary, depending on their education and credentials.

2-5 Describe the role of a medical assistant in the clinical laboratory.

2-6 Explain the focus of CLIA '88, and why it was developed.

2-7 Demonstrate understanding of the levels of laboratory testing designated by CLIA '88.

2-8 Identify the laboratory professionals qualified to perform the various levels of laboratory testing as allowed by CLIA '88.

2-9 Identify the agencies responsible for overseeing CLIA '88 compliance.

CAAHEP/ABHES STANDARDS

 CAAHEP Standards

IX.C.5: Discuss licensure and certification as it applies to healthcare providers.

IX.C.8: Compare criminal and civil law as it applies to the practicing medical assistant.

 ABHES Standards

4.b: Medical Law and Ethics: Federal and State Guidelines
4.f: Medical Law and Ethics: Health laws and regulations
Graduates. f: Comply with federal, state and local health laws and regulations.

KEY TERMS

Ambulatory care	Credentialed	Provider-performed microscopy procedures (PPMPs)
CLIA '88	High-complexity tests	
CLIA-waived	Labile	U.S. Department of Health and Human Services (HHS)
Centers for Medicare & Medicaid Services (CMS)	Moderate-complexity tests	U.S. Food and Drug Administration (FDA)
COLA	Phlebotomist	
	Proficiency testing	

Medical assistants are in a unique situation, as the diverse training they receive allows them to assume numerous roles in an ambulatory setting. A medical assistant may have an opportunity to interact with various health-care agencies and related entities, such as radiology clinics, insurance companies, physical therapy offices, specialty physician offices, or pharmacies. In addition, the duties of the medical assistant will most likely include communication with the laboratory, and many medical assistants also perform laboratory testing in physician office laboratories. It is important to understand who makes up the workforce of the medical laboratory so that effective communication may be established. It is also vital that medical assistants understand the regulations controlling laboratory testing as they apply to the scope of practice in the physician office laboratory to remain compliant. This chapter provides an understanding of how to keep the physician office laboratory operating within the boundaries of the regulations. It will also provide insight into the clinical laboratory by identifying which career paths are available to a medical assistant.

LABORATORY PROFESSIONALS

Laboratory professionals pay a critical role in quality health care. The test results they generate improve patient care by providing information to the physician that cannot be discovered in any other way. Even though many processes in the laboratory have become automated, it is important for those performing the testing procedures to have adequate background knowledge for appropriate interpretation of the test results. It is also imperative that laboratory employees are knowledgeable about the procedures necessary to ensure quality testing methods in the laboratory, laws and regulations governing laboratory processes, and how all the laboratory departments work together.

Personnel in the Laboratory Setting

The personnel involved in laboratory testing are classified according to their education and credentials. Table 2-1 provides a list of the laboratory professionals that may play a role in laboratory testing, including their credentials and education. The basic classifications include the following:

- **Pathologists:** These are board-certified physicians who have specialized training in disease and laboratory interpretation. A pathologist may function as the laboratory director for sites that perform all levels of laboratory testing, and is generally affiliated with hospital and reference laboratories.

- **Physicians:** A physician without any laboratory specialty training may function as the laboratory director of a physician office laboratory. Dentists may also serve as laboratory directors if they perform laboratory testing in their clinics. Physicians may not serve as directors for hospital or reference laboratories unless they have additional credentials specifically qualifying them for this setting.

- **Nurse-practitioners or physician assistants:** These are known as midlevel health-care providers, and they may function as directors of physician office laboratories. Nurse-practitioners have at least 6 years of education; physician assistants generally possess at least a 4-year degree, as well as additional focused medical education. These midlevel providers are not usually employed in a reference or hospital laboratory.

- **Medical laboratory scientists:** Personnel with this title often work in a reference or hospital laboratory as testing personnel or as supervisors. They must have at

TABLE 2-1

Laboratory professional title, education, and credentials

Laboratory Professional Title	Education	Credentials
Pathologist	Doctorate with at least 8 years of education	MD or DO, board certified as pathologist
Physician	Doctorate with at least 6 years of education	MD or DO
Physician assistant	Bachelor's degree	PA
Nurse-practitioner	Master's degree	NP or ARNP
Clinical laboratory scientist	Bachelor's or master's degree	CLS, certified by National Certification Agency for Medical Laboratory Personnel (NCA)
Medical laboratory scientist	Bachelor's degree	MLS, certified by the American Society for Clinical Pathology (ASCP) or MT if certified by the American Medical Technologists (AMT), or International Society for Clinical Laboratory Technology (ISCLT)
Medical laboratory technician	Associate degree	MLT, certified by the American Society for Clinical Pathology (ASCP) or American Medical Technologists (AMT)
Clinical or registered laboratory technician	Associate degree	International Society for Clinical Laboratory Technology (ISCLT)
Medical assistant	1-year certificate or associate degree	May be certified by the American Association of Medical Assistants (CMA) or registered by the American Medical Technologists (RMA)
Phlebotomist	Varies by state	May be nationally certified by various agencies; not always required; some states may allow training on-the-job with no formal education

Note: Those with an associate degree or higher are generally required to have certification (credentials) to work in the laboratory. Those below this level of education are not necessarily required to have formal certification.

least a 4-year degree in laboratory medicine, and are credentialed by the American Society for Clinical Pathology. Those qualified with a 4-year degree may also be known as medical technologists if they received their certification through the American Medical Technologists.

- **Medical laboratory technicians:** These employees usually perform testing procedures in a hospital or reference laboratory. They may also be employed in physician office laboratories. Medical laboratory technicians must have completed at least an associate degree in laboratory medicine, and are nationally certified through the American Society of Clinical Pathology or through the American Medical Technologists.

- **Medical assistants:** Medical assistants may work in a physician office laboratory, but they can also be employed in a reference or hospital laboratory if the

tasks they perform are within their lawful scope of practice. Medical assistants have completed a medical assisting program that included at least an introduction to laboratory procedures. Medical assistants are not required to be certified to work in a laboratory, but if they choose to pursue a certification, they may test through the American Association of Medical Assistants to become a certified medical assistant (CMA), or through the American Medical Technologists to become a registered medical assistant (RMA).

- **Phlebotomists:** A **phlebotomist** may be a medical assistant, but there are also phlebotomists trained in short-term programs, either at technical colleges or on the job, specifically to draw blood and process laboratory specimens. Phlebotomists are primarily employed in physician office laboratories and hospital laboratories. Phlebotomists must have at least a high school diploma (or general equivalency diploma [GED]) and have documented training to draw blood. They may become certified nationally, and some states require additional state certification as well.

> **Test Your Knowledge 2-1**
>
> May a physician assistant serve as a laboratory director?
> (Outcome 2-2)

Those laboratory professionals that are **credentialed** have completed the required education for their specific classification, and they have also successfully passed a comprehensive assessment examination as required by their credentialing agency. To keep their credentials current, these professionals must participate in continuous education every year. Some states also require that laboratory personnel pass an additional state examination in order to work in a laboratory setting.

When entering a clinical laboratory, it may be difficult to tell by observation which employees have which type of credential, as they are all wearing lab coats and all performing what appear to be similar tasks. Figures 2-1 and 2-2 are representative of the personnel structure in a reference laboratory, a hospital laboratory, and an **ambulatory care** setting (such as a physician office laboratory). Laboratory testing may be performed by a variety of classifications, such as medical laboratory scientists, medical or clinical laboratory technicians, medical assistants, or phlebotomists.

> **Test Your Knowledge 2-2**
>
> May a medical technologist serve as a supervisor in a reference laboratory?
> (Outcome 2-3)

> **Test Your Knowledge 2-3**
>
> What type of credentials must a phlebotomist possess to work in a laboratory setting?
> (Outcome 2-4)

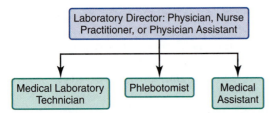

Figure 2-1   The personnel structure of the laboratory professionals working in a CLIA-waived physician office laboratory.

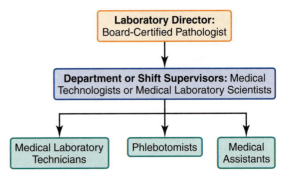

Figure 2-2   The personnel structure of the laboratory professionals working in a hospital or reference laboratory.

POINT OF INTEREST 2-1
Name changes

When working in a large laboratory (such as a reference or hospital laboratory), it is possible that you may encounter various credentials for individuals who are performing the same tasks. This is not unusual, but a recent merger of credentialing agencies may make this even more confusing!

Prior to 2009 there were three widely recognized credentialing agencies for laboratory personnel. They were the Board of Registry for the American Society of Clinical Pathology (ASCP), the National Credentialing Agency for Laboratory Personnel (NCA), and the American Medical Technologists (AMT). In October 2009, the NCA and the ASCP credentialing agencies decided to merge. Those who were previously credentialed by the NCA are now part of the ASCP organization, and those who were already part of the ASCP have not seen very many changes in their credential renewal processes. The certifying agency for the ASCP is now called the Board of Certification.

What has changed, however, are the terms used by these organizations for the various personnel classifications.

- **Baccalaureate degree–level personnel:** The ASCP previously used the designation *medical technologists* to describe this classification, and the NCA used *clinical laboratory scientist*. Now, the new title for those with a 4-year degree in medical technology that have successfully passed the examination is that of medical laboratory scientist, with the abbreviation MLS (ASCP).
- **Associate degree–level personnel:** The ASCP previously used the designation *medical laboratory*

technician to describe this classification, and the NCA used *clinical laboratory technician*. When the two agencies merged, they retained the designation *medical laboratory technician* for those with a 2-year degree who successfully pass the examination, and the abbreviation used for their credential is MLT (ASCP).

Medical Assistants in the Laboratory

As introduced in Chapter 1, medical assistants may play numerous roles in the clinical laboratory environment. Their education enables them to draw blood, assist with collection of other types of specimens, process specimens for testing, and perform simple or moderately complex test procedures. They may perform these tasks in the physician office laboratory, in a hospital laboratory, or in a reference laboratory. Medical assistants may also work in the microbiology or pathology department within a hospital or reference laboratory assisting with specimen preparation, answering phones, or entering specimens into the computer.

Some laboratory settings, especially a specialist or hospital laboratory, need their medical assistants to do more than draw blood or process specimens. In these settings they may be taught how to perform arterial blood draws, and also may learn how to assist with bone marrow aspirations or bronchoscopy specimen collection. In some situations, medical assistants may be running tests on automated instruments and performing urine microscopy examinations and manual differential procedures on normal blood smears. These specialized tasks require additional documented training beyond that offered in a traditional medical assisting education program, and the qualifications of the personnel performing these tasks may be regulated by state or local laws.

Test Your Knowledge 2-4

Are medical assistants only allowed to draw blood in a laboratory setting, or can they perform other duties?

(Outcome 2-5)

CLINICAL LABORATORY IMPROVEMENT AMENDMENTS OF 1988

CLIA '88 is an acronym for the Clinical Laboratory Improvement Amendment of 1988. This regulation establishes quality standards for all aspects of human medical laboratory testing, with the exception of those tests performed for research only. It was designed to ensure that all laboratory tests, regardless of where they are performed, would produce accurate reliable results and be performed in a timely manner.

History of the Regulation

The original Clinical Laboratory Improvement Act was enacted in 1967. It affected only private laboratories (federal and state laboratories were exempt) that received specimens via interstate commerce. This means that the only laboratories affected by the original act were those that provided services across state borders. These laboratories had to be licensed if they processed more than 100 interstate specimens per year. This act also improved laboratory quality standards overall by adding a requirement for **proficiency testing** to these licensed laboratories. Proficiency testing is used to verify that the results reported for a certain test are accurate. Because this Clinical Laboratory Improvement Act had such a small focus, there were many laboratories that were not affected by these requirements, especially physician office laboratories. It was estimated that of 200,000 laboratories in business in the United States, only about 12,000 were regulated.

In 1987, the *Wall Street Journal* published two articles expanding on the poor quality of laboratory testing in the United States. At that time, there was very little structured supervision of the quality of testing performed in laboratories that were not affected by the Clinical Laboratory Improvement Act of 1967. Specifically, the articles expanded on several situations in which Papanicolaou (Pap) smear tests showed false-negative results, allowing cases of cervical cancer to become advanced before a correct diagnosis was made. The cytology laboratories that were reporting these results were poorly staffed, and the technicians were overworked. Both the U.S. House of Representatives and the U.S. Senate held hearings to investigate the inaccurate Pap smear reports and other laboratory errors. As a result of these hearings, questions began to form about how laboratories functioned and about what kind of quality assurance was in place for the results reported. Therefore, it was decided that more federal oversight was necessary, and on October 31, 1988, the Clinical Laboratory Improvement Amendment of 1988 (CLIA '88) was enacted. Since that time, there have been several revisions, allowing more tests to be included in the **CLIA-waived** category, and giving the **U.S. Food and Drug Administration (FDA)** the responsibility to determine the level of complexity for laboratory tests.

Levels of Laboratory Testing Defined by CLIA '88

CLIA '88 requires that all laboratories performing tests on human specimens must register with the **Centers for Medicare & Medicaid Services (CMS).** The registration process, and title of the certificate granted to the laboratory, is based on the type of testing performed. The classification of the testing is based on the complexity of the testing procedure and the clinical significance of the results from the test, among other factors. This amendment classifies all tests into one of three categories:

- **CLIA-waived tests:** These are tests that are so simple and accurate that the likelihood of misinterpretation is minimal. This classification also requires that the tests will pose no reasonable risk of harm to the patient if the test were accidentally performed incorrectly. CLIA-waived tests also include procedures that have been cleared for home use, such as glucose testing performed by diabetics at home. Examples of CLIA-waived tests are streptococcal screens, urine pregnancy

tests, and mononucleosis testing. Many CLIA-waived tests are performed in physician office laboratories, but they may also be done in hospital or reference laboratories. Table 2-2 lists the types of tests that are CLIA-waived at this time. This list has grown significantly since CLIA '88 first went into effect, and will continue to change.

- **Moderate-complexity tests:** These tests are more complex than CLIA-waived tests. The complexity designation is based on a grading scale that takes into account the difficulty of test performance, the maintenance and troubleshooting required for the instrument used for the test, the amount of knowledge necessary to correctly interpret the results, and other specific aspects of the testing process. Some physician office laboratories perform moderate-complexity testing, but there are restrictions on the personnel performing the tests. Employees must be properly trained in these more advanced concepts in order to meet the requirements of the regulation. These tests also have more requirements for quality control and quality assurance documentation, and laboratories are required to participate in proficiency-testing programs to validate their test results. **Provider-performed microscopy procedures (PPMPs)** are also included in this classification, which concern the microscopic examination of **labile** specimens in the office performed by licensed health-care providers. Labile specimens are those that must be examined shortly

TABLE 2-2		
CLIA-waived tests		
Test Type	**Test Name**	**CPT Code**
Chemistry	Blood glucose by glucose monitoring devices cleared by the FDA for home use	82962
Urine and stool testing	Fecal occult blood	82270 GO 107
	Dipstick or tablet reagent urinalysis—nonautomated; for bilirubin, glucose, hemoglobin, ketone, leukocytes, nitrite, pH, protein, specific gravity, and urobilinogen	81002
	Urine pregnancy tests by visual color comparison	81025
	Ovulation tests by visual color comparison for human luteinizing hormone	84830
Hematology	Hemoglobin by copper sulfate—nonautomated	83026
	Erythrocyte sedimentation rate—nonautomated	85651
	Blood count; spun microhematocrit	85013

Note: This chart recognizes only the original CPT codes and test names listed as waived tests in 1988. There are numerous tests and testing methods that have been added to this list, which can be accessed at http://www.fda.gov/cdrh/clia/cliawaived.html

after collection because the appearance of the specimen will change rapidly after collection. Provider-performed microscopy procedures may include urine microscopic examinations, semen analysis for the presence or absence of sperm, nasal smear examinations, and other types of analysis that need to be performed on fresh specimens.

- **High-complexity tests:** This category of testing is performed almost exclusively in hospital and reference laboratories by highly trained laboratory professionals. These tests require substantial knowledge of the significance of the test results, complex testing procedures, and stringent requirements for calibration of instruments and quality control procedures to ensure the accuracy of the results.

Laboratories may perform multiple levels of testing; some may perform only CLIA-waived tests, whereas others may perform high-complexity tests as well as waived tests. All laboratories must register and pay a fee to CMS that is based on the complexity of the tests that they perform. Failure to register or follow all the regulations associated with the specified level of testing may result in significant fines (thousands of dollars per day of noncompliance) and potential closure of the laboratory.

Test Your Knowledge 2-6

Describe the minimum level of education required to perform the following types of laboratory testing:
   a. CLIA-waived tests
   b. Moderate-complexity tests
   c. High-complexity tests   (Outcome 2-7)

Test Your Knowledge 2-7

What factors are taken into account when assigning the different levels of complexity to the various laboratory tests?   (Outcome 2-7)

Employee Qualifications for Performance of CLIA Testing

The CLIA '88 regulations are very specific about the training necessary to perform the different levels of testing that are identified in the amendment:

- **CLIA-waived testing:** Minimum personnel requirements include a high school diploma or a GED, and thorough, documented training for the processes performed by the individual in the laboratory. Those performing CLIA-waived testing must follow the

manufacturer's directions provided with the kit used exactly as they are written, and appropriate training for all individuals performing the laboratory test must be documented. These tests may be performed by phlebotomists, medical assistants, or those with more laboratory education.

- **Moderate-complexity testing:** The minimum education requirements are very similar to those of the CLIA-waived category. Moderate-complexity tests are more complicated to perform, and they may have much more clinical significance if they are performed or interpreted incorrectly, so the training must be comprehensive if the individual performing the test has limited formal laboratory education. This additional documented training must include numerous areas of the laboratory, such as quality control testing procedures, maintenance of the testing instruments, clinical significance of the tests, and validity of the test results. In most circumstances, this level of testing is performed by a medical laboratory technician or medical technologist, but it is possible to appropriately train a medical assistant to perform at this level as well.

- **High-complexity testing:** In order to perform tests in the clinical laboratory that have been established as high complexity by the CLIA standards, the laboratory professional must possess at least an associate degree in laboratory science. He or she must also have documented training on site for quality control procedures, maintenance and troubleshooting of the instruments used for the procedures, and more in-depth knowledge of the test parameters. These high-complexity tests usually comprise numerous performance steps, and the results have a high level of clinical significance. High-complexity tests are performed only in larger laboratories such as hospital and reference laboratories, and generally are performed by clinical or medical laboratory technicians, clinical laboratory scientists, or medical technologists.

Test Your Knowledge 2-8

What levels of laboratory testing may a clinical laboratory scientist with 4 years of education perform?   (Outcome 2-8)

Oversight of CLIA Laboratories

Various agencies are involved with the enforcement of the CLIA '88 regulations. These include the FDA, the CMS, and the **U.S. Department of Health and**

Human Services (HHS). The HHS has the overall responsibility for laboratory quality assurance as designated in CLIA '88, but it has delegated various parts of the process to other agencies. The FDA is responsible for determination of the levels of complexity for the various laboratory tests. After the level of complexity has been determined, laboratories that perform these tests must apply for the appropriate certificate that allows them to perform these tests. The laboratory may qualify only for certain testing procedures based on the qualifications of their personnel. They apply to CMS for this certificate, whether it is a **Certificate of Waiver** (allowing them to perform CLIA-waived testing only) or another type of certificate that allows them to perform tests of higher complexity. A laboratory can only begin testing after receiving CMS certification. Compliance is monitored by the CMS or, in some situations, by state or private agencies that have regulations that are at least as stringent as those of the CMS, and have an agreement with CMS to monitor compliance. Some laboratories are affiliated with **COLA,** an independent company that accredits laboratories. COLA uses various educational methods to help laboratories meet the requirements for CLIA compliance, and CMS recognizes COLA as an accrediting agency. If a laboratory retains its accreditation with COLA, it will be assumed that that laboratory is meeting the CLIA requirements and will be granted the certificate that is appropriate for the level of complexity tested without site inspection requirements from the CMS. COLA is most commonly associated with physician office laboratories, but the organization is recognized by larger laboratories for accreditation purposes as well.

The CLIA certificate types are based on the complexity of the tests performed. Here is a summary of the available certificates for laboratories:

- **Certificate of Waiver:** Allows laboratories to perform only CLIA-waived tests.
- **Certificate of PPM:** Allows the licensed health-care providers in an organization to perform designated microscopic examinations.
- **Certificate of Compliance or Certificate of Accreditation:** Allows the laboratory to perform CLIA-waived tests, PPMPs, moderate-complexity tests, and high-complexity tests. These certificates are granted after the laboratory has been inspected. If the inspection was performed by a governmental agency, the laboratory receives a Certificate of Compliance. If the inspection was performed by a private accreditation

company, the laboratory receives a Certificate of Accreditation.

> **Test Your Knowledge 2-9**
>
> Which federal agency assigns the CLIA categories to laboratory tests?   (Outcome 2-9)

SUMMARY

Within a typical laboratory setting you will find professionals with various credentials and educational levels. Those who work in a hospital or reference laboratory may have different qualifications than those who work in a smaller physician office laboratory. There are regulations that dictate who can perform which type of testing, and what training and supervision must be involved for each test. CLIA '88, applies to all laboratories in the United States that perform testing on human specimens, except for federal laboratories and those that perform only research testing. Every testing site must register and pay a fee to comply. This regulation has established three levels of testing: CLIA-waived tests, moderate-complexity tests, and high-complexity tests. The levels have different requirements for testing personnel, quality control procedures, instrument maintenance, and laboratory supervision. The FDA makes the decision about which complexity level each test will have. Medical assistants with appropriate additional training may perform CLIA-waived or moderate-complexity tests, but those who perform high-complexity testing must have more specialized laboratory training in order to be compliant. All laboratories must register with CMS to legally perform laboratory testing at any level.

TIME TO REVIEW

1. A labile substance is one that: Outcome 2-1
   a. Is not fixed and is easily destroyed
   b. Is not fixed but can be stored for an extended period of time
   c. Is fixed with some sort of preservative
   d. Can easily be transferred to a reference laboratory

2. True or False: Ambulatory care   Outcome 2-1
   refers to the care provided to those transported to the hospital as an emergency transport.

3. Which laboratory settings may employ a medical assistant?   Outcome 2-2

   a. POL
   b. Hospital laboratory
   c. Reference laboratory
   d. None of the above
   e. a, b, and c

4. True or False: Pathologists serve as directors in reference laboratory settings.   Outcome 2-3

5. A laboratory professional with an associate degree in laboratory science may work in which laboratory setting?   Outcome 2-4

   a. Reference laboratory
   b. Hospital laboratory
   c. Physician office laboratory
   d. None of the above
   e. a, b, and c

6. List three duties that may be performed by a medical assistant in a hospital or reference laboratory.   Outcome 2-5

7. CLIA '88 stands for: Outcome 2-6

   a. Clinical Laboratory Incident Act #88
   b. Clinical Laboratory Improvement Amendment of 1988
   c. Consistent Laboratory Improvement Amendment of 1988
   d. Continual Linear Improvement Act of 1988

8. Choose the types of laboratory testing that may be performed by a medical assistant.   Outcome 2-7

   a. CLIA-waived testing
   b. Moderate-complexity testing
   c. Provider-performed microscopy procedures
   d. High-complexity testing

9. True or False: Those performing CLIA-waived testing do not need to follow the manufacturer's directions; they may write their own procedures as needed.   Outcome 2-8

10. What role does the Centers for Medicare & Medicaid Services play in CLIA '88 enforcement?   Outcome 2-9

    a. It is not involved
    b. It inspects each laboratory
    c. It handles all the laboratory registration procedures
    d. It determines the level of complexity for all laboratory tests

Case Study 2-1: CLIA quiz

Rose is starting at a new job in a physician office laboratory today. As part of her orientation, the physician who is in charge of the laboratory asks her a few questions to test her understanding of the laboratory organization. He asks her to answer the following questions about CLIA '88. How should she answer these?

1. Was CLIA '88 created to protect employees or patients?
2. Is it still necessary to be trained in the performance of CLIA-waived test procedures, or can these be performed without documented training?
3. Do laboratories have to be formally registered in order to legally perform testing on human specimens?

RESOURCES AND SUGGESTED READINGS

American Medical Technologists
   Certifying agency for laboratory professionals
   http://www.amt1.com
American Society for Clinical Pathology
   Membership and certification information for laboratory professionals, as well as continuing education information
   http://www.ascp.org
Centers for Disease Control and Prevention CLIA-related publications from the Federal Register and the Code of Federal Regulations
Excellent reference for the actual CLIA regulations presented in a time line that is easy to follow
   http://wwwn.cdc.gov/clia/chronol.aspx
Centers for Disease Control and Prevention CLIA Subpart A General Provisions
   Provides various details about CLIA '88, including compliance requirements
   http://wwwn.cdc.gov/clia/regs/subpart_a.asp#493.1
Tests waived by the FDA from January 2000 to present
   List of all CLIA-waived tests. Updated regularly.
   http://www.accessdata.fda.gov/scripts/cdrh/cfdocs/cfClia/testswaived.cfm
Information about the COLA accreditation services and education products. Also includes online education programs that may be used to fulfill continuing education requirements.
   http://www.cola.org

Chapter 3

Laboratory Safety and Preventing the Spread of Disease

Constance L. Lieseke, CMA (AAMA), MLT, PBT(ASCP)

CHAPTER OUTLINE

Learning Outcomes
After reading this chapter, the successful student will be able to:

3-1 Define the key terms.

3-2 List the major types of infectious agents.

3-3 Restate the difference between pathogenic and nonpathogenic microorganisms

3-4 Describe the various shapes of bacteria presented in the text.

3-5 Compare and contrast bacteria and viruses.

3-6 Describe medical asepsis.

3-7 Explain what the chain of infection concept refers to, and describe how the chain may be broken.

3-8 Explain how the CDC Standard Precautions are used in a laboratory setting.

3-9 Analyze the importance of proper hand-washing procedures and appropriate use of personal protective equipment.

3-10 Explain appropriate procedures for hand sanitization for health-care workers.

3-11 Examine the fundamental concepts included in the OSHA Hazard Communications Standard.

3-12 List the required components on a Material Safety Data Sheet.

3-13 Explain how a chemical label provides safety information.

3-14 Describe how a laboratory employee may protect themselves from other physical dangers in the laboratory.

3-15 Identify who is protected by the OSHA Blood-borne Pathogens Standard.

3-16 Interpret the key terms included in the OSHA Bloodborne Pathogens Standard.

3-17 List the essential components of an exposure control plan.

3-18 Discuss the appropriate use and disposal of sharps in the laboratory environment.

3-19 Define biohazardous waste and explain proper disposal methods for this type of laboratory waste.

3-20 Compare and contrast the major bloodborne pathogens that are considered to be a threat in the laboratory environment.

3-21 Detail the appropriate follow-up procedure in case of an accidental bloodborne pathogens exposure.

CAAHEP/ABHES STANDARDS

 CAAHEP 2008 Standards

III.P.4. Perform Handwashing
III.C.III.3. Discuss Infection Control Procedures
III.C.III.5. List major types of infectious agents
III.P.III.2. Practice Standard Precautions
X.C.XI.1: Describe Personal Protective Equipment
X.C.XI.3: Describe the importance of MSDS in a health-care setting
X.C.XI.4. Identify safety signs, symbols and labels
X.C.XI.8. Discuss Fire safety issues in a healthcare environment

 ABHES 2010 Standards

- Clinical: Apply principles of aseptic techniques and infection control
- Clinical: Use standard precautions

KEY TERMS

Aerobic	Carriers	Fecal-oral route
Acquired immune deficiency syndrome (AIDS)	CD4 cells	Fomites
Anaerobic	Centers for Disease Control and Prevention (CDC)	Fungi
Asepsis	Cirrhosis	Hazard Communication Standard
Asymptomatic	Cocci	Health care–associated infection
Bacilli	Contagious	Hepatitis
Bacteria	Contaminated sharps	Hepatitis A (HAV)
Biohazard symbol	Diplococci	Hepatitis B (HBV)
Biohazardous waste	Disinfection	Hepatitis C (HCV)
Bloodborne pathogen (BBP)	Electron microscope	Hepatitis D
Bloodborne Pathogens Standard (1910.1030)	Engineering controls	Human immunodeficiency virus (HIV)
Carcinogenic	Epidemiology	Infection
	Exposure control plan	Infection control

Infectious	Other potentially infectious materials (OPIMs)	Spores
Material Safety Data Sheets (MSDS)	Parasites	Standard Precautions
Medical asepsis	Parenteral exposure	Staphylococci
Microorganisms	Pathogens	Sterilize
Mucous membranes	Percutaneous	Streptococci
Mycotic	Personal protective equipment (PPE)	Surgical asepsis
National Fire Protection Association (NFPA)	Postexposure prophylaxis (PEP)	Susceptible
Nonintact skin	Protozoa	Transient bacteria
Normal flora	RACE	Transmissible
Nosocomial infection	Regulated waste	Universal Precautions
Occupational exposure	Resident bacteria	Vector
Occupational Safety and Health Administration (OSHA)	Sanitization	Viruses
Opportunistic pathogen	Spirilla	Window period
		Work practice controls

INFECTION CONTROL AND LABORATORY SAFETY

Pathogens, infection, and *contamination* are words that most of us have heard at home or in our communities. What do they really refer to? What impact may they have on our laboratory environment, our health, and the health of our patients? The laboratory setting has stringent safety precautions that must be observed in order to keep our health-care workers safe as they perform their daily routines. Laboratory professionals use various chemicals and equipment that put them at risk for injury. In addition, specimens taken from the human body present a unique challenge as they are naturally **infectious**, or capable of transmitting disease to others. **Infection control** is the term used to describe the process of protecting health-care workers and the patients they serve from the infectious agents in our facilities. In addition, because all the hazards faced in the laboratory are not from infectious agents, further safety methods must be employed to protect our laboratory professionals. It is imperative that as a medical assistant working in a laboratory environment you understand the hazards you may encounter, the laws that are designed to protect you and the patients you serve, and the appropriate use of the safety equipment that is available to you.

CORE CONCEPTS OF INFECTION CONTROL

In recent years, we all have become more aware of the infections that may be transmitted through the water, through the air, or with casual contact in our communities. Severe acute respiratory syndrome (SARS), the Asian flu, *Escherichia coli* outbreaks, and other pathogens such as the monkeypox virus remind us that we are very vulnerable. The presence of AIDS and hepatitis C is further proof of how our world has changed in the past 35 years. Be very mindful of the fact that almost any transmissible infection could find its way into your laboratory at any moment, as it may be present in your community, and you won't be aware of it. An ill patient may come into the office for medical services with an infectious condition, a specimen may be dropped off that is capable of transmission, or a salesperson may arrive and offer her hand, which is covered with bacteria, for a greeting.

Microorganisms

Diseases that may be encountered in your medical office or laboratory (even without any blood exposure) include varicella (chickenpox), tuberculosis, viral respiratory infections, conjunctivitis (pinkeye), gastrointestinal infections, and measles. Sometimes these infections affect the personnel, and sometimes they affect other patients within the facility. They are all caused by **microorganisms,** living organisms that are too small to be seen without a microscope. Most microorganisms are harmless to humans. However, a small percentage of **bacteria**, **viruses, fungi, protozoa,** and **parasites** are capable of causing disease in the human body. These disease-causing organisms are known as **pathogens.** An **infection** is the invasion of the body by pathogens that then cause disease symptoms. Not all microorganisms are pathogenic, and some are only capable of causing disease when they enter a part of the body where they don't normally reside. A disease is **contagious** or **transmissible** if it can be spread to other people directly or indirectly.

Test Your Knowledge 3-1

Staphylococcus aureus is a type of bacteria that sometimes functions as a pathogen. What other types of microorganisms may cause disease in humans?   (Outcome 3-2)

Test Your Knowledge 3-2

Do all microorganisms cause disease?   (Outcome 3-3)

Types of Microorganisms

Bacteria. Bacteria are single-celled organisms that have a cell wall in addition to the cell membrane that our human cells possess. (This is an important property when identifying different types of bacteria with special stains, as is discussed in Chapter 10.) Of all the bacteria known to exist, approximately 4% are known to cause disease in humans. Bacterial infections are treated with medication that will kill the microorganisms or keep them from multiplying, (antibiotics), but for effective treatment, identification of the causative agent is often necessary.

An initial step of the identification process is to examine a sample under the microscope so that the bacteria can be classified according to one of three basic shapes, as seen in Figure 3-1. **Cocci** are round bacteria, which can then be classified further by their appearance when examined microscopically. Cocci that grow in grape-like clusters are **staphylococci,** those that grow in chains are **streptococci,** and those that grow in pairs are **diplococci.** Diseases caused by cocci include streptococcal sore throat, pneumonia, abscesses, food poisoning, gonorrhea, and meningitis.

Long, slender, rod-shaped (oval) bacteria are called **bacilli.** These are especially prevalent in the soil and the air. Many types of bacilli are able to form **spores,** which is a dormant form of the bacteria that is resistant to changes in heat, moisture, and disinfectants. Bacilli cause diseases such as botulism, tetanus, diphtheria, tuberculosis, and salmonella food poisoning. *E. coli* is a normal bacilli that is present on our skin and in our intestines, but if we come in contact with a specific strain, *E. coli* O157:H7, it may lead to serious food poisoning, and may even be fatal.

Spirilla are curve-shaped or spiral bacteria. This type of bacterium is less frequently isolated in specimens from the human body, but the infections may be quite serious when they occur. *Treponema pallidum* is a spirillum that causes syphilis, and cholera is caused by another type of spirillum. This category may also be described as curved rods and microbiologists may subdivide it further into those bacteria that only have a slight curve and those that are tightly wound like a spring.

Test Your Knowledge 3-3

How are staphylococci and diplococci different?
     (Outcome 3-4)

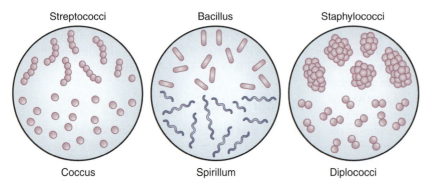

Figure 3-1 Types of bacteria, including cocci, staphylococci, streptococci, diplococci, bacilli, and streptococci.

> ### Test Your Knowledge 3-4
> Describe the appearance of bacilli viewed under the microscope.   (Outcome 3-4)

Viruses. Viruses are another common type of pathogenic microorganism. They are the smallest infectious agent, and are not really cells. Viruses are either made up of RNA or DNA surrounded by a protein capsule, and require a host cell to survive and replicate. Viruses cannot be observed using a simple microscope such as is found in most laboratories; they require use of an **electron microscope** for visualization. They invade the cells of our body, and use our own structures to make more virus particles. Viruses cause many of the diseases for which we are vaccinated, including measles, mumps, and chickenpox. The **human immunodeficiency virus (HIV)** is the causative agent of AIDS, and is an example of a retrovirus. Antiviral medications are available for some viral infections, but because of the way virus particles use human cells, the treatment may be quite damaging to the host as well as to the virus. Antibiotics are not effective against viruses.

> ### Test Your Knowledge 3-5
> List two ways that viruses are different from bacteria.   (Outcome 3-5)

Fungi. Fungi are plant-like organisms that flourish in an environment that is dark and damp. Yeast is a type of fungus, and fungal infections on the body are called **mycotic** infections. Athlete's foot and ringworm are examples of fungal infections.

Parasites. Parasites are similar to viruses because they require a living host to survive. A genus of bacteria known as *Rickettsia* is parasitic. Parasites take their nourishment from the host and require their host cells to reproduce, but they do not utilize the human cell in the same way that a virus does. Malaria is an example of a parasitic disease; the malaria parasite actually works into the red blood cells of the host and causes the patient to become ill. The word *parasite* may also be used to refer to larger, multicellular organisms such as tapeworms, which live inside the human host and use the body to survive.

Protozoa. Protozoa are complex single-cell microorganisms, most of which are nonpathogenic. However, there are a few species that can cause very serious infections in humans. Protozoa live in the soil and water.

Microorganism Growth Requirements

Because we have so many microorganisms present in our environment, we must find ways to eliminate as many as possible, with an emphasis on the removal of pathogens that could cause harm. However, it is impossible and impractical to **sterilize** our environment in the laboratory, which would involve the elimination of all microorganisms. **Sanitization** reduces the number of microorganisms on a surface with cleaning. Heat or chemicals are often used for sanitization in the healthcare environment. **Disinfection** is the process by which a medical assistant applies a chemical to a surface to kill the pathogenic microorganisms that may be present. Sanitization is often performed before an item is disinfected, so that the majority of the microorganisms are already removed before the pathogens are targeted. Items such as examination tables, countertops, and equipment are disinfected on a regular basis. Skin may also be disinfected, as it is impossible to sterilize the skin by eliminating all the microorganisms. Seventy percent isopropyl alcohol or povidone-iodine solutions are used for skin disinfection. Work surfaces and equipment are often disinfected in the laboratory with a freshly prepared 10% bleach solution.

Asepsis means that a surface is without infection. In the medical environment, there are two types of asepsis. **Surgical asepsis** means that all the pathogenic organisms have been destroyed before they enter the body. Invasive procedures such as venipuncture, injections, and urinary catheterization require surgical asepsis to be in place so that pathogenic microorganisms aren't introduced into the body of the patient. Equipment used for these types of procedures must be sterilized, and special care is used to avoid infection. **Medical asepsis** is a term used to describe a procedure or an environment that allows a patient to be treated without exposure to pathogenic microorganisms. For noninvasive procedures and the majority of care provided in the medical office, medical asepsis is adequate to protect the patients from potential infection. The items that are used for this type of care are clean and have been disinfected, but sterility is not necessary. To disinfect the environment appropriately and achieve medical asepsis, we must understand what elements microorganisms need for survival. These include the following:

- **Temperature:** The optimum temperature for each microorganism will vary. Human pathogens tend to prefer our body temperature, so they grow best at approximately 98.6°F.
- **pH:** A neutral pH is best suited for most microorganisms. This is why many disinfectants and cleaning

agents are basic or acidic, as they will kill the microorganisms by making their environment inhospitable.

- **Darkness and moisture:** Most microorganisms like darkness or dim light, and they all need moisture to survive.
- **Nutrition:** The type of nutrition varies depending on the type of microorganism, but they all need something in their environment to use as a food source.
- **Oxygen: Aerobic** microorganisms need oxygen present for survival. **Anaerobic** microorganisms are best suited for environments that have an absence or low levels of oxygen.

Good aseptic practices for the medical setting will attempt to eliminate the elements necessary for pathogenic microorganisms to survive. These practices may include the following:

- Disinfect work areas (using an appropriate disinfecting agent for the health-care environment) between patients.
- Take appropriate respiratory precautions while working with patients with potentially infectious respiratory conditions. Provide masks and tissues to the patients, and enforce their use by employees as well.
- Close the door of the treatment or blood-draw area if possible when an infectious disease is suspected.
- Limit access of nonessential personnel and visitors to patient care areas.
- Keep the laboratory and waiting room area well lit, well ventilated, and free of dirt and dust.

Test Your Knowledge 3-6

Brittany, a phlebotomist working in the laboratory, is cleaning up at the end of her shift. She uses the disinfectant provided by her employer and some paper towels to thoroughly clean the area where she has been drawing blood from patients. Is this work area now sterile?   (Outcome 3-6)

Chain of Infection

Figure 3-2 is a representation of the way pathogens are transmitted from person to person. This is represented as a chain, because all the parts of the circle are sequential and linked to one another. To stop the transmission of disease, the chain must be broken. A medical assistant working in a laboratory environment must practice good infection control techniques to achieve medical asepsis and break the chain. The potential infection needs to be

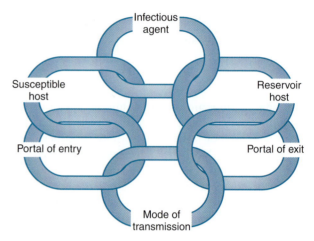

Figure 3-2   Chain of infection.

stopped at the source before it can be transmitted. The essential parts of the chain include the following:

- **Infectious agent:** A pathogenic microorganism. This may be a virus, bacteria in the environment, or pathogens that are carried in the bloodstream. There may also be microorganisms that are only pathogenic in specific situations. For instance, if an individual is taking antibiotics for an extended period of time, she may develop a yeast infection, because the yeast is taking advantage of the body's imbalance created with the antibiotic use. The yeast would be an **opportunistic pathogen.**
- **Reservoir host:** Someone who is infected or "carrying" the infectious agent. This may be a person or an animal that may or may not have symptoms of the infection. A reservoir host provides the necessary environment for the pathogen to grow.
- **Portal of exit:** The means by which the pathogen leaves the host body, either through the eyes, mouth, ears, intestinal tract, urinary tract, respiratory tract, reproductive tract, or broken skin. Another portal of exit may be through the blood or other body fluids capable of transmitting pathogens.
- **Mode of transmission:** This describes how the pathogen moves from one person to another. It may be transmission through the air as moisture droplets after a sneeze or a cough, other direct transmission occurs as one person touches another or via an insect or other **vector.** Vectors are living organisms that take in the pathogen, allow it to live and multiply in or on their bodies, then transmit it to another host without becoming ill with the pathogen during the transport. Dirty hands are a very common mode of transmission.

Pathogens may also be transmitted by inanimate objects, known as **fomites.** Doorknobs, telephones, countertops, and writing instruments are common fomites in the laboratory environment. Contaminated food or water may also function as a mode of transmission.

- **Portal of entry:** The pathogens enter the body in the same ways that they leave the body. The **mucous membranes** that line the external openings of our bodies are a common portal of entry and exit for pathogenic microorganisms.
- **Susceptible host:** A susceptible host is not protected from the pathogen as it enters his or her body. The pathogen to grow and multiply within the susceptible host. Age and illness can affect the susceptibility of a patient or an employee. A potential host will protect him- or herself (become less susceptible) in various ways. Protection may include vaccinations against certain viruses or bacteria, appropriate nutrition, or proper use of personal protective equipment.

In addition to understanding the chain of infection, it is important to realize how the chain may be broken by health-care staff members. Appropriate infection control practices and patient education are effective means of breaking the chain. Specifics include the following:

- **Infectious agent:** Although health-care professionals may not always be able to break the chain at this link, it is important to remember that an infectious agent may be eradicated if a patient takes all of his or her antibiotics as directed. Patient education in this area is critical.
- **Reservoir host:** Health-care personnel are sometimes tempted to go to work when they are ill. They are essentially a reservoir host at this time, and if they are not in the facility when they are ill, the chain is broken. In addition, if there is a patient in the waiting room with a suspected illness that is highly contagious, removing the patient from the vicinity of other patients may break the chain at this point.
- **Portal of exit:** Providing respiratory protection and tissues to patients may contain the infectious agent as it leaves the body. Keeping infected wounds covered may also affect this link of the chain.
- **Mode of transmission:** The simplest and most important action that health-care personnel can take to break the chain of infection is washing their hands. In addition, contaminated surfaces should be cleaned immediately after care is provided, and often throughout the workday. Patients should be educated about how to protect themselves if they live in the same household

with another family member who is ill. Hand sanitization is also critical for family members and patients to eliminate an opportunity for the pathogens to be transported to another susceptible host.

- **Portal of entry:** Those who are working with patient specimens must wear appropriate protective equipment (such as a face shield to provide mucous membrane protection, gloves, and a laboratory coat) to protect the common portals of entry. Health-care personnel working with patients who have respiratory symptoms should protect their own respiratory passages with a mask. All broken skin should be covered when working with patients, and there should be no eating, drinking, chewing gum, or applying makeup in the area where specimens are collected or processed.
- **Susceptible host:** Health-care personnel should always keep their vaccinations up to date to keep them from being susceptible to vaccine-preventable diseases. In addition, a balanced lifestyle with good nutrition and adequate rest will reduce susceptibility. Patients should be encouraged to keep vaccinations up to date, and those who have impaired immune systems should be cautioned about protecting themselves while in the community.

Test Your Knowledge 3-7

How might a medical assistant break the chain of infection at the mode of transmission link?   (Outcome 3-7)

Test Your Knowledge 3-8

Cally Jones just completed a set of vaccinations to protect her from hepatitis A. Where has she broken the chain of infection for this disease?   (Outcome 3-7)

Standard Precautions

We have discovered that there are numerous microorganisms in our environment that have specific requirements they need to survive. Some of these microorganisms are pathogens, meaning that they can cause infection in the human body. A **health care–associated infection** is one that is acquired in a health-care facility, such as a hospital, long-term care facility, physician office, or laboratory. If a patient in an inpatient facility enters without any evidence of infection, and develops signs of one more than 48 hours after being admitted, the infection is then investigated as a health care–associated infection. This type of infection may also be known as a **nosocomial infection**. Health care–associated infections are more common in inpatient facilities in which patients are in close proximity to one another, but it is also possible to acquire an infection in an ambulatory care setting. For example, chickenpox is highly contagious and can be spread from one person to another via droplets in the air after an infected individual coughs or sneezes. If a susceptible patient is in the same waiting area for an extended period of time with someone who is infected, the patient may develop chickenpox as a health care–associated infection.

Health care–associated infections have become more prevalent, more dangerous, and more expensive to treat in the past few decades. In response, the **Centers for Disease Control and Prevention (CDC)** has developed a set of **Standard Precautions** to assist health-care facilities with their infection control efforts. This standard is based on the premise that every person is potentially infectious with a microorganism that could be transferred to someone else in the health-care setting. Appropriate hand-washing techniques are stressed in the standard, as it has been found that this is the most effective action taken by medical staff to stop the spread of infection. Appropriate use of personal protective equipment, equipment disinfection, good respiratory hygiene, appropriate use of sharps, correct disposal of linen, and environmental cleaning practices are also addressed in the standard. For those working in inpatient facilities, the standard includes information about different types of precautions to be taken in isolation situations. The Standard Precautions expand and enhance the **Universal Precautions** developed in the 1980s, which specifically addressed infections transmitted through contact with blood and other potentially infectious materials. The premise of the Universal Precautions was that everyone was potentially infectious for bloodborne pathogens and that the same care should be used to treat every specimen.

Test Your Knowledge 3-9

According to the CDC recommendations for Standard Precautions, who is to be considered infectious?

(Outcome 3-8)

Test Your Knowledge 3-10

What is the most effective action a health-care worker can take to stop the chain of infection?   (Outcome 3-8)

Centers for Disease Control and Prevention Hand-Washing Recommendations

Even though research has shown that the hands of health-care personnel are one of the most common modes of transmission for pathogens, there are still issues with hand-washing compliance. The CDC recognized that this issue needed to be addressed, and the guidelines recently released now recommend the use of alcohol-based hand rub for routine decontamination of the hands in many situations, which may be quicker and easier for health-care professionals to use than washing the hands with soap and water. Either hand washing and decontamination using alcohol-based hand rubs remove or kill **transient bacteria,** viruses, or other types of microorganisms that may be present on the hands. Transient microorganisms, which attach themselves to our hands during our day-to-day activities, are responsible for most of the contamination and potential infection as health-care workers move from patient to patient. **Resident bacteria,** or **normal flora,** are bacteria living on and in between the deeper layer of our skin cells, and are not removed during routine hand cleaning. Here are some of the specific recommendations for hand hygiene:

1. Avoid any unnecessary touching of surfaces surrounding the patient.
2. If your hands are visibly dirty or contaminated with blood or other materials, wash them with soap and water. (It is not important at this point whether it is an antimicrobial soap that is used.)
3. Hands should be washed before eating and after using the restroom.
4. If hands are not visibly soiled, or if they were washed with a soap that was not antimicrobial, it is recommended that an alcohol-based hand rub be used. It may be used instead of the soap and water wash, or in addition to hand washing after a nonantimicrobial soap is used.
5. Hands should be decontaminated (washed or cleansed using the alcohol-based hand rub) in these situations:
   a. Before and after direct contact with patients, even if the patient has intact skin
   b. After contact with blood, body fluids or excretions, mucous membranes, nonintact skin, or dressings used for open wounds
   c. If the health-care provider will be going from a contaminated body site to a clean body site on the same patient
   d. After contact with any objects, such as equipment, in the immediate area of the patient
   e. After removing gloves

5. It is also recommended that artificial nails be avoided if the duties of the health-care provider include direct contact with patients at high risk for infection. Keep natural nails less than one-fourth-inch long.
6. Minimize jewelry on the hands, as bacteria may be present underneath or in jewelry and is not removed during normal hand-washing techniques.
7. Refilling of soap pump dispensers is discouraged. If a refill is necessary, the dispenser should be rinsed thoroughly before more soap is added. Bacterial contamination may be present in the small amount of soap at the bottom of the container.

> **Test Your Knowledge 3-11**
>
> What is an acceptable alternative to hand washing in the laboratory in most situations?   (Outcome 3-9)

> **Test Your Knowledge 3-12**
>
> Describe three situations in which a health-care worker should decontaminate their hands.   (Outcome 3-10)

Acceptable Medical Hand-Washing Procedures

The CDC recommendations outline specific practices to be employed when washing or disinfecting hands because this is such an important part of infection control practices. These procedures are explained in detail in Procedures 3-1 and 3-2.

> **Test Your Knowledge 3-13**
>
> Why would a clean, dry paper towel be used to turn off the water faucets after hand washing?   (Outcome 3-10)

Procedure 3-1: Perform Hand Washing

TASK

Perform hand washing appropriately, using the recommended technique for medical personnel.

CAAHEP/ABHES STANDARDS

 CAAHEP 2008 Standards

III.P.4. Perform Handwashing

 ABHES 2010 Clinical

- Apply principles of aseptic techniques and infection control
- Use standard precautions

CONDITIONS

- Antibacterial soap
- Running water
- Paper towels
- Manicure brush and stick

Procedure	Rationale
1. Remove all rings, and make certain that lab coats, watches, and bracelets are pushed up above the wrist area.	It is not possible to clean appropriately under rings, so they should be removed. Watches and bracelets need to be moved above the wrists so that the wrists can be cleaned.
2. Adjust the water temperature until it is warm but not hot.	Hot water leads to skin breakdown, and should be avoided.
3. Wet the hands and wrists.	To provide the best sudsing action with the soap, the hands should be wet before applying the soap.
4. If using a soap dispenser, use a clean paper towel to dispense the amount of soap recommended by the manufacturer. This is usually 3–5 mL or 1–2 pumps. If an automatic soap dispenser is used, the paper towel is not necessary.	A push-top soap dispenser or an automatic dispenser is recommended. If bar soap must be used, the bar of soap must be kept in the hands until they are thoroughly covered with suds, and a drainable soap dish must be in use to avoid pooling of dirty water around the bar of soap.

Continued

Procedure 3-1: Perform Hand Washing—cont'd

Procedure	Rationale
5. Rub the hands together vigorously for at least 10–15 seconds. All surfaces of the hands should be covered with soapsuds, as well as between the fingers and up over the wrist area. Keep the hands lower than the elbows.	The friction created helps to minimize the amount of bacteria on the hands. The hands must remain lower than the elbows to avoid having the water run up to the elbows, causing contamination farther up on the arm.

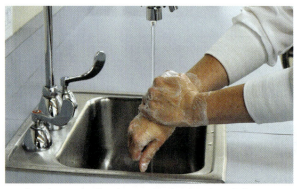

Hand washing with all surfaces covered with suds, including wrists

Procedure	Rationale
6. Avoid touching the lab coat or scrubs on the front of the sink, and avoid touching the hands to the inside of the sink while scrubbing.	If the lab coat or scrubs touches the front of the sink, it will become contaminated with dirty water. The inside of the sink is considered to be "dirty," so should not be touched during the hand-washing procedure.
7. Clean the top of the fingernails with the brush and clean under the fingernails with the manicure stick.	The cuticle area and the skin surrounding the fingernails harbor bacteria, so special care needs to be taken to clean this area thoroughly. The manicure stick should be used under the fingernails to remove as much contamination as possible.
8. Rinse the hands under the warm water, keeping the hands lower than the elbows.	The hands need to remain below the elbows to avoid contamination. All soap must be rinsed from the hands.

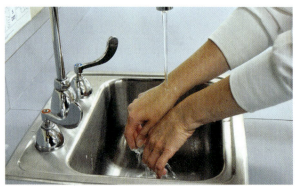

Rinsing of hands with fingertips pointing downward.

Procedure	Rationale
9. Dry the hands thoroughly with paper towels. Dispose of the paper towels in an appropriate receptacle.	Hands should be dried thoroughly before continuing. Special care should be given to the area between fingers.
10. Using another clean, dry paper towel, turn off the water faucets. Dispose of the paper towel in the appropriate receptacle.	A clean, dry paper towel must be used rather than using the damp one that was used to dry the hands. The moisture on the paper towel may draw the bacteria present on the faucets back onto the clean hands.

Procedure 3-2: Sanitize Hands With an Alcohol-Based Hand Sanitizer

TASK

Sanitize hands using an alcohol-based hand sanitizer.

CAAHEP/ABHES STANDARDS

CAAHEP 2008

III.P.III.2. Practice Standard Precautions

 ABHES 2010 Clinical

- Apply principles of aseptic techniques and infection control
- Use standard precautions

CONDITIONS

Alcohol-based hand sanitizer containing 60% to 95% alcohol

Procedure	Rationale
1. Remove all rings, and make certain that laboratory coats, watches, and bracelets are pushed up above the wrist area.	It is not possible to clean appropriately under rings, so they should be removed. Rings contain microorganisms that can cause infection. Watches and bracelets need to be moved above the wrists so that the wrists can be cleaned.
2. Verify that the sanitizer to be used is alcohol based.	The CDC recommendations sanction only the use of alcohol-based sanitizers.
3. Dispense the manufacturer's recommended amount of the product in the palm of the hand.	Do not dispense less than is recommended or the hand sanitization will be incomplete. Do not apply more than is recommended or the dry time will be increased.
4. Cover all surfaces of the hands and fingers with the sanitizer solution, and continue to rub these surfaces until the product is completely dry. Don't forget the areas around and under the fingernails, as well as between the fingers and the wrist area.	The skin around the fingernails and cuticles harbors a lot of microorganisms, so pay close attention to this area.
5. Allow the hands to air-dry. Do not use a paper towel to dry hands.	If the hands are not allowed to air-dry, the sanitization process is incomplete. The microorganisms will continue to be destroyed while the solution dries on the hands.

Proper Use of Personal Protective Equipment

Later in this chapter you will learn about the **Occupational Safety and Health Administration (OSHA)** Bloodborne Pathogens Standard, which is a comprehensive policy addressing **bloodborne pathogen (BBP)** exposure in health-care settings. A key component of this standard, as well as the Standard Precautions, is proper use of **personal protective equipment (PPE).** Personal protective equipment helps to protect the employee from bloodborne pathogens (those pathogens that are transmitted via direct contact with blood and other infectious body fluids), and in addition it helps to protect them from the pathogens in their environment that are not bloodborne. In order to be effective, personal protective equipment must be worn at appropriate times, removed when not needed, and disposed of properly. When considering PPE for a task, the employee must decide what type of exposure is reasonably anticipated while performing that task. Policies must be in effect by the employer to guide these decisions for PPE use.

The most important personal protective equipment in the medical laboratory is properly fitting gloves (see Fig. 3-3). Employers are responsible for providing PPE to employees, and gloves are no exception. Most facilities no longer use latex gloves; latex allergies have become too widespread to continue with this practice. Latex alternatives (such as nitrile gloves) are readily available. Gloves should be worn when contact with blood, mucous membranes, or nonintact skin could be anticipated when performing a certain task. Gloves should also be worn when contact with **other potentially infectious materials (OPIMs)** is anticipated. OPIMs are those that are capable of transmitting bloodborne pathogens.

It is not necessary to wear gloves when touching a patient with intact (unbroken) skin for routine care, such as taking vital signs and helping a patient into the procedure chair. Hands should be washed before and after each glove use, and gloves should always be removed after caring for a patient. The same pair of gloves should never be used for the care of more than one patient. Do not wash gloves. Gloves should not be worn after patient care when leaving that immediate area, as they may be contaminated with unseen microorganisms that will be deposited on door handles, telephones, and the like. Also, do not touch your face or hair while caring for a patient and wearing gloves. Do not wear the same pair of gloves for a patient if you are going from a dirty body site to a clean body site; remove the gloves, wash your hands, and put on a clean pair. Remember, gloves cannot prevent a needlestick injury, but they can prevent a pathogen from entering your body through a small break in your skin under the glove, and they can protect you from transient microorganisms that you may be exposed to while working in the health-care environment.

Test Your Knowledge 3-14

Marni is working hard to successfully draw blood from a patient who has very fragile veins. As she works, the phone keeps ringing. She finally obtains a sample, and just as she completes the draw and has the patient put pressure on the site, she reaches out with her gloved hand and answers the phone. What has she done wrong in this scenario?   (Outcome 3-9)

Gloves should be removed promptly after use. The method of removal is critical, as the gloves may be contaminated with unseen microorganisms that must not be spread to the surrounding area. Procedure 3-3 explains the steps involved in aseptic glove removal.

Personal protective equipment also may also include masks, goggles, face shields, or respirators (Fig. 3-3). A mask may be worn to protect others from droplets that may be generated when coughing or sneezing. Masks may be given to patients to wear while they are in the facility, or health-care professionals who have an upper respiratory infection or allergies may wear masks. Remember to keep the mask tight to the face so that it is effective. Masks with goggles or face shields may be worn to protect the employee's eyes, mouth, and nasal passages from moisture droplets or aerosols in the laboratory environment.

Respirators are required when working with patients with pulmonary tuberculosis or when dealing with certain types of specimens considered potentially infectious for airborne transmission. Respirators must also be worn when working with certain chemicals used as preservatives in the laboratory. Respirators must be fit properly to the face of the employee to be effective, and the filters must be maintained as directed.

Gowns may be used when additional protection is required during patient care (Fig. 3-3). These are especially important when entering isolation areas of the hospital or when working in a nursery environment with newborns. Care must be taken to keep the interior side of the gown free of contamination to protect the employee. Gowns are usually made of light, disposable material, and must be disposed of immediately after use. Generally

Procedure 3-3: Removal of Contaminated Gloves

TASK

Properly remove and dispose of contaminated gloves.

CAAHEP/ABHES STANDARDS

 CAAHEP 2008

III.P.III.2. Practice Standard Precautions

 ABHES 2010 Clinical

- Apply principles of aseptic techniques and infection control
- Use standard precautions

CONDITIONS

- Nonlatex gloves
- Biohazard waste container

Procedure	Rationale
1. Grasp the palm of the glove on the nondominant hand. Keep the gloves away from the body and the hands pointed toward the floor.	Grasping the palm will allow a firm hold as this glove is removed. Keeping the hands away from the body pointed toward the floor will minimize the risk of splatter in the eyes or mucous membranes.
2. Pulling on the palm of the glove, turn it inside out as it is removed from the nondominant hand.	If the glove is inside out, it will not be able to contaminate the bare skin, as the soiled area will be on the inside of the glove.
3. Crumple up the contaminated glove into the other gloved hand.	This allows the contaminated glove to be held safely while the other glove is removed.
4. Insert two of the ungloved fingers under the cuff, against the wrist of the gloved hand.	Be careful not to touch the contaminated side of the glove with the bare hand.
5. Pulling down with these fingers, turn the second glove inside out over the other glove while slipping it off the fingers.	This method will allow the contaminated surfaces to remain inside the glove bundle.
6. Dispose of the gloves in a biohazard waste container.	Visible contamination on the gloves means that they need to be disposed of as biohazardous waste.
7. Wash hands.	Hands must always be washed after removing gloves because gloves are not foolproof and hand contamination is still possible. It also helps to remove any powder residue that may be left behind on the hands.

there is a disposal area just inside or outside the room where the gowns were worn.

Laboratory coats are also used when there is a potential for splashing or soiling of the clothing worn by laboratory professionals. These should be OSHA approved as fluid resistant to offer the best protection. The coats must have tight cuffs, and should button or snap up to the neckline when worn. Clean laboratory coats should not be stored with dirty coats, and employees must not wear their contaminated laboratory coats into eating areas or the restroom. Laboratory employees are also not to take their coats home to be laundered, as this could contaminate their home environment. If laboratory coats are required at the facility where an employee works, OSHA regulations dictate that the facility is responsible for providing the coats and cleaning them commercially after use.

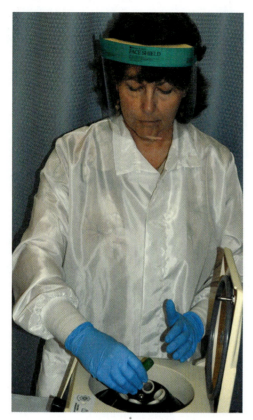

Figure 3-3 Medical assistant wearing OSHA-approved laboratory coat, appropriate face protection, and gloves.

Laboratory professionals should never apply makeup, chew gum, eat, or drink when working with blood or OPIMs. Also, food must never be stored in the same refrigerator with specimens or medications, regardless of how it is packaged.

Test Your Knowledge 3-15

What type of personal protective equipment should be worn when a medical assistant is performing a routine blood draw?

(Outcome 3-9)

POINT OF INTEREST 3-1
Bloodborne facts

The U.S. Department of Labor, Occupational Safety, and Health Administration (OSHA) has published a series of fact sheets that cover various aspects of the Bloodborne Pathogens Standard. This standard may be difficult to understand and therefore compliance may be complicated. These fact sheets are excellent tools for offices that are struggling to develop their plans appropriately or for anyone who is trying to update knowledge of the subject. They cover many subjects, including the hepatitis B virus, vaccine, and postexposure follow-up, and proper use of personal protective equipment. Single copies may be obtained by contacting the OSHA Publications Office, Room N-3101, 200 Constitution Avenue, NW, Washington, DC 20210.

LABORATORY SAFETY

The laboratory environment is unique because of the types of hazards present. As we have already discussed in this chapter, laboratory professionals are surrounded by potential pathogens as they perform patient care and work with specimens. In addition, employees are using or are in the vicinity of chemicals of various types, as well as electrical testing equipment. Laboratory professionals are also exposed to bloodborne pathogens, as needle use and handling fluids from the human body are part of the daily duties in this environment. All of these potential risks make safety in the laboratory workplace somewhat complicated. This chapter has already provided information about protection from exposure to pathogenic microorganisms in the environment and basic infection control practices. Now we will emphasize chemical safety, physical safety, and bloodborne pathogen safety in the laboratory.

Chemical Safety

Numerous chemicals are present in the clinical laboratory. Some of these are used as cleaning agents or disinfectants, whereas others may function as preservatives for laboratory specimens. Hydrochloric acid (HCl), for example, is often used as a preservative for 24-hour urine specimens, and bleach is used as a recommended method for cleaning surfaces exposed to blood and other potentially infectious materials. Both acidic and alkaline substances can cause severe burns, and mixing various chemicals may have disastrous effects. To protect the employees using these chemicals, OSHA created the **Hazard Communication Standard.** This standard gives all employees the right to know about the potential hazards associated with the chemicals in their workplace. The required components addressed in this standard include the following:

- A hazard communication program to be developed and used within the facility
- Current inventory of all hazardous chemicals used in the workplace

- Appropriate labeling of those chemicals designated as hazardous
- Material Safety Data Sheets
- Documented training for employees

> **Test Your Knowledge 3-16**
>
> Who is the OSHA Hazard Communication Standard designed to protect?   (Outcome 3-11)

The Hazard Communication Standard establishes comprehensive guidelines for labeling chemicals. These guidelines include the name of the chemical; contact information for the manufacturer; physical and health hazards of the chemical; safety precautions; and information pertaining to the storage, handling, and disposal of the chemical. The original container, as well as any transfer containers for the same chemical must be labeled in this manner.

> **Test Your Knowledge 3-17**
>
> The laboratory assistant who is working the evening shift notices that the laboratory is almost out of a disinfectant that staff members use to clean some of the instruments. He wants to be sure that the supervisor orders the same product that is now in use. Where can he look to find the name of the manufacturer to tell his supervisor?   (Outcome 3-13)

A **Material Safety Data Sheet** (**MSDS**) must also be available for every hazardous chemical in use. This is a document provided by the manufacturer that provide even more details about the chemical than those printed on the label. A current MSDS must be kept on file for any chemical in use that is considered potentially hazardous, and these sheets must be accessible to employees at all times (Fig. 3-4). The standard requires that the following information be provided on all Material Safety Data Sheets:

- **Identification:** Must include the generic and brand name, as well as the name, address, and emergency phone number for the manufacturer, and the date the MSDS was prepared.
- **Composition of ingredients:** List of the ingredients, and how much of the chemical is considered to be safe for exposure.
- **Physical and chemical properties:** Includes items such as appearance, odor, boiling point, specific gravity, pH, etc.

- **Fire and explosion data:** Will this chemical catch fire or explode if used incorrectly? If so, how should you extinguish the fire?
- **Reactivity data:** How does this chemical react with other chemicals? What types of interactions should be avoided?
- **Health hazards:** Includes information such as the route of entry, signs and symptoms to be aware of in case of overexposure, medical conditions that might be worsened when this chemical is used, and acute or chronic health hazards that may develop with regular exposure to the chemical. This section of the MSDS is very important to the health-care professional who uses this chemical as part of his or her daily tasks. There is also information presented about the **carcinogenic** (cancer-causing potential) classification of the chemical.
- **Emergency first-aid procedures:** What should you do if overexposure occurs as a first aid measure while help is on the way?
- **Precautions for safe handling and use of the chemical:** Includes instructions for handling a chemical spill, how to store the chemical, and how to dispose of the chemical and or container.
- **Control measures:** Includes the personal protective equipment and safety apparatus that should be used when dealing with the chemical.

> **Test Your Knowledge 3-18**
>
> How many required components must be present on a Material Safety Data Sheet?   (Outcome 3-12)

The last required component of the Hazard Communication Standard is employee training. All employees who might be exposed to hazardous chemicals at work must be provided information about the chemicals and their potential hazards prior to the beginning of their employment in the area where the chemicals are used, and again whenever the hazard may change with the addition of new chemicals or new duties. There must be documentation of each training session, and the education must be continuous; not only offered at the time of initial employment. There must also be assurance that the employee understood the information presented. The required training elements include the following:

- A general overview of the right to know standard, explaining all the components involved, where to find the inventory of hazardous chemicals in use, and where the written hazard communication program is kept for that facility

The Clorox Company 1221 Broadway Oakland, CA 94612 Tel. (510) 271-7000	Material Safety Data Sheet

I Product:	CLOROX REGULAR-BLEACH
Description:	CLEAR, LIGHT YELLOW LIQUID WITH A CHARACTERISTIC CHLORINE ODOR

Other Designations	**Distributor**	**Emergency Telephone Nos.**
Clorox Bleach EPA Reg. No. 5813-50	Clorox Sales Company 1221 Broadway Oakland, CA 94612	For Medical Emergencies call: (800) 446-1014 For Transportation Emergencies Chemtrec (800) 424-9300

II Health Hazard Data

DANGER: CORROSIVE. May cause severe irritation or damage to eyes and skin. Vapor or mist may irritate. Harmful if swallowed. Keep out of reach of children.

Some clinical reports suggest a low potential for sensitization upon exaggerated exposure to sodium hypochlorite if skin damage (e.g., irritation) occurs during exposure. Under normal consumer use conditions the likelihood of any adverse health effects are low.

Medical conditions that may be aggravated by exposure to high concentrations of vapor or mist: heart conditions or chronic respiratory problems such as asthma, emphysema, chronic bronchitis or obstructive lung disease.

FIRST AID:

Eye Contact: Hold eye open and rinse with water for 15-20 minutes. Remove contact lenses, after first 5 minutes. Continue rinsing eye. Call a physician.

Skin Contact: Wash skin with water for 15-20 minutes. If irritation develops, call a physician.

Ingestion: Do not induce vomiting. Drink a glassful of water. If irritation develops, call a physician. Do not give anything by mouth to an unconscious person.

Inhalation: Remove to fresh air. If breathing is affected, call a physician.

III Hazardous Ingredients

Ingredient	Concentration	Exposure Limit
Sodium hypochlorite CAS# 7681-52-9	5 - 10%	Not established
Sodium hydroxide CAS# 1310-73-2	<1%	2 mg/m[1] 2 mg/m[2]

[1]ACGIH Threshold Limit Value (TLV) - Ceiling

[2]OHSA Permissible Exposure Limit (PEL) – Time Weighted Average (TWA)

None of the ingredients in this product are on the IARC, NTP or OSHA carcinogen lists.

IV Special Protection and Precautions

No special protection or precautions have been identified for using this product under directed consumer use conditions. The following recommendations are given for production facilities and for other conditions and situations where there is increased potential for accidental, large-scale or prolonged exposure.

Hygienic Practices: Avoid contact with eyes, skin and clothing. Wash hands after direct contact. Do not wear product-contaminated clothing for prolonged periods.

Engineering Controls: Use general ventilation to minimize exposure to vapor or mist.

Personal Protective Equipment: Wear safety goggles. Use rubber or nitrile gloves if in contact liquid, especially for prolonged periods.

KEEP OUT OF REACH OF CHILDREN

V Transportation and Regulatory Data

DOT/IMDG/IATA - Not restricted.

EPA - SARA TITLE III/CERCLA: Bottled product is not reportable under Sections 311/312 and contains no chemicals reportable under Section 313. This product does contain chemicals (sodium hydroxide <0.2% and sodium hypochlorite <7.35%) that are regulated under Section 304/CERCLA.

TSCA/DSL STATUS: All components of this product are on the U.S. TSCA Inventory and Canadian DSL.

VI Spill Procedures/Waste Disposal

Spill Procedures: Control spill. Containerize liquid and use absorbents on residual liquid; dispose appropriately. Wash area and let dry. For spills of multiple products, responders should evaluate the MSDS's of the products for incompatibility with sodium hypochlorite. Breathing protection should be worn in enclosed, and/or poorly ventilated areas until hazard assessment is complete.

Waste Disposal: Dispose of in accordance with all applicable federal, state, and local regulations.

VII Reactivity Data

Stable under normal use and storage conditions. Strong oxidizing agent. Reacts with other household chemicals such as toilet bowl cleaners, rust removers, vinegar, acids or ammonia containing products to produce hazardous gases, such as chlorine and other chlorinated species. Prolonged contact with metal may cause pitting or discoloration.

VIII Fire and Explosion Data

Flash Point: None

Special Firefighting Procedures: None

Unusual Fire/Explosion Hazards: None. Not flammable or explosive. Product does not ignite when exposed to open flame.

IX Physical Data

Boiling point..approx. 212°F/100°C
Specific Gravity (H₂0=1) .... ~ 1.1 at 70°F
Solubility in Water .... complete
pH ....~11.9

©1963, 1991 THE CLOROX COMPANY
DATA SUPPLIED IS FOR USE ONLY IN CONNECTION WITH OCCUPATIONAL SAFETY AND HEALTH   DATE PREPARED 08/09

Figure 3-4 MSDS information sheet for Clorox Bleach. *Courtesy of Clorox.*

- An explanation of what an MSDS is, where it may be found in the workplace, and how to use one
- Identification of the specific chemicals used in the work area for that employee, with instructions for the protective measures to be employed, including the personal protective equipment that is appropriate for that specific chemical
- The meaning of the labels and symbols used on hazardous chemicals
- Emergency measures to be taken in case of a spill or exposure

To ensure the safe use of chemicals, remember always to wear the appropriate personal protective equipment and safety equipment for the task at hand. Also, never use a chemical in a fashion other than that for which you were trained to use it. Do not transfer chemicals to unlabeled containers, and do not reuse containers that have been used previously. Remember that mixing chemicals may have disastrous effects; adding even water to some chemicals can be very dangerous. Finally, every employee should know the location of the eye wash station and emergency shower in the vicinity of their work area.

Physical Safety

As is the case with any business, there is always the chance that things will go wrong in the laboratory. This could include a chemical exposure, but it could also be a fire, an electrical emergency, or other personal injuries.

A laboratory professional needs to be aware of all hazards in the workplace, and also needs to be ready to respond to emergencies appropriately.

It is always essential for any business to have a plan of action in case of an emergency, but it is even more critical for a health-care facility such as a laboratory. Employees are not only responsible for themselves, but also for the patients in their presence at the time of the incident. Appropriate training and careful planning may dictate the difference between a positive or negative outcome of an emergency situation. This includes posting of emergency numbers (such as 911 or another internal number in a large facility for emergency response), maps showing the closest exit from various places within the building, employee training on use of fire extinguishers, and hazard identification.

The **National Fire Protection Association (NFPA)** has developed a labeling system that provides general information to employees and rescuers about the health, flammability, or reactivity hazard of chemicals. These categories are represented by blue, red, yellow, and white diamonds, each containing a number. The colors of the diamonds represent the different types of hazards, and the number contained within each diamond indicates the severity of the hazard. The blue diamond represents the respective health danger with exposure to the chemical. The red diamond indicates flammability hazard, and the yellow diamond indicates the reactivity potential for the chemical if exposed to increased heat or other conditions. There is also a white diamond, which

may include a special symbol, indicating whether a chemical is radioactive or reacts with water (Fig. 3-5).

Test Your Knowledge 3-19
How do the NFPA fire labels protect employees?
(Outcome 3-14)

Fire Safety

In order to keep themselves and those around them as safe as possible, all employees should know the procedures to follow in case of fire in their facility. Fire safety basics such as Stop, Drop, and Roll (in the case of clothing that has caught on fire) are likely familiar concepts. However, when in the workplace, there are more aspects to consider: Where are the fire extinguishers? How do I use them? What can I do if there is not one nearby? Where is the nearest exit? How do I call for help? These are all questions that should be answered in initial training, and the procedures should be reviewed on a regular basis.

According to the National Fire Protection Association, there are four classifications used to describe fires, each of which has its own type of fire extinguisher to be used. Multipurpose extinguishers are also available to use for Class A, B, or C fires.

- **Class A:** Class A fires involve common household materials such as wood and paper. Water or a water-based

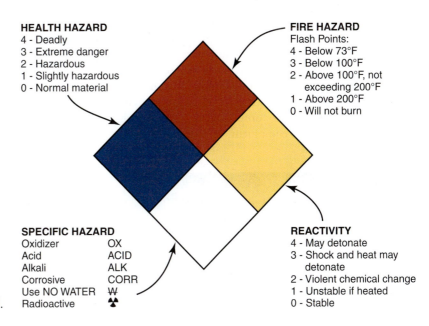

HEALTH HAZARD
4 - Deadly
3 - Extreme danger
2 - Hazardous
1 - Slightly hazardous
0 - Normal material

FIRE HAZARD
Flash Points:
4 - Below 73°F
3 - Below 100°F
2 - Above 100°F, not
    exceeding 200°F
1 - Above 200°F
0 - Will not burn

SPECIFIC HAZARD
Oxidizer   OX
Acid   ACID
Alkali   ALK
Corrosive   CORR
Use NO WATER   W̶
Radioactive   ☢

REACTIVITY
4 - May detonate
3 - Shock and heat may
    detonate
2 - Violent chemical change
1 - Unstable if heated
0 - Stable

Figure 3-5   NFPA chemical fire symbol.

solution is needed to put out this type of fire, and these are contained in a Class A extinguisher.

- **Class B:** Class B fires generally involve flammable liquids and/or vapors, and they need to be smothered to be put out. The Class B extinguishers contain chemicals, carbon dioxide or foam.
- **Class C:** Class C fires are related to electrical equipment, so special care must be used to extinguish them. If the solution used to extinguish the fire conducts electricity, the fire will not be extinguished. The Class C extinguishers use chemicals or other types of substances that do not conduct electricity.
- **Class D:** Class D fires frequently lead to explosions, as they occur with reactive metals such as sodium or potassium. They are very difficult to control, and there is not a fire extinguisher available in most sites to extinguish this type of fire. Sand or other dry powder agents work best for this type of fire.

Fast action is critical when a fire is discovered to keep those in the workplace as safe as possible. A common acronym recommended to help those facing a fire remember what to do is **RACE:** Rescue, Alarm, Confinement, Extinguish. Table 3-1 lists the letters and expands on the meaning.

Test Your Knowledge 3-20

What is designated by the different letters assigned to fire extinguishers?   (Outcome 3-14)

Electrical Safety

We are surrounded by electrical equipment in the laboratory environment, so that fire and electrical shock are definitely potential hazards. Most hazards can be minimized by appropriate maintenance and service of the equipment and the electrical outlets. The use of extension cords and overloading of electrical outlets should be avoided. Also, only qualified personnel should service electrical equipment. In case of electrical

TABLE 3-1	
RACE: The steps to take in the event of a fire	
R	Rescue individuals in danger
A	Activate the alarm system
C	Confine the fire by closing windows and doors
E	Extinguish the fire using an appropriate fire extinguisher

shock, remember that you must stay safe in order to help those who have been injured. Shut off the source of the electricity immediately, if possible. Do not touch the victim if you are unable to shut off the source of the electricity. Call for emergency assistance immediately. If the source of electricity has been eliminated, evaluate the victim and begin cardiopulmonary resuscitation (CPR) if necessary.

Body Mechanics

As a medical assistant working in a laboratory environment, you may be performing numerous venipunctures each shift. These procedures often require bending over the patient sitting in the phlebotomy chair, or perhaps in a hospital setting, bending over the bed of a patient. This bending can cause a great deal of stress to the muscles of the back and neck, resulting in pain. There are additional duties in the laboratory that may require lifting or carrying equipment trays or supplies. A laboratory professional may need to assist a patient with transfer from a wheelchair to an examination table or other chair. In all these situations, it is important to keep your back as healthy as possible. Stretches and regular exercise help, as well as staying close to an ideal body weight. Remember to use the muscles in your legs when lifting heavy objects, and when carrying heavy objects keep them close to your body and avoid twisting motions. Change your position as often as possible; avoid sitting or standing for prolonged periods without a break. If patient transfer is part of the duties for a medical assistant in your work environment, appropriate techniques should be part of the initial training for employees.

Bloodborne Pathogen Safety

Many of you who are reading this textbook have never lived in a world without the presence of HIV and **acquired immune deficiency syndrome (AIDS).** However, it was not that long ago that these diseases were not yet known. Prior to 1980, there was not a lot of information available about potential bloodborne pathogen exposure in health care. **Hepatitis B (HBV)** was discovered in 1967, but research on the methods of transmission were still in progress for many years. With the discovery of the HIV in 1983, change came quickly. It became evident that health-care workers needed to be protected from the hazards of working with blood and other potentially infectious materials. Studies performed in the 1970s showed that the rate of hepatitis B infection for health-care workers was ten times that of the general population. A reliable vaccination was created and released to the general public in 1982, but compliance was voluntary, and many health-care workers had already been exposed to the virus. After HIV was identified, data were gathered to see how many health-care workers were potentially infected as a result of occupational exposure, and although the numbers related directly to exposure on the job were low, they were too high to be ignored.

Bloodborne pathogen is a term used to describe any pathogenic microorganism found in human blood that can cause disease in humans. These diseases are spread through direct contact with the bloodstream of another individual. This means that there must be a piercing of the skin (**parenteral exposure**), direct blood-to-blood contact as might occur when **nonintact skin** touches the blood of another individual, or mucous membrane exposure, as occurs with sexual activity or accidental splashes into the eyes or mouth. These diseases are not carried only in the bloodstream of the infected individual. Other potentially infectious materials include semen, vaginal secretions, cerebrospinal fluid, synovial fluid, pleural fluid, pericardial fluid, peritoneal fluid, amniotic fluid, saliva when dental procedures are being performed, and all body fluids that are visibly contaminated with blood. If it is impossible to tell which type of fluid you may be working with, it is also to be assumed that it is a potentially infectious material. Tears, feces, urine, sputum, nasal secretions, sweat, and saliva (spit) are not considered to be infectious unless they are grossly contaminated with blood.

Universal Precautions

Bloodborne pathogen exposure in health care was first addressed by recommendations from the CDC in 1982, specifically referring to the information about the newly identified HIV. In 1985, the CDC published a recommendation to adopt Universal Precautions when dealing with blood or other potentially infectious materials. The concept of universal precautions recognized the fact that it was impossible to identify all patients who may be infected with HIV or other bloodborne pathogens by taking a health history and performing an examination. The recommendation was that all patients (and all specimens of an infectious nature) were to be considered infectious for HIV and other bloodborne pathogens, and the same precautions were to be taken in all situations. Prior to this, gloves were not mandatory in health-care settings, mouth pipetting was still performed in the laboratory, and laboratory coats were not required. Special precautions were taken only if a specimen or patient was labeled as

infectious. Currently, the CDC standard precautions have expanded universal precautions to include all means of infection.

> ### Test Your Knowledge 3-21
> What are some examples of OPIMs?   (Outcome 3-16)

Bloodborne Pathogens Standard

In 1988, OSHA strengthened this recommendation of Universal Precautions with the publication of the **Bloodborne Pathogens Standard (1910.1030).** This standard provided a rigorous policy to protect health-care workers who had **occupational exposure** to blood or other potentially infectious materials in the workplace. This standard had special significance for those who worked in a laboratory environment, because the amount of potential exposure was quite high for this population. This regulation required that all employers with potential occupational exposure to bloodborne pathogens in their workplace develop an **exposure control plan.** An exposure control plan must include the following components:

- **Exposure determination:** The plan requires that all employers determine which classifications of employees have risk of exposure, and during what types of duties that the risk exists.
- **Methods of exposure control compliance:** Exposure control compliance means that all employees are to be taught how to practice universal precautions by implementing appropriate personal protective equipment. It also required that the employer use and train the employees to use **engineering controls** and **work practice controls** to minimize their risk of exposure. Engineering controls are physical devices (such as needle safety devices or stationary safety shields) that are used by the employees to make their environment safer as they perform their duties. Work practice controls are ways that employees might alter the manner in which they perform a task to minimize the risk of bloodborne pathogen exposure. These include rules banning eating or drinking in an area where there is potential exposure, bandaging cuts before application of gloves, wearing gloves and other PPE appropriately, wearing close-toed shoes, and disposing of **biohazardous waste** and **contaminated sharps** correctly. Biohazardous waste is a classification used to describe substances contaminated with liquid or semiliquid blood or other potentially infectious materials. Contaminated sharps

are needles or other materials capable of piercing the skin that have been used with blood or other potentially infectious materials.

- **Hepatitis B vaccination** (or documented declination of the vaccine by the employee) must be made available for all employees with occupational risk of bloodborne pathogen exposure.
- Communication of hazards to all at-risk employees, which must occur initially upon assignment, and at least annually. (Retraining must also occur if there are changes to the procedures or hazards in a specific area of the facility.) Records for this training must be kept for at least 3 years. Initial training must include:
- Information about the **epidemiology,** signs, symptoms, and methods of transmission of bloodborne pathogens.
- Instruction about the specific methods employed by that facility (their exposure control plan) to protect their employees, as well as general preventative procedures.
- Information about the hepatitis B vaccine
- An explanation of the procedure to follow for an exposure incident

---

Test Your Knowledge 3-22

True or False: The OSHA Bloodborne Pathogens Standard was created to protect patients.   (Outcome 3-15)

Test Your Knowledge 3-23

List two key components required in an exposure control plan.   (Outcome 3-17)

Appropriate Sharps Use and Disposal. Unfortunately, more health-care professionals are exposed to bloodborne pathogens by contaminated needles or other sharp devices than through any other route. This means that safety must be considered at all times when using and disposing of contaminated needles, glassware, or any other instruments that have come into contact with infectious materials. In 1999, there was an update to the Bloodborne Pathogens Standard requiring that employers constantly evaluate new safety equipment for invasive procedures to be certain that they are using the safest methods and products. The addendum also requires that employees who actually use the products on a daily basis have input as to which product is most efficient and easiest to use before the choices are made for which item to purchase. There are many choices available for needle

safety devices, and no excuse not to use them. Keep in mind the following when considering sharps safety:

1. Always make sure that employees are trained on the appropriate use of the needle safety device in use. Many of these devices are designed to be "one handed," and if the employee tries to use two hands, he or she is at great risk for a puncture with a contaminated needle.
2. Contaminated needles are never to be recapped with the original needle cover, bent, or broken off. They must be disposed of immediately after use.
3. A biohazard sharps container should always be within reach when drawing blood or giving injections so that the needle can be disposed of immediately. These containers must be rigid and puncture-proof, and should be snapped closed and disposed of when they are three quarters full.
4. If contaminated glassware is broken, use mechanical means to clean up the mess, and then dispose of the glassware in a biohazard sharps container. A small disposable broom and dustpan may be designated for this type of situation, or tweezers may be used to pick up the pieces of glass. Thicker industrial gloves that are puncture resistant may also be used. Clean the area with an appropriate disinfectant (10% bleach solution allowed to sit for 20 minutes) to eliminate potential bloodborne pathogen exposure.
5. When performing capillary blood draws from the finger or foot of a patient, always use a capillary puncture device that recoils into the original holder. Do not try to reuse these devices.
6. Use plastic tubes and other containers instead of glass whenever possible.

Test Your Knowledge 3-24

Are all needle safety devices operated in the same way?   (Outcome 3-18)

Regulated Waste and Housekeeping. In a health-care setting, there is a need to sort the waste generated by the facility. Some of the waste may be disposed of in the same way as household trash. Other waste is regulated, and requires special attention for disposal. The OSHA definition of **regulated waste** is quite long. Essentially, the term refers to any liquid blood or other potentially infectious materials. It also refers to contaminated items that are soaked with blood to the extent that the blood could be released if the item were compressed, or items caked with blood so that the blood could be released if the item were handled. Regulated waste also refers to contaminated sharps and any other microbiological wastes that may contain blood or OPIM.

Regulated waste must be disposed of in containers that are clearly identifiable as biohazardous. The containers (or bags) must either be red or must be marked with a **biohazard symbol** (Fig. 3-6). When using bags to collect regulated waste other than sharps, care should be taken to avoid adding items to the bag that are not biohazardous in nature. All bags must be closed securely when full, to be enclosed in larger containers for disposal by a regulated waste facility. All sharps containers will also be picked up by regulated waste facilities for disposal. Only companies that are licensed to carry biohazardous waste are allowed to transport and incinerate this type of refuse.

Other housekeeping guidelines in the laboratory include disinfection of counters at the beginning and end of each shift (at a minimum) with a fresh 10% bleach solution or an OSHA-approved disinfectant that is designed to kill the hepatitis B virus and HIV. Also, remember all biohazardous spills must be cleaned up using a spill kit that is designed for this purpose.

Test Your Knowledge 3-25

Is all laboratory waste considered to be biohazardous?

(Outcome 3-19)

DISEASES CAUSED BY BLOODBORNE PATHOGENS IN THE LABORATORY SETTING

The OSHA Bloodborne Pathogens Standard is very comprehensive, and is designed to protect employees who work with blood and other potentially infective body fluids. But what exactly are the employees being protected from, and how serious are the diseases?

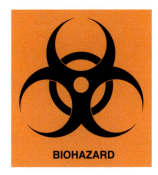

Figure 3-6   Biohazard symbol.

Hepatitis

Any discussion of bloodborne pathogens usually includes the topic of hepatitis. Essentially, **hepatitis** means "inflammation of the liver." When we discuss hepatitis in relation to bloodborne pathogens, we are referring to hepatitis that is caused by a viral infection. There are numerous types of the hepatitis virus that have been isolated, and not all of them are bloodborne. The ones that we are most concerned with are hepatitis B and hepatitis C, as these viruses are bloodborne pathogens, and they can cause serious illness. Table 3-2 lists details about the different types of hepatitis and other bloodborne pathogens.

Hepatitis B Virus (HBV)

Hepatitis B was first identified as a unique virus in 1967. It was formerly known as serum hepatitis, because there was a high prevalence of infection with the hemophiliac population who had received blood products as part of their treatment. The hepatitis B virus targets the liver, and it is the most serious hazard facing those in the health-care industry. HBV may be present in the blood and other potentially infective fluids of the body. Unfortunately, it may survive on surfaces in dried blood for up to 1 week. Hepatitis B may be transmitted in a health-care setting through needlesticks or other contaminated sharps, by contact with contaminated surfaces, or through mucous membrane exposure with aerosols or splatters created while handling infectious specimens. For those not employed in health care, transmission usually is the result of sharing contaminated needles, or through sexual contact.

Hepatitis B causes flu-like symptoms, and the affected patient may appear jaundiced. The symptoms of infection often do not appear until months after the virus has entered the body. Most of those who are infected recover, but approximately 2% of those infected will develop chronic infection, which causes **cirrhosis** of the liver or cancer. There are also patients that may be **carriers** of the hepatitis B virus who do not know it. These patients often have had no definitive symptoms of the infection, but they are capable of passing it on to others. Fortunately, a series of vaccinations may prevent hepatitis B infection. OSHA requires that these vaccinations be offered free of charge to all employees who have bloodborne pathogen exposure in the workplace.

There is also a newly discovered form of hepatitis virus that affects only those who are already hepatitis B positive. This appears to be a mutant or variant form of HBV, but it is unique enough to be identified as its own

TABLE 3-2

Comparison chart for various types of viral hepatitis and HIV

	Method of Transmission	Symptoms?	Long-term Effects?	Vaccination or Prevention	Comments
Hepatitis A	Fecal-oral route, contaminated food/water. Not bloodborne	Vomiting, abdominal pain, jaundice, flu-like symptoms	Not usually. Symptoms usually resolve within months	Vaccinations available; appropriate personal hygiene will eliminate transmission in many situations	May spread even in situations with appropriate personal hygiene if drinking water becomes contaminated
Hepatitis B	Bloodborne	Symptoms often delayed after initial infection; include abdominal pain, vomiting, jaundice	A small percentage become chronically infected; leads to cirrhosis and death	Vaccinations available; also avoidance of high-risk activities	Greatest bloodborne pathogen risk for health-care workers due to nature of the virus
Hepatitis C	Bloodborne	May be asymptomatic; if symptoms present, less obvious than HBV infection and also delayed after initial infection	Many infected individuals develop chronic infection; slowly causing permanent liver damage	No vaccination available	
HIV	Bloodborne	Initial infection may produce flu-like symptoms; as disease progresses, symptoms change	Infection is fatal when the patient develops AIDS	No vaccination available; avoidance of high-risk activities is essential	

virus. This is known as **hepatitis D**. There currently is no vaccination available for hepatitis D.

Hepatitis C Virus (HCV)

You may have heard of **hepatitis C (HCV)** as the new "epidemic" disease of the world. This statement is misleading. Although there are millions of cases of hepatitis C infection that have been diagnosed over the past decade, these patients did not necessarily have a recent infection. Hepatitis C infection is usually **asymptomatic,** so most of those who are now being diagnosed with the disease were actually infected more than a decade ago. For many years researchers knew that there was another form of hepatitis virus that was different from both HBV and HAV. They just couldn't isolate it as a unique strain of the virus. In 1989, technology finally allowed the hepatitis C virus to be identified as another cause of post-transfusion hepatitis. The hepatitis C virus is a bloodborne pathogen, and many of those who are diagnosed today shared dirty needles for drug use, received blood transfusions or other blood products, or had tattoos applied prior to the mid-1980s. If there are any symptoms of the HCV infection, they are usually milder than those of hepatitis B, so are often misread as being symptoms of the flu. Unlike hepatitis B, in which it is uncommon to advance to the chronic form of the disease, those with hepatitis C infection usually progress to the chronic stage (approximately 80% to 85% of patients). Of these, a small percentage develop permanent liver damage and/or liver failure. Transmission of the hepatitis C virus in a health-care setting usually requires a larger accidental exposure than would be necessary to transmit HBV. There is no vaccination for HCV.

Hepatitis A Virus (HAV)

Although the **hepatitis A (HAV)** virus is not a bloodborne pathogen, it is important to understand how it is transmitted. HAV attacks the liver of infected patients and causes inflammation just like the other forms of viral infections that we have discussed. The hepatitis A virus is very contagious, and is transmitted by the **fecal-oral route.** The virus is shed in the feces of infected individuals, often before they even know they are infected. The fecal material containing the virus can then be passed on to others through direct contact (such as touching another individual) or indirect contact through food, water, or inanimate objects. Patients with HAV usually show symptoms sooner than those with HBV or HCV, and are often initially more severely ill. However, the hepatitis A virus rarely progresses to cause chronic infection or permanent liver damage. There is a series of vaccinations available to protect against hepatitis A infection.

> **Test Your Knowledge 3-26**
>
> Are all forms of hepatitis considered to be bloodborne pathogens?
> (Outcome 3-20)

> ### POINT OF INTEREST 3-2
> #### Pathogenic microorganisms
>
> In most situations, the discussion of bloodborne pathogens focuses on hepatitis B, HIV, and hepatitis C. However, the OSHA Bloodborne Pathogens Standard is not only designed to protect employees from infection with these viruses. The standard actually includes any pathogenic microorganisms that may be present in blood or other potentially infectious materials. Examples of other diseases that may be transmitted by direct contact with blood of infected individuals include malaria, syphilis, babesiosis, brucellosis, leptosporosis, Creutzfeldt-Jakob disease, and viral hemorrhagic fever.

Human Immunodeficiency Virus

The human immunodeficiency virus (HIV) attacks the immune system of our bodies. The HIV infection may eventually lead to AIDS. Viruses need the genetic information in our cells to survive and replicate, and HIV is no different. It attacks a type of white blood cells in our body known as **CD4 cells.** This type of blood cell fights infection in our bodies. Those infected with HIV are **susceptible** to opportunistic infections. These infections are caused by microorganisms that would not normally infect individuals who have healthy immune systems. HIV infection also makes the infected patients more prone to develop certain types of cancer.

When patients are infected with HIV, they undergo several stages. Initially, they may have swollen glands, or they might have slight flu-like symptoms. This generally lasts from weeks to months. Also, initially, because the amount of virus particles in the infected patient's body is still low, an HIV test result would be negative. HIV tests are designed to detect antibodies to the virus, and in the early stages of infection, the level of antibodies in an individual are not high enough for detection. The patient is still capable of passing on HIV during this time through blood-to-blood contact or sexual activity. This is known as the **window period** of infection, and may last up to 6 months.

The second stage of infection is generally asymptomatic. The infected patient may still not know that he or she is HIV positive. This stage can last for months or even years.

When patients reach the third stage, they often contract one or more opportunistic infections. This can be the first time many patients find out that they are HIV positive. Their symptoms will vary, depending on the infection that they are experiencing.

The final stage of HIV infection is what we know as AIDS. At this stage, the HIV-positive patient has been diagnosed with an opportunistic infection or disease that has been classified by the CDC as an AIDS indicator. These diseases include esophageal thrush, cytomegalovirus infection, a type of cancer known as Kaposi's sarcoma, and invasive cervical cancer in the HIV-positive patient. An AIDS diagnosis may be made based on the number of CD4 cells present in a blood sample as well. Remember, HIV infection causes AIDS, but an infected patient does not have AIDS until he or she reaches this final stage and contracts one of the indicator diseases, or is diagnosed with AIDS because of the blood count.

For many infected individuals worldwide, HIV infection is fatal. The treatment regime has changed significantly in the past 25 years, and more HIV-positive patients than ever before are able to live long lives without acquiring AIDS. Fortunately, HIV is not a very hearty virus; it dies immediately when it comes into contact with air, and the amount of virus necessary for an infection to occur from an accidental exposure has to be quite high. Hepatitis B infection is a much more serious risk from accidental health-care worker occupational exposure than HIV infection. Phlebotomy procedures are most often responsible for HIV exposure that occurs in a health-care setting. As of 2000, the CDC had processed 56 claims in which it appeared that a health-care professional had contracted HIV from an accidental exposure. At this time, there is no vaccination for the human immunodeficiency virus, and accidental infection is battled with rapid administration of antiviral medications.

Test Your Knowledge 3-27

What are two characteristics that hepatitis B and HIV have in common?   (Outcome 3-20)

POSTEXPOSURE FOLLOW-UP PROCEDURE

You have taken all the appropriate precautions, read all the training manuals, worn all the right personal protective equipment . . . but your patient jerks his arm right at the end of the phlebotomy procedure, and you are punctured by a contaminated needle. Now what? The Bloodborne Pathogens Standard carefully spells out what type of follow-up care employers must offer to their employees (free of charge) if there is an accidental exposure to blood or other potentially infectious materials in the workplace. Remember, an exposure can be **percutaneous** (through the skin) as in the scenario above, but it may also be a mucous membrane exposure through a splash in the eyes or in the mouth. Here are the steps to follow if there is an accidental exposure:

1. Wash the site thoroughly with soap and water. If it is a mucous membrane exposure, thoroughly flush the exposed area with water.
2. The incident must be reported immediately to the appropriate manager or other contact person within your health-care facility. Many of the antiviral medications used for treatment after an exposure should be started within a few hours, so an immediate report is critical.
3. Fill out an incident report form. The route of exposure and the circumstances surrounding the incident are very important and are required by law.
4. Identification of the source individual needs to be determined as soon as possible. Consent should be obtained for the source individual to be tested for HBV, HCV, and HIV, unless his or her status is already known for these diseases. If the individual refuses to consent for the test, the employer must document that a refusal was made. If allowed by local law, the test will be performed regardless, so that the employee can be treated effectively. The results of these tests will be made available to the exposed employee. A blood sample will also need to be obtained from the exposed employee to test for a baseline level for HBV, HCV, and HIV.
5. The exposed employee will have the opportunity to seek medical attention as soon as possible after the initial report has been completed. **Postexposure prophylaxis** is most effective if initiated rapidly after the exposure. This means that preventive medication (such as antiviral medicine) should be administered within hours of exposure. The health-care professional providing the follow-up care will be provided with information about how the accident happened, any laboratory testing results that might be available,

and all medical records for the employee that might be relevant (such as vaccination records). The health-care professional also must be provided a copy of the Bloodborne Pathogens Standard.

6. The health-care professional performing the follow-up care will determine whether postexposure prophylaxis is necessary for HBV, HCV, or HIV, depending on the risk evaluation. The route and amount of exposure, the vaccination status of the employee, and the circumstances of the exposure will be taken into consideration. The treatment for the employee often consists of a combination of drugs for an extended period of time.

7. Follow-up blood tests are generally performed on the exposed employee, at a minimum interval of 6 weeks, 12 weeks, and 6 months. It is possible that this series may be extended up to 12 months.

8. The exposed employee also must be offered counseling and reminded that confidentiality must be retained in reference to the source individual. All medical follow-up for the employee is also retained confidentially.

Test Your Knowledge 3-28

What should happen immediately if an employee splashes blood in her eyes? (Outcome 3-21)

Test Your Knowledge 3-29

True or False: All employees who are victims of a blood-borne pathogen exposure will be sent to see a health-care provider for follow-up care. (Outcome 3-21)

SUMMARY

The world we live in is a complex place, with new health hazards constantly emerging. As health-care workers, we must protect ourselves from potential pathogens in our environment, our patients, and our workplace. There are several government regulations that have been designed to protect employees in a health-care or laboratory environment. Education concerning these regulations, and careful adherence to their principles, are essential steps to working safely in this unique environment. Standard Precautions have been developed to assist with infection control efforts. The Hazard Communications Standard establishes guidelines to protect employees

from chemicals in the workplace, and the Bloodborne Pathogens Standard educates health-care employees about the risks they face from bloodborne pathogens as they perform their duties. Medical assistants must be familiar with the details contained in these documents to use safety materials in their workplace and to be prepared for accidents when they happen.

TIME TO REVIEW

1. A bacteria that is aerobic needs _____ to survive and replicate: (Outcome 3-1)
   a. Nitrogen
   b. Oxygen
   c. Carbon dioxide
   d. Water

2. True or False: A substance that produces or causes cancer is carcinogenic. (Outcome 3-1)

3. The types of microorganisms listed in this chapter that may be human pathogens include: (Outcome 3-2)
   a. Protons, neutrons, and electrons
   b. Bacteria, viruses, and parasites
   c. Bacteria, viruses, fungi, and parasites
   d. None of the above

4. True or False: Most of the types of bacteria present in our environment are pathogenic. (Outcome 3-3)

5. True or False: The presence of bacteria anywhere in our bodies is always an infection. (Outcome 3-3)

6. A round-shaped bacteria that appears in pairs when viewed under the microscope is known as a: (Outcome 3-4)
   a. Cocci
   b. Spirilla
   c. Bacilli
   d. Diplococci

7. Which type of infection is best treated by antibiotic use? (Outcome 3-5)
   a. Viral
   b. Bacterial
   c. Viral and bacterial
   d. None of the above

8. True or False: In a medically aseptic   Outcome 3-6
environment, bacteria may still be present on
surfaces.

9. How does the "chain of infection"   Outcome 3-7
have to be broken to keep a pathogen from causing
disease?

   a. It must be broken at multiple points to keep the
   pathogen from causing disease
   b. Only vaccinations will break the chain of
   infection
   c. The chain of infection must only be broken at
   one point to discontinue the spread of infection
   d. The pathogen must be killed before the chain
   will be broken

10. What are the elements addressed in   Outcome 3-8
CDC Standard Precautions document?

   a. Appropriate use of personal protective equipment
   b. Equipment disinfection procedures
   c. Respiratory hygiene
   d. Sharps use
   e. All of the above

11. True or False: Hand washing is   Outcome 3-9
designed to remove the normal (resident) flora from
our skin.

12. When using an alcohol-based hand   Outcome 3-10
rub to disinfect the hands, it is important to:

   a. Put on gloves while hands are still damp
   b. Rub the solution thoroughly on all parts of the
   hands and wrists
   c. Use only a drop of the solution
   d. Always wash the hands first before using

13. The OSHA Hazard Communications   Outcome 3-11
Standard addresses:

   a. The use of personal protective equipment
   b. The formal education required by everyone in
   the laboratory before they can be hired to perform certain tests
   c. What type of fire extinguisher to use for various
   types of fires
   d. The brand of hand sanitizer endorsed by the federal government

14. Which of the following components   Outcome 3-12
are required for any Material Safety Data Sheet?

   a. Identification of the chemical
   b. Color of the chemical

   c. Health hazards
   d. a and c
   e. All of the above

15. True or False: Laboratory employees   Outcome 3-14
may protect themselves from occupational back
injuries by using appropriate bending techniques
when lifting heavy objects.

16. Why was the OSHA Bloodborne   Outcome 3-15
Pathogens Standard created?

   a. To protect employers from lawsuits
   b. To create a revenue source for OSHA
   c. To educate and protect employees from the
   hazards of bloodborne pathogens
   d. To protect patients from bloodborne pathogens

17. What is an example of parenteral   Outcome 3-16
or percutaneous bloodborne pathogen exposure?

   a. A respiratory infection contracted when working
   with a patient with pneumonia
   b. Touching a patient's blood with a bare hand with
   unbroken skin
   c. An accidental needlestick with a needle contaminated with the blood of a patient
   d. Splashing urine on the arm while pouring a
   specimen

18. True or False: The OSHA Blood-   Outcome 3-17
borne Pathogens Standard requires the development
of an exposure control plan. Part of this plan
requires that all employees who have occupational
exposure to blood or other potentially infectious
materials are offered an opportunity to receive a
series of hepatitis C vaccinations at no charge.

19. True or False: When using a needle   Outcome 3-18
to draw blood, it is okay to lay it down on the table
next to the drawing chair right after the blood draw,
and come back later to activate the safety device and
dispose of it correctly.

20. Who must transport biohazardous   Outcome 3-19
waste?

   a. Employees of the laboratory that have been
   appropriately trained
   b. The local municipal garbage disposal company
   c. A certified, licensed biohazardous waste disposal
   company
   d. None of the above

21. What do hepatitis A, hepatitis B, hepatitis C, and HIV all have in common? Outcome 3-20

    a. They are all caused by viruses
    b. They are all caused by bacteria
    c. They all have vaccinations to prevent infection
    d. None of them have vaccinations to prevent infection.

22. Are blood tests part of the follow-up procedure for health-care workers who are are percutaneously exposed to blood in the workplace? Outcome 3-21

Case Study 3-1: Too tired to think

Jackie was really tired. She had been up all night with her 3-year-old daughter who had an ear infection. When she reported to her job at the GI clinic the next morning, she was relieved to find out that she would be working in the laboratory, as this meant that she would be on her feet a bit less than if she were working as the MA for one of the physicians. It was Friday, which was usually a slow day in the laboratory.

In the middle of the morning, Jackie had drawn three glass red-top blood tubes from Mr. Sifton. She was fighting back a yawn, and when she turned around to put the blood in the rack on the counter, she accidentally tapped one of the tubes against the edge of the counter with a great deal of force. The tube flew from her hand and broke against the refrigerator a few feet away.

Jackie was flustered. Mr. Sifton had already left, and she knew that she would have to call him and ask him to return for another blood draw. In addition, she had quite a mess to clean up, as the blood had splattered a great deal. She knew that the bloody mess had to take precedence, because other patients would be entering the laboratory at any time.

Jackie was already wearing her nitrile gloves, so she bent down and started to pick up the pieces of the tube that had broken. Suddenly she felt a sharp pain in her finger, and realized that she had punctured her glove and her finger with a slice of glass.

1. What are two things that could have been done to avoid the parenteral exposure to the patient's blood?
2. What is the first thing that Jackie should do now? What else needs to happen as soon as possible?

RESOURCES AND SUGGESTED READINGS

OSHA Hazard Communication Standard
  OSHA regulation for chemical safety in the workplace http://www.osha.gov/SLTC/hazardcommunications/standards.html
Small Business Handbook
  General reference tool to verify that the OSHA Standards are in place properly at your worksite http://www.osha.gov/Publications/smallbusiness/small-business.html#hazsub/
National Fire Protection Association
  National Fire Protection Association website that includes information about fire, electrical, and building safety http://www.nfpa.org
Updated directives for OSHA Bloodborne Pathogens Standards, 1991
  Additional information added to the OSHA Bloodborne Pathogens Standards in 1991 1910.1030- 29CFR http://www.osha.gov/pls/oshaweb/owadisp.show_document?p_table=standards&p_id=10051
"Viral Hepatitis"
  Excellent information about the different forms of viral hepatitis presented by the Centers for Disease Control and Prevention http://www.cdc.gov/hepatitis/index.htm
Hepatitis B Foundation, "Meet Dr. Blumberg"
  Facts concerning the discovery of hepatitis B, and Dr. Blumberg who was awarded a Nobel Prize in 1976 for this discovery http://www.hepb.org/about/blumberg.htm

Chapter 4

Assuring Quality

Constance L. Lieseke, CMA (AAMA), MLT, PBT(ASCP)

CHAPTER OUTLINE

Learning Outcomes   *After reading this chapter, the successful student will be able to:*

4-1   Define each of the key terms.

4-2   Compare and contrast quality assurance and quality control.

4-3   Explain why quality is essential for laboratory testing.

4-4   Describe circumstances when a medical assistant may need to perform quality control testing in the laboratory.

4-5   Classify the types of quality control specimens used in the laboratory.

4-6   Explain the concept of troubleshooting and list various actions that may be taken when quality control samples are not in range.

4-7   Demonstrate the ability to correctly log quality control results with appropriate documentation techniques.

4-8   Provide examples of the ways that quality may be assured with laboratory testing procedures.

CAAHEP/ABHES STANDARDS

 CAAHEP 2008 Standards

I.P.I.11. Perform quality control procedures
I.A.I.2. Distinguish between normal and abnormal test results
II.C.II.7. Analyze charts, graphs and/or tables in the interpretation of healthcare results
II.P.II.2. Maintain laboratory test results using flow sheets

 ABHES Standards

Medical Laboratory Procedures 10.a: Quality Control, and Graduates: a. Practice Quality Control

KEY TERMS

Accuracy	External quality control specimens	Quality assurance (QA)
Analyte	Internal quality control indicators	Quality control (QC)
Calibration	Mean	Quantitative results
Calibration verification	Oncologist	Reference ranges
Clinical significance	Panic results	Shift
Competency testing	Precision	Trends
Critical results	Proficiency testing	Troubleshooting
Electronic quality control devices	Qualitative results	Valid

ASSURING QUALITY IN THE LABORATORY

Laboratory results are extremely important to patient diagnosis and treatment. However, the results reported back to the physician are only as good as the testing methods themselves. This chapter explains various ways that the quality of the testing process can be monitored, so that the patient results reported will be correct. Quality control (QC) and quality assurance (QA) will be covered in detail, as well as documentation techniques and troubleshooting. Other procedures that are part of overall test quality assessment will be explored, such as proficiency testing and competency assessments, and the rules for quality performance of CLIA-waived tests will be reviewed.

QUALITY CONTROL AND QUALITY ASSURANCE

The terms *quality assurance* and *quality control* seem so similar; you may be wondering why it is important to know the difference. Essentially, they are both part of a plan to provide excellent quality care to the patients we serve. Quality control is part of the quality assurance process, but with a more specific focus.

Try to remember the last time you visited a health-care provider or laboratory to have your blood drawn and tested. How was your experience? Did you receive the information you needed to prepare for the blood draw appropriately? Did you feel that the person who drew your blood was trained adequately? How confident were you that the testing process was done in a way that accurate and valid results were obtained and reported

back to your physician? Did your physician contact you in a timely manner with your results? These impressions, even though they were very personal to you, are all part of a quality assurance program at that facility.

Quality assurance (QA) includes all the policies and procedures necessary to provide excellent quality in laboratory testing. Chapter 1, introduced the three parts of laboratory testing: preanalytical, analytical, and postanalytical processes. A good quality assurance program acknowledges every part of the testing process to ensure that the laboratory staff members are doing all they can to contribute positively to the welfare of the patient in a timely manner. Quality assurance may be thought of as the big picture and it may include policies and procedures for collection, patient education, training for those performing the testing, maintenance and record keeping of instruments, monitoring of ordering and storage procedures for testing kits or reagents, and monitoring of turnaround times for results to be available to the health-care provider. Box 4-1 shows more detailed components of a quality assurance plan.

Quality control (QC) practices are used in the laboratory to ensure the quality of the testing process and the accuracy and precision of the results. Although the focus of quality control is specifically on the testing process, these practices are not limited to the details of how the test was performed. A good quality control program includes appropriate employee training, documentation of storage and shipping of reagents or testing kits used for testing, adherence to the manufacturer's instructions, correct interpretation and documentation of results, and verification that the results being reported are accurate and reliable. Quality control focuses on the second part

BOX 4-1 QA processes

Preanalytical Phase

Requisition appropriately filled out

Patient preparation

Patient identification

Sample identification; three identifiers must be used

Correct sample collection techniques; venipuncture performed correctly, etc.

Correct storage and transportation of sample

Correct storage of testing kits and quality control materials

Appropriate training of personnel

Preparation of standard operating procedures and policy manuals for reference

Retention of current package inserts for correct instructions

Analytical Phase

Valid test kit; not expired and stored correctly

Instrument properly maintained and calibrated

Proper mixing/preparation of quality control samples

Proper mixing/preparation of patient samples

Following manufacturer instructions exactly as written for CLIA-waived tests

Proper documentation of quality control results; verification of acceptable QC values before patient sample is analyzed

Order/perform confirmatory tests as recommended by manufacturer

Postanalytical Phase

Appropriate documentation of patient results

Appropriate units reported with test results

Results transmitted to health-care provider in timely manner

All critical results called immediately

Include correct reference ranges with laboratory results

Report all test results to authorities as required by law

Properly dispose of used testing materials

TABLE 4-1

Quality assurance versus quality control

Quality Assurance	Quality Control
Addresses procedures in all phases of laboratory process; includes quality control	Focuses specifically on the testing process, or analytical phase of the laboratory process
Comprehensive plan including patients, employees, and employers	Includes processes performed by employees and influenced by policies of employers
Plan developed by the employer and the quality assurance officer	Policies often established by the manufacturer; also may be developed by the employer
Requires comprehensive and detailed documentation	Requires detailed documentation
Requires critical thinking and analysis to design the plan and keep it current	Requires critical thinking and analysis to decide if the patient sample can be reported based on the quality control results

of the laboratory testing process: the analytical phase. Anything that relates directly to the testing process may be part of quality control. Table 4-1 shows how quality assurance and quality control compare to one another.

Test Your Knowledge 4-1

List two ways that quality assurance and quality control are alike. (Outcome 4-2)

WHAT IS QUALITY?

The laboratory environment is no different from that of any other business. Customers are essential to the survival of the laboratory, and the testing provided is a service that the customers need. Who are the customers? This is not quite as easy to answer as it might seem at first. The laboratory serves patients; that is pretty clear. The patients may be varied in age, socioeconomic class, race, and gender, but laboratory results are a critical part of their care. However, the laboratory can serve the patients only if the quality of the laboratory performance meets the expectations of the health-care provider who sends the patient (or the specimens from the patient) to a specific laboratory for testing. Therefore, the health-care providers are also laboratory customers.

The performance of the laboratory must be of very high quality to serve both of these types of customers efficiently. Consider this scenario:

*A new **oncologist** opens a practice in your community. He specializes in providing care to patients with cancer, and is very concerned that the laboratory* *testing available will be sufficient to meet his needs. Within the first week, he orders several screening tests for ovarian cancer to be performed on his patients. The analyzer used to perform these tests breaks down on Monday, and no one in the laboratory contacts the physician to let him know of the delay. He finally receives his screening tests on Friday, and one of the results is positive. He is very upset about the time that it took for him to receive this result in his office, and decides to send all his testing requests to another laboratory.*

This is an example of a breakdown in quality assurance. If the physician had been notified of the expected delay for his results, he may still have been upset, but at least the lines of communication would have been open. Another alternative would have been sending the samples to another laboratory while the machine was serviced; the delay would most likely have been minimized, and the physician would have received his results in a timely manner.

Other examples of poor quality performance are incorrect results, improper patient preparation, reporting the wrong **reference ranges** (a range of expected values for a healthy individual for a specific test) for a specific patient's gender and age, or even improper billing practices. All aspects of the customer experience in the laboratory must be of high quality, as the test results may have significant impact on the treatment for the patient. A patient may be put on antibiotics when they are not needed because a streptococcal screen was incorrectly interpreted as positive. Another patient result may show a false elevation in potassium levels when a specimen is mishandled, and the physician may change their medication based on these results. This could be a life threatening situation.

It may be helpful to consider laboratory quality as a series of "Rights":

- Right result
- Right time (both specimen collection and reporting of results)
- Right specimen
- Right patient
- Right reference range for result interpretation
- Right price for the services provided

Test Your Knowledge 4-2

How do incorrect laboratory results affect patient care?

(Outcome 4-3)

The Medical Assistant's Role in Assuring Quality Results

Most medical assistants working in a laboratory environment will be performing Clinical Laboratory Improvement Act–waived (CLIA–waived) tests. These are tests that are very simple to perform with results that are easy to interpret. As introduced in Chapter 3 of this text, laboratory tests are categorized under CLIA regulations based on the complexity of the process. Some of the tests are categorized as "waived" tests because they are exempt (or waived) from many of the regulatory procedures of the laboratory tests that are more complex in nature. This does not mean, however, that they are exempt from quality control procedures. Even before the testing process begins, the medical assistant can be checking the sample collection devices (such as swabs or blood tubes) for outdates, and participating in necessary training to be ready for the procedure.

The first opportunity that a medical assistant might have to be involved in quality control is when the testing kit or reagents arrive in the laboratory. Storage instructions are printed on the outside of the box, and these need to be followed precisely to provide accurate test results. Reading the package insert is critical, as the procedure specified by the manufacturer must be followed carefully. When the box is opened, this package insert should be stored in a safe place. Many laboratories have a binder for these sheets, and it is the medical assistant's responsibility to verify that the insert has not changed since the last one was placed in the binder. Laboratories may also keep multiple copies that have the date of receipt documented for reference.

Types of Quality Control Specimens

When the kit (or the reagent) is opened for use, it will be necessary to test a quality control specimen as recommended on the package insert. Some testing procedures may call for two types of quality control specimens to be analyzed. There are three general categories used to describe quality control specimens:

1. **External quality control specimens:** This may be a reference solution that comes with the kit, or a swab that has been treated with material that will cause the test to read positive or negative. External quality control materials may also need to be purchased separately from the testing materials. Regardless of how the materials are provided, the most important concept to follow is that of the analysis of the quality

control specimens exactly as directed by the test manufacturer, and the comparison of the results from the specimen to the data provided to be sure that the test performance is as expected. These may be **qualitative results** for tests that provide a positive or negative result, or they may be **quantitative results** with a range of expected results. Quantitative tests provide results as numbers indicating the concentration of certain substances. If the results of the external quality control specimen are not as expected, the kit or reagent cannot be used to test patient samples until the problem has been identified and solved.

2. **Internal quality control indicators:** These are quality control indicators that are part of the individual testing kits. They show that the test process was **valid,** but they do not provide a test result. An internal quality control measurement is usually a color indicator, and in the package insert there will be an explanation of acceptable performance before a test result can be reported. Internal quality control specimens are most common in qualitative testing procedures. Remember, if the test is not valid (the indicator does not develop properly), you may not report the patient test result. Figure 4-1 shows how an indicator might appear.

3. **Electronic quality control devices:** Electronic quality control devices are reusable, and are used to verify the function of an instrument used for analysis. The electronic quality control devices are commonly test strips or cuvettes. The devices come with an expected numerical range of results, and it is imperative that the results fall within this range when tested, or no patient results may be reported until the problem has been identified and solved.

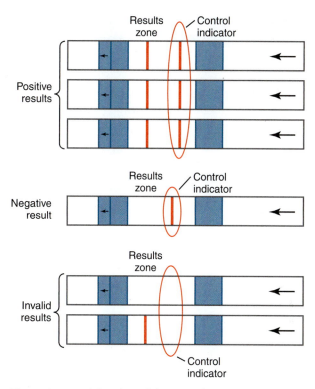

Figure 4-1 Valid and invalid test results.

Medical assistants may also perform tests that have been classified as CLIA moderate-complexity procedures. These procedures may require quality control procedures to be performed with more frequency than the CLIA-waived tests, and there is more training and documentation required for the employee who is performing the tests. Laboratories that perform these moderately complex tests are required either to follow the recommendations for quality control included in the package insert from the manufacturer, or process at least two levels of quality control materials with each analytical run. The CLIA regulations state that the laboratory must use the more stringent option of the two. Tests of moderate complexity utilizing instruments also require calibration, calibration verification, and proficiency testing. These concepts are discussed later in this chapter.

What Happens When Things Are "Out of Control"?

It is very important to recognize the importance of quality control specimens as an indicator of the reliability and accuracy of the testing method to be utilized for

---

Test Your Knowledge 4-3

Do electronic QC devices let you know whether a test is valid? (Outcome 4-3)

Test Your Knowledge 4-4

If a medical assistant is using a machine to analyze a blood sample for a test result, what type of QC may she be required to use?
   a. External
   b. Internal
   c. Electronic
   d. a and c (Outcome 4-4)

Procedure 4-1: Documentation of Qualitative Quality Control Values

TASK

Properly perform quality control testing and document qualitative QC values on a chart.

CAAHEP/ABHES STANDARDS

 CAAHEP 2008

I.P.I.11. Perform quality control procedures
I.A.I.2. Distinguish between normal and abnormal test results
II.C.II.7. Analyze charts, graphs and/or tables in the interpretation of healthcare results
II.P.II.2. Maintain laboratory test results using flow sheets

ABHES Standards

Medical Laboratory Procedures 10.a: Quality Control, and Graduates: a. Practice Quality Control

CONDITIONS

- CLIA-waived test kit
- External quality control material
- Quality control chart
- Pen

Procedure	Rationale
1. Open the CLIA-waived test kit and secure the package insert.	It will be necessary to have the package insert available for reference as the quality control specimen is analyzed.
2. Verify which type of quality control specimen your laboratory uses for this testing procedure. Find the directions in the package insert for that type of specimen.	The quality control specimen may be one that is provided with the kit or it may be a commercial one that is purchased separately. It is important that the correct procedure be used for the testing process.
3. Wash hands and apply gloves.	Appropriate personal protective equipment should be used when testing quality control materials just as it would be used for testing samples.
4. Following the directions in the package insert, perform the testing procedure using the positive quality control specimen. Repeat with the negative quality control specimen.	The performance of the testing procedure should be verified with both a positive and negative control specimen as recommended by the manufacturer.
5. Verify that the positive and negative quality control specimens provide the appropriate results.	Tests must be valid and the results must be as expected for the test kit to be considered "in control."
6. Remove gloves, dispose of them appropriately, and wash hands.	Gloves should be removed before documenting results.
7. Record the results on the log sheet. Include these factors: a. Date and time of test and employee ID b. Analyte tested (what type of test was performed?) c. Type of quality control (external); brand name if a commercial control was purchased separately	All these factors are very important documentation, and any form should allow for the recording of complete information.

Procedure	Rationale
from the kit, and lot number of quality control material. **d.** Result (positive or negative) **e.** Was result acceptable? **f.** Corrective action taken, if necessary	
8. Put away testing supplies and disinfect work area.	

Procedure 4-2: Documentation of Quantitative Quality Control Values

TASK

Properly perform and document quantitative quality control values on a chart. Determine whether the values are acceptable according to laboratory protocol.

CAAHEP/ABHES STANDARDS

 CAAHEP 2008

I.P.I.11. Perform quality control procedures
I.A.I.2. Distinguish between normal and abnormal test results
II.C.II.7. Analyze charts, graphs and/or tables in the interpretation of healthcare results
II.P.II.2. Maintain laboratory test results using flow sheets

 ABHES Standards

Medical Laboratory Procedures 10.a: Quality Control, and Graduates: a. Practice Quality Control

CONDITIONS

- Quantitative testing method
- External quality control material
- Quality control chart with established acceptable ranges provided
- Pen

Procedure	Rationale
1. Consult the instructions for the testing method if necessary before continuing with the process.	With automated testing procedures, the manufacturer's recommendations usually do not change as often as they might with the CLIA-waived test kits. However, consulting the instructions is always appropriate.
2. Verify which type of quality control specimen your laboratory uses for this testing procedure.	The quality control specimen may be one that is provided with the testing method, or it may be a commercial product that is purchased separately.
3. Wash hands and apply gloves.	Appropriate personal protective equipment should be used when testing quality control materials just as it would be utilized for testing samples.
4. Following the directions in the package insert or the laboratory procedure manual, perform the testing procedure using the quality control specimen. Repeat with a second quality control level if recommended by the manufacturer.	The performance of the testing procedure should be verified with both a high and low level quality control specimen as recommended by the manufacturer.

Continued

Procedure 4-2: Documentation of Quantitative Quality Control Values—cont'd

Procedure	Rationale
5. Put away quality control material.	Many quality control specimens must remain refrigerated, so this should occur immediately after use.
6. Remove gloves, dispose of them appropriately, and wash hands.	Gloves should be removed before documenting results.
7. Record the results on the log sheet by placing a dot at the line at which the date and specimen result intersect. In addition, document the time of the test and your identification. Verify that the correct control level brand and lot number are on the log sheet.	All these factors are very important documentation, and any form should allow for the recording of complete information.
8. Verify whether the quality control is within the established ranges and whether there is a pattern developing that needs attention, such as a trend or a shift in the results. If there is a problem or if the quality control is out of range, do not process patient samples.	Careful documentation of the results and observation of any quality control patterns are absolutely necessary. Patient samples cannot be processed if the sample is out of range or if there is an undesirable pattern forming in the results.
9. Repeat the test if results are out of range. If the condition persists, begin troubleshooting the problem. Document the repeat and also if there are troubleshooting steps taken.	Troubleshooting may include opening a new bottle of quality control material, cleaning the instrument, verifying the instructions for performing the test, verifying that the quality control chart is for the correct lot number, etc.
10. If the troubleshooting is not successful, do not allow the instrument to be used for patient samples, and contact a supervisor or the manufacturer for further action.	It is essential that the problem be resolved as soon as possible to continue with quality patient care.

patients. When the QC results are not as expected, the person running the test or operating the instrument must not report any patient results until the problem has been solved. The systematic process of identifying the problem with the testing procedure is called **troubleshooting.** There are times when the quality control specimen does not provide a positive result as expected, or when the test results appear invalid when running a pregnancy test QC specimen. The medical assistant performing the test must immediately try to identify the problem with the testing procedure before the process can continue. Here are some actions to take when troubleshooting a testing process:

1. Check the expiration dates of the reagents, kit, and quality control reagents in use. If any of these supplies are outdated, document the discrepancy, discard the expired item, and perform the test again using materials that are not past their expiration date.

2. Verify how the specimen, kit, reagent, or quality control material has been stored. Were the manufacturer's recommendations followed? If there is evidence that the storage instructions were not followed, the results provided by this testing method may be inaccurate. The testing component that was mishandled must be discarded, with appropriate documentation of the issue.

3. Verify the specimen type required for the testing procedure. Sometimes a kit is designed to work only with certain types of body fluids. The acceptable specimen type will be provided as part of the package insert.

Tests performed on body fluids not indicated as acceptable may provide inaccurate or invalid results.

4. Was the control material well mixed and at the correct temperature for the test? The quality control material may require warming to room temperature before use or vigorous mixing prior to testing. These instructions must be followed carefully.

5. Refer to the current package insert. Are you aware of skipping a step, or doing the procedure incorrectly? Has the package insert or instructions changed since you last performed the test?

6. If an instrument was used for the test, is it clean? Check the maintenance documentation, and see if the recommended schedule has been followed for routine instrument care. If needed, perform the recommended maintenance, after which the QC can be analyzed again.

7. Read the troubleshooting portion of the manufacturer's instructions. There is valuable information here that may help to solve the problem.

Usually the problem may be identified by following these suggestions. If the problem is still not apparent, a new quality control specimen should be obtained for a retest. If it is an internal control and the quality control specimen comes with the kit, open a new kit and try the test again. Finally, documentation of the details and troubleshooting process is critical. If there seems to be a pattern emerging, it is imperative that everyone knows what has occurred, and the steps that have been taken to solve the problem. Details also help while communicating with a manager or supervisor about the problem. Sometimes the medical assistant may need to contact the manufacturer for advice, and these details will be necessary to continue the troubleshooting process.

Test Your Knowledge 4-5

Cindy Lou has recently been trained to perform pregnancy testing in the physician office laboratory (POL) where she is employed. She receives a blood specimen from the physician who asks her to test it to see if a young patient is pregnant. Cindy follows the pregnancy testing procedure exactly as she was taught, but the test results show that it is an invalid test. What are two possible explanations?   (Outcome 4-6)

Documentation of Quality Control Results

Quality control requirements are different for CLIA-waived tests than they are for those of moderate or high complexity. Many of the waived tests are qualitative in nature, which means that the result provided is either positive or negative, rather than a measurement reported as a number or percentage. The quality control assessment for these qualitative tests may be built in to the individual testing devices or the laboratory may purchase other quality control specimens to verify the performance quality for the **analyte** (substance being tested). Whether the QC is internal or external, it must be documented, and this record must be kept for at least two years. As with any document in the laboratory or in a patient's chart, the results on the quality control chart must be documented in pen, not pencil. This provides a permanent record that is not easily changed. One of the most common sources of laboratory error is that of transcription; it is very important to carefully document all laboratory data. Figure 4-2 is an example of a quality control log sheet to be used for a qualitative test. At a

Date and time of test/ Employee identification	Analyte tested	Type of quality control specimen used; external or internal?	For external quality control; brand and quality control lot numbers	Quality control result	Results acceptable? (yes or no)	Corrective action taken

Figure 4-2   Log used to record quality control results for a qualitative test.

minimum, the documentation should include the following:

- **The date and time of the quality control test.** Remember, the frequency that the QC is tested must be at least as often as the manufacturer recommends.
- **The quality control material lot number and level.** If it is internal control, this would be documented as additional information. If the testing device has a color change that occurs to verify the validity of the test, this needs to be recorded as well.
- **The lot number for the testing kit in use.** If this test kit was just opened, the kit should also have the date and the initials of the person who opened it written on the test kit box.
- **Results of the quality control test.** This is often just positive or negative for qualitative CLIA-waived tests.
- **Documentation of whether the kit or test can be used to test patient samples.** Remember, this decision is based on whether the quality control results were within the established acceptable ranges.
- **Documentation of troubleshooting or corrective action, if required.**
- **Initials or signature of employee performing test.**

> **Test Your Knowledge 4-6**
>
> Why is it important to document the date of a quality control test?   (Outcome 4-7)

Various moderate-complexity tests, as well as some that are CLIA-waived, will provide quantitative results. This means that the quality control results for these testing methods will also be reported as a number, rather than merely a negative or positive result indicating the presence or absence of a substance. Because the results reported for these tests are to fall within an established range, it is very important that the quality control results are monitored closely to verify the method's performance. A common tool used to record these quantitative results is a Levey-Jennings chart, used to monitor the quality control performance over a set time interval. The acceptable quality control ranges are either established by the laboratory before patient samples are analyzed with the kit or instrument, or they are established by the manufacturer and adopted by the laboratory. The values obtained each time the quality control is processed are charted (in pen) according to the date and the value obtained. The chart also has spaces to document the analyte being tested, the QC level, the lot numbers of the kit and the quality controls, and other information that may be necessary for that particular laboratory. Levey-Jennings charts will also include the **mean** (average) expected value, as well as limits for acceptable QC testing results. If an individual quality control test falls outside of these ranges, patient testing cannot continue until the problem has been addressed. This type of graph can also be monitored for **trends** in the data, which show a progressive change in the results from day to day that continue to move gradually in one direction. **Shifts** will also be evident, and can be identified on the graph as a set of results that suddenly move significantly, but still remain within an acceptable range. Sometimes a shift will be evident when the results move from one side of the mean to the other, but a shift may also be evident even if the results remain on the same side of the mean. Both of these situations must be addressed, because they are indicative of a problem with the quality control procedure, the testing method, the operator, or a combination of these factors. Figure 4-3 is an example of a quantitative Levey-Jennings quality control chart.

> **Test Your Knowledge 4-7**
>
> Is a Levey-Jennings chart used to document qualitative QC test results? Why or why not?   (Outcome 4-7)

Accuracy and Precision

The Levey-Jennings chart can be a useful tool to verify whether a testing method is demonstrating accuracy and precision. These are very important concepts to keep in mind in the laboratory environment. **Accuracy** is a word used to define how close the result produced for that test is to the real value. This can be visualized by thinking of a bull's-eye target. The true value for a test procedure is at the center of the target. If the test is accurate, then each time the test is performed the results will be near the center of the target.

Precision describes the reproducibility of results. This can also be thought of as a measurement of whether the results are close together if the test is run multiple times on the same specimen. Visualizing the bull's-eye target again, a test shows good precision if the results are all clustered closely together when the test is run multiple times.

A test can be precise but not accurate. This means that the results for a certain test may all be close to the same value, but not near the true value for that test. The goal for laboratory testing is to have results that are both

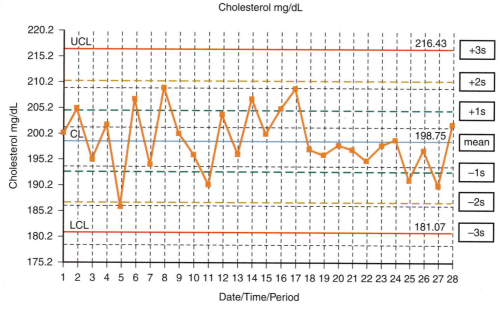

Figure 4-3 Levey-Jennings chart used to record quantitative quality control results.

accurate and precise, and quality control measures help to identify problems in these areas before they affect the quality of the patient results for that test.

OTHER METHODS OF ASSURING LABORATORY QUALITY

All laboratory results have **clinical significance,** meaning that a health-care provider may change the treatment or assign a diagnosis for a patient based on the laboratory results. In addition, there are established **reference ranges** for all laboratory tests. These are the expected values for patients in a normal population for a certain analyte. In order to feel confident that the laboratory results reported are accurate and reliable, all facets of quality assurance must be taken into consideration. The best way to understand how these all fit into patient care is to consider a patient scenario with a negative outcome:

Mr. Butler has developed an atrial arrhythmia and is being treated with the drug digoxin to help increase the efficiency of his heart muscle and correct problems with the electrical impulses that pass through his heart. Mr. Butler visits the laboratory monthly to have his drug level checked, as digoxin has serious side effects if the concentration is too high in the bloodstream. When the laboratory tests the digoxin level, a higher-than-normal level is discovered for someone being treated for his condition, and the result is well outside the reference range. When Mr. Butler's physician receives the report, he calls his patient, verifies his health status, and tells him that he needs to decrease his digoxin dose for a few days. The physician asks Mr. Butler to go to the laboratory to have another specimen drawn at the end of the week. On day three after decreasing his dose, Mr. Butler has his drug level rechecked. This second draw is extremely low, well below the reference range. The result is drastically different from what it was a few days earlier, and is much lower than it should be with the minor medication adjustment based on the previous high result.

Of course, Mr. Butler's health-care provider is eager to find out how the results for the digoxin could be so different in just a few days. He contacts Mr. Butler and confirms that he followed the dosage changes as directed. The physician then contacts the laboratory that performed the testing on the first sample. The laboratory staff rechecks the sample, and finds the result is close to the first reading: still high above the reference range. However, when their quality assurance officer steps in to resolve the issue, she finds that the quality control results for the digoxin test have been slowly reading higher and higher for a few days prior to the test date. This trend has gone unnoticed by the personnel performing the tests, because the results were all within the acceptable range.

POINT OF INTEREST 4-1
Statistics used for quality control assessment

Statistics is a specific branch of mathematics that deals with the collection, analysis, and interpretation of numerical data. We use statistics in the laboratory to analyze the quantitative data derived from quality control testing. The entire process is quite complicated, but developing an understanding of a few key terms can benefit the medical assistant as he or she works with these data.

To establish acceptable ranges for qualitative QC testing procedures, the mean, standard deviation, and variance must be established.

- **Mean:** The mean is the numerical average of a set of numbers. To calculate the mean, find the sum (total) of a set of values (numbers), then divide that sum by the number of values in the set. For instance, if you were to analyze a specimen ten times for a potassium level, you might generate these numbers: 4.5, 4.4, 4.2, 4.6, 4.5, 4.1, 4.3, 4.6, 4.5, and 4.7 mmol/L. The mean of these values would be calculated by adding them all together, then dividing by 10, because there were ten results used for the calculation. The mean result for these numbers would be 4.4 mmol/L.

- **Variance:** The variance is a bit more complicated to calculate. It gives a numeric indication of how much the values in the set vary or deviate from the mean. The variance is calculated after the mean for the set of numbers has been established. Each number is subtracted from the mean, and this difference is squared, which means to multiply it by itself one time. The sum of the squares is then established, and this sum is divided by the total number of values minus one. (The term used for this calculation is $n - 1$.) Therefore, for our scenario presented above, we would follow these steps from the calculate mean of 4.4 mmol/L:

The sum of the deviations squared is 0.34, and this number divided by $n - 1$ (9 in our example) is 0.036. The variance for this set of numbers is 0.036.

Value	Potassium Deviation; How Far from the Mean of 4.4?	Deviation Squared; Multiplied by Itself
4.5	0.1	0.01
4.4	0.0	0.00
4.2	0.2	0.04
4.6	0.2	0.04
4.5	0.1	0.01
4.1	0.3	0.09
4.3	0.1	0.01
4.6	0.2	0.04
4.5	0.1	0.01
4.7	0.3	0.09

- **Standard deviation:** The standard deviation provides a measurement of how the values we are working with are placed or scattered around the calculated mean for the values. The standard deviation uses the variance that was calculated in the previous step, and is calculated by taking the square root of the variance. For the potassium scenario that we are working with, the standard deviation would be calculated by calculating the square root of 0.036. The standard deviation would be 0.061 mmol/L for this set of potassium results.

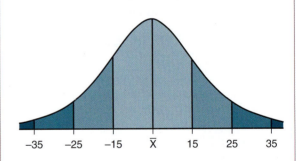

The previous calculations are used to establish acceptable values or allowable standard deviation for their qualitative laboratory results. If the potassium values were analyzed for 100 people who were considered to be of normal health, we would find that their values could be plotted on a graph to form a Gaussian curve (see above), which is sometimes known as a bell curve or normal distribution curve. In a normal curve, half of the values are greater than the mean and half of the values are less than the mean for that test result. Statistically, it has been shown that 68% of the results in a normal population will be within one standard deviation above or below the mean, and 95% will be within two standard deviations above and below the mean. Ninety-nine percent of the results will fall within three standard deviations of the mean.

Normally, when establishing acceptable ranges (also known as confidence limits) for a laboratory procedure, the quality control results must fall within a range of two standard deviations above or below the mean in order to be an acceptable result. For our potassium scenario, if this was a quality control material that was tested ten times, the results would need to fall within two standard deviations of the mean. The mean was 4.4, and the quality control results would need to be 4.4 plus or minus 0.122 to be within range. This means that the acceptable ranges for this quality control sample would be 4.28 to 4.52 mmol/L.

She also checks the maintenance logs for the instrument used for digoxin testing, and finds that the machine has not been serviced as recommended by the manufacturer. This is a very serious situation, especially because Mr. Butler may not have been the only patient affected by the instrument's performance.

The QA officer begins to make a plan to correct the issues. The first part of her plan is to have the overdue maintenance performed on the instrument. This includes cleaning the internal components of the machine and changing some tubing and reagents. After the maintenance has been performed, the machine has to be calibrated. **Calibration** is a standardization of the instrument for a specific analyte, meaning that a calibration sample (generally ordered from the manufacturer) is processed using the instrument. If the reading does not come out exactly as it should, the instrument is adjusted (according to manufacturer's instructions) until it does measure the calibration sample at precisely the predetermined level.

Once the calibration is complete, quality control assessment must be performed again. This is called **calibration verification.** The calibration and subsequent verification show that the testing instrument has been reading the digoxin specimen results several increments higher than they really were. This caused Mr. Butler's reading to appear falsely elevated; his specimen was tested once again after the calibration and verification and found to be at the high end of the expected reference range. His dosage should not have been altered. This

change in medication may have put his health at risk unnecessarily.

To follow up on this incident, the QA officer documents all that has occurred. Her follow-up includes reeducation of the personnel responsible for the quality control and maintenance for the testing instrument. She develops a plan to follow up with these employees to see if the intervention and retraining were successful. The QA officer also notifies the laboratory director and any other required personnel in the organization who need to be notified of a testing system problem leading to a bad patient outcome.

If the patient's health had been negatively affected by the medication change in response to the first digoxin test result, the laboratory would be at risk for legal action. As a result of this situation, it is likely that the physician may decide to send his specimens to a different laboratory for analysis.

As this scenario draws to a close, the QA officer feels confident that the digoxin levels reported from that instrument are now accurate and reliable. She also has to go back and follow up on reported results for other patients tested close to the time that Mr. Butler had his test performed.

However, another question still exists: How well do the digoxin results from this laboratory compare to others that are performing the same test with the same instrument? This is the final step of assuring quality for the laboratory. It is like taking a standardized assessment to see if the results produced in a certain laboratory compare well to those of others across the country. **Proficiency testing** is a means to measure the performance of a laboratory externally. For laboratories performing moderate- or high-complexity testing, federal regulations require that proficiency testing is performed at least three times yearly. The laboratories are sent specimens from a provider that has been approved by their licensing agency, and these specimens must be tested exactly as a patient sample would be tested. The laboratories then report their results back to the approved provider, and they are compared to other laboratories that perform the same test using the same method. If a laboratory's results are too different from the others used for the comparison, that laboratory may be told that it can no longer offer that specific test until the problem is identified and solved. In addition, if a laboratory is not successful with its proficiency testing, there will usually be a site visit performed by those who certify or license this laboratory for operation.

For proficiency testing to be valid, it is important to stress that the samples provided are to be run precisely the same as patient samples. Laboratories are not allowed to run the samples in duplicate unless the patient samples would be treated in this way. Proficiency testing is a powerful tool, providing verification for a laboratory that their results are comparable to others performing the same test across the region or country.

By law, laboratories that perform only CLIA-waived tests are not required to participate in proficiency testing. However, they may choose to voluntarily participate. The Centers for Medicare & Medicaid Services (CMS) still recommends that some sort of external quality verification is performed periodically, whether it is through a commercial agency or informally. Informal verification of quality may include splitting a patient sample and sending some of it to another laboratory to see what its result is, or asking for another laboratory to share its patient's samples for the same reason. Many laboratories also perform internal proficiency testing in which they pool patient samples, run them numerous times to get an acceptable range for the results, and then use these to supplement their commercial quality control materials throughout the day. These patient pool specimens are usually separated into small samples and frozen until they can be tested. The internal patient quality control samples are a nice way to supplement the commercial quality control in the laboratory, but they do not help with comparisons to other laboratories unless they are shared.

There is one more recommended method to assure quality in the laboratory. This process is known as **competency testing.** Competency testing actually evaluates the personnel who perform the laboratory tests, by direct observation, or by introducing mock specimens with known values into the patient load and evaluating the results and documentation after the test is complete. This evaluation process can be especially critical with the CLIA-waived tests, as often the person who performs the test has little or no formal laboratory training, and he or she may not realize the significance of cutting corners by not following the procedure exactly as the manufacturer recommends it to be performed. Many laboratories have designed a program in which competency testing of some sort is performed annually for each employee, in which a supervisor provides samples of known results for personnel to test. If the documented results do not fall within the established ranges, then additional training needs to be integrated into the laboratory environment.

Test Your Knowledge 4-8
How is the process of calibration different from running a quality control specimen?   (Outcome 4-8)

Test Your Knowledge 4-9
Is proficiency testing required for all laboratories?
(Outcome 4-8)

The CMS has performed site visits at CLIA-waived laboratories across the United States over the course of the past few years and the results have been very informative. Because the regulatory requirements for laboratories that perform only CLIA-waived tests are minimal, there is concern for the quality of the services provided by these laboratories. The following is a summary of the issues identified in the site visits:

- The employees performing the tests were inadequately trained. Training must be provided by a qualified person who has knowledge of the test performance, and the actual performance of the test should be evaluated as the trainer observes.
- There were high turnover rates for testing personnel, especially medical assistants.
- CLIA-waived testing sites were performing tests that were not CLIA waived, using personnel who were not adequately educated or trained to perform the procedures. This could be a potentially dangerous situation for patients, as the procedures may not be performed correctly and the testing personnel may not be able to identify significant issues with the testing process due to lack of training.
- Many of the sites did not have the most recent manufacturer's procedural instructions for the tests they were performing. Approximately 20% of the sites reported that they did not routinely check the manufacturer's package inserts to see if there were recommended changes in the procedure. There were also cost-cutting measures in effect in some laboratories, in which urinalysis testing strips or fecal occult blood slides were being cut in half to increase the number of specimens tested per kit. This destroys the integrity of the testing process, and means that the laboratory is noncompliant with the CLIA regulations.
- Quality control testing was not performed as specified by the manufacturer by many of the sites, and units of measure were incorrectly reported with patient results.

- Problems were identified with expiration dates and storage methods for the testing kits, as well as documentation of the lot numbers and control results for the kits once they were opened. There were also issues with inadequate performance of instrument maintenance and calibration.
- Approximately 6% of the laboratories visited did not perform follow-up confirmatory tests as recommended by the manufacturer.
- Some of the sites were testing specimens that were not acceptable for that waived method. For instance, some tests are designed to be performed on urine, but the laboratory was testing plasma instead.

In 2005, the Centers for Disease Control and Prevention (CDC) published a report summarizing the results of site visits mentioned above. (You can find the link to the report in the Resources and Suggested Readings section at the end of this chapter.) In addition to the summary, the report also includes recommendations for good laboratory practices for waived testing sites. The majority of these recommendations have been included in this chapter. They include specific considerations for all three parts of the laboratory testing procedure: preanalytical, analytical and postanalytical phases.

1. Be certain that there is a written request or requisition for all tests performed.
2. Follow the written instructions for collection methods carefully, and verify what type of specimen is needed for the test ordered before collection.
3. Properly identify the patient and specimen, and store the specimen properly until the testing process begins.
4. Check the kit expiration date.
5. Know the product insert; be sure that copies are kept current at all times, and refer to them often. A sample package insert is reproduced in Figure 4-4.
6. Follow the procedure provided by the manufacturer exactly as written.
7. Run controls often, at least as often as is recommended by the manufacturer.
8. Repeat the test if there is a problem, and troubleshoot if the problem continues. Always verify that the test result is valid if there is an indicator present on the testing device.
9. Accurately record the results; use the correct units and be sure that the reference ranges reflect the population and sample type that you are reporting.
10. Sign and date your results wherever they are recorded in your laboratory setting.
11. Notify the health-care provider that ordered the tests in a timely manner. Be aware of **panic** or **critical results.** These are test results that are far enough outside of the reference ranges that they may be considered to be life threatening, and must be reported *immediately* to the ordering physician or another appropriate responsible party. When notifying the physician's office of these results, document who was notified, what was reported, and when it was reported, and sign and date this documentation.

Test Your Knowledge 4-10

What is the most important step that a medical assistant can take to ensure that he or she is performing a CLIA-waived test for mononucleosis correctly?

(Outcome 4-8)

SUMMARY

Quality assurance in the clinical laboratory is like a big umbrella covering numerous aspects of the process. A good QA plan should address issues such as education of the providers and patients concerning appropriate patient preparation before testing, initial and ongoing education of all personnel, written procedures, thorough documentation of all testing, quality control and maintenance procedures, and plans for how to follow up on problems that may develop. Quality control focuses more on the testing process itself, and includes specimen and testing kit or reagent storage, following directions, and reporting results appropriately. Other means of assuring quality in the laboratory may include calibration, external proficiency testing, and competency testing. The most important aspect of all these measures is to assure quality results for the patients we serve so that they can be cared for appropriately.

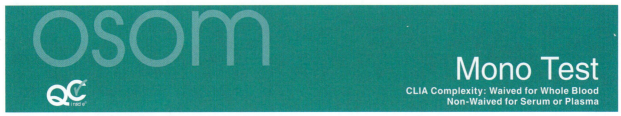

FOR LABORATORY AND PROFESSIONAL IN VITRO DIAGNOSTIC USE ONLY.

INTENDED USE
The OSOM® Mono Test is intended for the qualitative detection of infectious mononucleosis heterophile antibodies in serum, plasma or whole blood as an aid in the diagnosis of infectious mononucleosis.

SUMMARY AND EXPLANATION OF TEST
The diagnosis of infectious mononucleosis (IM) is suggested on the basis of the clinical symptoms of fever, sore throat and swollen lymph glands. The highest incidence of symptomatic IM occurs during late adolescence (15–24 years of age). Infectious mononucleosis is caused by the Epstein-Barr Virus (EBV).[1,2] The laboratory diagnosis of IM is based on the detection of IM heterophile antibodies. These heterophile antibodies are directed against antigens found in bovine, sheep and horse erythrocytes. The OSOM Mono Test utilizes an extract of bovine erythrocytes to give the required sensitivity and specificity.

KIT CONTENTS AND STORAGE
25 Test Sticks in a container
25 Test Tubes
25 Transfer Pipettes
25 Capillary Tubes with 1 Capillary Bulb
1 Diluent (contains buffer with 0.2% sodium azide)
1 Mono Positive Control (contains rabbit anti-beef stroma in tris buffer with 0.2% sodium azide and 0.05% gentamycin sulfate preservatives)
1 Mono Negative Control (contains goat albumin in tris buffer with 0.2% sodium azide)
1 Work Station
1 Directional Insert
2 Additional test sticks have been included in the kit for external QC testing
Note: Extra components (tubes, pipettes, capillary tubes and capillary bulb) have been provided for your convenience.
Store the Test Sticks and reagents tightly capped at 15°–30°C (59°–86°F).
Do not use the Test Sticks or reagents after their expiration dates.

MATERIALS REQUIRED BUT NOT PROVIDED
Specimen collection containers.
A timer or watch.

PRECAUTIONS
• For in-vitro diagnostic use only.
• Follow your laboratory safety guidelines in the collection, handling, storage and disposal of patient specimens and all items exposed to patient specimens.
• The Diluent and Controls contain sodium azide which may react with lead or copper plumbing to form potentially explosive metal azide. Large quantities of water must be used to flush discarded Diluent or Controls down a sink.
• The Capillary Bulb contains dry natural rubber.
• Do not interchange or mix components from different kit lots.

SPECIMEN COLLECTION AND PREPARATION
Serum, Plasma, or Whole Blood Sample
Obtain specimens by acceptable medical technique. Collect whole blood samples using a tube containing EDTA or heparin as an anticoagulant. Other anticoagulants have not been tested. Serum and plasma specimens may be refrigerated (2°–8°C; 36°–46°F) and tested within 48 hours; serum and plasma specimens held for longer times should be frozen (below –10°C; 14°F) and tested within 3 months. Test whole blood specimens within 24 hours. Specimens must be at room temperature (15°–30°C; 59°–86°F) when tested.

Fingertip Whole Blood
Hold the capillary tube horizontally while collecting the sample. Touch the end of the capillary tube to the drop of blood on the patient's finger. Fill the capillary tube completely. Place the small end of the black bulb onto the capillary tube. Place your fingertip over the opening in the bulb. Squeeze the bulb to dispense the whole blood sample into the test tube.

QUALITY CONTROL
External Quality Control
For external QC testing, use the controls provided in the kit. Add one free falling drop of control to the Test Tube and then proceed in the same manner as with a patient sample. Quality Control requirements should be established in accordance with local, state and federal regulations or accreditation requirements. Minimally, Genzyme Diagnostics recommends that positive and negative external controls be run with each new lot and with each new untrained operator. Some commercial controls may contain interfering additives. The use of these controls is not recommended.

Figure 4-4   Package insert. *Courtesy of Genzyme Diagnostics.*

Internal Quality Controls
The OSOM Mono Test provides two levels of internal procedural controls with each test procedure.

• The red Control Line is an internal positive procedural control. The Test Stick must absorb the proper amount of test material and be working properly for the red Control Line to appear.
• A clear background is an internal negative procedural control. If the test has been performed correctly and the Test Stick is working properly, the background will clear to give a discernible result.

If the red Control Line does not appear, the test may be invalid. If the background does not clear and interferes with the test result, the test may be invalid. Call Genzyme Diagnostics Technical Assistance if you experience either of these problems.

LIMITATIONS
• As with all diagnostic assays, the results obtained by this test yield data that must be used as an adjunct to other information available to the physician.
• The OSOM Mono Test is a qualitative test for the detection of IM heterophile antibody.
• A negative result may be obtained from patients at the onset of the disease due to heterophile antibody levels below the sensitivity of this test kit. If symptoms persist or intensify, the test should be repeated.
• Some segments of the population with acute IM are heterophile antibody negative.[1]

EXPECTED VALUES
A heterophile antibody response is observed in approximately 80–90% of adults and children with EBV-caused IM. This percentage drops to approximately 50% for children under four years of age.[1]

While the incidence of IM reflects wide seasonal, ethnic and geographical variation, a large epidemiological study noted that the highest incidence of symptomatic IM occurred during late adolescence (15–24 years of age)[2].

PERFORMANCE CHARACTERISTICS
A total of 439 specimens (183 serum, 176 plasma and 80 whole blood) were evaluated by two clinical labs in a clinical study. Test results of the OSOM Mono Test were compared to results obtained with a commercially available latex particle agglutination test for the qualitative determination of infectious mononucleosis heterophile antibodies. Discrepancies between the results given by the OSOM Mono Test and the latex particle agglutination test were resolved by Epstein-Barr Virus (EBV) specific serological assays. In these assays, the specific antibodies to the EBV capsid antigen (IgM) and EBV nuclear antigen-1 (IgM and IgG) were determined.

Serum Specimens: Comparative Test

OSOM Mono Test		+	−
	+	74	8*
	−	0	101

*6 out of 8 tested postitive by EBV testing

Whole Blood Specimens: Comparative Test

OSOM Mono Test		+	−
	+	30	3*
	−	0	47

*1 out of 3 tested postitive by EBV testing

Plasma Specimens: Comparative Test

OSOM Mono Test		+	−
	+	67	15*
	−	0	94

*8 out of 15 tested postitive by EBV testing

All Specimens: Comparative Test

OSOM Mono Test		+	−
	+	171	26*
	−	0	242

*15 out of 26 tested postitive by EBV testing

When compared to a commercially available latex particle agglutination test for infectious mono-nucleosis heterophile antibodies, the OSOM Mono Test showed a sensitivity of 100% and a specificity of 90.3%. The overall agreement was 94.1%.

Fifteen of the 26 discrepant samples were determined to be recent or acute EBV infections by EBV serological testing, in which case the sample was considered positive. Including the samples confirmed positive by EBV serological testing, the overall clinical study specificity of the OSOM Mono Test is 95.9% and the overall sensitivity is 100%.

POL Studies
An evaluation of the OSOM Mono Test was conducted at three physicians' offices or clinical laboratories where testing was performed by personnel with diverse educational backgrounds. Each site tested the randomly coded panel consisting of negative (5), low positive (3) and moderate positive (4) specimens for three days. The results obtained had 99.1% agreement (107/108) with the expected results.

Figure 4-4   Cont'd

TIME TO REVIEW

1. *Analyte* means: Outcome 4-1

   a. A similarity between two things
   b. A substance being tested
   c. A method used for testing samples
   d. A type of proficiency testing

2. True or False: The mean of a set of   Outcome 4-1
   results is the average of the results.

3. A quantitative testing procedure   Outcome 4-1
   provides results as:

   a. Numbers or measurements
   b. Positive or negative
   c. Descriptive analysis by a pathologist

4. Which concept focuses specifically   Outcome 4-2
   on the analytical phase of laboratory testing?

   a. Quality control
   b. Quality assurance
   c. Documentation
   d. Personnel training

5. Which of these statements   Outcome 4-3
   describes how the details of the postanalytical phase
   of laboratory testing affects quality assurance?

   a. The postanalytical phase of laboratory testing is
      not considered to be part of quality assurance
   b. When results are reported promptly to the physi-
      cian as part of the postanalytical process, patient
      care is positively affected
   c. Postanalytical processes such as appropriate pa-
      tient education are critical for quality patient care
   d. Postanalytical processes such as performing the
      test procedures using the manufacturer's inserts
      are critical for quality patient care

6. True or False: If a medical assistant   Outcome 4-4
   performs only CLIA-waived testing, will it be necessary for her to perform quality control?

7. When is troubleshooting performed?   Outcome 4-5

   a. Daily
   b. Quarterly
   c. As needed
   d. When directed by the package insert for the
      test kit

8. Please provide three examples of   Outcome 4-6
   data that must be documented when logging quality
   control for a qualitative test.

9. What is the purpose of   Outcome 4-8
   calibration verification?

   a. Calibration verification is performed to see if the
      internal quality control is working correctly
   b. Calibration verification is performed to see if
      calibration is necessary for an instrument
   c. Calibration verification is performed when a new
      reagent lot number is put into use for the first
      time
   d. Calibration verification is performed after a
      calibration has been completed on an instru-
      ment to verify that the calibration was success-
      ful and that the instrument is ready for patient
      testing

10. True or False: Competency testing   Outcome 4-7
    addresses only test results.

11. Where do laboratories obtain   Outcome 4-7
    samples for proficiency testing?

    a. From the test kit manufacturer
    b. From approved providers
    c. From the CMS
    d. From the CDC

Case Study 4-1: An unexpected delay

A 3-year-old child is brought into the office with a potential urinary tract infection. The mother of the child
goes into the restroom and helps with the collection of
a very small amount of urine to run a urinalysis test. The
physician wants the test run as soon as possible so that
the child can be started on antibiotics, as she is very uncomfortable and cries whenever she has to urinate.

The medical assistant turns on the urinalysis instrument, and takes out the quality control material from the
refrigerator. While the instrument is performing an internal electronic check, she notices that the quality control
material has a printed expiration date that has already
passed, but only by a couple of weeks.

1. Would it be acceptable to use this quality control
   material? What are potential outcomes of this
   decision?
2. What is one step that could be taken before inform-
   ing the physician of the situation?

RESOURCES AND SUGGESTED READINGS

"CDC Report Assesses the State of Proficiency Testing"
A summary of a recent report released by the CDC addressing laboratory quality
http://www.aacc.org/publications/cln/2008/June/Pages/cover1_0608.aspx

"Clinical Laboratory Improvement Amendments Overview"
A written overview of CLIA policies and procedures, and numerous links for more specific information http://www.cms.hhs.gov/CLIA/

"CDC Report on Good Laboratory Practices for Waived Testing Sites"
Summary of site visits to CLIA-waived testing sites, as well as recommendations for quality practices. Also available as a printed document. http://www.cdc.gov/mmwr/preview/mmwrhtml/rr5413a1.htm

"Tests Waived by the FDA From January 2000 to Present"
List of all CLIA-waived tests. Updated regularly. http://www.accessdata.fda.gov/scripts/cdrh/cfdocs/cfClia/testswaived.cfm

"Laboratory Quality Control"
Good information about basic quality control standards http://www.virology-online.com/presentations/index.htm

"Good Laboratory Practice With Waived Systems"
Great information from the WA State Department of Health about laboratories that perform only waived tests http://www.doh.wa.gov/hsqa/fsl/LQA_Home.htm

"Recommended Elements of a Laboratory Quality Assurance Plan"
Recommendations based on Environmental Protection Agency (EPA) procedures for development of a QA plan http://www.umass.edu/tei/mwwp/files

"Abbott Diagnostics Practical Application Quality Control Guide"
Summary of the practical application of quality control principles http://www.abbottdiagnostics.com/Your_Health/Thyroid/Testing/quality.cfm

"Westgard Rules: What Are They?"
Summary of the Westgard Rules interpretation of Levey-Jennings QC charts; the Westgard system for defining quality control limits http://www.westgard.com/mltirule.htm

Chapter 5

Legal and Ethical Issues

Constance L. Lieseke, CMA (AAMA), MLT, PBT(ASCP)

CHAPTER OUTLINE

Learning Outcomes

After reading this chapter, the successful student will be able to:

5-1 Define the chapter key terms.

5-2 Explain the difference between law and ethics.

5-3 Distinguish between informed and implied consent, and describe when consent may be refused.

5-4 Express the principles presented in the Consumer Bill of Rights and Responsibilities.

5-5 Explain who has a right to a patient's medical information, and in what circumstances that right may be waived.

5-6 Compare and contrast intentional and unintentional torts.

5-7 Describe the liability assumed by a medical assistant in the laboratory, and why personal malpractice insurance is recommended.

5-8 Explain what is meant by scope of practice, and how these limitations are established for medical assistants.

5-9 Explain the acronym HIPAA, and explain how it affects the daily activities of a medical assistant in the laboratory environment.

5-10 Define *ethics* and explain the difference between personal and professional ethics.

5-11 Describe several ways that a medical assistant working in the laboratory may be part of risk management for his or her workplace.

CAAHEP/ABHES STANDARDS

 CAAHEP Standards

IX.C.1: Discuss legal scope of practice for medical assistants
IX.C.5: Discuss licensure and certification as it applies to healthcare providers

 ABHES Standards

#4: Medical Law and Ethics, b: Federal and State Guidelines, f: Health Laws and Regulations
Graduates: f: Comply with federal, state and local health laws and regulations

KEY TERMS

Assault	Implied consent	Patient identifier
Battery	Informed consent	Privacy Rule
Department of Health and Human Services (HHS)	Intentional tort	Protected health information (PHI)
Disclosure	Laws	Reportable condition
Duress	Liability	Risk management
Emancipated	Libel	Scope of practice
Ethics	Malfeasance	Slander
Expressed consent	Malpractice	Standard of care
Fraud	Misfeasance	Statutes
Health Insurance Portability and Accountability Act (HIPAA)	Negligence	Tort
	Nonfeasance	Unintentional tort

LEGAL AND ETHICAL ISSUES IN THE LABORATORY ENVIRONMENT

Most of us understand that it is important to obey the law and that there may be consequences if we make the wrong choices. However, in our daily lives, we realize that there are factors other than laws that affect our actions. These factors may include our personal values and ethics. In addition, as health-care employees, medical assistants must adhere to a set of professional laws and ethics to perform our duties as we should. In this chapter, you will learn the difference between law and ethics, and examine how these concepts define the professional actions of those employed in a health-care environment.

LAWS AND ETHICS

Laws are essentially rules of conduct that have been created by government at the local, state or national level. An established rule or law may also be known as a **statute.** Laws are enforced by appointed authorities. For instance, the Occupational Safety and Health Administration has created rules to uphold the federal laws developed to safeguard employees. Generally, laws protect the public by prohibiting activities that may be harmful, and establishing some form of consequences that would discourage those that continue to pursue these activities. Health-care laws are designed to protect the rights of the patients, the employees, or the employers.

Ethics are like laws because they dictate or determine appropriate behavior for individuals. They are different from laws because they are not created by governmental agencies. Personal ethics are behavioral guidelines that an individual develops throughout a lifetime, guided by personal values and morals, and influenced by upbringing. Professional ethics are developed by a well-recognized professional organization, with the anticipation that those working in that profession will use them as a guide for appropriate conduct.

LEGAL CONCEPTS AFFECTING PATIENT INTERACTIONS

There are numerous laws and statutes that play a role in a health-care setting. In addition to federal laws, each state has a medical practice act that dictates the delivery of health-care services in that state. Medical assistants act as agents of the physician office or laboratory where they are employed, which means they have a responsibility to abide by the laws that dictate their actions as they perform health-care procedures and deal with patient information. In order to follow the established rules, it is vital to learn some general legal concepts.

Consent

The law requires that there is consent, or permission, given before any treatment occurs. The consent may be given verbally, in writing, or nonverbally by behavior. **Implied consent** means that the patient's actions send a message of agreement to the treatment offered. For instance, when a patient offers his or her arm for a blood draw, the consent for the procedure is implied by this action. Implied consent also dictates care that occurs in an emergency situation. If the patient is not able to refuse consent, or if there is no legal document stating that emergency care should not be offered, emergency medical assistance may be rendered. It is assumed (implied) that the patient would want to be saved.

Informed consent is necessary whenever the treatment involved includes an invasive surgical procedure, experimental drugs, or any treatment that could be a significant risk to the health of the patient. This may also be known as **expressed consent.** Informed consent requires that the patient is advised of the following details:

- The name of the procedure to be performed and the health-care provider that will perform the procedure
- Risks of the procedure
- Risks involved if the procedure is *not* performed
- Alternatives to the treatment offered

It is essential that the patient understand the components printed on the consent form, as it is a legal document. The patient must sign and date the consent form,

and this must be witnessed. As in all situations concerning consent, the responsibility for explaining the procedure and the risks belongs to the health-care provider (such as a physician or nurse-practitioner) but the medical assistant may be asked to verify that the form is filled out correctly, as well as witness the signature of the patient.

Minors generally are not allowed to sign an informed consent. There are exceptions to this rule, which may vary from state to state. The exceptions generally involve requests for birth control or treatment of sexually transmitted infections. There are also exceptions for **emancipated** minors, and those in the armed forces who are still under the legal age of consent. Emancipated minors have been declared by the court to be independent and capable of making their own medical decisions. All other minors must have a parent or legal guardian sign the consent form for them.

A patient has the right to refuse consent at any time. Patients may decline treatment for any reason, based on personal beliefs, cultural differences, or financial considerations. If consent is refused, the patient should fill out and sign a form declining the procedure. This documentation can be very important if there is a negative outcome based on the patient's decision to refuse treatment.

Release of Information and Patient Rights and Responsibilities

Every patient who seeks medical care has certain rights and responsibilities. Medical personnel should always be conscious of these principles when dealing with patients, so that they can stay within appropriate boundaries in their interactions. Patient responsibilities include providing the physician with accurate information about his or her medical history and current condition, following the physician's instructions for treatment and follow-up care, and providing appropriate compensation to the health-care provider for services provided.

Patient rights have been addressed numerous times through the years. In 1998, the President's Advisory

Commission on Consumer Protection and Quality in the Health Care Industry issued a Consumer Bill of Rights and Responsibilities. This document addresses seven distinct areas of patient care:

1. *Information disclosure:* Patients have the right to know the details of their health-care plan, their health-care professionals, and the facilities they may use for care. This means that an interpreter must be provided if needed for understanding.
2. *Choice of providers and plans:* Patients have the right to evaluate different providers and/or health coverage plans to make the best choices for their needs.
3. *Access to emergency services:* If an emergency need arises, a patient has the right to receive services wherever needed without prior authorization. (However, this does not mean that the patient will not have to pay for these services if they are not covered specifically by their health-care plan.)
4. *Participation in treatment decisions:* All patients need to know about their treatment options and have the right to participate in decisions about their medical care. This also means that they have the right to refuse care if they choose.
5. *Respect and nondiscrimination:* All patients have the right to receive respectful treatment from their health-care providers that is considerate of their feelings and without discrimination.
6. *Confidentiality:* Patients have the right to expect their health-care information to remain confidential.
7. *Complaints and appeals:* All patients have the right to an objective review of any complaints they have about their health-care provider or health-care plan. This can include any part of their experience, including billing, accessibility of the building for those with special needs, operating hours, and so on. Of course, the right to review and appeal also pertains to the quality of care experienced.

Even though patients have the right to expect their health-care information to remain confidential, there are limitations. The physical medical record (where the information is documented; also known as "the chart") belongs to the health-care provider, but the information in the record belongs to the patient. Patients have the right to request their medical information, and they also have the right to control who has access to their medical records in most situations. The information contained in the medical record may be requested by numerous parties, such as insurance companies, family members, and legal representatives. Later in this chapter we will learn more about the law which details how personal information may be protected.

There are some situations where the **disclosure** (sharing) of the patient's information is required, even without consent. For instance, if a patient is diagnosed with a **reportable condition,** state and federal laws require that the laboratory or the health-care provider contact the local health department or the Centers for Disease Control and Prevention (CDC). Reportable conditions are diseases or conditions that have been deemed to be dangerous to the general public health. The statistics accumulated by the state or federal agencies allow the prevalence of the disease in the population to be tracked. Examples of reportable conditions include HIV infection, Lyme disease, cholera, hepatitis, measles, and gonorrhea infection. If a laboratory test is positive for these conditions, the result must be passed on to the appropriate authorities as soon as possible. The patient does not have the right to stop this report process, although in some situations he or she may have the right to request anonymity to protect his or her identity.

Test Your Knowledge 5-3

Lily Lee is moving to another city to attend college. She would like to get a copy of her medical records to take with her as she establishes a new physician relationship in her new home. Does she have the right to a copy of her medical record? Is it appropriate for her to take the entire original record from the office?

(Outcome 5-4 and Outcome 5-5)

Test Your Knowledge 5-4

If someone is assaulted, was he or she touched or physically injured? (Outcome 5-1)

Tort Law

Torts are wrongful acts that are committed against a person or property that result in harm. The harm caused by the tort may be physical or emotional. This type of act does not include those that involve violation of a contract. Torts may be classified as intentional or unintentional. In the case of an **intentional tort,** it must be apparent that the action was deliberate and intended to cause harm. Intentional torts include the following:

- **Assault:** An assault involves threatening an individual, or making a person fear harm.

- **Battery:** Battery is the act of touching another without that person's permission. A person may be committing battery even if the touch does not cause harm.
- **Duress:** If a patient is forced or coerced into an act (such as signing a consent form or undergoing a procedure against his or her will), that person may claim duress.
- **Libel:** If a health-care professional makes a false written statement about a patient (or someone else), he or she may be accused of libel. This is especially a problem when the false statement causes a problem with the victim's reputation or employment.
- **Slander:** Slander is false statement made about someone else orally.
- **Fraud:** Fraud is a dishonest or deceitful act that is performed with the intent to hide the truth.

Unintentional torts are situations in which the harm was the result of an accident. The accuser must believe that the employee was performing his or her job in good faith when the patient was harmed, and the incident was not deliberate. **Negligence** is often involved in unintentional torts, as it means that a professional did not take reasonable care to prevent harm. The term **malpractice** is used if a health-care professional is shown to be negligent in his or her duties. Malpractice accusations are the most common reason for claims against health-care professionals, and the legal decisions are based on the **standard of care** (minimum safe professional conduct) for a reasonable professional with the same training who might be facing a similar situation. Malpractice may be classified in one of three ways:

1. **Malfeasance:** In this situation, the treatment provided was wrong and unlawful.
2. **Misfeasance:** If treatment was provided, but it was performed in an improper manner, it is known as misfeasance.
3. **Nonfeasance:** When the health-care professional fails to perform a necessary act or delays treatment excessively, the act is known as nonfeasance.

Test Your Knowledge 5-5

What is the difference between an intentional and unintentional tort? (Outcome 5-6)

Liability

Health-care professionals assume a certain amount of **liability** in everything that they do, meaning that they are legally obligated to perform their duties to the best of their ability. Liability exists in all areas of our lives: driving a car or while walking the dog, for example. We are responsible for our actions, and obligated to drive the car to the best of our ability, as well as keep our dog on a leash and under control while on the walk. For health-care professionals, their liability insurance is actually malpractice insurance, as they may be held responsible for an intentional or unintentional tort if they make a mistake or they don't perform their jobs to the best of their ability. Anyone who works in a medical office is liable for all interactions with the public, whether performing an invasive procedure, taking a blood pressure reading, or participating in a phone call with a patient. A malpractice suit may be filed against any or all of the employees in an office or laboratory.

In most health-care facilities, the malpractice insurance coverage for the physician or health-care provider generally includes coverage for the medical assistant working for them. Many medical assistants don't pursue their own malpractice insurance coverage. This may be a mistake. If a patient sues the practice (specifically naming each individual involved), for malfeasance, for example, the best outcome for the physician may be to settle out of court. This means that the incident will still be on the record for the medical assistant, who was not part of the decision to settle in this way. For medical assistants (or other allied health-care professionals) who work in the laboratory setting, it is especially important to have appropriate personal coverage. Even though the physician may have malpractice insurance that appears to be adequate, it is possible that when drawing blood or performing laboratory tests outside of the direct supervision of the physician, the medical assistant may be found to be solely responsible for malpractice. In addition, if a physician is sued for malpractice because of a venipuncture or other procedure performed by his or her medical assistant, the physician can even file suit against the medical assistant for financial damages incurred as a result of the incident.

Test Your Knowledge 5-6

Is a medical assistant working in a laboratory liable for his or her actions while working with patients? Is it possible for him or her to be sued for malpractice? (Outcome 5-7)

Scope of Practice

Scope of practice is a term used to describe the activities that an employee in a specific profession can and cannot perform. These limitations are different for each of the health-care professionals present in a physician office or laboratory environment. The scope of practice is dictated by licensure and training, and may vary according to the state in which a professional offers his or her services.

Medical assistants are not licensed, meaning that they are required to work under the license of another qualified health-care professional, such as a physician, nurse-practitioner, or physician's assistant. These health-care professionals have a responsibility to train the medical assistant and to establish his or her duties and limitations within the practice. Many states have statutes in place that limit the duties that a medical assistant may perform. Although certification is not mandatory, medical assistants may take a comprehensive examination to become nationally certified by the American Association of Medical Assistants or registered through the American Medical Technologists. In addition, some states require very specific certification or registration for allied health professionals who perform invasive procedures.

Educational programs for medical assistants vary. Some may be just a few months in length, whereas other programs offer a 2-year associate degree. In addition, each state may have different laws that dictate the tasks that may be legally performed by medical assistants. This means that the scope of practice for a medical assistant is based on his or her education and training, as well as the limitations that may be in effect by the state in which he or she practices.

In general, the scope of practice for medical assistants includes the following limitations:

- Medical assistants are not able to make independent medical assessments or diagnose, or give advice independently.
- It is the physician's responsibility to be aware of the medical assistant's scope of practice, whether based on state laws or the medical assistant's training.
- Medical assistants are not able independently to write prescriptions or give out medication samples without specific documented orders from a qualified health-care professional.
- Medical assistants cannot independently interpret test results or treat patients.

In most states, the following are tasks that medical assistants are allowed to perform:

- Assisting with various clinical and patient care procedures
- Carrying out administrative procedures such as answering phones, working with charts, and performing billing and coding

- Obtaining medical histories
- Explaining treatment procedures to patients (within the guidelines established by the facility)
- Preparing and assisting with various routine and specialty examinations
- Collecting specimens, including venipuncture and capillary puncture
- Performing electrocardiograms (ECGs)
- Administering medication
- Assisting with prescription refills
- Performing Clinical Laboratory Improvement Act–waived laboratory tests or those of moderate complexity
- Assisting with various disease management programs, such as tracking laboratory results for a patient on medication
- Administering injections

> **Test Your Knowledge 5-7**
>
> Is the scope of practice the same for medical assistants anywhere in the United States?   (Outcome 5-8)

HEALTH INSURANCE PORTABILITY AND ACCOUNTABILITY ACT

Earlier in this chapter, we discussed the Consumer Bill of Rights and Responsibilities. One component addressed the confidentiality of a patient's health record. This is a very complex issue, and it has been addressed in various ways, as the protection of personal health information is one of the most important duties of a health-care professional. It is impossible to establish a good working relationship with a patient if there is no trust in the professional's ability to keep private information secure. Patients share information with those in health care that they do not divulge to anyone else, and the expectation is that this information will only be shared if it is absolutely necessary for patient treatment.

In the early 1990s, it became evident that there were areas of health care that needed reform. Congress passed the **Health Insurance Portability and Accountability Act (HIPAA)** to provide guidelines for this reform. This act was originally designed to improve the efficiency and effectiveness of the health-care system by focusing on the following areas:

- Improvement of the health benefit options for covered workers who leave or change jobs
- Standardization of electronic health data

- Creation of unique health identifiers for the various entities involved in health-care services
- Development of security standards for handling **protected health information (PHI),** which includes anything in the patient's health record that could be used to identify the patient

One of the standardization methods for handling health data was to increase the use of computers for transmission of health information. This created more concerns about the unauthorized access to personal information that may occur with electronic transmission. To address these confidentiality issues, the **Department of Health and Human Services (HHS)** developed the **Privacy Rule,** which is an expansion of the original HIPAA mandate that applies to confidentiality of health information, and the rights of patients to control access to their own records. This rule went into effect April 2003, and it carries significant monetary consequences for noncompliance. This is the first federally mandated set of rules for the protection of health information.

Test Your Knowledge 5-8

Does HIPAA impact only confidentiality of medical information? (Outcome 5-9)

The Privacy Rule outlines very specific precautions that are to be practiced in every health-care facility. There are several standard provisions that all medical assistants should keep in mind, regardless of their specialty of practice:

1. Any document that includes a **patient identifier** must be treated as protected health information. These identifiers include demographic information such as name, address, and phone number, but also include photos, Social Security numbers, birth dates, and other types of unique information that may be linked back to that specific patient. Documents must have all patient identifiers removed before they can be discarded, or they must be destroyed in such a way that this information is not available after disposal.
2. Patients have a right to know how their PHI has been shared, even if it was necessary for treatment.
3. Patients have a right to review and/or to request copies of their medical records. This law does not state that they have the right to walk out of an office with their physical chart, nor does the office have to allow review or copies to be available at any time. A patient can submit a request for the records, with the

understanding that it may take some time to process the request and copy the records.
4. Health information cannot be shared with others without the patient's consent. This does not apply to reporting that may be required by law.
5. When any patient information is shared, it is important that it is limited to data that are essential for that situation. This is especially important when dealing with labor and industry claims for injured employees or insurance claims, as the health-care professional should include only records about a specific treatment if it is in question, but not the entire chart.
6. The Privacy Rule also requires every office to have a privacy notice and to train all employees about HIPAA and the Privacy Rule. All patients must receive a copy of the office's privacy notice, and patients must give written consent or permission to disclose their health-care information. A privacy or HIPAA compliance officer must be assigned for every institution to oversee the process within that office.

The HIPAA regulations still allow health-care providers to share information with family members who are directly responsible for the care of a patient, or to other providers or members of the health-care team (such as radiology services, laboratory professionals, etc.) when it is necessary for patient care. Also, the regulations recognize that sometimes it is impossible for oral privacy to be assured in all areas of a practice; there has to be evidence that this has been addressed to the full extent of the facility.

The Impact of the Health Insurance Portability and Accountability Act on the Medical Assistant

The privacy section of the HIPAA regulations may affect phone conversations with or about patients, discussion of patient issues within earshot of the waiting area in a clinic, or the visibility of patient information to visitors in an office. Laboratory requisitions that contain PHI cannot be left where patients may have access to them, computer screens should not be visible to patients as they walk to and from the treatment area, and patient schedules that contain names should not be posted where they are visible by those who are being treated. Fax numbers used to transmit laboratory results must be carefully monitored, as these results need to end up in a secure location once received. Complications arise when protected health information is shared via e-mail, although this method of transmitting information may be more efficient for patient care within a large organization or between providers. The need for electronic security measures is great. Also, many clinics have changed the way they call patients from the waiting room for treatment; they now call the patients by the first or the last name, but not both. It is the responsibility of the designated HIPAA compliance officer to decide the specific methods used by an office for compliance with the regulations, and to ensure that appropriate training is provided for all employees.

It is also illegal to gossip about patients, even if it is in a private area where other patients cannot hear. Discussions about patient care are to be limited to those that are necessary for providing quality health care. As health-care professionals, medical assistants are not allowed to share any protected health information with family or friends. Sometimes this is difficult, as health-care professionals may have knowledge about a family friend or relative that others would want to know. It is illegal to share this information, so care must be taken to keep it private.

Another example of illegal action is idle searching of the database within a health-care facility to see who might have had services provided. There were recent reports in the news of employees who lost their jobs and of facilities that were fined significantly when an employee searched for the records of a celebrity rumored to be in a certain facility. Even if this information is not shared with anyone else, it is a HIPAA violation to perform the search. It can (and will) be tracked back to the responsible individual.

ETHICS

Most of the information in this chapter is based on laws and legal terms that dictate the actions of health-care professionals. But there are also ethical decisions that must be made every day in order to interact appropriately with patients, coworkers, and other members of the health-care team. Ethics are standards that define our actions, but they are not created or enforced by governmental agencies. As was explained at the beginning of this chapter, there are two types of ethics that define our actions while at work. We must adhere to a set of personal ethics that are defined by our own sense of what is right and wrong. Professional ethics also define our actions. These are based on the standards of our professions, and although they are not laws, there are consequences to unethical behaviors.

Personal ethics begin to develop in childhood. We generally understand what our parents and community define as acceptable behavior by the time we enter grade school. These are based on our morals and values, and become refined as we approach adulthood. Personal values such as the desire to help others will make a health-care professional much better at performing his or her job. Empathy, honesty, responsibility, and respect for others are also part of our personal ethics; this is often known as our *work ethic*. Remember, if there is something that you are doing at work that you are not proud of, it is probably unethical at the personal level for you.

Professional Behaviors

Professional ethics are standards established by the profession, and usually sponsored by a professional organization that represents the profession. Physicians have several codes of ethics that define their actions, such as the Hippocratic Oath and the Code of Medical Ethics defined by the American Medical Association. One ethical theme present in both codes is the show of respect for patients and to show compassion for those served, while staying within legal limits of practice. By utilizing these standards, physicians may remind themselves why they chose this profession, and also remember what their patients may expect from them.

The American Association of Medical Assistants also has a code of ethics (Box 5-1). These guidelines also include respect for patients and the laws that guide the medical assisting profession, as well as service to the community and lifelong learning. At a minimum, professional ethics for medical assistants must put patients first by honoring their right to confidentiality and by being honest in all professional situations. If this code is supported by a strong set of personal ethics, a medical assistant will be a valuable asset to the profession.

Remember that there are ethical dilemmas that develop. Many times there may be a situation that arises that is not illegal, but it is unethical. This may include situations in which the medical assistant does not agree with the actions of the employer, even though these actions are not illegal. Usually these issues involve disrespect for patients or a poor quality of care due to the attitude of the physician. The medical assistant will need to make choices about whether she can continue employment with this practice.

> **Test Your Knowledge 5-9**
> List two professional standards included in the AAMA Code of Ethics.   (Outcome 5-10)

BOX 5-1 American Association of Medical Assistants code of ethics

American Association of Medical Assistants (AAMA) Code of Ethics

Members of AAMA dedicated to the conscientious pursuit of their profession, and thus desiring to merit the high regard of the entire medical profession and the respect of the general public which they serve, do pledge themselves to strive always to:

A. Render service with full respect for the dignity of humanity;

B. Respect confidential information obtained through employment unless legally authorized or required by responsible performance of duty to divulge such information;

C. Uphold the honor and high principles of the profession and accept its disciplines;

D. Seek to continually improve the knowledge and skills of medical assistants for the benefit of patients and professional colleagues;

E. Participate in additional service activities aimed toward improving the health and well-being of the community.

POINT OF INTEREST 5-1
Medical assisting scope of practice

There is a lot of confusion among medical assistants as well as physicians, nurse-practitioners, physician assistants, and other health-care providers about the scope of practice for the medical assistant. The confusion is well earned; the scope of practice for each state differs widely. For those medical assistants who move from one state to another, it can become even more difficult to know what they are allowed to do in any given state.

Governing Agencies

Just finding the regulations for each state can be difficult. A good resource may be the program director for the local CAAHEP or ABHES accredited medical assisting programs. These program directors should have up-to-date information about the scope of practice for the medical assistants in their area, and should be able to provide information about which governing body oversees medical assistants in their state. In many states the department of health oversees the unlicensed members of the health-care teams. In other areas, medical assistants may be part of the state nursing board.

Registration or certification

Medical assistants are nonlicensed members of the health-care team. There is no license available in any state for medical assistants. However, most states do require some sort of registration process for the medical assistants in their jurisdiction. This may include a testing process by which they are registered and certified to perform in that state, or the state may require only that the medical assistant fill out certain paperwork and submit a fee to become registered. Some states require the medical assistant to bear the burden of registration fees, whereas other states require that the medical assistant be registered each time she or he changes employers and the employer is responsible for the fee.

Many medical assistants are under the impression that if they become Certified Medical Assistants through the AAMA or Registered Medical Assistants through the American Medical Technologists that this will cover them regardless of their state of residence and that these credentials somehow expand their scope of practice. This is not true. Many states will grant registration (or certification) if the medical assistant is nationally certified, or they may require those who are not nationally certified complete a state certification process. However, this varies from state to state, so it is very important to find out what the regulations are in your state of residence. Usually the office manager or physician you are working for knows the rules, but occasionally they have decided not to work with the state to register their medical assistants. This is not a safe environment to work in, as the medical assistant may be operating outside of his or her scope of practice and unlawfully performing tasks, which place him or her at risk for legal actions.

Allowable tasks

Every state has limitations for the tasks that can be performed by the medical assistants. The following are some of the tasks that may be limited:

- **Invasive procedures:** Some states allow medical assistants to draw blood, but this task is still limited in a few areas. Many states (e.g., New York) do not allow medical assistants to administer medication through any route, including by injection. It is important to clarify this before performing injections or venipuncture.

Continued

- **IV access:** Most states limit the IV access of nonlicensed health-care personnel. In some areas, the medical assistant is allowed to stop the IV or remove the catheter when it is no longer needed, but most areas prohibit much more than this.
- **Placement of urinary catheters:** This is an area where many medical assistants are currently operating outside of their scope of practice. Most states prohibit the placement of a urinary catheter by a nonlicensed health-care professional.
- **Administering oral medications:** Although medical assistants are allowed to give injections in most states, the administration of oral medication may still be limited. Washington State, for example, has a list of oral medications that can be administered by health-care assistants, which include medical assistants.
- **Working in a hospital setting:** Some states prohibit medical assistants from working in a hospital or inpatient setting if they are performing clinical procedures. This decision is based on the presence (or absence) of health-care providers in the vicinity while invasive procedures are performed.
- **Suture removal:** Most states allow medical assistants to remove sutures, but there are limitations in a few areas.
- **Botox administration or assisting with other cosmetic procedures:** Medical assistants generally cannot operate laser equipment or administer Botox or other injections that are not considered to be medications.

RISK MANAGEMENT AND THE MEDICAL ASSISTANT

After reading through this chapter, it may appear that the legal aspects of the medical profession are overwhelming. There is a lot of information to remember, but as a medical assistant, there are many things that you can do to avoid risk of harm to yourself, your patients, and your practice. This concept is called **risk management.** These risks may be legal in nature, as in a case in which a malpractice suit is filed for poor quality of care; financial in nature, as in a case in which a laboratory or physician office chooses not to accept patients with specific insurance coverage because of the potential for low levels of reimbursement; or physical in nature, as in a case in which a medical assistant might not use the appropriate technique to perform a capillary blood draw, or when an office staff doesn't notice the puddle inside the front entrance to the clinic and a patient slips and falls.

Because a medical assistant may be the member of the health-care team in an office or a laboratory who spends the most time with a patient, it is important that he or she keep the following risk management techniques in mind to avoid potential harm or legal action:

- Act within the defined scope of practice
- Use all available training to be certain that techniques are performed with the highest level of skill possible
- Use current, up-to-date equipment as available
- Perform regular performance checks on any testing equipment used for patient samples
- Follow the manufacturer's instructions exactly for all laboratory testing performed
- Consult resources (other employees or reference materials) if you have questions
- Verify the identity of every patient before you begin interactions
- Chart when patients call to inquire for test results, and when they are notified of the results
- Be certain that all laboratory results are handled in a timely manner
- Practice confidentiality at all times
- Always practice universal precautions and keep your environment medically aseptic
- Treat all patients with respect and overcome personal biases to treat them all equally
- Act as a chaperone when needed for procedures
- Obtain informed consent when necessary
- Be vigilant for potential safety hazards in the clinic environment
- Document promptly and thoroughly
- Log all phone call correspondence
- Remember not to criticize other members of the health-care team or other health-care providers
- Do not give advice that has not been approved by the office policy
- Do not be afraid to ask for help if you are feeling overwhelmed by the number of patients you are assisting or by the tasks at hand.

> **Test Your Knowledge 5-10**
>
> After drawing the blood from a patient, medical assistant Krissy Clark takes the time to document the blood draw site, the date, and the time of the draw on the laboratory requisition. Is this an example of risk management?   (Outcome 5-11)

SUMMARY

The majority of the time, the relationship between a patient and the health-care team is an amicable one in which both parties are satisfied with the care provided. However, there are unfortunate situations that may arise as a patient is treated that damage this relationship. Sometimes these result in charges of malpractice, and sometimes they may require legal actions because a member of the health-care team ignored the legal guidelines that define their scope of practice. In order to protect ourselves from these situations, it is important to stay insured as a means of protecting our financial security. It is also important to be aware of the legal boundaries for each profession. Ethics play a role as well, as not all inappropriate actions in a medical office or laboratory are illegal. Risk management is a way to provide care defensively; avoid problems before they start!

TIME TO REVIEW

1. What is a statute?   Outcome 5-1

   a. A personal set of rules dependent on an individual's sense of right and wrong
   b. A law established by the legislative branch of a government entity
   c. Behavioral standards established by a professional organization

2. If a newspaper article prints   Outcome 5-1
   information about a local physician that is untrue, what legal term might be used to describe this action?

3. What is the meaning of the acronym   Outcome 5-1
   HIPAA?

4. Who establishes laws that affect   Outcome 5-2
   health-care organizations?

   a. Professional organizations
   b. Governmental agencies
   c. Local groups of practitioners
   d. Local health departments

5. The_____   Outcome 5-3
   _____ is responsible for explaining the details of a procedure to the patient before the informed consent paperwork is signed.

6. Which of these principles are not   Outcome 5-4
   addressed in the Consumer Bill of Rights?

   a. The right to insurance coverage
   b. The right to emergency services when needed
   c. The right to be treated without discrimination
   d. The right to an interpreter if needed

7. What is a reportable condition?   Outcome 5-5

8. True or False: It is not necessary for a   Outcome 5-7
   medical assistant to carry her own malpractice insurance.

9. Referring to the medical assisting   Outcome 5-8
   scope of practice explained in this chapter, which of these duties would be outside the guidelines?

   a. Offering medical advice based on personal experiences
   b. Documentation of procedures performed
   c. Assisting with a Pap smear specimen collection
   d. Scheduling appointments

10. True or False: It is a HIPAA violation   Outcome 5-9
    to fax medical information to a health-care specialist who is functioning as a consultant for a patient's complicated medical condition.

11. Personal ethics are defined by: Outcome 5-10

    a. Professional standards of the profession
    b. Local statutes
    c. Experiences and guidance beginning in childhood
    d. HIPAA

12. True or False: Risk management   Outcome 5-11
    should be a part of the routine for everyone working in the health-care environment.

Case Study 5-1: Too much talk

Amy Conner is the receptionist who greets patients at the front desk for a family practice physician. A 17-year-old young man comes in to have his blood drawn a few days after seeing the physician. He enters the reception area by himself, and gives Amy his requisition. She notices that in addition to several routine chemistry tests, the physician has ordered an HIV screen to be performed. Amy puts the laboratory orders into the computer system, and hands the labels to the medical assistant to perform the blood draw.

After the young man leaves the facility, Amy steps into the hallway behind the reception area and starts

Continued

a conversation with the medical assistant. She tells the medical assistant how sad it is that an HIV test has to be done on someone so young, and expands her conversation to include all the potential ways that he could have contracted HIV. After a few minutes she hears someone at the front desk and steps back to her work area.

The 17-year-old patient is now at the front desk again, with his mother standing next to him. He appears to be uncomfortable, and the mother starts to ask questions about the conversation that Amy was having in the hallway.

a. Are Amy's actions in violation of the law?

b. Should Amy assume that the mother knows all about the blood tests that were ordered for her son?

c. How should this situation have been handled?

RESOURCES AND SUGGESTED READINGS

"Office for Civil Rights—HIPAA"
    Detailed reference for the HHS Privacy Rule
    http://www.hhs.gov/ocr/Health InformationPrivacy
"What Is Ethics?"
    Article published by Santa Clara University about the meaning of ethics, and how personal and professional ethics differ http://www.scu.edu/ethics/practicing/decision/whatisethics.html
"Quidel Rapid Diagnostic Products"
    Links to the Quidel point-of-care test kits, including CLIA-waived tests. http://www.quidel.com/products/product_list.php?cat=1&by=brand&group=1
"Reportable Diseases"
    Information about reportable diseases that must be reported to the local authorities or the Centers for Disease Control and Prevention http://www.nlm.nih.gov/medlineplus/ency/article/001929.htm

Chapter 6

Laboratory Equipment

Constance L. Lieseke, CMA (AAMA), MLT, PBT(ASCP)

CHAPTER OUTLINE

Learning Outcomes

After reading this chapter, the successful student will be able to:

6-1 Define the key terms.

6-2 Describe the different types of microscopes introduced in this chapter.

6-3 Identify the different parts of a compound microscope.

6-4 Describe maintenance procedures for a compound microscope.

6-5 Explain how to correctly focus a microscope to examine a specimen on a slide.

6-6 Explain the role of a medical assistant in a physician office laboratory that performs microscopic examinations of specimens.

6-7 Explain how to operate and maintain a centrifuge.

6-8 Describe how temperature must be monitored for a laboratory refrigerator.

6-9 Explain why an incubator is sometimes used in a laboratory environment.

6-10 List several advantages of providing CLIA-waived testing in a physician office laboratory.

6-11 Demonstrate understanding of the basic principles used for measurement in laboratory instruments.

6-12 Explain why automated urine analyzers are used.

6-13 Describe similarities between the different types of coagulation testing instruments available for CLIA-waived testing.

6-14 List several types of instruments used for CLIA–waived chemistry testing.

6-15 Describe the operation of an instrument used to measure hemoglobin in a whole blood specimen.

6-16 List the types of hematology instruments presented in this chapter.

6-17 Describe some of the types of glassware found in the laboratory, and how to correctly measure the liquid level in glassware.

CAAHEP/ABHES STANDARDS

None

KEY TERMS

Agglutination	Electrolyte	Meniscus
Anemia	Electron microscope	Monocular
Aperture	Eyepiece	Objective lenses
Arm	Fecal occult blood	Ocular lens
Balanced	Fine adjustment knob	Oil immersion lens
Base	Flask	Pipette
Beaker	Glass slides	Plasma
Binocular	Glucose	Prothrombin time test
Centrifugal force	Glycosylated hemoglobin monitoring	Protime
Centrifuge		Reagent strips
Cholesterol	Graduated cylinder	Revolving nosepiece
Coarse adjustment knob	Hemoglobin	Rotations per minute (rpm)
Compound microscope	Incubator	Serum
Condenser	International normalized ratio (INR)	Spectrophotometer
Cover slips		Stage
Cylinder	Iris diaphragm	Stereo microscope
Diluent	Laboratory thermometer	Tachometer
Dissecting microscope	Light source	Water baths
Electrical impedance	Lysed	

LABORATORY EQUIPMENT

Laboratories use many types of instruments to process, store, and analyze specimens. As the complexity and variety of tests offered by a laboratory expand, so do the number of instruments in use. Because medical assistants are generally working in laboratory environments performing Clinical Laboratory Improvement Act (CLIA)–waived tests, they don't usually use a wide variety of instruments. This chapter focuses on equipment commonly used for specimen processing and storage, as well as performance of CLIA-waived testing procedures.

Selected instruments used for laboratory tests of moderate complexity are also presented.

Microscopes

There are several types of microscopes available. These vary by the amount of magnification, the manner by which the image is viewed, and the light (energy) source used. A typical laboratory setting will use a **compound microscope,** and some laboratories may also use a **dissecting microscope,** especially if the laboratory performs blood bank procedures. Specialty laboratories may also have personnel trained to operate an electron microscope to create three-dimensional images of the specimens. All microscopes provide magnification so that microscopic structures or organisms that are too small to be seen with the naked eye can be identified or quantified in a specimen. Sometimes it is necessary to apply stain to a specimen before viewing, and sometimes the specimen is viewed in its natural state.

Compound Microscopes

The compound microscope is the most common type used in a general laboratory setting. The magnification for this type of microscope is compounded, or increased by two different sets of lenses. The energy source is a replaceable bulb that sits in the base of the microscope and shines very brightly. Adjustments may be made for the amount of light used for viewing, as well as the strength of the magnification, which makes this microscope very versatile. Compound microscopes are often used to visualize stained blood smears, urine sediment, and various microbiology specimens.

Test Your Knowledge 6-1

What is the most common type of microscope used in the clinical laboratory?
  a. Dissecting microscope
  b. Electron microscope
  c. Fluorescent microscope
  d. Compound microscope   (Outcome 6-2)

Figure 6-1 shows a compound microscope with its component parts identified. It is important that medical assistants working in the laboratory know how to set up a microscope properly, focus a slide for viewing, and maintain the microscope appropriately after the procedure. To perform these procedures correctly, the medical assistant must be able to identify the parts of the microscope. Although at first glance the microscope itself may appear complex, its parts may be broken into categories to help you to remember their names and understand their function.

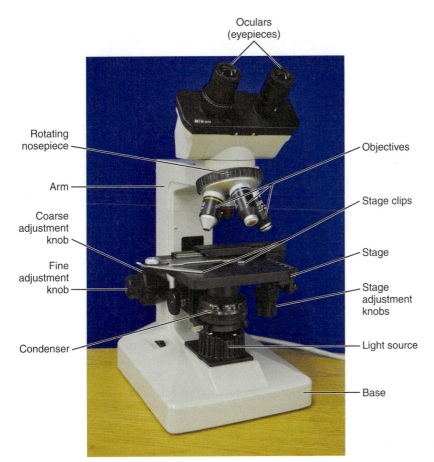

Figure 6-1   Parts of a compound microscope.

Supportive Structures. The more delicate parts of the microscope are supported by a **base** and an **arm.** The base sits on the surface (tabletop or laboratory bench) to keep the microscope secure. The microscope arm is a curved metal support, and is to be gripped when it is being carried. It is important to remember to use two hands whenever moving the unit; one should grip the arm, and one should be placed under the base.

Another supportive structure is the **stage,** which is the surface on which the slide sits for viewing. Most compound microscopes have metal clips that hold the slide securely in place on the stage and allow the slide to be moved around for viewing by turning a mechanical control knob, located under the stage.

> **Test Your Knowledge 6-2**
>
> On a compound microscope, what is the name of the surface where the slide is placed for observation?
>
> (Outcome 6-3)

Structures Used for Specimen Viewing. To view a specimen with the microscope, there are two types of structures used. Some of the structures are designed to provide the necessary light to see the specimen, whereas others are necessary to provide various amounts of magnification. To visualize the specimen as clearly as possible, it is very important that the light and the magnification are both at the correct setting.

Light Sources The **light source** is located in the base of the microscope. The bulb can be turned on and off with a switch or knob, which is usually located on the base toward the back of the microscope. The bulb should not be touched with the bare hands when changing the light source, as the natural oils present on the skin may be transferred to the bulb, and these will overheat when the bulb is turned on, causing the bulb to shatter. The light will come up from the bulb at the base of the microscope, through the **condenser,** then up through the specimen on the stage and finally through the optical magnification components to be viewed.

The condenser is designed to focus the rays of light on the specimen for a clearer image. It may be raised or lowered, depending on the density of the specimen viewed. The knob to adjust the condenser height is on the side under the stage. An **iris diaphragm** is located on the front or just underneath the condenser. The iris diaphragm may be adjusted to increase or decrease the *amount* of light reaching the slide. The amount of light needed to view a specimen depends on its density;

generally, the denser the specimen, the more light will be needed. In addition, as the magnification increases, there is more need for light, so the condenser and iris diaphragm need to be adjusted for better viewing.

> **Test Your Knowledge 6-3**
>
> What is the purpose of the condenser on the compound microscope?
>
> (Outcome 6-3)

Magnification The compound microscope has two different points of magnification. The first magnification is encountered as the light passes through the specimen from below the stage, and flows into one of the **objective lenses.** These lenses are located on a **revolving nosepiece** and are identified with their respective power of magnification: 4X, 10X, 40X, and 100X. The different objectives also vary by rings of different colors on each, and by the length of each objective tube. When using the microscope, the operator starts with the objective marked with the lowest magnification, and proceeds through the various levels as needed to view the specimen. If the 100X objective is used, a thin layer of oil is placed between the objective and the specimen on the slide to further focus the light and make the image as sharp as possible. This objective is known as the **oil immersion lens.**

The second point of magnification available in a compound microscope is located within the **eyepiece** at the very top of the microscope. An internal mirror actually reflects the image from the slide through this **ocular lens** (eyepiece) where an additional 10X magnification is accomplished. This means that if the 100X oil immersion lens is used to examine a specimen, the object is actually viewed as 1,000 times larger than it would be without magnification. A **binocular** microscope is one that has two ocular lenses (or eyepieces), and a **monocular** microscope is one that has only one ocular lens used to view the specimen.

Focus on the specimen is achieved by using the **coarse adjustment knob** and the **fine adjustment knob**. These knobs project out from the side of the microscope arm. The larger of the two knobs is the coarse adjustment, and is used when the specimen is first being brought into focus at a low magnification. The fine adjustment is the smaller knob, and is used to fine-tune the focus. The fine adjustment knob is used with the higher magnification levels.

Microscope Maintenance Procedures. A microscope must be handled and maintained properly in order to keep it functioning as it should. The following are a few guidelines for handling and maintaining a compound microscope that a medical assistant should adhere to:

1. Keep the microscope covered with a plastic cover when not in use. This protects the delicate microscope and lenses from excess dust and potential damage.
2. Always use two hands (as described earlier) to carry a microscope.
3. Do not touch the light source or the lenses with your fingers. The light source may overheat and burst because of the transferred oils, and fingerprints on the lenses can be very difficult to remove.
4. The optical lenses and eyepieces should be kept clean at all times. These may be cleaned *only* using lens paper, as the glass surfaces are very delicate and will be scratched if Kimwipes or other tissues are used. Xylene may be used to assist with removal of oil or other buildup. A small amount should be placed on the lens paper before gently rubbing the lens.
5. When cleaning the objectives, remember always to clean the 100X optical lens last. This one is used with oil immersion, and if cleaned first, the lens paper used may contaminate the other lenses with oil as they are cleaned. Do not apply pressure to the lenses when cleaning.
6. Keep the stage clean between uses.
7. When moving from one objective to another during use or cleaning procedures, always use the nosepiece to change the powers. Do not push against the tubes directly to move them.
8. Slides should be removed or added to the stage only when the lowest power objective is turned down toward the light source. Do not attempt to remove or add slides when the higher power objectives are in place (pointed down toward the specimen), as the objective lenses may be damaged during the process, and/or the slide may be broken.

Test Your Knowledge 6-4

True or False: The 100X objective (oil immersion objective) should be cleaned first when performing maintenance on the compound microscope.   (Outcome 6-4)

Test Your Knowledge 6-5

What should be used to clean the eyepieces on a microscope?
   a. Kleenex or a similar facial tissue
   b. Laboratory tissues such as Kimwipes
   c. Lens paper
   d. None of the above   (Outcome 6-4)

Procedure 6-1: Microscope Use

TASK

Correctly use a compound microscope to obtain specimen focus with all objectives.

CAAHEP/ABHES STANDARDS

None

CONDITIONS

- Compound microscope
- Lens paper
- Specimen slide
- Immersion oil
- Laboratory tissue such as Kimwipes
- Gloves (if needed)

Procedure	Rationale
1. Wash hands and gather necessary supplies. Apply gloves if the specimen is infectious and unfixed (without preservative).	Gloves are not necessary if the specimen is fixed with chemicals that will kill the microorganisms on the slide. If dealing with unfixed specimens (such as vaginal smears or unstained urine) gloves must be applied.
2. Remove the microscope from storage, if necessary. Be sure to use one hand on the arm and one under the base of the microscope.	The microscope may be kept on the countertop, or it may be stored in a drawer or on a shelf. Always support the microscope with two hands to avoid hitting it against surfaces that could damage the instrument.

Continued

Procedure 6-1: Microscope Use—cont'd

Procedure	Rationale
3. Plug in the microscope to the electrical outlet. Verify that the excess cord does not hang over the edge of the counter.	The cord needs to be behind the microscope to avoid catching the cord and accidentally pulling the microscope from the counter.
4. Use lens paper to clean the eyepieces and the objectives. Start with the eyepieces, after which each objective should be cleaned starting with the lowest power and finishing with the 100X objective. Only the optical surface should be cleaned with the lens paper.	The eyepieces should be cleaned before the objectives to avoid possible transfer of oil to the eyepieces from the objectives. It is also important to remember that the 100X objective should be cleaned last because it is used with oil that could be transferred to the other objectives.
5. Turn on the light source and adjust the light to a low level.	The light should be at a low level as you begin to focus the specimen. More light will be required later as the objectives are changed to higher levels.
6. Adjust the eyepieces to be the same width as your eyes. With some models, it may be possible to adjust the eyepieces individually for a sharper focus.	Both eyes should be used at the same time when looking through a binocular microscope. This will be best accomplished when the width of the eyepieces matches that of your eyes.
7. Rotate the nosepiece to bring the lowest power objective straight down where it is pointing at the slide. There should be an audible click when this objective is in the proper position. Watch the stage and objective closely to avoid touching the stage with the objective. The lowest power objective may have a 4X or a 10X printed on it.	Focus always starts with the lowest power objective. Some microscope models may have a 4X objective, but most will have 10X as the lowest possible magnification.
8. Using the coarse adjustment knob, move the stage until it is at the lowest point possible.	The coarse adjustment knob is the larger knob at the back of the microscope. Moving the stage down will allow space to put the slide in place without potentially touching the objective with the slide.
9. Place the slide on the stage with the specimen side up. If the compound microscope used has stage clips, use these to secure the slide in place. Using the stage adjustment knob, position the slide so that the area on the slide to be viewed is directly over the hole where the light will shine through the specimen.	If the slide is not faceup, it will be very difficult to reach optimum clarity when viewing the specimen. It is especially important to center the slide where the specimen viewing area is focused over the hole where the light comes through when the specimen covers only a small area on the slide.
10. If the microscope has a condenser, adjust the condenser all the way up, using the adjustment knob to the side of the condenser. Using the adjustment lever on the diaphragm, open the iris diaphragm to allow the maximum amount of light to be utilized for viewing the specimen. This will be adjusted to a lower level as you work through the focusing process.	As the specimen focus process begins, it is essential to have as much light as possible available. The condenser may be moved farther from the specimen, and the diaphragm may be adjusted as the specimen is brought into closer focus.

Procedure	Rationale
11. While looking through the eyepieces, slowly turn the coarse adjustment knob until the specimen comes into approximate focus. It may not be possible to bring the specimen into complete focus using only the coarse adjustment knob.	The coarse adjustment knob allows for an approximate focus.
12. Without moving the slide or the objective, use the fine adjustment knob to bring the specimen into complete focus.	The fine adjustment knob is to be used only after approximate focus has been accomplished with the coarse adjustment knob.
13. Adjust the amount of light entering the specimen by moving the condenser down and by adjusting the diaphragm until the specimen appears in crisp, clear focus.	Too much light at a low magnification may cause the specimen to appear washed out, and some of the formed elements may be overlooked. Too little light does not allow for enough contrast to identify some of the structures.
14. Use the stage adjustment knob to move the object viewed directly into the center of the field of vision while looking in the microscope.	If this step is not performed, you may not be able to find the object again after changing to the next level of magnification, especially if the specimen only covers a small portion of the slide.
15. Use the nosepiece to swing the next objective so that it is pointing directly down at the slide. As before, the objective should click into place.	Always watch the objective as you move it into place to avoid touching anything with the objective lens.
16. Use the fine adjustment knob to bring the object into focus. It may be necessary to adjust the amount of light entering the specimen to see the object clearly.	With the objectives above 10X, do not use the coarse adjustment knob for focus.
17. If desired for the type of specimen viewed, continue this process, using the fine focus and adjusting the available light as the objectives are changed to higher levels of magnification.	Some specimens do not require higher levels of magnification if the structures can be identified at the lower levels.
18. If the oil immersion lens (the lens marked with the 100X and a ∞ symbol) is to be used, it will be necessary to place one or two drops of immersion oil on the slide before rotating the objective into place. a. Use the nosepiece to move the current objective out of the way, but do not lower the 100X objective until the oil has been added. b. Keep the slide as it was with the previous objective and place the drop(s) of oil on the slide right over the light source. c. Then, use the nosepiece to lower the 100X lens into place and adjust the focus as needed with the fine adjustment knob.	Resist the urge to make more room for this objective before moving it into place. This objective will be very close to the slide; it will appear that it is going to touch the slide, but if the proceeding steps were performed correctly, it will not touch the slide. The oil will seal the objective with the slide to keep the light focused on the specimen with clarity.

Continued

Procedure 6-1: Microscope Use—cont'd

Procedure	Rationale
19. After the specimen has been analyzed as needed, lower the stage to the lowest possible point, and remove the slide from the stage clips.	The stage should always be at the lowest point during storage to avoid potentially damaging the objectives.
20. Using the nosepiece, adjust the objectives so that the lowest power is pointing down toward the stage.	This allows the focusing to start appropriately when a new slide is put on the microscope, and also helps to avoid potential damage to the objectives.
21. Turn off the light source, and clean the eyepieces and objectives using lens paper. Remember to clean the 100X objective last, if applicable. Xylene can be used on the lens paper if needed for excessive soiling of the lenses.	Only lens paper should be used for this, as any other type of tissue will scratch the sensitive lenses. If the 100X objective is cleaned first, the rest of the lenses may be contaminated with oil. If xylene is used, be sure to follow appropriate protective measures as described by the manufacturer and the workplace.
22. Wipe off the stage and the rest of the microscope using a laboratory tissue such as Kimwipes. Moisten the tissue if necessary to remove dust. The stage should be disinfected periodically by using an alcohol wipe.	The slides, specimens, and oil can easily soil the stage.
23. Unplug and secure the electrical cord, and put the plastic cover back on the microscope. Be certain to move the microscope to the appropriate storage area as directed by office policy.	Be sure to use two hands when transporting the microscope.
24. Discard the slide or place it in the appropriate storage area as dictated by office policy.	Stained specimens are often stored for a period of time for future study. Slides should be treated as a "sharp" and disposed of in a puncture-resistant biohazard container.
25. Remove gloves (if used for the procedure) and wash hands.	Hands should be washed before and after each procedure in the laboratory setting.

Test Your Knowledge 6-6

Which adjustment knob should be used first when the specimen on the microscope is initially brought into focus?

(Outcome 6-5)

Test Your Knowledge 6-7

Is the microscope stage moved when objectives are changed for higher magnification of a specimen?

(Outcome 6-5)

Other Types of Microscopes

A dissecting microscope may also be utilized in the laboratory to view specimens that need to be seen in their natural state without compression or those that are too thick to be viewed effectively with the compound microscope. This type of microscope may also be known as a **stereo microscope** because the microscope is designed to allow a slightly different view from each of the eyepieces, providing an image with depth and dimension. The light source for this type of microscope is not focused in the same way that the compound microscope is focused; it is diffused or reflected onto the image rather than shone directly through it. The magnification ability of the dissecting microscope is not as extensive as that of the compound microscope, as it is usually only capable of enlarging the specimen by 40 or 100 times its normal size. Dissecting microscopes are often used for blood bank procedures when the technologist is examining different serum and cell combinations to look for **agglutination** of the specimen. Dissecting microscopes may be used for a variety of other purposes in the clinical laboratory when fine, detailed work needs to be performed with some magnification.

An **electron microscope** allows for much greater magnification of specimens, and also provides a three dimensional image. Electrons are utilized to "excite" the specimen, and the resulting interaction with the atoms present in the specimen will produce an image to be recorded and studied. This image is more of a picture that is defined by the properties of the specimen, rather than a true image seen by the eyes while viewing the specimen. The image created by the excitation of the sample is stored and viewed on a computer. Electron microscopes may be used to visualize specimens that are far too small to be seen with a compound microscope, such as viruses and the interior structures of cells. This type of microscope is not routinely found in clinical laboratories, as the user requires specialized training to operate it and interpret the images created with examination.

Test Your Knowledge 6-8

What type of microscope may be used to see viruses?
  a. Compound microscope
  b. Electron microscope
  c. Dissecting microscope
  d. Fluorescent microscope   (Outcome 6-2)

How Do Medical Assistants Use Microscopes?

The majority of the time, a medical assistant will not perform microscopic examinations for diagnostic purposes. There are a few microscopic procedures that have been classified as CLIA moderately complex procedures, and these can be performed by medical assistants with appropriate documented training. These include urine microscopic analysis (see Chapter 22) and normal blood cell differential counts (see Chapter 12). These are the exceptional cases in specialized offices such as urology offices or physician office laboratories with minimal staffing. Most commonly, a medical assistant's use of a microscope is limited to focusing the specimen for the health-care provider, as well as performing maintenance procedures. It is of great benefit for a medical assistant to

be capable of focusing the microscope, as this allows the health-care provider's valuable time to be spent examining the specimen rather than performing the original setup process. Medical assistants may be focusing stained blood smears, urinalysis sediment specimens, vaginal smears, nasal smears, Gram-stained microbiological specimens, and microscopic examinations for the presence of fungal elements on the microscope for examination. Remember, if the health-care provider does perform microscopy examinations, the laboratory must register as a CLIA site that provides this type of service.

Test Your Knowledge 6-9

Is a medical assistant properly trained to perform microscopic identification procedures?   (Outcome 6-6)

Centrifuges

A **centrifuge** is an instrument used to prepare blood (or other liquid specimens) for transport or testing. Blood is made up of cells that are suspended in a liquid substance called **plasma.** Chemical analysis is often performed on the plasma, and in order for the results to be accurate, the cells must be removed from the liquid portion of the blood as soon as possible after the specimen is obtained. A centrifuge is used to force the separation of the cells from the fluid portion of the blood (plasma).

If a blood specimen is allowed to sit for an extended period of time in a tube, gravity causes the cells to settle to the bottom of the tube, as they are denser (heavier) than the surrounding fluid. A centrifuge creates a powerful "artificial" gravity source, called **centrifugal force.** The force is formed as the specimen spins around an axis hundreds to thousands of times per minute. When a specimen is processed by a centrifuge, the separation of the different components of the blood is accelerated; the cells are pushed to the bottom of the tube within minutes. This allows the plasma to be removed from the cells in a timely manner so that chemical analysis can be performed. Urine specimens may also be centrifuged to bring the suspended elements (such as blood cells, bacteria, etc.) to the bottom of the tube so that they can be examined under a microscope.

There are various types of centrifuges available for use in a laboratory. Some of the benchtop models are designed to spin 8 to 10 samples at a time for a maximum of 10 minutes each cycle. Others are units the size of a dishwasher, capable of processing hundreds of tubes in each cycle for extended periods of time. The decision about which type of centrifuge to use is based on several factors, including the volume of samples to be processed, the requirements for the liquid portion of the blood after separation, and the amount of separation required. The decision may also be based on the recommended maintenance procedures for the centrifuge model of choice, as well as cost. Some centrifuges generate a lot of excess heat as they operate, due to the rapid turning of the unit around the axis. These models require built-in refrigeration to decrease the temperature to keep the specimens from becoming overheated.

Centrifuge Maintenance

Maintenance of all centrifuge models is similar. It is important that the interior and exterior of the machine stay clean and that there is nothing impeding the rotation of the unit around the axis. The **rotations per minute (rpms)** must also be checked at least quarterly using a **tachometer.** If the rotations have changed significantly since the last check, the instrument should be serviced, as there may be a problem that needs to be addressed. Many centrifuge models have a brushed drive motor, and these brushes must be changed at intervals recommended by the manufacturer. All metal components of the centrifuge should be checked for cracks at least once a month. As with all electrical equipment, the electrical cord should also be checked for wear periodically.

> **Test Your Knowledge 6-10**
> List two maintenance procedures to be performed on a centrifuge.   (Outcome 6-7)

Centrifuge Safety

- All medical centrifuges should have a cover that must be locked in place when in operation. Figure 6-2 shows an example of a centrifuge. The cover keeps the operator safe from potential aerosol formation or splashing that may occur if a specimen breaks or if a tube becomes uncovered during the cycle.
- It is also important that the centrifuge is **balanced** before starting. This means that for every tube inserted into the centrifuge, a tube with the same weight of fluid must be placed directly across from it in the unit. This additional tube may be filled with the same fluid as the specimen (another blood tube filled to the same level, for example), or it may be a balance tube that is filled with the same amount of water. This is a critical step, no matter what type of specimen is to be centrifuged. If the unit is not balanced, it is possible that the centrifuge will rock while operating (like an

off-balanced washing machine), fall off the countertop, and break the specimens as they are spinning.
- Be certain that all specimens are capped securely before starting the centrifuge.
- It is very important to follow the manufacturer's recommendations concerning length of cycles and specific maintenance.
- Remember never to open the centrifuge before it stops spinning completely. Never use your hand to try and slow down the final spin; this can be very dangerous.

> **Test Your Knowledge 6-11**
> What does it mean to balance a centrifuge?
>   (Outcome 6-7)

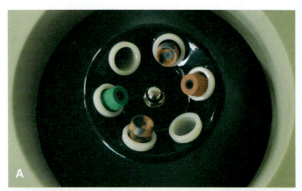

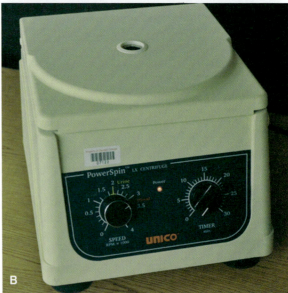

Figure 6-2   The inside (A) and outside (B) of a typical benchtop centrifuge.

Procedure 6-2: Operating the Centrifuge

TASK

Use a benchtop centrifuge to successfully separate plasma from cells in a blood specimen.

CAAHEP/ABHES STANDARDS

None

CONDITIONS

- Gloves
- Benchtop centrifuge
- Blood specimen in tube
- Balance tube
- Spacers to go inside slots in centrifuge if necessary
- Water and transfer pipette
- Test tube rack
- Disinfectant wipe

Procedure	Rationale
1. Wash hands and gather necessary supplies. Apply gloves.	Hands should be washed before and after performing any procedures in the laboratory, and gloves must be worn whenever handling blood specimens.
2. Verify that the centrifuge is plugged into an electrical outlet. Open the lid and verify that all the slots in the centrifuge are empty.	Occasionally the previous user will have left a tube or a spacer in one of the slots within the centrifuge, which can cause it to become unbalanced while processing the specimen. Care should also be taken to verify that there is no liquid in the bottom of the receptacles in the centrifuge, as this could also cause the centrifuge to become unbalanced.
3. Pick up the blood specimen and hold the tube at eye level. Fill the balance tube with water until the two tubes have an equal volume of fluid.	The tubes must have the same fluid volume for the centrifuge to be balanced. This can also be accomplished with two tubes of blood that are the same and are filled to the same level.
4. Verify that the original rubber cap is on the blood tube securely. The balance tube should also be capped with the original rubber cap.	To avoid aerosol formation, all specimens processed in the centrifuge should be securely capped.
5. For some centrifuge models, it may be necessary to place a rubber spacer or adapter in the centrifuge slot to accommodate the size of tube spun. Consult the manufacturer's recommendations.	The spacer or adapter will allow the blood tube to remain high enough in the centrifuge to be removed after spinning, and it may also allow for a tighter fit within the slot to avoid the breakage from vibration that is possible when the tube does not fit securely.
6. Place the two tubes in slots within the centrifuge that are across from each other. The centrifuge can be operated if the other slots are empty, as long as the two tubes are across from each other.	Balance is essential to keep the centrifuge from vibrating excessively while operating. An unbalanced centrifuge can cause the tubes to break, and it also can cause the centrifuge to fall off the countertop due to the excessive motion.
7. Close the lid securely. Turn on the timer on the centrifuge to the appropriate time for spinning a blood specimen. This will be indicated on the front of the centrifuge or in the manufacturer's insert.	Larger tubes may require a higher rate of centrifugation or a longer time in the centrifuge to achieve the desired separation of cells and plasma.

Continued

Procedure 6-2: Operating the Centrifuge—cont'd

Procedure	Rationale
8. Monitor the centrifuge for at least 20 to 30 seconds after it has been turned on to see if the instrument is vibrating excessively. If so, turn off or unplug the centrifuge immediately.	An unbalanced centrifuge can be dangerous if it vibrates on the countertop and moves from its original position.
9. Do not attempt to open the centrifuge until it has come to a full stop.	Opening the centrifuge prematurely or placing a hand into the unit while it is still spinning can be very dangerous.
10. When the centrifuge has come to a complete stop, open the lid and carefully remove the tube of blood. Place the blood in a rack for further processing.	Care needs to be taken when removing the tube of blood so that the plasma and cells do not become mixed.
11. Remove the balance tube and the spacers and adapters if used. The balance tube may be discarded or reused for another specimen. The spacers and adapters are to be stored for use with the next centrifuge load.	Some laboratories keep a set of balance tubes close at hand to be used for additional centrifugation. Be sure that the tube cap is securely fastened if using the balance tube again.
12. Use a disinfectant wipe to wipe down the exterior and interior of the unit.	If excessive contamination is evident, it may be necessary to clean the unit to a greater extent. In many units, the slots in which the tubes are placed are removable so that they can be washed if necessary.
13. Remove gloves and wash hands.	Hands should be washed before and after performing any procedures in the laboratory.

POINT OF INTEREST 6-1
"Sally Centrifuge"

In many areas of the world health-care providers do not have access to electricity or funds for purchasing traditional instruments used for diagnosis. The presence of anemia contributes significantly to the diagnosis and subsequent treatment of disorders such as malnutrition, HIV/AIDS, tuberculosis, and malaria. Blood specimens collected from the patients in these areas must be shipped to larger health-care facilities for testing, which is expensive and time consuming.

In 2010, two Rice University college students created an inexpensive centrifuge that allows the cells to be separated from the plasma in microhematocrit tubes in 10 to 20 minutes without the use of electricity. Lauren Theis and Lila Kerr created the centrifuge as a class project, using materials that included combs, yogurt containers, and a salad spinner. The centrifuge cost approximately $30 to build, and it can process 30 samples of 15 microliters each at one time. The centrifuge must be pumped by hand for 10 to 20 minutes, at which point it reaches speeds of approximately 950 rotations per minute and successfully separates the blood cells from the plasma in the tubes. The tubes then can be compared to a reference chart to obtain the hematocrit result, used to diagnosis the presence of anemia.

These students are part of a Rice University program, Beyond Traditional Borders. As part of this program, the students used the centrifuges in several remote locations during the summer of 2010 to test their ability to withstand traditional use in a health-care setting. If successful, "Sally Centrifuge" could have a profound impact on the ability to deliver affordable, timely health care in many locations across the globe.

Laboratory Refrigeration

Many specimens must be maintained at reduced temperatures to provide reliable test results when analyzed. The instructions for specimen collection and processing for a particular test may include refrigeration of the specimen, or possibly freezing of the plasma or **serum.** To ensure that the specimens are at the correct temperature, the refrigerators or freezers in the clinical laboratory should be monitored each day; in large laboratories with multiple shifts, they may be monitored more than once a day.

A **laboratory thermometer** is used to obtain accurate, reliable temperature readings. Laboratory thermometers are usually made of a measurement device that has the end designed to register the temperature while submersed in a container filled with liquid. The employee who is monitoring the temperature will open the door of the refrigerator or freezer, read the temperature on the thermometer, and record the result on a log sheet nearby. To keep the temperature as stable as possible, the door for the refrigerator or freezer should be opened only long enough to read the thermometer. Some thermometers are designed with systems that allow them to be monitored by a device that is outside of the refrigerator. This is advantageous because it is not necessary to open the door of the unit to take the temperature. In either case, a range of acceptable readings for each refrigerator or freezer must be established, and if the results fall outside this range, corrective action must be taken immediately. The specimens in the unit must be transferred elsewhere until the temperature reading is within the acceptable range again.

In laboratory situations in which refrigeration temperature is especially critical, an alarm system may be installed that sounds whenever there is a fluctuation in the temperature readings. Blood bank facilities have a very small range of acceptable storage temperatures for units of blood, and must have processes in place for critical monitoring of all their refrigeration units. These special refrigerators often have battery backups that activate a cooling system in case of power failure, as well as remote monitoring systems and audible alarms. The temperature for these units must be monitored more frequently than other refrigerators; often there is a continuous recording of temperatures.

Some refrigerators and freezers in physician office laboratories may be used to store specimens as well as vaccines or other medications. These products will have very specific storage requirements, so monitoring of the temperature used for storage will be especially critical. If the unit falls outside the acceptable storage ranges, the medication and vaccines may need to be discarded. Quality control materials may also be stored in refrigerators or freezers with specimens, and these materials will also have specific storage requirements that must be followed.

It is imperative that all refrigeration or freezer units in a laboratory setting are properly maintained to avoid excessive moisture or ice buildup. The refrigeration coils at the back of the unit should be kept free of dust buildup, and the interior and exterior of the unit should be kept as clean as possible. *No food or drink is to be stored in laboratory refrigerators where specimens are kept.* This is a safety precaution designed to protect employees from potential contamination of their food, as well as an Occupational Safety and Health Administration (OSHA) regulation that must be followed.

Test Your Knowledge 6-12

If specimens are to be kept at a certain reduced temperature, how often should the refrigerator temperature be monitored? What other precautions should be in place?   (Outcome 6-8)

Incubators

When microbiology specimens are collected from a human for analysis, the pathogens that may be present are reproducing at body temperature. This temperature is approximately 25° to 27° Celsius or 95° to 99° Fahrenheit. To keep these pathogens alive until they can be identified, it is necessary to keep them at this temperature for a few days. A laboratory **incubator** is used for this purpose. The temperature for an incubator must be monitored at least daily, and the results must be documented on a log sheet. Much like a laboratory refrigeration unit, there is a limited acceptable range for these temperature readings, and if the incubator falls outside of that range, the unit must be serviced.

In addition, **water baths** or other types of heating units may be used in a laboratory. Water baths may be used to heat specimens as part of specific testing procedures. Other heating units may be used to "fix" a specimen to a slide, or to sterilize inoculation devices in the microbiology laboratory.

EQUIPMENT USED FOR AUTOMATED CLIA-WAIVED LABORATORY TESTING

Many medical offices choose to perform automated CLIA-waived tests in their own laboratory on site. Performance of these tests in the office environment rather than in a reference laboratory may benefit the patient in various ways:

- On-site testing may assist the health-care provider to assign a definitive diagnosis quickly. This allows a plan of treatment to be established before the patient leaves the office. The patient and health-care provider can discuss the plan, and an opportunity is provided for face-to-face communication. This can be especially critical for patients who are acutely ill and those with chronic health conditions requiring frequent laboratory testing to monitor the progress of their treatment.
- CLIA-waived tests performed in the physician's office may be less expensive for the patient. Many times insurance coverage is limited for laboratory testing, so a reduced charge is definitely a benefit.
- Performance of testing on site may allow patients to minimize visits; they can have their specimen collected and tested at the same location that they see their health-care provider, without going to a separate destination for collection and/or testing. This helps improve patient compliance rates.

CLIA-waived automated testing may also be performed in larger laboratories for tests that do not require more advanced methods of analysis. These laboratories may employ medical assistants or phlebotomists to perform these testing procedures with appropriate oversight by other laboratory professionals. Automated methods for CLIA-waived tests include chemical urinalysis, chemistry testing, and hematology testing.

Test Your Knowledge 6-13

List one advantage of performing automated CLIA-waived tests in a physician office laboratory.   (Outcome 6-10)

Testing Methodology

Chemistry analyzers may test the liquid portion of the blood (plasma) or the whole blood specimen. Hematology instruments are designed to perform various measurements on the cells present in the specimen. Automated analyzers used for CLIA-waived hematology, coagulation, urinalysis, and chemistry testing (as well as advanced instruments used in more complex testing procedures) are often used to provide quantitative results of substances or cells present in the specimens. Other testing instruments may provide qualitative results, such as those used for **fecal occult blood** testing or urine drug screening. In this case, the presence or absence of a specific analyte provides

the necessary information for the health-care provider to develop a plan of action.

Most of the CLIA-waived chemistry testing methods explained in this textbook use reagents that change color when they are exposed to the chemicals present in the specimen. This color change is measured by a **spectrophotometer,** an instrument that measures light intensity. A specific wavelength of light enters a sample, and depending on the amount of color change, a certain amount will continue through the sample to be measured on the other side. The measurement of the intensity of the light at the end of the process is directly related to the concentration of the chemical substances present in the solution. The light intensity measurement may be changed by absorption of the light by the specimen, or by reflecting or scattering the light so that it is not measured directly at the end of the reaction.

Hematology testing often uses **electrical impedance,** a process for counting cells in the whole blood specimen and differentiating them by size. For this type of test, whole blood specimens are added to a **diluent** (a liquid used for dilution of a specimen) that is capable of conducting electricity. An electrical current is applied to the mixture of specimen and diluent as it passes through a small opening, called an **aperture.** Because the blood cells do not conduct electricity, they break the current between the electrodes on either side of the aperture. The amount of impedance (interference of the electrical signal) caused by a certain cell will allow the instrument to count the cell and approximate the size and other physical properties. A similar type of measurement uses the amount of light scattered by a specimen to measure the cell numbers and cell sizes in a hematology specimen.

Hematology instruments (such as those that test only **hemoglobin**) may also use spectrophotometers to measure a specific substance. In this case, the cells must be broken, or **lysed** prior to the testing procedure, so that the hemoglobin present inside the cells may be measured.

When using an instrument to perform any of these tests, it is imperative that the manufacturer's instructions are followed concerning frequency and extent of quality control testing and calibration of the instrument. These procedures must be performed as directed to verify that the instrument is operating as it should before patient samples are analyzed. The reagents used with the analyzers often have storage requirements and expiration dates that must be monitored as well, and quality control samples must be prepared and processed as directed to produce meaningful results.

Test Your Knowledge 6-14

Electrical impedance is a common term used to describe how the number of cells in a specimen are measured. What process occurs to allow the cells to be counted by the instrument?   (Outcome 6-11)

Instruments Used for Chemical Testing of Urine Specimens

Urine specimens are analyzed in various ways. One of the methods used to evaluate the specimen is a chemical analysis to detect and/or quantify the presence of substances in the urine specimen that may indicate disease. Quite often, this analysis will be performed manually in a physician office laboratory, but this analysis may also be performed using an instrument and **reagent strips** that are imbedded with small squares designed to change color when exposed to specific chemicals present in the urine specimen. Although the exact number and types of chemicals analyzed in the specimen may vary according to the manufacturer of the unit, common chemical substances detected include the following:

- pH levels
- protein
- glucose
- blood
- leukocytes
- specific gravity
- bilirubin
- glucose
- ketone
- urobilinogen
- nitrite

The process of reading the reagent strips is time and color sensitive. The chemical measurements are based on changes in color that develop in response to the presence of certain chemicals. These changes do not all occur at the same rate, which means that the reagent pads on the strips must be read at specific time intervals after the strip has been exposed to the urine specimen. Automated urine analyzers are designed to move the strip through the measuring device with the appropriate speed to read these reagent pads at the correct time.

A similar procedure is used for testing urine using any of these machines. Essentially, the reagent strip is immersed in the urine specimen, blotted to remove excess specimen, then applied to a tray that feeds the reagent strip into the instrument for analysis. The instrument times the advance of the strip appropriately for the different reagent pads to be analyzed for color changes. The amount of color change is directly related to the concentration of the chemical substances in the urine, and once analyzed, the results are printed on a strip that may be kept as a permanent record. Some of the instruments are also capable of transmitting the results directly to a computer so that they may be stored electronically. Urine analyzers are quick and easy to use, and eliminate the need for the employee to monitor the reaction of the different areas of the reagent strip for the full time needed for color development.

Common urine analyzers include the Clinitek Urine Analyzer, manufactured by the Bayer Corporation, and the Urisys 1100 Analyzer, manufactured by Roche. Henry Schein also manufactures the One Step Plus Analyzer (Fig. 6-3). The automated chemical analysis testing that is performed with these instruments is CLIA-waived, as long as the manufacturer's directions are followed exactly as printed. Quality control and maintenance for this type of equipment may include the use of commercial quality control specimens of different levels, calibration of the instrument, and cleaning of the instrument at regular intervals. Some general aspects to keep in mind

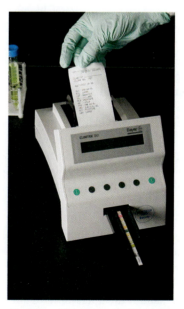

Figure 6-3   One Step Plus Urine Analyzer. *Courtesy of Henry Schein, Inc.*

when performing urine testing with an automated instrument include the following:

- Reagent strips do outdate. *Always* check the expiration date before using the strips.
- Reagent strips must be protected from moisture, so the bottle must be closed immediately after removing the necessary strips for testing.
- Automated urinalysis instruments may produce erroneous results in situations in which the urine is discolored by medications or dyes used for diagnostic purposes. The employee performing these tests must keep this in mind and follow the manufacturer's recommendations and the office policy for confirmatory testing before reporting results on discolored specimens.
- As with all testing procedures, documentation of the quality control and maintenance procedures is critical, as well as the appropriate documentation of all patient results.

Instruments Used for Coagulation Testing

Coagulation testing is used to screen patients for blood clotting issues. It may also be used to monitor patients who have been placed on anticoagulant therapy, such as warfarin (Coumadin). As presented in more detail in Chapter 15, coagulation testing is commonly performed as a CLIA-waived test in the physician office laboratory environment. The most common test used for screening or monitoring is the **prothrombin time test.** This test is more commonly known as a **protime,** and it measures the length of time necessary for a blood specimen to form a clot when reagents are added. The result is reported in seconds. Protimes may also be performed in larger laboratories using testing methods that are not CLIA-waived. When the protime test is performed, an **international normalized ratio (INR)** is usually reported in addition to the test result. The INR is a calculation provided by dividing the protime result for the patient by the normal control value for the lot of reagents currently in use for that system.

Protime testing on the CLIA-waived instruments is accomplished by inserting a reagent strip or cartridge into the instrument, then adding one or more drops of blood to the designated area of the strip. The blood specimen is usually obtained from a capillary puncture, and a drop is placed directly onto the testing device or transferred from the finger using a capillary transfer device. There are specific timing and quantity requirements, and if the operator does not follow these guidelines, an error code will result and the test must be repeated with a fresh specimen. Some of these

coagulation analyzers provide a printout, others can be connected to an external printer for result documentation, and still other instruments may be interfaced to the computer for the results to be stored electronically. The units do have a display screen where the operator can read the result.

Various CLIA-waived methods and instruments may be used to perform the protime test. These include the ITC ProTime-3 as well as Roche Diagnostic's CoaguChek S, XS, and XS Plus. Other CLIA-waived protime systems include the Hemosense Inratio system, and several products produced by the Lifescan Corporation. Figure 6-4 shows a Roche CoaguChek S with reagents and necessary to perform a protime test. Each type of instrument has instructions that are a little bit different, but all the testing systems share some of the following characteristics:

- All CLIA-waived or home use systems have test strips that are packaged individually so that one test is performed at a time.
- Each lot of test strips has a unique product code that must be entered into the machine to perform the test. Some products have a computer chip with the product code, and this must be inserted into the analyzer prior to the sample testing process.
- All instruments have quality control procedures; some are built-in internal controls that run automatically during the testing process, while other instruments use liquid commercial control materials that are run as

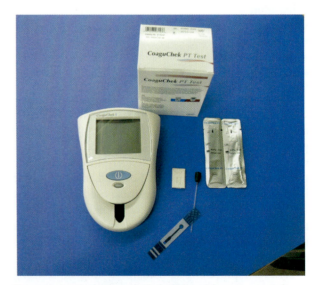

Figure 6-4   Roche CoaguChek S Plus with reagents and quality control materials.

patient samples. As always, the quality control (QC) values must be documented and interpreted as recommended by the manufacturer.

- The reagents all have specific storage requirements, although these vary from brand to brand.
- All CLIA-waived methods require whole blood samples for testing, and the test is designed to be run on capillary blood. A lancet is used to pierce the skin for the sample.
- Many of the testing methods recommend use of a microcapillary tube with a bulb or a collection cup to assist with obtaining adequate sample volume.
- The blood sample is applied directly to the reagent strip for all methods; generally there is a window or circle that must be covered completely with blood.
- The instruments require very little maintenance. Most have batteries and some also have A/C adapters. The batteries must be changed periodically, and should be removed from the device if it will not be used for an extended period of time. The analyzers should also be kept clean. The instrument (especially the sample application area) may be cleaned with a cotton-tipped applicator moistened with isopropyl alcohol or a 5% bleach solution.
- None of the instruments should be immersed in water or any other liquid.
- All manufacturer's instructions for the testing process must be followed exactly as written.

Test Your Knowledge 6-15

What type of specimen is needed for handheld coagulation instruments?

   a. Plasma
   b. Serum
   c. Urine
   d. Whole blood   (Outcome 6-13)

Test Your Knowledge 6-16

Are results for CLIA-waived coagulation testing available at the completion of the test?   (Outcome 6-13)

Instruments Used for Chemistry Testing

CLIA-waived automated chemistry testing procedures are now available for a variety of analytes. Some of the most common tests performed in the physician office laboratory are **glucose** measurements and **glycosylated hemoglobin monitoring** for diabetes screening and treatment. **Cholesterol** studies and **electrolyte** measurements are also quite

common. Many instruments now have the capability of performing chemistry panels that include three or more tests, providing the health-care provider a more comprehensive set of information to work with as they develop a treatment plan. The test results are usually available within an hour of the test onset, and many of the instruments are capable of transmitting these results directly to a computer for documentation. Calibration of these analyzers may be performed internally or with an external cartridge, and many methods include an internal method of quality control that eliminates the need to purchase separate liquid controls. Also, because the CLIA-waived status for these instruments applies to whole blood specimen testing, most of the instruments require only a few drops of blood, which can be accomplished with a capillary blood draw.

There are more CLIA-waived glucose testing methods than any other type of chemistry analyzers. Many of the glucose instruments used in the physicians' office laboratory are also in use as home testing devices. These instruments have become more technologically advanced, and use even less blood for analysis than in the past. It is no longer required to use fingertips for all samples; innovative lancets and reduced specimen volume requirements have allowed the sites for specimen collection to vary. Devices used at home and in the office allow for test results to be stored, and some also may interface directly with a computer system to allow for closer monitoring and better communication with the health-care provider.

Glucose analyzers utilize reagent strips or cassettes that are inserted into the instrument. A capillary blood specimen is obtained and a few drops are placed directly onto the appropriate area of the reagent strip. The strip may be advanced into the instrument, or the specimen may be analyzed through the application area at the front of the instrument. The analyzer includes a display screen on which the operator may view the results, and (as is the case for the other instruments already covered in this chapter) the analyzer may be capable of printing results or transmitting them directly to a computer for electronic storage. Some instruments are even capable of charting or graphing patient data to provide a historical overview of results over a period of time.

Glucose analyzers found in the physician office laboratory may include the Roche Diagnostics Accu-Chek, the Abbott iStat, and the Hemocue Glucose 201 Microcuvette. There are many CLIA-waived glucose analyzer methods, and more information may be found for any specific type by visiting the website for that manufacturer. It is important to remember that each brand of analyzer has unique reagent strips and quality control materials; these are not interchangeable.

Other chemistry tests may be performed using CLIA-waived automated testing procedures in a physician office setting or other small laboratory. These include measurements for electrolytes, blood urea nitrogen (BUN), triglycerides, cholesterol, and calcium. Instruments used for testing these analytes use individual testing cartridges, which are self-contained. A capillary blood sample may be obtained in some situations, or in others the entire tube of blood collected by venipuncture may be placed in the instrument to be sampled. Because each testing cartridge is self-contained, the blood sample is added to every cartridge individually. The addition of the sample may be performed within the instrument using an automated method, or the person performing the test may add the sample to each cartridge by hand. Results are usually available within 30 minutes, even if the patient has several tests performed at once. The results are printed out on a slip that may be added to the patient record, and many models are also capable of transmitting the information electronically to a computer system.

The CLIA-waived automated chemistry instruments that use individual cartridges are more expensive to operate per test than the large chemistry analyzers found in reference and hospital laboratories, because of the high cost of the individual cartridges. Larger instruments have reagents that cost less per assay, but they are not CLIA waived for operation. The low sample volume and limited variety of testing procedures ordered in a physician office laboratory are served well by the instruments that use the self-contained individual cartridges.

The Abbott iStat Chem 8+ Cartridge analyzer is a common CLIA-waived chemistry instrument that may be used for point-of-care testing in an emergency room, at the bedside of a patient in the hospital, or in a physician office laboratory. It uses whole blood, and can be used to produce results for a variety of tests. Cholesterol testing may be performed using the Cholestech LDX, but this instrument may not be used for very many other types of tests. The Abixis Piccolo Xpress blood chemistry analyzer has a good deal of flexibility, uses tubes of whole blood, and doesn't take up very much space on a countertop. A comprehensive list of the CLIA-waived automated chemistry testing instruments may be found on the U.S. Food and Drug Administration (FDA) website listed in the Resources and Suggested Readings section at the end of this chapter.

Test Your Knowledge 6-17

What is a common chemistry analyzer used in small laboratories to test cholesterol levels?   (Outcome 6-14)

Instruments Used for Hemoglobin Measurements

Hemoglobin is the molecule within the red blood cells that carries oxygen to the tissues of the body. Iron is necessary to build this molecule, so the hemoglobin level of the blood is directly related to the oxygen-carrying capacity of the cells, as well as the iron levels of the individual. Hemoglobin (Hgb) is commonly performed as a screening test for **anemia,** and it may also be ordered as a test to monitor progress when a patient is being treated for anemia.

Because hemoglobin is part of the red blood cell structure, the cells must be broken or lysed before the hemoglobin level can be measured. In CLIA-waived automated hemoglobin testing instruments, the cells are lysed within the individual cuvette when the blood is added. For instance, in the HemoCue hemoglobin testing method, the inside of the individual cuvette used for the test is coated with a chemical (sodium deoxycholate) that destroys the red blood cell membranes, allowing the hemoglobin to be measured.

Test Your Knowledge 6-18

Is hemoglobin measured from intact red blood cells?
(Outcome 6-15)

Regardless of the type of instrument used, hemoglobin testing is always performed using whole blood. CLIA-waived systems use capillary samples, and the blood is usually applied directly to the cuvette (or testing device such as a strip) from the capillary puncture site. Proper capillary technique must be used to provide an appropriate specimen. One test is performed at a time, and the individual testing device may be placed in the instrument after the blood has been added, or it may be necessary to place it in the machine prior to the addition of the sample. (Check the manufacturer's recommendations for details.) The instruments will have a display screen on which the progress of the test may be monitored once the blood has been added; generally the results are available within one minute. Some of the instruments may be capable of printing the results, whereas others may also be able to send the results electronically to a computer system for documentation.

The CLIA-waived hemoglobin systems are equipped with electronic calibration methods. The HemoCue system has a standardized cuvette with known values that should be checked at regular intervals to be certain that the instrument is operating correctly. The ITC Hgb Pro has an internal calibration that is performed every time a test is performed. If the internal calibration process does not show that the instrument is working correctly, an error will result and the instrument cannot be used for patient testing until the calibration is successful. Liquid commercial quality control specimens may also be utilized to verify that any hemoglobin instrument is operating appropriately.

Other Hematology Instruments

Many physician office laboratories use hematology instruments that have been classified as moderately complex according to CLIA regulations. Common manufacturers are Beckman Coulter and Abbott. Remember, when performing tests of moderate complexity, it is necessary to perform quality control and calibration procedures more frequently, and there are more regulations for personnel training.

> ### Test Your Knowledge 6-19
> Is a glucometer an example of an instrument used for hematology testing? (Outcome 6-14)

Glassware and Other Miscellaneous Laboratory Equipment

Physician office laboratories don't have as much glassware as larger laboratories, and in many cases, glassware is now replaced by plastic disposable containers. However, there are a few standard items that may be found in the laboratory setting, regardless of the size of the facility:

- **Pipettes:** Pipettes are used to move liquid from one place to another. It is similar to the turkey baster that you may find in your kitchen. Some pipettes are designed to measure small amounts of liquid very accurately. Others are used just to transfer liquids from one place to another, without measurement. Pipettes come in varied sizes, and are often plastic and disposable.
- **Beakers** and **flasks:** Beakers and flasks are both containers that may be used to store, transfer, or heat liquids. Beakers generally are wide at the top and have a flat base, whereas flasks have a narrow opening at the top and a rounded bottom that is much larger than the top.
- **Glass slides** and **cover slips:** Glass slides are still used in the laboratory, even though many items are now made of plastic. Slides made of glass are still the best item to use when viewing items under the microscope, as they do not distort the view in the manner that some plastic slides may. Slides may be completely clear, or they may be frosted partially or completely for specialized uses. Some slides may have a depression in the

center for certain types of specimens. Cover slips are small panes of glass or plastic placed on top of liquid specimens on the glass slides before viewing. Cover slips are often used when the specimen is viewed in a natural state without any preservative or staining.
- **Cylinder:** A cylinder is a slim, round container that is used to measure liquids. A **graduated cylinder** is marked with specific units to allow for accurate measurement.

Because glassware is often used to accurately measure liquid in the laboratory setting, it is important to know the correct way to read the amount of liquid present. Liquid in a glass container is not completely flat at the top, because liquid is "attracted" or pulled up or down the sides of the container to form a curve. This curved surface of the liquid is known as the **meniscus.** In a narrow container, the meniscus will be more curved than it will be in a wide container. When measuring liquid in glassware, always perform the measurement at the lowest or highest point of the meniscus; this principle applies whether removing liquid to obtain a certain volume, or adding liquid to a container. Figure 6-5 shows how to measure liquid correctly in glassware using the meniscus.

> ### Test Your Knowledge 6-20
> The curved area at the top of a column of liquid in a glass cylinder is called the:
> a. Photometer
> b. Diaphragm
> c. Flask
> d. Meniscus (Outcome 6-17)

SUMMARY

Various types of automated instruments may be found in the clinical laboratory. These instruments may be used to process samples for analysis, examine specimens under the microscope, or analyze body fluids utilizing CLIA-waived automated testing techniques. Medical assistants need to know the correct way to use and maintain equipment for specimen processing, focus microscopes, and perform automated testing appropriate to their level of training. It is also important that medical assistants familiarize themselves with the other equipment used in the laboratory setting, such as refrigerators, incubators, and various types of glassware. Care should be taken to maintain all equipment appropriately, and follow the manufacturer's directions to perform testing procedures exactly as directed.

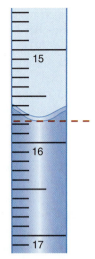

Figure 6-5   Reading the liquid volume using the meniscus. Many liquids curve at the edges of glass containers because of the attraction of the molecules to the glass. This curvature at the top of the liquid is called the *meniscus*. The level is to be measured at the horizontal center of the curvature. Some liquids curve upward instead of downward from the edges of the container, in which case the liquid level is to be read at the top of the curvature. Always hold the container at eye level when measuring.

TIME TO REVIEW

1. What disorder might be monitored   Outcome 6-1
   by performing periodic glycosylated hemoglobin tests?
   a. Diabetes
   b. Hypertension
   c. Hyperlipidemia
   d. Hypokalemia

2. A device used to transfer small   Outcome 6-1
   quantities of liquids is a:
   a. Pipette
   b. Cuvette
   c. Cylinder
   d. Beaker

3. True or False: A tachometer is a   Outcome 6-1
   type of thermometer used to measure temperatures in the laboratory environment.

4. True or False: The objective is a   Outcome 6-1
   device that can be adjusted to control the amount of light that enters a specimen on a microscope.

5. How many eyepieces does a   Outcome 6-1
   binocular microscope have?
   a. One
   b. Two
   c. Three
   d. Four

6. True or False: Centrifuges are   Outcome 6-7
   used to process all laboratory specimens before testing.

7. What are two tasks that a   Outcome 6-6
   medical assistant may be asked to perform with a microscope?
   a. Maintenance and cleaning of the microscope
   b. Prepare and focus specimens on the microscope for examination by the health-care provider
   c. With appropriate training, examination of urine sediment
   d. All of the above

8. True or False: Automated urine   Outcome 6-12
   analyzers are used to test for bacteria and other suspended objects in urine specimens.

9. What are two types of   Outcome 6-14
   CLIA-waived chemistry instruments presented in this chapter?

10. Which company is mentioned   Outcome 6-16
    in the text as a common manufacturer of hematology instruments?
    a. Bayer
    b. Dimension
    c. Beckman Coulter
    d. Piccolo

11. Why is a cover slip used?   Outcome 6-17
    a. To view specimens that have been preserved with an additive
    b. To view specimens in their natural state
    c. To view large specimens without the use of a slide
    d. To view chemical reactions

Case Study 6-1: This test won't work!

The manager for the internal medicine office where Cindy Lou is employed as a medical assistant is on vacation. In her absence, the lead medical assistant has placed a few orders for laboratory supplies, including some test strips for the glucometer used for glucose testing.

On Tuesday morning, Cindy knows that a patient is scheduled for diabetes monitoring. This usually involves a blood glucose level to be performed during his visit. Cindy decides to process the quality control specimens for the glucometer first thing in the morning so that she can be ready for the patient's arrival.

Cindy turns on the instrument, allows it to perform the internal verification that it always goes through, and inserts a test strip to process the quality control specimen. The test strip seems to fit in the instrument a bit differently from the way it has before, but she continues with the process. After inserting the strip and adding the QC material, the display screen flashes an ERROR code, and no result is displayed for the test. Cindy removes this strip and inserts another one, but receives the same result. She checks the QC material to see if it might be expired, and finds that it is not. Once more Cindy attempts to process a QC specimen of a different level (high glucose level) but receives the same code.

1. What is the most probable explanation for the ERROR code?
2. Can Cindy Lou process a patient specimen despite the ERROR codes?

RESOURCES AND SUGGESTED READINGS

"US Centrifuge Systems: Frequently Asked Questions"
Frequently asked questions about how a centrifuge works, and types to choose from http://www.uscentrifuge.com/faq.htm
"The Clinical Laboratory Improvement Act and the Physician's Office Laboratory"
Various educational modules and mini quizzes for CLIA waived hematology and chemistry tests http://www.medicine.uiowa.edu/CME/clia/default.asp
"Tests Waived by the FDA From January 2000 to Present"
List of all CLIA waived tests; updated regularly http://www.accessdata.fda.gov/scripts/cdrh/cfdocs/cfClia/testswaived.cfm
"Principles of Spectrophotometry"
Great explanations about how spectrophotometry works http://www.ruf.rice.edu/~bioslabs/methods/protein/spectrophotometer.html
"Welcome to HemoCue"
Information about the various products manufactured by HemoCue http://www.hemocue.com
"Glossary of Microscope Terms"
Explanations for many of the terms used with microscope use http://www.microscope-microscope.org/basic/microscope-glossary.htm

Case Study 6-2: Lack of focus

Lucille has been working in the laboratory at the local obstetrics and gynecology office for several years. She routinely performs blood draws and several different CLIA-waived laboratory tests. The providers in the office have decided that they want to start performing microscopy procedures in the office to better serve their patients.

To perform the microscopy procedures, the providers in the office ask Lucille to demonstrate how well she can focus the microscope. Lucille has not worked with a microscope since she was in medical assisting school, but she does her best to remember the steps involved. She is successful with the initial focus using the 10X objective, but can't seem to bring the specimen into focus when she switches to the 40X objective.

1. What are two possible explanations for the lack of focus with the 40X objective?

Overview of the Laboratory
What Does It All Mean?

The purpose of this section is to introduce you to global aspects associated with the clinical laboratory and laboratory testing. As this section clearly indicates, laboratory testing is crucial to the diagnosis and monitoring of patient diseases and conditions, as well as to rule out any diseases and conditions. This being said, an alert medical assistant will have a comprehensive understanding of these aspects. Further, the medical assistant will use appropriate corresponding techniques and procedures to ensure proper laboratory sample collection for testing by appropriately trained and educated individuals. Our Case in Point for this section explores some of these important concepts and serves as a review of the section content.

Case in Point

As noted in this case, during the first week of your student practicum you are introduced to the clinical laboratory by your clinical instructor, Doris. Your patient, Mr. Hershey, presents to Maple Grove Clinic for evaluation. After examining Mr. Hershey, Dr. Pueblo determines that he requires laboratory testing to determine his condition. This situation gives you and Doris a wonderful opportunity to discuss important concepts associated with both the clinical laboratory and laboratory testing. Highlights of this discussion follow for your review and consideration.

There are numerous ways in which laboratories are structured and organized based on a number of factors, including the environment in which the laboratory exists (it may be a small rural hospital or large commercial reference laboratory). Each laboratory determines what tests it will run, what instrument it will use for the tests, and the values considered as normal for the typical patient population the laboratory serves. There are three phases of laboratory testing: preanalytical, analytical, and postanalytical. Every laboratory test passes through all three phases. An error in any of the three phases may adversely affect the laboratory results generated. Most of the problems encountered in laboratory testing occur during the preanalytical testing phase because of a variety of issues, for example, collecting the sample on an individual other than the targeted patient.

Laboratory tests are categorized based in part on the difficulty of the procedure required to obtain the results. Health-care support individuals, including medical assistants, are allowed under government regulations to perform select testing under strict guidelines. Handling every sample using universal precautions is an important point to emphasize, as doing this contributes to the validity of the test results obtained. In addition to running the laboratory tests, quality control samples must also be tested on a regular basis to ensure that the test is working properly. Laboratory test results can only be released (in laboratory jargon this is called "turned out") to the patient's chart if the quality control samples test properly. In the event that quality control results are not in range, investigation and resolution of the problem must occur before patient results can be considered valid. Individuals vary in many ways. Variations in laboratory test values (as well as quality control samples) are no exception. Because of this, laboratory test results considered as being normal fall within a range of values.

In conclusion, laboratory tests provide physicians and other primary care providers with valuable information. In fact, many sources have reported that some 70% to 80% of diagnosis and treatment decisions are based on laboratory results. As this section clearly suggests, there are many important aspects to laboratory structure and testing, all of which contribute to the bottom line: accurate laboratory tests performed in a timely manner.

On the Horizon

It has been widely documented that as many as 70% to 80% of all patient treatment decisions are based on laboratory test results. Similarly, there is strong evidence to support the fact that laboratory test results are only as good as the sample from which the testing occurs. Specimen collection and processing, also known as the preanalytical phase (meaning the steps before actual analysis occurs) of testing, is thus a very important factor that contributes to the reliability of the laboratory test results obtained. Results from such samples collected and/or processed improperly cannot be considered valid and thus are of no benefit to the patient. There is widespread evidence that most laboratory testing errors occur in during the collection and processing of specimens.

Relevance for the Medical Assistant (Health-Care Provider)

Medical assistants and other health-care support personnel are often called upon to assist in the collection of, perform the collection of, instruct patients on the collection of and process samples for laboratory testing. To ensure the most reliable results for the patient, an in-depth understanding of specimen collection and processing is of paramount importance.

Case in Point

After a relatively smooth morning, your first patient after lunch is Wilma F., a 70-year-old woman. After reviewing Wilma's file, you notice that she was seen and treated 3 weeks ago, on what just happened to be on your day off, for a urinary tract infection. As you help Wilma get onto the scale to weigh her and then again when you place the blood pressure cuff on her arm, you notice that she is very hot to the touch. Your suspicions are confirmed when you take her temperature and it is 101.5°F! You ask Wilma to identify all symptoms she has been experiencing. She tells you that in addition to feeling hot all the time, she has a burning sensation and pain during urination. You document these details and tell Wilma that the doctor will be in to see her shortly and you leave the examining room. After the doctor examines Wilma, he asks you to collect her blood and assist Wilma in collecting urine for urinalysis and culture.

Questions for Consideration:

- What special considerations must be addressed to collect the blood in an appropriate manner in this case?
- What special equipment do you need to collect this blood sample?
- What type of urine sample should you assist Wilma to collect?
- How is this type of urine sample collected?
- Why are the blood and urine collection processes so important to implement in this case?

Section II
Specimen Collection and Processing

As one might imagine, there are many things that must be considered in this situation to ensure that laboratory specimens are properly collected and processed. That being said, this section is divided into four chapters, each with a targeted focus.

Chapter 7: Overview of Specimen Collection and Processing consists of an in-depth discussion of the proper ordering and documentation associated with specimen collection. The name of the laboratory test(s) being ordered, methods of collection, patient preparation, and proper information for specimen labeling are all addressed. Specimen collections that involve a process known as the chain of custody are identified and described.

Chapter 8: Collection and Processing of Blood Samples explores the anatomy and physiology of the cardiovascular system as well as body sites both suitable and unsuitable for the collection of blood. The equipment and procedures for successful venipuncture and capillary puncture specimens and the process of creating peripheral blood smears is detailed.

Chapter 9: Collection and Processing of Urine Samples introduces the reader to the most common types of urine samples, including but not limited to catheterized, midstream-clean catch, first morning collection, and timed collection. The purpose of each specimen type is identified.

Chapter 10: Collection and Processing of Samples for Microbial Studies covers the general requirements for proper collection of samples for microbial studies. Samples described include throat swabs for strep screen and culture, sputum, urine, blood (using aseptic technique), wounds, and stool. Samples for saline wet preps and KOH preps are also described. Processing supplies, particularly media and techniques used to support growth of microorganisms, are covered.

Chapter 7

Overview of Specimen Collection and Processing

Constance L. Lieseke, CMA (AAMA), MLT, PBT(ASCP)

CHAPTER OUTLINE

Specimen Ordering
    Required Items for All Laboratory Tests
    Test Specifics
        Medicare-Approved Panels
        Standing Orders
        Reflexive Testing
Patient Identification
    Verification of Patient Identity
        Acceptable Patient Identifiers
        Electronic Bar Codes

Patient Preparation
Specimen Collection at Home
Items That Must Be Documented With Specimen Collection
Labeling Information
Chain of Custody
Summary
Time to Review
Resources and Suggested Readings

Learning Outcomes
After reading this chapter, the successful student will be able to:

7-1 Define each of the key terms.

7-2 List the required items necessary for ordering any laboratory test.

7-3 Compare and contrast organ- or disease-specific panels that are approved by the Centers for Medicare & Medicaid services (CMS) to custom panels created by some laboratories.

7-4 Explain how standing orders are used in the laboratory.

7-5 Describe reflexive testing and explain how it may benefit patients.

7-6 Describe acceptable methods used to verify patient identity.

7-7 Demonstrate understanding of the importance of proper patient preparation prior to specimen collection.

7-8 Instruct patients in how to fast for a laboratory test.

7-9 Explain the importance of timing for peak and trough medication levels.

7-10 Explain why thorough documentation of specimen sources is so important.

7-11 Describe what to include when documenting specimen collection.

7-12 Describe appropriate labeling procedures for laboratory specimens.

7-13 Describe the critical aspects involved in a specimen collection that requires a chain of custody.

CAAHEP/ABHES STANDARDS

 CAAHEP Standards Met

IV.P. Psychomotor Skills, Concepts of Effective Communication, #6: Prepare a patient for procedures and/or treatments.

 ABHES Standards

10. Medical Laboratory Procedures, Specimens

KEY TERMS

1 or 2 hr postprandial (1 or 2 hr pp)	First morning void	Random specimen
Chain of custody	Glucose challenge	Reflexive testing
Fasting	Glucose tolerance test	Standing orders
	Peak collection level	Trough collection level

Proper specimen collection and processing are critical components of laboratory testing as part of the pre-analytical phase. As introduced in Chapter 1, certain factors in the collection and processing of specimens are universal: clear, concise patient preparation instructions, verification of patient identification, labeling procedures, and source documentation are all utilized for specimen collection procedures, regardless of the specimen source. To have a positive impact on patient treatment and outcomes, health-care employees who collect specimens or instruct patients to prepare for specimen collection must be knowledgeable about the techniques required for quality procedures.

SPECIMEN ORDERING

Laboratory testing begins with orders for specimens to be collected. Sometimes this step may ambiguous. Communication from the health-care provider may be unclear for various reasons. Examples of potential problems include verbal orders that are misunderstood, the use of nonstandardized abbreviations, and handwritten orders that are difficult to read. It is imperative that everyone involved with the process understand how critical the initial data used to order a test may be.

Required Items for All Laboratory Tests

A laboratory requisition form is used to order specific laboratory testing procedures, but the requisition is also used to provide information needed for reimbursement

for these procedures. In addition, the test ordered must always be documented in the patient's chart.

Laboratory requisition forms may vary; some are organized with the tests listed in alphabetical order, whereas others may be organized with the tests listed in categories. Regardless of the organization of the laboratory requisition form, there are certain items that are essential for the collection process to be carried out appropriately. Many of these items are introduced in earlier chapters in the textbook. At a minimum the requisition form should include the following:

1. Complete demographic information for the patient. This includes the full name and birth date, the patient's gender, and the billing information.
2. Name of ordering health-care professional and documentation of any other additional agencies or health-care professionals that should receive copies of the laboratory report.
3. Date for the test collection. A specific date may be a critical factor, or there may be a bit more flexibility for the collection date. For instance, sometimes a laboratory test will be ordered to be checked for a medication blood level after the patient has been on that particular medication for several days; this date should be noted on the requisition form so that the patient knows when to have his or her blood drawn.
4. Specific documentation for the tests ordered. Each test must be marked carefully and completely with an X or a circle around the test. Each test will be accompanied by a current procedural terminology (CPT)

code (printed on the requisition form next to the test), which may help with definitive choices when a provider is unsure of which test to order.

5. Diagnosis codes (in the form of an ICD-9 code) must be included with all laboratory tests ordered. Each test must have a diagnosis code specifically assigned to it, rather than one or two codes written randomly on the requisition form, as they may not apply to all the tests ordered. A diagnosis code is required for reimbursement.

6. If a test may be performed on more than one type of body fluid, it is very important to specify which fluid is to be used for the analysis. For instance, cortisol levels may frequently be performed using serum or urine; if the source is not documented correctly, then the patient may be required to return to resubmit the specimen.

7. When a medication level is ordered, the time of the last medication dose should be included on the requisition form, or the time of the requested blood draw should be specified. This may be critical for appropriate interpretation of the results.

8. If a wound culture is required, the source must be documented carefully. Specimen processing for microbiological specimens will vary depending on the site of the collection and the type of sample.

9.

> **Test Your Knowledge 7-1**
>
> List three items that must be present on a laboratory requisition form when ordering a specimen collection. (Outcome 7-2)

Test Specifics

Laboratory tests may be ordered in several ways. If a health-care provider feels that only one analyte needs to be tested to assist with diagnosis and treatment, he or she will order a single test, such as a glucose level for a patient who is being screened for diabetes, a potassium level for someone who is taking diuretics, or a hematocrit test for someone who is being treated for anemia. However, it is often beneficial for the health-care provider to order a group of tests that have been designed to enable providers to make more accurate diagnoses. These groups of tests may be *custom panels* that have been designed by a specific laboratory or specialty. A thyroid panel, for instance, may include three different tests that measure different aspects of thyroid function. These custom panels are not universal in nature; what is included in a custom panel by one laboratory will not necessarily be the same as those included in a panel by the same name with another laboratory.

Medicare-Approved Panels

Health-care providers must be careful when ordering panels, especially for those patients who have Medicare coverage for their payment source. The Centers for Medicare & Medicaid Services (CMS) has adopted several organ- or disease-specific panels that were designed by the American Medical Association (AMA). These panels will be the same no matter which laboratory uses them. These are the *only* panels that are always covered by Medicare without the need of an Advanced Beneficiary Notice of Noncoverage (ABN), even though some of the tests included in the panel have limited Medicare coverage. Care must be taken, however, to ensure that all the tests in the panel are really necessary for the treatment of the patient. If there is no documentation in the patient's chart to show necessity for the entire panel, the health-care provider may be held responsible for fraudulent ordering practices. The Medicare-approved organ- or disease-specific panels are the following:

- Basic Metabolic Panel(s); with or without ionized Calcium
- Electrolyte Panel
- Hepatic Panel
- Hepatitis Panel
- Comprehensive Metabolic Panel
- Renal Function Panel
- Lipid Panel

Laboratories must follow strict reimbursement rules for tests that are included in panels. The total cost of the panel may not exceed the totals of the separate tests included in the panel. Table 7-1 itemizes the tests included in the CMS-approved panels.

TABLE 7-1	
Medicare-approved panels	
Test Name	**CPT Code**
Comprehensive Metabolic Panel (CPT 80053)	
Albumin	82040
Bilirubin, total	82247
Calcium	82310
Carbon dioxide	82374
Chloride	82435
Creatinine	82565
Glucose	82974
Alkaline phosphatase	84075

Continued

TABLE 7-1–cont'd
Medicare-approved panels

Test Name	CPT Code
Potassium	84132
Total protein	84155
Sodium	84295
Transferase, alanine amino (ALT, SGPT)	84460
Transferase, aspartate amino (AST, SGOT)	84450
Blood urea $$	84520
Hepatic Function Panel (CPT 80076)	
Total protein	84155
Albumin	82040
Alkaline phosphatase	84075
Transferase, aspartate amino (AST, SGOT)	84450
Transferase, alanine amino (ALT, SGPT)	84460
Bilirubin, total	82247
Total protein	84155
Basic Metabolic Panel With Ionized Calcium (CPT 80047)	
Glucose	82974
Potassium	84132
Sodium	84295
Blood urea nitrogen	84520
Calcium, ionized	82330
Carbon dioxide	82374
Chloride	82435
Creatinine	82565
Basic Metabolic Panel With Calcium (CPT 80048)	
Glucose	82974
Potassium	84132
Sodium	84295
Blood urea nitrogen	84520
Calcium	82310
Carbon dioxide	82374
Chloride	82435
Creatinine	82565
Renal Function Panel (CPT 80069)	
Glucose	82974
Potassium	84132
Sodium	84295
Blood urea nitrogen	84520
Calcium	82310
Carbon dioxide	82374
Chloride	82435
Creatinine	82565
Phosphorus	84100
Lipid Panel (CPT 80061)	
Cholesterol, total	82565
Triglycerides	84478
Electrolytes (CPT 80051)	
Potassium	84132
Sodium	84295
Carbon dioxide	82374
Chloride	82435

Current Procedural Terminology © 2011 American Medical Association, All Rights Reserved.

Test Your Knowledge 7-2
How are custom panels similar to the Medicare-approved panels? (Outcome 7-3)

Standing Orders

Frequently health-care professionals will establish a set of **standing orders** for a patient, meaning that the patient is to have a specific test performed at a certain time interval for a period of time. For instance, a patient may need to have a potassium level checked every 3 months to monitor progress while on a certain medication. To set up the standing order, the physician will submit a requisition form to the laboratory with the initial potassium level ordered, but the requisition form may also include additional orders to repeat this test every 3 months. Some laboratories may also have a separate form used to transmit information about standing orders, rather than using the initial requisition form. Standing orders may not be continued for more than a year without a new order being written by the health-care provider. Recently, the practice of using standing orders has been questioned. In 2007, there was a change to the Physician Fee Schedule update, which specified a need for a separate order for every blood glucose test performed for patients in certain settings; the rule emphasized that a standing order was not sufficient for documentation of necessity for these patients. Even though this ruling addressed only blood glucose, it does serve as a warning for future policy changes in reference to standing orders.

Reflexive Testing

Another practice that may be used in a clinical laboratory is **reflexive testing.** In this situation, additional testing is automatically performed in response to certain abnormal results. An example of reflexive testing is the antibiotic sensitivity testing performed on culture samples. If a culture specimen has a positive result, an antibiotic sensitivity is automatically performed to provide the physician with additional knowledge about the best way to treat the infection. Without this reflexive option, it would be necessary to contact the physician and request a separate order for this sensitivity to be performed, which would delay patient treatment.

The addition of reflexive tests allows the ordering physician to receive additional information in a timely manner rather than waiting until the initial sample result is transmitted back to the physician and another order is placed for a new sample to be collected. In order for reflexive testing to be performed within the guidelines necessary for reimbursement, it is essential that the ordering physician is made aware of the tests included in the reflexive testing panel, and it is also necessary that the physician be offered the opportunity to order these secondary tests separately without the reflexive option if needed. These reflexive tests are to be documented clearly on the requisition form.

PATIENT IDENTIFICATION

As presented in Chapter 1, the medical assistant or phlebotomist responsible for collecting samples for analysis plays a critical role. Appropriate patient identification and documentation of the collection procedures used are very important components of this preanalytical process.

Verification of Patient Identity

Whenever a patient presents for specimen collection, it is imperative that the person performing the collection verify the identity of the patient. This is the most important procedure in the specimen collection process. A minimum of *two* unique identifiers must be used to verify patient identification. Incorrect identification of the patient may result in specimen collection on the wrong patient, and misdiagnosis of the patient because of incorrect laboratory values. Drawing the wrong patient may even have fatal consequences if the treatment plan developed is incorrect.

Acceptable Patient Identifiers

- **Name:** It is always best to ask the patient to state his or her name; do not ask, "Are you Mrs. Smith?" as many patients may say "Yes" without actually hearing or understanding what was asked. Ask the patient to state his or her name, and spell the last name.
- **Birth date:** The patient must also state his or her birth date. It is possible to have two patients with the same first and last name, but improbable that they will also share the same birthday.
- **Social Security number or patient ID:** The use of the Social Security number is no longer recommended in most cases, with the exception of those who are receiving care in a government facility. A patient ID may have been assigned to the patient (especially in the case of managed care clients or hospital settings) and this may serve as a unique identifier.
- **Driver's license or other picture identification:** For legal specimens or those that are associated with employment, a picture ID is necessary for definitive identification. It is an acceptable means of identification in all situations, but not always necessary. In many office settings, the picture ID is part of the patient's permanent health record.

In hospitals or other settings in which the patient may not be able to converse with the collector, it is especially important that the identity of the patient is established before the specimen is collected. Never use the name written or printed above the bed as that of the patient. If the patient has an armband that has been placed on the wrist, this may be used if the patient is not capable of verifying his or her identity verbally. Never use an armband for identification if it is not securely placed on the patient's arm. If the patient is not wearing appropriate identification, it will be necessary to locate the health-care professional responsible for this patient (usually one of the nursing staff) and ask him or her to reband the patient and provide definitive ID before collecting the specimen. In this situation, be sure to document the name of the person who provided the identification.

Test Your Knowledge 7-5

Should an armband taped on the side of a hospital bed not be used for patient identification?   (Outcome 7-6)

Electronic Bar Codes

Most likely, not many of us remember a time when we didn't have bar codes on our groceries and other items that we purchase in retail stores. Bar codes allow for more specific identification of the product purchased, and provide an efficient way to update prices and product inventory. The health-care industry has also found that the use of electronic bar codes helps to streamline the process of ordering laboratory tests. Using labels with electronic bar codes on the individual tubes and specimen containers helps to assure specimen identification and patient confidentiality, and allows for automated sorting and distribution of the specimens in large laboratory settings. It is especially important to verify identification in situations in which bar codes are used, because the individual specimen containers do not necessarily include the patient's name. The individual specimens may only be identified with the bar code or specimen ID label that represents that patient in the electronic system.

PATIENT PREPARATION

In addition to the verification of patient identity and demographic information, the medical assistant responsible for specimen collection must also verify whether the patient prepared appropriately for the test ordered prior to collection of the specimen. The reference ranges for laboratory tests are based on specific parameters, and if these were not in place for the patient being tested, their results may appear to be abnormal. Examples of specific preparation procedures include the following:

- Fasting: A **fasting** specimen may be required for tests such as blood glucose levels or lipid testing. Fasting means that the individual must go without food and any liquid other than water for 12 hours prior to the blood draw. The patient usually can take medication that has been prescribed if it poses a health risk to skip or postpone a dose until after the period of fasting. If the patient did take medication during this fasting period, it must be documented on the requisition form.

- 1 or 2 hr postprandial: A **1 hr pp or 2 hr postprandial** (**1 or 2 hr pp**) blood draw means that the specimen is collected 1 or 2 hours (respectively) after the individual eats a meal. These pp samples are usually used for blood glucose testing.

- Glucose challenge: When patients are screened for diabetes (especially for pregnant women) a **glucose challenge** may be ordered. In this situation the patient is given a drink that contains 50 g of glucose to ingest. One hour after the sweetened drink is consumed, the patient has his or her blood drawn again for a glucose test.

- Glucose tolerance test: A **glucose tolerance test** has several steps, and is usually only ordered if the fasting blood sugar, postprandial blood sugar, or glucose challenge results are abnormal. In this situation, a blood sample is drawn from the fasting patient. (The patient usually provides a urine specimen as well.) The patient is then asked to drink a solution that contains 100 g of glucose. Subsequent blood draws are performed every half hour for a period of 3 to 6 hours. (This process is presented in more detail in Chapter 17.)

- Timed drug levels: Reference ranges for blood medication levels are based on the rate at which different drugs are metabolized. Some types of medication peak in the bloodstream relatively quickly after ingestion, while others are slow acting. The medical assistant or phlebotomist needs to verify (and document) when the patient last took their medication before performing the collection. Some drugs may have therapeutic ranges that are very close to the levels where the drug may harm the body, and the timing of the draw is essential to determine whether the dosage should be changed. Drugs may also be ordered as **peak** or **trough collection levels**. These terms mean that the specimen is to be drawn when that particular drug is at the highest level (peak) and/or the lowest level (trough) in the bloodstream. Because each medication is absorbed and cleared from the body differently, the time after the last dose of the medication for the peak and trough draw will vary. The peak levels are generally obtained 1 to 2 hours after a drug is given; the trough levels are usually just before the next dose is due. With peak and trough levels, if the medical assistant does not verify the time of the last dose, the result may appear to be abnormal when in actuality the specimen was just drawn at the wrong time.

- Restricted diets for specimen collection: Some laboratory tests performed on blood, stool, and urine require that the patient restrict his or her diet before and/or during collection. Examples may be avoidance of rare meat for a few days before the collection of a stool specimen for fecal occult blood testing, or avoidance of certain foods during the collection time for a 24-hour urine specimen.

- Random specimens: **Random specimens** do not require special preparation before collection. The concentration of many chemical substances and cellular components present in the bloodstream does not change throughout the day, and can be collected at any time. This term is also used to describe urine specimens used for basic urinalysis testing, as well as many microbiology specimens.
- First morning void: During sleep, the body continues to create urine as the blood circulates through the kidneys. The **first morning void** specimen may be requested for specific urine chemistry tests, as the concentration of the analyte will be elevated in this specimen because it has been in the bladder all night. A microalbumin test is an example of a test that is often ordered as a first morning void specimen.

Test Your Knowledge 7-6

Mr. Rider comes in for a blood draw as part of his annual physical. The physician has ordered a fasting blood glucose level. Just as the medical assistant begins to prepare for the blood draw, she notices that the patient has a coffee mug in his hand. What should she ask him before she begins the draw?   (Outcome 7-8)

SPECIMEN COLLECTION AT HOME

Urine, stool, and microbiology specimens are often collected by patients in the privacy of their homes and delivered to the laboratory soon after. With this type of collection, special care must be taken to educate the patient properly in reference to specimen collection and storage. Information for patient use should be offered verbally and in writing to ensure understanding and compliance. Collection and storage techniques should be verified again before accepting the specimen at the laboratory. For instance, a urine specimen collected at home should be collected using a sterile container, and the specimen must be refrigerated and transported to the laboratory as soon as possible after collection. In contrast, stool specimens collected for culture are not to be refrigerated, but should arrive at the laboratory within 2 hours of collection. Some specimens must

remain protected from light, whereas other specimens need to be added to containers with preservatives immediately after collection. It is the responsibility of the medical assistant who accepts these specimens from the patient to verify that the collection and processing have been performed correctly. Prior patient education is critical for quality specimens.

ITEMS THAT MUST BE DOCUMENTED WITH SPECIMEN COLLECTION

Documentation does not end with the collection of the specimen. It is essential that details about the collection are recorded on the requisition form, as these details help to provide critical information that may affect the test results.

- **Who?** The initials (or other unique identification, such as an employee ID) for the person who collected the specimen must be documented on the requisition form. This information may be critical if there are any problems with the specimen. This information is also placed on the blood tube after collection while in the presence of the patient.
- **What?** What type of specimen was collected? For blood specimens, there should be documentation of the type of specimen collected because venous, arterial, and capillary samples may have different reference ranges for a specific analyte. Reimbursement for the collection may also vary with the type of blood specimen. For urine specimens, there should be documentation as to whether the sample is a random or timed urine collection, and the method used for the collection process. (This is further clarified in Chapter 9.) Body fluids (such as amniotic fluid or synovial fluid) are especially difficult to identify by sight, so clarification of the specimen type is essential at the time of collection; reference ranges are very different for each type of body fluid.
- **When?** Documentation of the date and time of collection is critical. The time must include a.m. or p.m., or military time may be used. Many chemical analytes change drastically with time once the blood has left the body, and these natural postcollection changes may be misidentified as part of a disease process if the specimen is not processed in a timely fashion. For timed collections, it is essential. The date and time of collection are added to the requisition form as well as the tube after a blood draw is complete.
- **Where?** The site of collection must also be documented. For blood draws, this does not need to be absolutely specific; a general location such as right

hand or left arm will do. This documentation can be very helpful if there are complications at the draw site. For culture specimens, documentation of the collection site should be as specific as possible, because the normal florae present in different areas of the body are not the same. The physical location of the culture collection site needs must be specified (right arm, left leg, opening of fistula, etc.) as well as the type of wound or collection procedure used. A superficial wound sample is different from that collected from a deep puncture wound, and a specimen collected by aspiration is different from a specimen collected by squeezing a pustule. For instance, bacteria that are common on the surface of the skin are *not* part of the normal florae in a deep wound, even if the specimens are both taken from the right great toe.

Test Your Knowledge 7-7

Why is it important to document that a blood specimen was obtained from a capillary puncture rather than a vein?   (Outcome 7-10)

LABELING INFORMATION

All collection containers must be labeled immediately after collection, meaning that the specimen must be labeled in an outpatient setting while in the presence of the patient and before another outpatient requisition form is accepted. In an inpatient setting, the specimen labeling process must be complete before the phlebotomist leaves the patient's room. Labeling may involve writing with an indelible pen directly on the preaffixed label on the tube after collection, or by applying a label that has been generated by a computer and adding a few items. Computer-generated labels often include bar codes that may be read by the instruments used for testing. Tubes should never be prelabeled before specimen collection, as this can lead to incorrect patient identification if the collection is unsuccessful and the tubes are not discarded, or if there is more than one patient present in a blood drawing area at the same time. Specimens that are mislabeled can potentially cause serious harm to patients when inaccurate patient results are generated.

The specimen label must include the following information:

- The name of the patient and a unique identifier number. The ID number is generated by the computer

at the time of the blood draw, or it may be part of the requisition form available as a small peel-off label. If the patient number is not available, the date of birth may be used instead. Two patient identifiers are required.
- Date and time of collection
- Initials (or other unique ID) for the person who performed the specimen collection
- Other required information may include documentation of a peak or trough draw, or at what time a specimen is taken for a glucose tolerance test. Even though the time of the draw should indicate which specimen is in the tube, it is a good idea to document this in more than one way to avoid any confusion.

For patients who collect their specimens at home, the person who accepts the specimen at the laboratory must verify that the specimen is labeled appropriately while in the presence of the patient. If a patient drops off a specimen that is not labeled and no one is present to accept the specimen, it will need to be recollected.

Test Your Knowledge 7-8

List two items that must be included on the label after a blood specimen is collected.   (Outcome 7-12)

CHAIN OF CUSTODY

Sometimes blood or urine is collected in situations in which the test results may be used as legal evidence. Blood may be collected for DNA analysis or blood alcohol level readings, whereas urine may be tested for drugs of abuse. The tests may be ordered in preemployment situations, in the case of on-the-job accidents or suspected drunk driving, or for some athletes. In these situations, it is imperative that medical assistants follow their facility's guidelines very carefully as they perform their duties. The specimens that are collected must have written documentation for their processing and storage from the point of collection through the testing and reporting process. It must be evident that a responsible individual had possession of the specimen, or had secured the specimen at every step of the process. The record of the individuals who have access to the specimen is called the **chain of custody**. A chain of custody is a physical object: a form that is filled out and signed each time that the specimen changes hands. An example of a chain of custody form may be found in Figure 7-1. Critical components of the process include the following:

1. **Identification of the patient:** This is the most important part of the process. Sometimes patients are not willing participants in the process, as they may have been placed under arrest, or may have been involved in some sort of incident at their place of work. If the patient is not able (or willing) to show appropriate identification, the arresting officer or supervisor must identify the patient and it must be documented on the form.

2. **Explanation of the process and witnessed signed consent form.**

3. **Secure collection area and standardized process:** Especially in the case of urine specimens, there are very specific procedures that must be followed to eliminate the opportunity for patients to add water or other substances to the specimen, or to substitute a specimen that they may have brought from outside the premises. For instance, the patient is not allowed to take any coats or purses into the restroom during the collection. The handles of the faucet in the collection area may be secured with tamper-evident tape, or the water supply may be shut off from outside the room. In addition, the toilet water always has a bluing agent added to avoid an opportunity to take water from the toilet unnoticed. The specimen temperature is documented immediately when the collection is complete as a means of quality assurance.

4. **Assignment of a sample number:** Legal specimens should not be identified by name after the initial collection process. This helps to protect the patient's confidentiality, and also limits the opportunities for someone to tamper with a specific specimen.

5. **Securing the specimen and protecting against tampering:** The specimen has a tamper-evident seal that is affixed at the time of collection. The patient and the collector initial this seal and the specimen is sealed in the presence of the patient. If this seal is broken when the sample is accessed for testing, the chain of custody is invalidated.

6. **Documentation of processing:** The specimen must remain in a secure location at all times. The chain of custody form provides an opportunity to document where the specimen was stored, and who placed it in that location at each step of transfer. Legal specimens must be kept in a locked location with limited authorized access until they are tested.

The documentation continues until the time that the specimen is disposed of.

There may be times when the medical assistant is called to testify about the collection process of a legal specimen. If the chain of custody process is followed carefully, there should be no problem with testifying regarding the specimen processing. Poor documentation may be reason for dismissal of a legal case, and could have serious repercussions.

Test Your Knowledge 7-9

What are two methods used to protect a legal specimen from potential tampering?   (Outcome 7-13)

POINT OF INTEREST 7-1
DOT drug screening

Urine may be tested for drugs of abuse for many reasons. The test is a common part of preemployment screening for many corporations. Most of the large retail store chains now require drug screening as a preemployment procedure, and some of them also use random drug screens as well.

There are also times when the federal government requires drug screen testing. The Omnibus Transportation Employee Testing Act of 1991 set a standard that requires drug and alcohol testing for employees who are employed in professions that the government has designated as "safety-sensitive." This regulation potentially affects more than 10 million individuals. These employees may be working in the following areas:

- Those in the trucking industry
- Railroad workers
- Bus drivers or other mass-transit employees
- Pilots and other aviation employees
- Employees in other types of public transportation
- Those who work on public pipelines

The U.S. Department of Transportation (DOT) has set standards concerning who will be tested, as well as the policies and procedures to be followed for these individuals. The collection process is even more critical in these situations, and the laboratory testing may be performed only at laboratories that have been approved by the DOT. Special chain of custody forms are used for the collection process, and the procedures for processing of the paperwork are very specific.

NON FEDERAL DRUG TESTING CUSTODY AND CONTROL FORM
                                18290
                SPECIMEN ID No.
STEP 1: COMPLETED BY COLLECTOR OR EMPLOYER REPRESENTATIVE

A. Employer Name, Address, I.D. No.
ABC Temporary Employment Agency 1 Main Street, Hollywood, NY 11111
B. MRO Name, Address, Phone and Fax No.
C. Doyel 6291 Park Ave, Hollywood, NY 11111

C. Donor Name   John A. Smith, Jr.   Donor SSN or Employee I.D. No.   123888
D. Reason for Test: ☐ Pre-employment   ☒ Random   ☐ Reasonable Suspicion/Cause   ☐ Post Accident
                    ☐ Return to Duty   ☐ Follow-up   ☐ Other (specify)_____
E. Drug Tests to be Performed: ☒ Hair 5 Drug Panel   ☐ Urine 5 Drug Panel   ☐ Other (specify)_____
G. Collection Site Address: 1 Main Street Hollywood, NY 11111

STEP 2: COMPLETED BY COLLECTOR

Read specimen temperature within 4 minutes. Is temperature between 90° and 100°F? ☐ Yes ☐ No, Enter Remark	Specimen Collection: ☐ Split ☐ Single ☐ Non Provided (Enter Remark)	☒ HEAD HAIR ☐ URINE

REMARKS   ☐ BODY_____

STEP 3: Collector affixes bottle seal(s) to bottle(s). Collector dates seal(s). Donor initials seal(s). Donor completes STEP 5 on Copy 2 (MRO Copy)
STEP 4: CHAIN OF CUSTODY - INITIATED BY COLLECTOR AND COMPLETED BY LABORATORY

I certify that the specimen given to me by the donor identified in the certification section on Copy Z of this form was collected, labeled, sealed and released to the Delivery Service noted in accordance with applicable Federal requirements.

                                                            AM
X   John Doe   2:00 PM   PM   **SPECIMEN BOTTLE(S) RELEASED TO:**
        Signature of Collector   Time of Collection
    John Doe   01/31/2012   UPS Next Day Delivery
    (PRINT) Collectors Name (First, MI, Last)   Date (Mo, Day, Yr)   Name of Delivery Service Transferring Specimen to Lab

RECEIVED AT LAB:	**Primary Specimen Bottle Seal Intact**	**SPECIMEN BOTTLE(S) RELEASED TO:**
X _____ Signature of Accessioner _____ (PRINT) Accessioner's Name (First, MI, Last) Date (Mo, Day, Yr)	☐ Yes ☐ No, Enter Remark Below	

STEP 5a: PRIMARY SPECIMEN TEST RESULTS - COMPLETED BY PRIMARY LABORATORY

☐ NEGATIVE   ☐ POSITIVE for: ☐ MARIJUANA METABOLITE   ☐ CODEINE   ☐ AMPHETAMINE   ☐ ADULTERATED
        ☐ DILUTE   ☐ COCAINE METABOLITE   ☐ MORPHINE   ☐ METHAMPHETAMINE   ☐ SUBSTITUTED
        ☐ REJECTED FOR TESTING   ☐ PCP   ☐ 6-ACETYLMORPHINE   ☐ INVALID RESULT

REMARKS_____
TEST LAB (if different from above)_____
I certify that the specimen identified on this form was examined upon receipt, handled using chain of custody procedures, analyzed, and reported in accordance with applicable Federal requirements.

X _____   _____   _____
        Signature of Certifying Scientist   (PRINT) Certifying Scientist (First, MI, Last)   Date (Mo, Day, Yr)

STEP 5b: SPLIT SPECIMEN TEST RESULTS - (IF TESTED) COMPLETED BY SECONDARY LABORATORY

	☐ RECONFIRMED ☐ FAILED TO RECONFIRM - REASON _____
Laboratory Name	*I certify that the split specimen identified on this form was examined upon receipt, handled using chain of custody procedures, analyzed, and reported in accordance with applicable Federal requirements.*
Laboratory Address	X _____ _____ _____ Signature of Certifying Scientist (PRINT) Certifying Scientist (First, MI, Last) Date (Mo, Day, Yr)

Figure 7-1   An example of a chain of custody form. The top copy contains the name of the patient, but this copy does not follow the specimen as it progresses to the testing phase. The copies that are used with the specimen after it is input into the computer are designated only by the specimen ID number.

SUMMARY

Specimen collection and processing are critical components of the laboratory testing. Care must be taken to fill out the request for testing in the proper manner, educate the patient appropriately for necessary preparation, and thoroughly document the collection procedure. It is also necessary to label the specimen using recommended procedures so that there are no potential problems with identification as the testing process continues. The type of collection, the type of specimen, and the date and time of collection are critical components that must be logged on the requisition form after collection. In legal situations, care must be taken to follow established procedures to ensure that specimens are kept safe from tampering until they are tested and the results are reported. This process uses a chain of custody form, which must be filled out by anyone who has access to the specimen during and after collection.

TIME TO REVIEW

1. When is a trough blood level drawn?   Outcome 7-1

2. Which of these items does not need to   Outcome 7-2
be included on a complete laboratory requisition form?

   a. ICD-9 code(s)
   b. Ordering physician's name
   c. Cost of tests
   d. Demographic information for the patient

3. How are CMS panels different from   Outcome 7-3
custom panels created by independent laboratories?

   a. The custom panels include fewer tests
   b. The CMS panels have been approved by the AMA
   c. The reimbursement rates are better for the custom panels
   d. They are essentially the same

4. True or False: Reflexive testing causes   Outcome 7-5
excessive time to be spent before results are available to the ordering health-care provider.

5. True or False: All medication is   Outcome 7-9)
absorbed and used by the body at the same rate.

6. List three items that must be   Outcome 7-11
documented on the requisition form after a specimen is collected.

7. True or False: It is acceptable to use   Outcome 7-12
a computer-generated label on a tube after collection as long as it includes the basic required information.

Case Study 7-1: Standing orders

Mr. Johnson comes into the laboratory to have his potassium level checked. He has a standing order to have this test performed every 3 months because of a medication that he takes for a heart disorder. When he arrives at the laboratory, the phlebotomist checks the records for Mr. Johnson in the computer system. He informs Mr. Johnson that he cannot draw his blood today because his standing order has expired.

1. What does the phlebotomist mean by stating that the standing order has expired?
2. What needs to occur before Mr. Johnson can have his blood drawn for the potassium test?

Case Study 7-2: Labeling

Cassy Jones is a medical assisting student who is training in the laboratory. She is trying very hard to get all the information correct for every situation, and she tells her trainer that she is working on anticipating the needs of the practice so that she can be better organized. When her trainer returns from lunch one afternoon, she finds that Cassy has labeled blood tubes for the expected blood draws for the afternoon. Cassy's trainer tells her that although she can see that her intentions were good, this is an unacceptable practice.

1. Why is the prelabeling of the tubes an unacceptable practice?

RESOURCES AND SUGGESTED READINGS

"University of Washington Laboratory Testing Policies"
Very specific information about testing and collection
processes designed for use by practitioners http://depts
.washington.edu/labweb/PatientCare/Policies/index.htm

"Errors in Laboratory Medicine"
Information about common laboratory errors including all
phases of the testing process http://www.clinchem.org/cgi/
content/abstract/48/5/691

"Laboratory Test Ordering and Documentation; List of Do's
and Dont's http://www.cap.org/apps/docs/pt_checkup/
pol_library/laboratory_test_ordering.pdf

Chapter 8

Collection and Processing of Blood Samples

Constance L. Lieseke, CMA (AAMA), MLT, PBT(ASCP)

Learning Outcomes   *After Reading this Chapter, the Successful Student will be able to:*

8-1 Define the key terms.

8-2 Explain the route used as blood moves through the heart.

8-3 Compare and contrast the qualities of veins and arteries.

8-4 Examine the ways that capillaries differ from veins and arteries.

8-5 Locate the most commonly used veins for drawing blood specimens, and explain why they are the best choice for this procedure.

8-6 Describe where capillary blood draws may be safely performed.

8-7 List the major contraindications for blood draws, as well as areas to be avoided.

8-8 List and describe the supplies necessary to perform successful venipuncture and capillary punctures.

8-9 Differentiate when the different methods of venipuncture (evacuated tube system, syringe system, or butterfly system) might be used.

8-10 Describe the significance of the tube stopper colors when drawing blood.

8-11 Explain the order of draw for specimen collection, and describe how it may be different with the various collection techniques.

8-12 Analyze techniques to be used with different age groups when performing venipuncture or capillary puncture.

8-13 Explain why capillary punctures may be preferred as a blood draw technique in some circumstances, and provide examples.

8-14 Summarize appropriate preparation techniques for blood draw procedures.

8-15 Successfully perform venipuncture and capillary puncture procedures using the process outlined in the textbook.

8-16 Demonstrate the ability to create a blood smear on a slide that would be suitable for staining, and explain why staining is important for examination of blood samples.

8-17 Explain how to process samples for various laboratory tests ordered.

8-18 Analyze the differences between serum and plasma.

8-19 Provide examples of inappropriate specimens, and describe how these issues may be avoided.

8-20 Describe how negative outcomes may be avoided when drawing blood.

CAAHEP/ABHES STANDARDS

 CAAHEP Standards:

I.C.I.4: List major organs in each body system
I.C.I.5: Describe the normal function of each body system
I.P.I.2: Perform Venipuncture
I.P.I.3: Perform Capillary Puncture
I.A.I.1: Apply critical thinking skills in performing patient assessment and care
III.P.III.3: Select appropriate barrier/personal protective equipment (PPE) for potentially infectious situations

 ABHES Standards

- Medical Office Laboratory Procedures: Collect, label and process specimens: Perform venipuncture
- Medical Office Clinical Procedures: Apply principles of aseptic techniques and infection control
- Medical Office Clinical Procedures: Use Standard Precautions

KEY TERMS

Antecubital area	Evacuated tube system	Plasma separator tubes (PST)
Anticoagulants	Flanges	Quality not sufficient (QNS)
Arteries	Gauge	Serum
Arterioles	Hematoma	Serum separator tubes (SST)
Basilic vein	Hemoconcentration	Sharp
Bevel	Hemolysis	Short draw
Butterfly system	Interstitial	Syringe system
Capillaries	Lipemia	Tourniquet
Capillary action	Lumen	Vacuum
Capillary puncture	Mastectomy	Vasodilation
Capillary tubes	Median cubital vein	Vasovagal syncope
Cardiovascular	Microcollection containers	Veins
Cephalic vein	Morphology	Venules
Clot activators	Multi-sample needle	Winged infusion set
Contraindications	Palpation	
Edema	Plasma	

The majority of laboratory testing is performed on blood specimens. As part of the preanalytical process, medical assistants and phlebotomists are responsible for greeting and identifying patients, verifying patient identification, making appropriate site selections for collection, using correct collection procedures, and processing specimens prior to the testing stage. It is essential that the health-care professional who performs these duties understands how to execute them correctly, as the potential impact of these processes is profound if they are performed improperly. This chapter provides details about how to collect and process various blood specimens, including necessary knowledge of the anatomy and physiology of the cardiovascular system, an introduction to the various tools used for obtaining blood, and information about how to avoid negative outcomes during the collection process. Procedures for processing specimens after collection are also presented.

ANATOMY AND PHYSIOLOGY OF THE CARDIOVASCULAR SYSTEM

In order to consider the various methods used to obtain blood specimens, it is important to understand the anatomy and physiology of the **cardiovascular** system. Essentially, all the body systems are connected, or linked, by the cardiovascular system, because it offers a means of transportation to and from all the cells of the body. *Homeostasis* is a state in which the body is healthy and in balance. For homeostasis to be maintained in our bodies, the cardiovascular system must transport water, nutrients, waste products, chemicals, and hormones everywhere within the body. The immune system is also dependent on the function of the cardiovascular system. In addition, circulation of the blood helps to keep the body's temperature within normal limits, contributing to homeostasis.

The Heart

The heart is the beginning and the end of the cardiovascular system, and is approximately the size of a closed fist. It is made of very strong cardiac muscular tissue. Within the structure of the heart are four chambers. The upper two chambers of the heart are the *atria* and the lower two chambers of the heart are the *ventricles*. The two sides of the heart are separated by a wall (called the *septum*) and the atria and the ventricles on each side of the heart are separated by *valves*, which keep the blood from flowing backward within the structure. Figure 8-1 allows us to follow the path of the blood flow through the heart and lungs.

1. Oxygen-poor blood flows into the right atrium through two large veins known as the superior vena cava and inferior vena cava.
2. As the heart contracts, the blood flows through the tricuspid valve (which separates the chambers) into the right ventricle.
3. From the right ventricle, the blood passes the pulmonary semilunar valve and enters the right and left pulmonary arteries. These arteries take the blood into the lungs for oxygenation. (These are the only arteries in the body that do not carry oxygenated blood.)
4. Once the blood has passed through the lungs, where it exchanges oxygen for carbon dioxide, the blood flows back onto the left atria through the right and left pulmonary veins. (These veins are the only veins in the body that carry freshly oxygenated blood.)
5. From the left atria, the blood passes through the bicuspid valve and enters the left ventricle. The left ventricle is the part of the heart where the muscular walls are the thickest, as the left ventricle is responsible for pumping the blood out of the heart into the arterial system to circulate through the body.
6. The blood passes through the aortic semilunar valve, finally exiting the heart through a very large artery, known as the aorta.

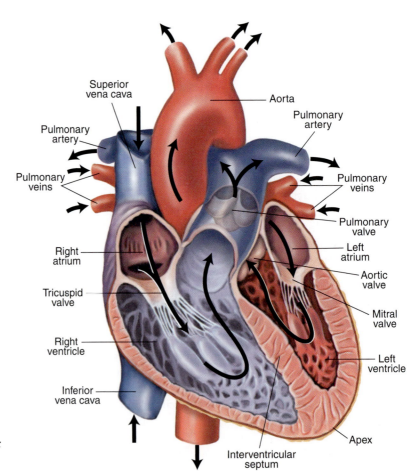

Figure 8-1   The pathway followed by the blood as it circulates through the heart, lungs, and vessels. *Reprinted with permission from Eagle S, Brassington C, Dailey C, and Goretti C:* The Professional Medical Assistant: An Integrative, Teamwork-Based Approach. *Philadelphia: FA Davis, 2009.*

7. In a single heartbeat, the heart goes through two stages: *systole* (the contraction of the heart muscle) and *diastole* (the relaxation of the heart muscle). During ventricular systole, the blood pressure increases, pushing the blood through the arterial system and adding pressure to the walls of the arterial vessels, causing them to expand. The diastolic (relaxation) phase allows the blood pressure to decrease and the arterial walls to adjust back to their normal size. We feel this increase and decrease in the blood pressure as a patient's pulse in the arteries of the body.

Blood Vessels

There are three types of blood vessels that make up the cardiovascular system: arteries, veins, and capillaries. Each type of vessel has unique characteristics that enable it to perform specific tasks. Blood specimens may be collected from any of these vessels. Figure 8-2 shows the relationship between the types of blood vessels that make up the cardiovascular system.

> **Test Your Knowledge 8-1**
> What organs and/or body systems make up the cardio-vascular system?   (Outcome 8-1)

Arteries

Arteries are the vessels that carry oxygenated blood away from the heart. Arterial walls are quite muscular and have more elasticity than do venous walls, and as the blood flows through the arteries (expanding and relaxing the vessels) it is felt as a pulse. There are three layers that make up the walls of both arteries and veins, but the walls of the arteries are thicker and stronger than those of the veins, and the arterial walls have more flexibility. Arteries get smaller and smaller as they branch through the body away from the heart. Smaller arterial vessels branch into **arterioles,** which then lead into capillaries. The blood that travels through arteries is brighter red than that which travels through the veins or capillaries due to the high level of oxygen present in the arterial red blood cells.

Veins

Veins carry blood back to the heart from the systemic circulation. Because this is not a process that actually follows the laws of gravity, the venous vessels have one-way valves that help to keep the blood from pooling in the extremities. The walls of the veins are made up of

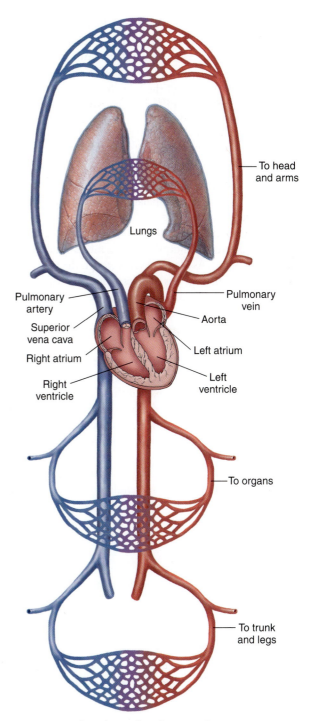

Figure 8-2   The relationships between the arteries, veins, and capillaries. *Reprinted with permission from Eagle S, Brassington C, Dailey C, and Goretti C: The Professional Medical Assistant: An Integrative, Teamwork-Based Approach. Philadelphia: FA Davis, 2009.*

three layers, but the layers are thinner and less muscular than are those of the arterial system. Veins require skeletal muscle movement to propel the blood back to the heart. Veins are smallest where they are attached to the capillaries; these tiny vessels are called **venules.** The veins become larger and larger as they approach the heart. The blood that travels through the veins has less oxygen than that in the arterial or capillary system, and is darker red in color. Veins do not have a pulse, and when palpated, veins feel less rigid than arteries.

Capillaries

Capillaries are so small that they can be seen only with a microscope. The walls of capillary vessels are made up of a single layer of epithelial cells. They are designed to link the arterial vessels to the venous vessels, and the blood that flows through the capillaries is a mixture of venous and arterial blood. As blood travels through the arteries to the arterioles, there is less and less room for the entire volume of blood to make it through the vessels. As the vessels get smaller, more fluids are pushed out of the vessel and into the **interstitial** spaces between the cells surrounding the blood vessels. By the time that the blood makes it to the capillaries, the size of the blood vessel has often reduced to the point that there is room for only one red blood cell at a time to make it through. The capillary beds are the only place in the body where exchange of nutrients, gases, and other molecules may occur, because the liquid portion of the blood is in direct contact with the cells around the vessels. As the capillaries join back with the venous system, they begin to get larger in diameter, and the vessels become venules, which gradually increase in diameter to become veins. Due to their small size, capillaries do not cause a pulse that can be felt.

Test Your Knowledge 8-2

What is one way that veins are different from arteries?

(Outcome 8-3)

Test Your Knowledge 8-3

Are capillaries approximately the same size as arteries and veins?   (Outcome 8-4)

SITE SELECTION

Appropriate site selection for venipuncture procedures is essential to obtain a blood sample that is acceptable for testing, and to avoid negative outcomes for the patient.

The most common area for venipunctures to be performed is the **antecubital area** of the arm, which is the area immediately in front of (the anterior side of) the elbow.

Most Commonly Used Veins

There are several veins in the antecubital area that may be successfully used for withdrawing blood. The **median cubital vein** (Fig. 8-3) is best for venipuncture because it is usually large and well anchored. This means that the median cubital vein doesn't usually move when the needle is inserted. The **cephalic vein,** which is located on the thumb (lateral side) of the antecubital area, and the **basilic vein,** on the little finger (medial side) of the antecubital area, may also be acceptable for venipuncture. If it is necessary to consider these two alternative venipuncture sites, the median cubital vein is the first choice; if this vein cannot be felt, the second choice would be the cephalic vein. The basilic vein is the last choice in the antecubital area because of its close proximity to the brachial artery and median nerve. The basilic vein is also not anchored as well as the other antecubital veins, so it has more of a tendency to move, or roll away, during the puncture.

When performing phlebotomy, finding a vein is one step that requires practice and experience. Applying a tourniquet may allow the vein to be more prominent. **Palpation,** which uses touch to feel for a vein, may be used with or without the tourniquet application to determine whether a vein is suitable for a blood draw. Sight may be helpful initially, but if a vein cannot be felt, that vein should not be used for a blood draw. Palpation is performed by using the tips of the gloved fingers (never the thumb) in a pushing manner as the fingers are moved across the arm. An acceptable vein should have some "bounce," like a soft rubber tube, when palpated. A tendon will feel flatter and harder than a vein, without

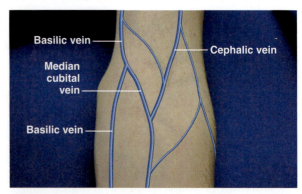

Figure 8-3   Antecubital area with vein selection; identification of the median cubital, cephalic, and basilic veins.

any elasticity, and an artery will feel like a taut rubber band. Veins may be differentiated from arteries because of the pulse that is felt in an arterial vessel. While feeling for the vein, it is important to establish the depth and size of the vessel, as well the direction of the vein. When the needle is inserted into the arm, it must follow the direction of the vein, and be inserted to the correct depth at which it will be in the vein rather than resting above or piercing through the vein. The angle of insertion is also very important to allow for the blood to enter the vein when it is pierced.

Venous patterns vary from person to person, as the anatomy of each patient is unique. In addition, some patients have vessels that are much more prominent in one arm than in the other. A venipuncture should not be attempted if the health-care professional is not sure whether the vein is suitable for the procedure or until the other arm has been checked for potential sites. If there is no suitable vein identified in the antecubital area of either arm, the back of the hand may also be considered for obtaining a sample. It is especially important to anchor the blood vessels of the hand before inserting the needle, as these vessels are located close to the surface of the skin and often roll away when the needle is inserted. The hand veins are also more prone to bruising and hematoma formation. Venipunctures should not be performed on the inside (or underside) of the wrist because of the presence of various nerves, tendons and ligaments, the close proximity of the radial artery, and the small size of the veins present in this area.

If an acceptable vein cannot be located, it may be necessary to encourage the vessels to become more prominent before venipuncture is attempted. To encourage **vasodilation,** a warm compress may be applied to the area, or the desired site may be massaged. Slapping, thumping, or flicking the draw site is not recommended. Lowering the arm down below the level of the heart may also allow the veins to become more evident. Tourniquet application is definitely beneficial, but it is important to remember that a tourniquet may stay on for a maximum of only 1 minute before it should be removed. A blood pressure cuff (stand-alone type) set at 40 mm Hg of pressure may also be useful in coaxing the veins to become more prominent.

Test Your Knowledge 8-4

What area of the arm should be the first choice for venipuncture?   (Outcome 8-5)

Appropriate Capillary Puncture Sites

Capillary blood draws (also known as dermal or skin punctures) may be used for blood collection when the required volume of blood needed for testing is small. The capillary beds in the fingers and heel are the sites generally used in the laboratory. The fingers are often used as sites for capillary punctures for adults and children over the age of 1 year. The puncture should be made on the fleshy central surface on the palmar side of the finger. Capillary draws should never be performed right on the tip of the finger, or on the extreme lateral side(s) near the fingernail, because of the close proximity to the bone. The capillary device should be oriented so that the puncture into the skin is perpendicular to the fingerprints; doing so means that the blood won't pool into the lines of the fingerprint during the collection process. Figure 8-4 shows where it is safe to perform a capillary puncture on a fingertip.

For infants (children below the age of 1 year) capillary blood draws are performed on the heel of the foot. The fingers on infants should not be used for capillary punctures, as there is not enough tissue to make this a safe choice while avoiding potential damage to the bone. The central area of the infant's heel, the arch of the foot, the ball of the foot, and the toes should *never* be used for blood draws. The capillary draw should be done only on the most medial and lateral section of the bottom of the heel. Figure 8-5 shows the safe areas for capillary punctures on an infant's heel. The bone of the foot may be damaged if the procedure is performed incorrectly and *osteomyelitis* (inflammation and/or infection of the bone and bone marrow) may result.

In all capillary draw situations, it is imperative that the site is warmed thoroughly before the process begins. It is also helpful if the hand or foot is held below the level of the heart. Massage may also benefit the process, as it

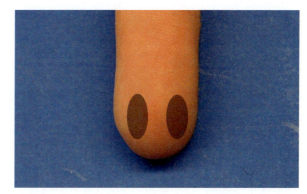

Figure 8-4   Locations for capillary draws for fingers.

Newborn screening

Each state provides newborn screening to detect disorders that would cause irreversible damage or death if undetected for an extended period of time. These disorders (for the most part) are not visible at birth; the babies appear to be healthy until the damage has already occurred. Irreversible neurological or musculoskeletal damage will result if these diseases are not detected. Most states require that the babies be tested prior to discharge from the hospital, with a recommendation for a second screening 7 to 14 days later. Examples of disorders that may be detected with screening include the following:

- Phenylketonuria
- Maple syrup urine disease
- Carnitine uptake deficiency
- Congenital hypothyroidism
- Cystic fibrosis
- Various hemoglobinopathies
- Galactosemia

The specimen collection usually includes a capillary sample taken from a heel stick. Blood may also be drawn from the veins on the back of the hand and applied to the collection paper. Special filter paper is used for the collection process, and the sample must be handled appropriately to avoid erroneous results or rejection of the specimen.

Test Your Knowledge 8-5

Are capillary draws always performed on the fingers?

(Outcome 8-6)

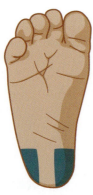

Figure 8-5   Locations for capillary draws in the heel of an infant.

will help to increase the blood supply to the area. When a capillary specimen is submitted for testing, it is important to document that the specimen came from a capillary draw rather than a venipuncture because the reference ranges for capillary blood samples are not the same as those for venous blood.

Blood used for capillary samples should be free flowing. It is important that the area immediately adjacent to the puncture site is not squeezed to increase the blood flow, as this will contaminate the sample with interstitial fluid. This fluid from between the cells has a different concentration of many chemical substances and will dilute the cell counts for hematology specimens. Massaging the finger well above the puncture site will help increase the blood flow. Specimens drawn from the heel may benefit from gentle pressure applied to the calf and ankle area.

CONTRAINDICATIONS AND AREAS TO AVOID

When considering an appropriate site for venipuncture, it is the responsibility of the health-care professional to use best judgment to avoid harming the patient unnecessarily. Also, as part of the preanalytical process, it is important to remember that any substances that may contaminate the specimen during the blood draw must be avoided. To accomplish these goals, there are certain **contraindications** and precautions for venipuncture to keep in mind.

Scars and Tattoos

Excessively scarred skin (as in the case of a burn) should not be used for venipuncture. Scarred areas are more susceptible to infection and often have reduced circulation; further, the veins underneath the scarred skin may be difficult to palpate and anchor. Skin that has been tattooed is also more prone to infection, and the dyes used in coloring the tattoo may cause test interference if they make their way into the specimen.

Mastectomy Considerations

If a patient has had a **mastectomy,** venipuncture should not be performed on the arm on the same side of the body as the procedure. Mastectomy procedures involve the removal of breast tissue. In addition, the lymph nodes surrounding the breast and under the arm also may be removed. The absence of these nodes can cause a decrease in the flow of the lymph fluid in the area, which puts the patient at an increased risk of lymphedema (accumulation of lymph in the tissues) and infection, even if the blood draw is not performed and only a tourniquet is applied. The opposite arm should be used for the blood draw. If a patient has a double mastectomy, the health-care professional who ordered the blood draw should be consulted to see what alternative sites may be used for blood collection.

Intravenous Fluids

Intravenous fluids are a potential source of contamination when drawing blood. In situations in which the patient is receiving IV fluids, it is preferable to use the opposite arm for venipuncture. If it is not possible to draw from the other arm, the IV flow must be discontinued (turned off) for at least 2 minutes (depending on the substance being infused) by a physician or other qualified health-care provider before the blood draw is attempted. After the IV fluid drip has been turned off, the tourniquet may be applied *below* the IV insertion site, and the blood draw may be drawn from below the IV site. Even with these precautions, the first 5 to 10 mL of blood withdrawn must be discarded to avoid potential contamination with IV fluid. If a coagulation test is part of the blood draw order, an additional 5 mL of blood should be drawn and discarded before this tube used for the coagulation testing is collected.

Veins that have been used for IV therapy are often irritated and damaged, even after the IV has been discontinued. Ideally, these sites should be avoided for venipunctures for at least 1 or 2 days after the catheter has been removed to allow for the vein to recover. *Phlebitis* (inflammation of the vein) may result if the area is not allowed to heal before venipuncture procedures are performed.

> ### Test Your Knowledge 8-6
> Is IV therapy always a contraindication for venipuncture? Why or why not?   (Outcome 8-7)

Bruising and Hematomas

Bruises and **hematomas** may occur as complications of venipuncture or IV therapy, and these sites should be avoided for subsequent blood draws. A bruise and a hematoma are similar in that each is a visible sign of damage to a vessel in which blood has escaped and entered the surrounding tissues. Hematomas result from damage to larger vessels such as veins and arteries, whereas a bruise may be the result of injury to a capillary

or a small blood vessel. A hematoma is often hard and swollen, and may be quite painful for the patient. If a blood draw is attempted in a bruised area or a hematoma site, it may cause additional discomfort for the patient and the integrity of the sample may be affected because of the pooling of old, dead cells in the area. Drawing from this area may also include the risk of infection due to inflammation of the tissues. If it is absolutely necessary to draw from an area with excessive bruising or a hematoma, the venipuncture should be performed below the injured site.

Varicose Veins

A *varicose vein* is one that is twisted and enlarged and very visible near the surface of the skin. These veins have lost their natural elasticity and integrity, and are prone to inflammation and blood clot formation. Varicose veins should not be used for venipuncture, as the blood flow through these areas has been adversely affected, increasing the chance for infection and bruising. These veins are also not very stable and will often roll away during the venipuncture.

Central Lines and Fistulas

Intravenous lines are used commonly to administer medication, fluids, or blood products, especially when there is a need for continued access for an extended period of time. There are times when a phlebotomist or medical assistant may be asked to withdraw blood from a *central venous catheter* or a *peripherally inserted central catheter* (PICC line). The central venous catheters are inserted into one of the major veins of the body, such as the subclavian, superior vena cava, or jugular vein. There is a piece of tubing extending out of the vein through the skin that is covered with a dressing. The central venous catheter is often left in place for an extended period of time to be used for administration of medication directly into the bloodstream.

A PICC is inserted into the cephalic or basilic vein of the arm or hand. These peripherally inserted catheters are fragile, as they are not inserted into a large vessel. Blood withdrawal from either of these devices generally requires injection of saline and/or a heparin solution into the catheter to clear the line before and after the blood is taken. It is essential to remember that anyone who withdraws blood from these types of lines must have specialized training, and in some states it is unlawful for a nonlicensed person to perform this function. In states where this is allowed, each facility must establish its own policy and training procedures.

Medical assistants and phlebotomists in most states are not allowed to perform this type of draw.

Another type of venous access device that may be in use is a *cannula*. This is a flexible tube that is used to gain access to the veins for *dialysis* treatment for those who have advanced kidney disease. The cannula is placed under the skin, and has a special port that is designed for insertion of a needle to withdraw blood for dialysis or for testing. A *fistula* is similar to a cannula, except that the device has been implanted in a way that it joins the arterial and venous system for hemodialysis procedures. The fistula is also under the surface of the skin, so it requires the skin to be punctured for access. It is recommended to use the other arm, rather than one containing the fistula. Blood draws should never be attempted from these implanted devices unless the practitioner has received specialized training. In many states, only licensed health-care providers may perform this procedure. In addition, a tourniquet should not be applied to the arm that contains a fistula or cannula.

POINT OF INTEREST 8-2
Arterial blood draws

Respiratory emergencies (such as advanced chronic obstructive pulmonary disease [COPD] or pulmonary edema) may require an arterial blood gas analysis for appropriate treatment to be started. In these situations the oxygen and carbon dioxide levels may be far outside the reference ranges, and the arterial blood pH may be increased or decreased to a life-threatening level. Arterial blood draws are similar to venipuncture procedures in that the site must be stabilized and cleansed properly before the needle is inserted. The angle of insertion, site selection options, and the way the blood enters the syringe are different from those of a venipuncture.

Arterial blood gases are commonly drawn from the radial artery; as a second choice, the brachial artery may be used as long as the patient is not being treated with anticoagulant drugs. The radial artery is easy to identify and secure because it is so near the surface of the body. To choose a site for an arterial blood draw, the health-care professional must palpate until the pulse is felt strongly. The site needs to be cleansed thoroughly, and the specimen needs to be drawn into a special heparinized syringe designed for this type of collection. A cup of wet ice also needs to be on hand, as the sample needs to be placed on ice immediately after the draw is complete.

The health-care provider should have his or her index finger on the pulse of the artery. The needle is inserted at an angle of approximately 45 degrees. The skin is pierced right next to the index finger. When the artery is entered, the blood will pump out through the lumen of the needle because of the pulse pressure. A flash is apparent immediately at the end of the needle attached to the syringe as the artery is pierced, and the blood will continue to fill the syringe without pulling on the plunger. (The plunger is pulled back before the needle is inserted to allow room for the blood in the syringe.) When the syringe is full, the safety device must be activated immediately on the needle. The needle will be removed and the end of the syringe will be plugged with a rubber stopper. The sample must be placed on ice immediately after labeling of the specimen. Firm pressure must be applied to the puncture site for a minimum of 5 minutes after the blood draw, or until the blood stops flowing from the site.

Due to the potential for arterial damage or nerve damage with arterial blood draws, intensive training is required for health-care professionals who perform this as part of their job. Training includes careful observation and supervised performance, as well as identification of risk factors associated with the process. Some states restrict this procedure to licensed personnel such as respiratory therapists or RNs.

Edematous Areas

In some clinical situations, patients may accumulate fluid in the intercellular spaces of the tissues. This accumulation of fluid is called **edema.** The presence of excess fluid may be widespread as a result of heart and/or renal failure, or it can be more localized from trauma or fluid leakage from an IV site. It will be very difficult to palpate a vein in edematous areas, because of the additional fluid in the tissues. If possible, these areas of the body should be avoided for venipuncture, because of the increased opportunity for infection and potential for contamination of the specimen with the additional fluids. If the edema is widespread, the medical assistant may need to apply gentle pressure to the site until the edema is displaced, then perform the venipuncture as quickly as possible. If this is not successful and alternative sites are not obvious, the phlebotomist or medical assistant who is drawing the specimen should notify the physician. Capillary collection procedures are often not an option when edema is present because of the excessive amount of fluid contamination.

> **Test Your Knowledge 8-7**
> Why is it important to avoid edematous areas when performing venipunctures?   (Outcome 8-7)

Obese Patients

Excessive body fat can make venipuncture very challenging. It may be very difficult to palpate veins in obese patients, and sometimes it is even necessary to use longer than normal needles to successfully reach the veins under the surface of the skin. Obese patients may be quite apprehensive about the blood draw process because of past experiences with unsuccessful venipunctures. The anxious attitude may make it even more difficult to carry out a successful blood draw. If the patient suggests a site where others have had success, it is best to attempt this site if there are no other prominent veins. Adipose tissue may also be displaced in some situations by applying gentle pressure with the fingers to "move" the tissue out of the way until the draw site has been established.

VENIPUNCTURE EQUIPMENT

There are various methods used to obtain blood from a vein. Each type of blood draw requires unique supplies and procedures. Blood may be withdrawn from a vein using the evacuated tube system, the syringe system, or the butterfly method. Regardless of the method chosen, tourniquets, gloves, sharps containers, alcohol and gauze pads, needles, and adhesive materials to be applied after the blood draw are necessary for the process.

Tourniquets

A **tourniquet** is a flexible band that is placed around the arm of the patient to make the veins more prominent. Most tourniquets found on the market today are stretchy and made of a nonlatex material. They are approximately 1 in. wide, and approximately 15 in. in length. Tourniquets are designed to apply pressure, which causes distention of the veins. The tourniquet must be placed approximately 3 in. above the site to be used for venipuncture. If it is placed closer, the ends of the tourniquet may interfere with the procedure. Remember, tourniquets are only a tool to help the vein to become more visible; there are times when it is not necessary to use a tourniquet, and some laboratory

tests prohibit the use of a tourniquet for the specimen collection.

Tourniquets should not be applied too tightly; this can cause pain for the patient, and may cause **hemoconcentration** in the veins because of the restricted blood flow. Hemoconcentration occurs when excessive pressure builds up in the veins below the tourniquet application site. The increased pressure in the veins will force water and small molecules out of the vessels into the surrounding tissues. Larger formed elements and molecules will remain in the venous blood, and become more concentrated. White blood cells, red blood cells, platelets, calcium, cholesterol, triglycerides, and bilirubin levels may all be affected by this venous concentration. Tourniquets that are left on for more than a minute may also cause hemoconcentration; therefore, the phlebotomist needs to remain aware of this as the venipuncture site is prepared. Extended tourniquet application time may also cause pain for the patient.

When applying a tourniquet, keep in mind that it should be applied in a way that it can easily be released with one hand. Tourniquets do not need to be applied to bare skin; they can be applied over the sleeve. Open wounds, scars, and bruises should be avoided when applying the tourniquet. Some tourniquets are disposable, and these should be discarded after each use. Others are designed to be used for multiple patients, and should be disinfected at least daily, and discarded if they are visibly soiled or lose elasticity.

Gloves

The Occupational Safety and Health Administration (OSHA) regulations designed to protect health-care employees specify that gloves are to be worn when collecting blood. After a blood draw, the gloves are removed, and the employee must sanitize his or her hands. For effective palpation and dexterity during the collection process, gloves should fit snugly. Except in very specific circumstances, it is not necessary for the gloves used for phlebotomy to be sterile. Most health-care settings no longer use latex gloves, due to the increase in latex sensitivity issues. A common substitute for latex gloves, nitrile gloves work well for phlebotomy. Vinyl gloves may also be worn, but they are not advised in all situations because of their tendency to break down when exposed to certain chemicals.

Sharps Biohazardous Waste Containers

A **sharp** is anything that has been exposed to blood (or other potentially infectious materials) that has corners, edges, or sharp projections that are capable of cutting or piercing the skin. In venipuncture, sharps include needles and capillary puncture devices. Glass slides may also be classified as sharps because they have sharp corners that may be hazardous. Sharps must be disposed of in a waste container that is specifically designed to be puncture resistant, leakproof on the sides and bottom, and labeled as biohazardous waste. These containers should be placed close to the site where the venipuncture is performed so that contaminated sharps may be disposed of immediately. Sharps waste containers come in various sizes, and should never be overfilled. If a sharps container is filled past the marked fill line, it is possible for injury to occur when an employee adds contaminated sharps to the container.

Alcohol and Gauze Pads

Seventy percent isopropyl alcohol is generally used for cleaning the venipuncture site. It may be applied by using a presoaked commercial square that is individually wrapped and packaged. Alcohol may also be applied by using a gauze pad that has been saturated just prior to use. Isopropyl alcohol is an effective antiseptic that can help to eliminate most transient and surface resident bacteria from the venipuncture site. The alcohol used to cleanse the site must be allowed to dry completely before the procedure is performed. If liquid alcohol is still present when the needle is inserted, it can cause a stinging sensation and irritation to the skin and/or the vein. Alcohol may also cause hemolysis of the red blood cells if it is introduced into the specimen.

When additional cleanliness is essential during the collection process (such as when blood cultures or arterial punctures are ordered), iodine or chlorhexidine gluconate may be used. Chlorhexidine gluconate is ideal for those who are allergic to iodine. Procedures used for drawing blood cultures are presented in more detail in Chapter 10.

Clean 2 x 2 gauze squares are recommended for venipuncture procedures. The gauze is applied after the needle has been removed from the arm and the collection is completed. Cotton balls should not be used because their excess fibers tend to stick to the wound and can cause bleeding to recur when the cotton ball is removed later.

Test Your Knowledge! 8-8

List three items that are needed for all venipuncture procedures, regardless of which technique used.

(Outcome 8-8)

Needles

Needles used to withdraw blood are always disposable and used only once. They are generally 1 to 1.5 in. in length. Figure 8-6 describes the different parts of a needle. The slanted part of the needle that creates the sharp tip is called the **bevel.** This slant helps the needle to enter the skin with a minimum amount of trauma and pain. There is a hole in the bevel where the blood enters the interior hollow portion of the needle, called the **lumen.** The **gauge** of the needle refers to the diameter of the lumen: the larger the needle, the smaller the number used to describe the gauge. Needles used for venipuncture are generally 20 to 23 gauge. Needles that are smaller than 23 gauge will cause **hemolysis** (breaking of the red blood cells with release of hemoglobin) as the blood cells are broken when they enter the small hollow cylinder that forms the lumen. Conversely, if the needle used is too large, hemolysis may also result because of the force at which the blood enters the tube or syringe through the large opening.

When removing the cap from a needle to prepare for venipuncture, it is important to inspect the needle for any defects such as burrs or a blunt tip. If there are problems present, the needle must be discarded immediately into a sharps container and a new one used for the procedure.

Needles used for the **evacuated tube system** are also known as **multi-sample needles.** They have sharp tips at both ends; the end with the beveled tip is designed to be inserted into the vein; the shorter, blunt tip at the opposite end is covered with a rubberized sleeve. The needle is designed to be screwed into a hard plastic holder that holds the tube and the needle. The needle

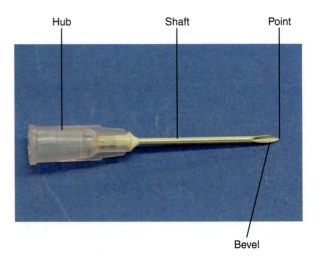

Figure 8-6 Identification of the different parts of a needle.

or the holder must be equipped with a safety device to protect the employee upon completion of the blood draw. A multi-sample needle and holder are shown in Figure 8-7.

When performing venipuncture utilizing the **syringe system,** a needle of similar length and gauge as that for the evacuated tube method is used (Fig. 8-8). These needles are designed to screw directly onto the syringe, so the needle only has one pointed end; the other end has a hub that attaches directly to the syringe. The needles or the syringe must be equipped with a safety device to protect the employee after the blood draw is completed. Examples of safety mechanisms include a cover that is pushed over the needle and locked in place after the draw, or a retractable needle that moves back into the syringe once the specimen is obtained.

The **butterfly system,** or winged infusion system, consists of a short needle with "wings" (Fig. 8-9). When used for venipuncture, the needle is generally 23 gauge, and is attached to a piece of plastic tubing that is approximately 12 in. long. The wings are held by the fingers while the needle is inserted into the vein. Butterfly needles are used for fragile veins (such as those in the hand) or pediatric draws. The butterfly tubing may be attached directly to a syringe, or an adapter may be used to attach the butterfly setup to a plastic evacuated tube holder. Proper activation of the safety devices included with the butterfly system is critical, as there are more accidental needlesticks attributed to the use of butterflies than there are in either of the other two systems.

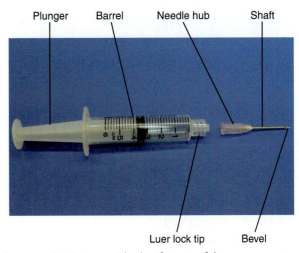

Figure 8-8 Syringe with identification of the various parts.

Test Your Knowledge 8-9

Are the needles used for all venipuncture techniques the same?   (Outcome 8-8)

Safety needles are required for all methods of venipuncture. The various safety devices are designed to be easily activated, using either a needle that withdraws into the device while still in the skin, or one hand activation of the safety device. Figure 8-10 shows various safety devices for evacuated tube systems, syringe needles, and butterfly needles. It is essential that the medical assistant performing venipuncture become comfortable

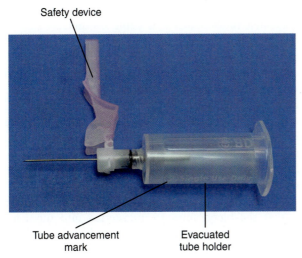

Figure 8-7 Multi-sample needle and holder with identification of parts.

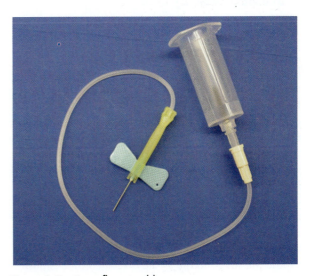

Figure 8-9 Butterfly assembly.

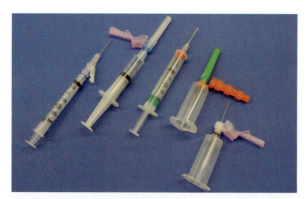

Figure 8-10 Safety devices for use with the evacuated tube system and syringe draws.

with the safety devices available to him or her so that the device can be activated quickly and safely for protection.

Additional Supplies

Blood spill cleanup supplies should be available near every phlebotomy station, and staff should be trained regularly on their use. In addition, because every tube should be identified while in the presence of the patient, it is important to have at least one functional pen available to identify the tube and document the blood draw information on the requisition. It is also necessary to have backup tubes and needles within reach for use when the procedure does not go as planned.

METHODS USED FOR VENIPUNCTURE

Evacuated Tube System

The most common and most efficient method of performing venipuncture is the use of the evacuated tube system. As described earlier in the chapter, blood is collected directly into an evacuated tube through a needle that has two pointed ends. This method is advantageous because there is no need to transfer the blood from one container to another after the draw, and also because multiple tubes of blood may easily and quickly be drawn with one skin puncture. The needle to be used with the evacuated tube system is screwed into an evacuated tube holder that is made of semirigid plastic. These tube holders are designed to be used only once; if the medical assistant tries to use them more than once, the needle may not screw in securely. The rubber cover covering the shorter, posterior end of the needle is pushed back to expose the sharp needle as the evacuated tube is pushed on during the blood draw. Evacuated tubes have the air

removed to create a vacuum, so as soon as the tube cap is pierced with the needle, the blood is pulled into the tube. When the blood draw is complete, the safety device for the needle must be activated, and the evacuated tube holder with the needle attached must be disposed of directly into a biohazardous sharps container.

The plastic evacuated tube holder has flared sections at the bottom, which are known as **flanges.** These are designed to be pushed against as the medical assistant changes tubes during the blood draw process. The flanges help to keep the venipuncture setup stable during the process of drawing blood. There is also a line marked on the tube holder; this is a "safe" mark that shows how far the tubes can be advanced into the holder before the vacuum will be affected. Some health-care personnel prefer to advance the tube to this mark before they begin the blood draw process, whereas others do not. If the tube is advanced past this mark, the vacuum will be affected and the tube may not fill as desired once the needle is in the vein.

Syringe Method

Health-care personnel may prefer to use the syringe method for venipuncture in patients having small or fragile veins. Use of a syringe to withdraw blood allows for more control of the vacuum used to withdraw blood from the vein, as the individual performing the venipuncture can control the speed and force used to pull on the plunger of the syringe. Syringe draws also allow the person performing the venipuncture to see the blood in the hub of the needle as the vein is entered, which can be reassuring when attempting a blood draw on a vein that is difficult to palpate or locate. This return of blood into the hub of the needle is called a "flash" of blood.

Syringes are made of a hollow plastic barrel with graduated measurements in cubic centimeters (cc) or milliliters (mL) printed on the side. Inside the barrel of the syringe is a plunger that is designed to fit tightly enough to create suction when the plunger is pulled backward. The sizes of syringes used for venipuncture may vary from 3 mL to 20 mL, with 5-mL or 10-mL syringes most commonly used. Any size needle may be attached to the syringe, but 20- to 23-gauge, 1-in. needles are most commonly utilized for venipuncture. Safety devices for the blood draw may be attached to the needle, or the syringe may be safety enabled.

One disadvantage of using syringes for venipuncture is that the blood must be transferred into tubes for further processing and testing after the blood draw. This must occur quickly so that the blood does not clot in the syringe. Transfer devices should be used to add the blood from the syringe to the necessary tubes (Fig. 8-11).

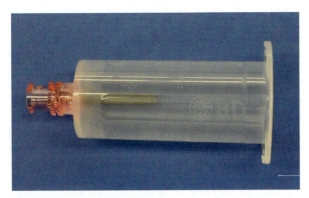

Figure 8-11 Transfer device.

Because the amount of blood obtained with one venipuncture is limited to the size of the syringe used, this must be taken into consideration before choosing the syringe method for blood collection. It may not be advantageous to use a syringe when there is an order that requires more than 10 mL of blood, as the sample may clot in the syringe before it can be successfully transferred to the correct blood tubes.

Winged Infusion or Butterfly Method

Winged infusion sets (also known as **butterfly systems**) are made up of a beveled needle that is attached to a length of tubing with a luer adapter on the opposite end. Just below the needle on the butterfly system are two "wings" that are made of hard plastic. The medical assistant will grasp these wings and use them to guide the insertion of the needle into the vein. Butterfly systems are often used for venipuncture in patients having very fragile veins, such as those in the hands. They are also used for many pediatric blood draws, small fragile veins in areas other than the hand, and sometimes for uncooperative patients. Butterfly sets are preferred in these situations because the needle can be maneuvered easily to gain venous access because of its decreased length. The angle used to enter the vein is smaller when using a butterfly setup. This can be especially important when attempting a blood draw from a superficial small vein, such as those in children. The attached flexible tubing allows for multiple tubes to be collected without danger of moving the needle in the vein. Butterfly systems may be used directly with evacuated tubes (utilizing a Luer adapter for this purpose), or they may be attached to a syringe when there is a desire to use very gentle pressure during the blood draw.

Venipuncture with a butterfly system has a higher risk of an accidental needlestick if the safety device is not activated properly before the medical assistant attempts

to process the specimen after the blood draw. Becton, Dickinson has a product with a push-button activation that withdraws the needle into a plastic reservoir before it is removed from the skin. Other products require activation of the safety device after the needle is removed from the patient, and it is imperative that the health-care professional performing the venipuncture follow directions for activation to avoid potential bloodborne pathogen exposure.

BLOOD COLLECTION TUBES

Evacuated tubes used for blood collection are available in several sizes, and are made of plastic with rubberized stoppers. (Glass collection tubes may still be available, but they are not recommended due to the potential for breakage and blood exposure for health-care personnel.) Evacuated tubes vary by diameter, length, and the additives present in the tubes. They are each designed to hold a specific amount of blood and vary from 2-mL tubes that may be used for pediatric or geriatric blood draws, to 15-mL tubes that are used when a high volume of blood is necessary for a particular assay. The medical assistant or phlebotomist drawing the blood will choose the tube size according to the age of the patient, the integrity of the vein, and the amount of blood needed for the test ordered. The different colors used for the stoppers are coded according to the additive contained within the tube.

These tubes are evacuated because the air within the tube has been removed to create a **vacuum.** This vacuum has been artificially created and calibrated by the manufacturer so that a very specific amount of blood will be drawn into the tube. The tube will never fill completely to the top, as they are not calibrated to hold that volume of blood. As long as the vacuum is still present within the tube, blood will continue to flow. If there has been a loss of vacuum in the evacuated tube, blood will not enter the tube, or it will fill incompletely. This is known as a **short draw** and often will require the specimen to be redrawn. Short draws are sometimes caused by dropping a tube prior to the venipuncture, pushing the tube too far onto the double-ended needle used for evacuated tube draws prior to the blood collection, or by accidentally pulling the needle out of the vein during the venipuncture process.

All blood tubes have an expiration printed on the label. There is an expectation that the vacuum and additives in the tube will function as expected until this date. The health-care worker who performs the blood draw is responsible for checking the expiration date on all tubes before they are used, and at the same time examining the tube for any obvious defects or breaks. Any tubes that are near expiration should be removed from the shelves before the printed date has passed.

Test Your Knowledge 8-10

Why are tubes used for blood collection called vacuum tubes?   (Outcome 8-8)

Color Coding of Tubes

Evacuated tubes are all sealed with a colored stopper. These closures are made of rubber and/or plastic and are designed to ensure the vacuum within the tube and provide a barrier to the blood once the tube is filled. Some tubes available on the market have a rubber stopper with an outside plastic cap of the same color. The plastic cap

provides protection for the employee when opening the tube, because the additional plastic cap hangs over the outside of the tube and forms a barrier to any aerosol formation from the blood in the tube. An example of this type of tube is the Hemogard tube, manufactured by Becton, Dickinson. See Figure 8-12 for an example of the Hemogard tube.

The stopper colors on evacuated tubes are color coded and used to indicate whether additives are present in the tubes, and if so, what types are present. Additives may function as **anticoagulants,** or **clot activators.** The additives may sometimes serve as preservatives of the integrity of the specimen. Anticoagulants will keep the blood from clotting in the tube so that the cells remain suspended in the plasma. Without the addition of anticoagulants, the blood will begin to clot in the tube immediately, and a visible solid clot will form within an hour. Clot activators, such as glass beads or silicone, are designed to speed up the clotting process so that the blood can be spun in the centrifuge within a shorter period of time after collection. Tubes may also contain a thixotropic separating gel that is designed to form a barrier between the blood cells and the liquid portion of the blood after it is centrifuged. The gel in these **serum separator tubes (SST)** or **plasma separator tubes (PST)** is in the bottom of the tube when the blood is collected, but as the tube is centrifuged, the cells move to the bottom of the tube and the gel travels up in the tube to form a barrier between the cells and the liquid. Figure 8-13 shows how the gel separates the sample after centrifugation.

The colors used for tube stoppers are similar from brand to brand, providing a uniform reference for the different types of additives. The type of anticoagulant present in the tube is printed on the label, along with the expiration date and the blood volume for the

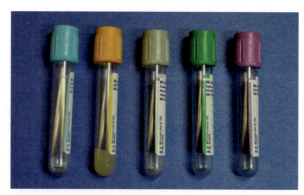

Figure 8-12   Vacuum tubes with Hemogard caps presented in the appropriate order of draw.

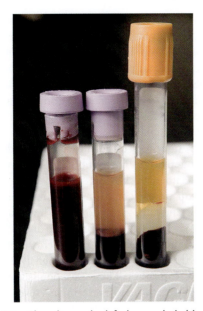

Figure 8-13 The tube on the left shows whole blood before centrifugation. The tube in the middle shows plasma sitting on top of clotted blood cells. The tube on the right is a tube with serum separator gel that has been spun in a centrifuge and shows serum sitting on top of clotted blood cells. *Reprinted with permission from Eagle S, Brassington C, Dailey C, and Goretti C: The Professional Medical Assistant: An Integrative, Teamwork-Based Approach. Philadelphia: FA Davis, 2009.*

tube. When using reference materials (such as laboratory requisition forms or laboratory directories) the specimen collection instructions will reference the stopper color needed for the test ordered or the additive present in the tubes. Each laboratory may have different tube requirements for a given test based on its testing methodology, so it is always best to verify the necessary tube before drawing the blood.

Test Your Knowledge 8-11

What is the significance of the different stopper colors used for the vacuum tubes?   (Outcome 8-10)

Types of Additives

Types of anticoagulants and/or additives present in the most common evacuated tubes are listed here with their respective color stoppers and summarized in Table 8-1.

- **Yellow:** Sterile tubes used for blood cultures. There are also specific yellow top tubes that contain a red blood cell preservative called acid citrate dextrose (ACD),

and these are used for special blood bank procedures. The sterile yellow tubes for blood cultures are by far more common.

- **Light blue:** Contains sodium citrate as an anticoagulant. Light blue top tubes are primarily used for coagulation studies. The ratio of blood to anticoagulant is critical for these tubes and they must always be filled completely to prevent potential dilution and erroneous results.

- **Red:** Glass red top tubes are sterile and contain no additives. Plastic red top tubes contain a clot activator. Red top tubes are used for a variety of tests in which serum is the preferred specimen.

- **Red/gray (tiger top) or gold:** Contains a silica clot activator that increases platelet activity and decreases the time necessary for a clot to form in the tube. Also contains thixotropic gel that separates the cells from the serum when the specimen is centrifuged. Used for chemistry and immunology testing in which serum is the preferred specimen.

- **Black:** Special tubes used only for Westergren sedimentation rates. Contain sodium citrate, but in a different concentration (blood to anticoagulant liquid 4:1) than the light blue top tubes. These tubes are not to be used for coagulation studies.

- **Green:** Contains heparin combined with sodium, lithium, or ammonium as an anticoagulant. These tubes are preferred for chemistry tests in which plasma is suitable for testing and the results must be obtained quickly, as the specimen does not need to clot before the sample may be spun in the centrifuge. Light green Hemogard tubes and those with green and black mottled stoppers contain thixotropic gel in addition to the anticoagulant, which separates the plasma from the cells after centrifugation.

- **Gray:** Contains sodium fluoride, which acts as a glucose preservative (called an antiglycolytic agent) keeping the glucose levels stable in the specimen for a period of time after collection. Also contains an anticoagulant; either potassium oxalate or sodium EDTA. Gray top tubes are not appropriate for general chemistry testing, but are used for glucose testing, as well as blood alcohol determinations.

- **Lavender:** Contains potassium EDTA (dipotassium ethylenediaminetetraacetic acid) as the anticoagulant. Prevents the use of calcium in the clotting process to prevent blood clotting and keep the blood cells suspended in plasma. Lavender top tubes are used for hematology testing because this preservative preserves the integrity and shape of the individual cells better than any of the other anticoagulants.

TABLE 8-1	
Table of common tube colors and additives	
Tube Stopper Color	**Additives**
Red top	None
Tiger top/ speckled top/ gold top	Clot activators/thixotropic gel
Green top	Heparin
Mint green top	Heparin and thixotropic gel
Light blue top	Sodium citrate
Lavender top	Potassium EDTA
Gray top	Sodium fluoride and potassium oxalate

ORDER OF DRAW FOR VENIPUNCTURE

The Clinical and Laboratory Standards Institute (formerly known as NCCLS) has recommended a specific order of draw for venipuncture specimens using the evacuated tube system, syringe collection method, or butterfly draws. There is a different recommended order of draw for capillary specimens. These recommendations were developed because of potential problems with additive carryover from one evacuated tube to another. Reports showed significant increases in potassium and some other analytes when a lavender top tube (containing potassium EDTA for an anticoagulant) was drawn just prior to the tube used for chemistry testing. Other potential carryover issues were also identified.

> **Test Your Knowledge 8-12**
> Why is the order of draw so important?
> (Outcome 8-11)

The recommended order of draw for the six most commonly used tubes:

1. **Blood culture specimens:** These may be yellow top tubes or a set of bottles used for blood cultures. They must be drawn first to avoid potential for contamination of the draw site.
2. **Light blue top citrate tube:** This tube is primarily used for coagulation studies, so it is important that additive crossover is avoided because of potential interactions. Previous recommendations always called for a red top tube to be drawn before the light blue top tube, but with the current CLSI recommendations,

this is no longer necessary. An exception is when a butterfly system is used to draw a light blue top tube; in this case, a red top tube is used as a "clear" tube because of the excessive air present in the tubing of the butterfly. The blue top tubes must be filled as far as the vacuum allows, and if the excess air from the tubing is introduced into the light blue top tube, the tube will not fill adequately.

3. **Red top, tiger top, or gold top tubes with or without clot activator:** These tubes are used when serum is the specimen of choice.
4. **Green top tubes:** These are both tubes that have gel separator and tubes that do not. They may be mint green or dark green. These are to be drawn before the EDTA tubes to reduce the risk of crossover that may increase the potassium levels when analyzed.
5. **Lavender top tubes:** These have potassium EDTA as the anticoagulant, and are primarily used for whole blood testing.
6. **Gray top tubes:** Gray top tubes are used for glucose testing, as well as a few other tests. They need to be drawn after the EDTA tubes because the additives present in the gray top tube could cause abnormal changes in the red blood cells to be analyzed if there is crossover. The gray top tube must be drawn after the tubes used for other chemistry testing, because the potassium oxalate present in the gray top tube could cause falsely elevated potassium results if the specimens were contaminated by the anticoagulant and this test was to be performed on the sample.

CAPILLARY PUNCTURES

Most blood collections are performed by puncturing a vein. However, there are times when a **capillary puncture** is a more appropriate method. During a capillary puncture, an incision is made in through the skin, which passes through the epidermis into the dermal layer. It is critical that the puncture reaches the dermal layer, as this is where the blood supply exists. Remember, the blood present in the capillary beds of the body is a mixture of venous and arterial blood. There is actually more arterial blood represented because of the increased arterial pressure forcing this blood into the capillary vessels. Because of the way that the skin layers are punctured, capillary samples may also include additional fluid from the space between the tissues and cells surrounding the capillary vessels. This is why it is very important to document the source of the blood specimen when collecting a capillary sample, as the reference ranges will be different from those used for venous blood.

Test Your Knowledge 8-13

Why is it important to document that a sample was capillary rather than venous?   (Outcome 8-13)

Capillary samples are never appropriate when the test ordered requires a large amount of blood, or if there are problems with the circulation for the patient. This technique should also be avoided if the patient has edema, as the excessive fluid may dilute the sample and cause erroneous results. CLIA-waived tests require very little blood, so capillary punctures are often performed for these tests. Some patients who are undergoing cancer treatment or dialysis may be better suited for capillary blood draws to allow their blood levels to remain stable. Capillary punctures are also appropriate for most children, some geriatric patients with fragile veins, and infants.

Capillary punctures should always be performed using retractable nonreusable lancets for the safety of the patient and the employee performing the puncture. These devices are calibrated to provide a uniform depth for the puncture, and they lock in place once the puncture has occurred so that they cannot be reactivated. The devices used for capillary punctures are color coded according to the depth of the blade. They vary from those used for infants, which must be less than 2.0 mm (to avoid potentially touching bone), to adult depths up to 3 mm, primarily used for finger punctures. Lancet devices that may be used for home testing or perhaps for an individual CLIA-waived test procedure usually will not provide a puncture that is feasible for collecting enough blood to fill a microtube for analysis. All puncture devices must be disposed of in a biohazardous sharps container.

During a venipuncture, a tourniquet is used to aid in the palpation and visualization of an appropriate draw site. Capillary draws do not require the use of a tourniquet, but it is very important that the site to be used is as warm as possible to help increase the blood circulation. This may be accomplished by soaking the appendage in warm (not hot) water; by using a warm, wet compress; or with use of a commercial hand warmer held on the skin until it is warm to the touch.

The capillary puncture also requires the use of clean gauze (usually at least two sets), 70% isopropyl alcohol to clean the site, and a bandage to be used after the puncture. The employee who is performing the capillary puncture should also prepare the site under the patients'

hand or foot by draping the area with an absorbent cloth or sheet to absorb any excess blood.

Capillary samples may be collected in various ways. **Microcollection tubes** may be utilized, which are smaller versions of the evacuated tubes used for venipuncture. These tubes are color coded in a way similar to the evacuated tubes, and many contain anticoagulants or other additives. **Capillary tubes** may also be used, especially for hematocrit testing. Capillary tubes are long, thin, hollow tubes designed to hold blood. The tubes are held horizontally with one end touching the drop of blood created by the capillary puncture. The tube fills with blood via **capillary action.** These tubes may be made of glass or plastic. They may be coated internally with heparin to keep the blood from clotting as it is collected, in which case the tube will have a red ring around it. Other capillary tubes do not include anticoagulant, and these plain tubes will have a blue ring around their diameter. Capillary tubes may also be part of a microcollection container setup, where the capillary action pulls the blood into the container. Figure 8-14 includes examples of devices used for capillary punctures.

Order of Draw for Capillary Puncture

The order of draw for the various microcollection containers using a capillary technique is different from the order used for venipuncture. The order is not the same because the capillary blood clots faster than the blood taken from a vein and because the potential for carryover

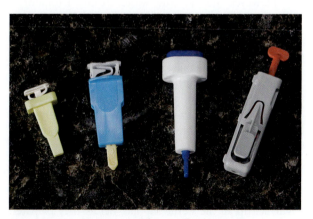

Figure 8-14 Devices used for capillary punctures. *Reprinted with permission from Eagle S, Brassington C, Dailey C, and Goretti C: The Professional Medical Assistant: An Integrative, Teamwork-Based Approach. Philadelphia: FA Davis, 2009.*

is not as high. For capillary draws, the order of draw is as follows:

1. **Lavender (EDTA) tubes are filled first.** It is imperative that these are well mixed during the process to avoid blood clot formation.
2. **Other additive tubes,** such as green top tubes or those with heparin and thixotropic gel, are collected next. Microcollection tubes are not used for coagulation studies, so there are no sodium citrate tubes to be filled.
3. **Nonadditive tubes are drawn last,** and will usually clot within 6 or 7 minutes.

Test Your Knowledge 8-14

Is the order of draw the same for capillary draws as it is for venipuncture specimens?   (Outcome 8-11)

POINT OF INTEREST 8-4
Waste reduction considerations

Unfortunately, specimen collection generates a lot of waste. Current practice prohibits reusing most items that are exposed to bloodborne pathogens because of the danger of exposure for subsequent patients. The contaminated waste must be disposed of and processed appropriately by a licensed biohazardous waste handler. The waste is packaged according to federal specifications, transported in a standardized manner, and finally incinerated.

However, not all the waste in the laboratory setting is contaminated. Lids from needles, plastic and paper packaging, and alcohol prep pad packages need to be added to the regular trash, not treated as biohazardous materials. Some of the packaging may be recyclable; this option should be employed whenever possible. Any paper may include protected personal information and so needs to be shredded before disposal to protect patients' privacy. Some recycling programs will process shredded paper.

To minimize waste, do not open sterile packaging until you are certain that you will be using a specific device for specimen collection. Many phlebotomists will set up all the sterile supplies before they palpate the vein of the patient. This may be a mistake, as it may become apparent that a different device is needed for the blood draw. The sterility has been compromised for the devices that were set out, so they will all need to be discarded, in addition to the devices actually used for the blood draw. Become aware of recycling options in the laboratory setting, and make use of this service whenever possible.

PREPARATION FOR BLOOD COLLECTION

Several steps are required in the blood collection process prior to the actual puncture of the skin. Specific procedures are utilized regardless of the method used to collect the sample. These critical aspects include the following:

- **A professional atmosphere:** A collection site where phlebotomy is performed should be clean, organized, well lit, and tidy. Many times this collection site is the only contact that the patient will actually have with the laboratory where the testing will be performed, and if they feel as if this is a professional environment, the patient will have more confidence with the testing process to follow.
- **Appropriate introductions:** When first approaching a patient, the health-care employee must identify him- or herself. Proper identification should also be worn, such as a name tag and/or uniform so that the patient feels in the presence of a qualified professional for the procedure.
- **Patient identification:** This is the most critical aspect of the collection procedure. The health-care employee should ask for the patient to give his or her entire name and birth date for verification of identification. This information should be checked against the requisition form for accuracy. It is important that the patient actually says, "I am Sally Smith," rather than the health-care employee asking, "Are you Sally Smith?" Many times patients will answer yes to such a question, even though they did not hear or understand the name given. If drawing blood from a patient in an inpatient setting, armbands may be used for identification, but in addition, the patient identity also needs to be verified in another way. The phlebotomist must document who provided the verification of the patient identity if it is not the patient.
- **Verification of orders and patient preparation:** The medical assistant or phlebotomist needs to verify what tests were ordered before continuing with the collection procedure. This can be accomplished by looking carefully at the requisition form or labels provided for the blood draw. The medical assistant is also responsible to see if patients are prepared properly for the test

ordered; for instance, if the test is a fasting blood sugar, the medical assistant must ask patients if they have been without food and drink (except water and necessary medications) for 12 hours. If the preparation was not followed appropriately, the specimen is not to be drawn. When drawing blood to test for a therapeutic drug level, the medical assistant needs to ask when the medication was last taken, and verify if that is an appropriate time interval for this particular test.

- **Hand sanitization:** The medical assistant must wash his or her hands (if they are visibly soiled from a previous procedure) or use hand sanitizer appropriately before touching the patient. Gloves must be worn during the venipuncture process and should not be applied until the hands are totally dry.

- **Site selection:** The medical assistant should always start in the antecubital area when looking for an appropriate venipuncture site. The first choice is the median cubital vein, the second choice is the cephalic vein, and the last choice in this area is the basilic vein. The medical assistant should always check the veins in both arms to make the best choice. The back of the hand may also be used for venipuncture if there are no suitable sites in the antecubital area. For a capillary draw on an adult, the middle finger or ring finger is used, and part of the preparation may be warming the site.

- **Preparation of necessary supplies:** It is not possible to prepare fully for the venipuncture before the site selection has been performed, because the choice of which method to use for the blood draw will be dependent on the integrity and size of the veins to be used for the blood draw. Once the site selection is complete, the medical assistant can prepare an evacuated tube setup, a syringe for the blood draw, or a butterfly setup. The tubes to be used should also be checked for expiration and/or defects, and laid out in order of draw close to the patient so that they can be easily reached during the procedure. Gauze and alcohol should be within reach as well.

Supplies may vary depending on the age and general health of the patient. An infant usually does not have venipuncture performed for most laboratory tests. Small children may need venipuncture, but a smaller volume of blood may be drawn using a butterfly and a 2- or 3-mL tube. Those patients who are over the age of 60 often present veins that collapse or roll easily, and due to complex health issues, it may be necessary to withdraw smaller volumes of blood for these populations. A syringe draw or butterfly setup will often be necessary.

- **Cleansing and support of the site:** Once the site has been selected, it must be cleaned. Seventy percent isopropyl alcohol is usually used to clean the site, and it is applied in a circular motion with the draw site at the center of the circle. The alcohol must be allowed to dry completely before the blood draw is performed. The site should not be repalpated after the alcohol has been used. If repalpation is absolutely necessary, the site should be cleaned again after being touched.

The venipuncture site should be well supported by using a chair that has arms or a cross support designed for blood-drawing procedures. It may be helpful to have the patient make a fist with the opposite hand and place this under the elbow, which helps to expose the antecubital area fully for inspection and offers additional support. For inpatients, the patient's arm should be settled on a pillow or rolled-up towel to help make the veins more accessible.

Support of the site may be complicated for small children. It may be necessary to ask the adult who accompanied the child to assist with the process by holding the child and securing the child's upper body for safety. A staff member may also be asked to assist in the process. The medical assistant should be ready for the blood draw as quickly as possible in this situation, and should not allow the child to see the needle for an excessive period of time before the venipuncture.

- **Patient communication:** Whenever the skin is to be punctured, remember to be honest with the patient about what will occur. *Never* tell a patient that the procedure won't hurt, or chastise the patient for expressing fear or discomfort with the procedure. Assure the patient that the procedure is necessary, and that it will be completed in as little time as possible. Try to adapt to the age of the patient by making appropriate small talk. Allowing the child to "blow away the pain" may be beneficial; the act of saying "ow" and blowing out may help to distract him or her from the process.

> **Test Your Knowledge 8-15**
>
> What is the most important aspect of patient preparation for blood collection procedures? (Outcome 8-14)

SPECIMEN PROCESSING

Once the blood specimen is collected, it may require further processing before it can be used for testing. The analysis may call for serum, plasma, or whole blood for

(Text continues on page 180)

Procedure 8-1: Venipuncture Using the Evacuated Tube System

The evacuated tube system is the method used most commonly for obtaining blood. It is fast and relatively safe, and allows for multiple tubes to be filled with one invasive procedure.

TASK

Successfully perform a venipuncture using the evacuated tube system. The process must be completed within 5 minutes.

CONDITIONS

- Hand-washing supplies and/or alcohol-based hand sanitizer
- Disposable gloves
- Tourniquet
- 70% isopropyl alcohol
- Double-pointed multi-sample needle
- Evacuated tube holder
- Laboratory requisition form or labels with specified test
- Evacuated tubes
- 2 x 2 gauze pads

- Adhesive bandage or wrap
- Test tube rack
- Biohazardous sharps container
- Biohazardous disposal bag

CAAHEP/ABHES STANDARDS

 CAAHEP Standards

I.P.I.2: Perform Venipuncture   **I.A.I.1:** Apply critical thinking skills in performing patient assessment and care   **III.P.III.3:** Select appropriate barrier/personal protective equipment (PPE) for potentially infectious situations

 ABHES Standards

- Medical Office Laboratory Procedures: Collect, label and process specimens: Perform venipuncture
- Medical Office Clinical Procedures: Apply principles of aseptic techniques and infection control
- Medical Office Clinical Procedures: Use Standard Precautions

Procedure	Rationale
1. Gather the requisition form and/or labels for the blood draw, and greet the patient. Identify yourself appropriately.	The requisition or labels are necessary to collect the correct type of specimen. It is always correct practice to identify yourself to the patient.
2. Wash hands (if they are visibly soiled) or apply hand sanitizer. Allow hands to dry completely.	Clean hands stop the spread of infection. Hands should be completely dry before attempting to apply gloves, or it will be difficult to put the gloves on the wet hands.
3. Verify the identity of the patient by asking for his or her name and at least one other unique identifier (such as the patient's birth date). Compare this information to the requisition form or labels.	Patient identification must always be verified using at least two unique factors.
4. Verify whether dietary restrictions were followed, and time of last medication dose, if needed.	Many laboratory tests require fasting specimens or other dietary restrictions. Drug dosage times are especially important for appropriate interpretation of the laboratory results.
5. Have the patient sit in the phlebotomy chair with appropriate arm support, and extend his or her arm to expose the antecubital area.	The arm should be supported for the venipuncture process, and the antecubital area will be the first area that is considered for the blood draw.

Procedure	Rationale
6. Apply gloves.	Gloves are required for procedures in which there is reasonable anticipation of exposure to blood or other potentially infectious materials.
7. Apply the tourniquet approximately 3 in. above the antecubital area (or above the wrist if a hand draw is necessary) and select an appropriate draw site using palpation. Use the tips of the ring finger and middle finger in a gentle probing motion as the antecubital area is examined. An appropriate vein will feel flexible and firm. Do not allow the tourniquet to remain on the arm for more than 1 minute.	The tourniquet needs to be placed high enough that it will not block the venipuncture site. Only blood vessels that can be palpated should be used for venipuncture; just looking at them is not sufficient. The thumb should never be used to feel for a vein, as there may be a pulse felt from the thumb that can be misleading. The thumb is also not as sensitive as the fingers.
8. While palpating, have the patient make a fist, but *do not* allow the patient to pump his or her hand.	Pumping the hand can cause erroneous test results due to hemoconcentration.
9. If an appropriate site is not identified on the first arm, examine the other arm. If the antecubital area is not appropriate on either arm, examine the back of the hands for other opportunities.	It is important to choose the best site before inserting the needle. If the first arm examined doesn't provide a vein that is appropriate, check the other arm. If necessary, the back of the hands may be considered as a blood draw site.
10. Once an appropriate site is selected, determine the direction of the vein; is it running straight up and down or at an angle across the arm? Establish a visible landmark (a mole or dimple in the skin, etc.) for reference.	The needle must be inserted in such a way that it follows the direction of the vein for the best chance of success. A landmark is helpful so that the chosen venipuncture site can be identified after cleaning the area.
11. Have the patient open the hand to relax the fist until the tourniquet is reapplied.	Relaxing the hand will help the blood to flow normally as the site is prepared.
12. Remove the tourniquet.	A tourniquet may not stay on the arm for more than 1 minute, or hemoconcentration may result.

Continued

Procedure 8-1: Venipuncture Using the Evacuated Tube System—cont'd

Procedure	Rationale
13. Apply 70% isopropyl alcohol to the area in a circular motion with the draw site at the center of the circle. Allow the site to air-dry.	70% isopropyl alcohol will kill most of the bacterial contaminants on the surface of the skin. Never blow or fan the site to speed up the drying process, as this recontaminates the clean area.

14. As the alcohol is drying, assemble the necessary supplies.
  a. Choose a needle of appropriate size and attach it to the evacuated tube holder. Do not remove the cap that covers the long end of the needle until right before the skin is to be punctured.
 	
  b. Arrange the necessary tubes for the tests ordered within easy reach of your nondominant hand, and have them set up in the correct order of draw.
  c. Verify that the tubes are not expired and that the anticoagulant is placed away from the rubber stopper within the tube. (You may need to shake the tube lightly to get the anticoagulant to move away from the stopper.) Check for any obvious defects in the tubes.
	Supplies need to be close by for ease of use and patient safety.
	This should always occur in the presence of the patient so that he or she is assured that the needle is sterile. The cap should not be removed until it is ready to be used to minimize the risk of contamination or possible injury. Needle sizes may vary according to the needs of the patient and the policy of the facility.
	The tubes may be laid out on the counter near the patient, or a small tube rack may work well for this purpose.
	
	Use of an expired tube may result in a loss of vacuum and an unsuccessful blood draw. Potential crossover of anticoagulant from one tube to another should be minimized as much as possible. Defective (such as cracked or chipped tubes) should be discarded immediately.

15. Verify that gauze pads and an adhesive bandage are within reach. Extra tubes should also be close by so that they can be used if necessary.	The gauze pads and adhesive bandages need to be ready for use immediately when the needle is removed from the skin. If the phlebotomist feels that there may be a chance that the vacuum is exhausted in the first tube, using a second one that is nearby may allow the venipuncture to be successful.
16. Once the alcohol is dry, reapply the tourniquet. Do not repalpate the venipuncture site, or if absolutely necessary, clean the end of the gloved finger with alcohol before touching the site.	If the site is touched after cleansing, it will need to be cleaned again before the venipuncture can begin.
17. Have the patient make a fist.	Forming a fist may help with the visualization of the veins once the tourniquet is reapplied.
18. Remove the cap to expose the end of the needle to be inserted into the arm. Do not allow this needle to touch anything before piercing the skin.	Touching this needle to any surface before it pierces the skin will cause contamination and possible introduction of bacteria into the vein.

Procedure	Rationale
19. Stabilize the chosen vein by anchoring it with the thumb of the nondominant hand about 2 in. below the draw site, and/or off to the side. Make sure that the skin is pulled taut over the vein.	It is important to stabilize the vein, but if the thumb is placed too close to the draw site, it will be in the way of the needle insertion and could cause interference with the angle used for the process and result in an unsuccessful blood draw. 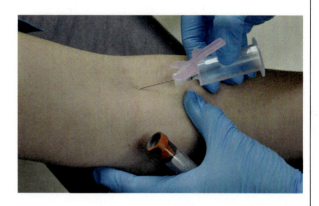
20. As you prepare to pierce the skin with the needle, it is good practice to warn the patient by saying something like, "Here we go; you will feel a stick."	If the patient is not expecting the skin to be pierced, he or she may be startled and move the arm or hand, causing an unsuccessful venipuncture.
21. Insert the needle at an angle of approximately 15 degrees, with the bevel up. The actual insertion site is approximately 1/4 to 1/2 inch below the identified draw site so that the needle is actually inserted into the vein at the chosen site.	If the angle is significantly less or more than 15 degrees, it may slide just above the vein or puncture through both sides of the vein rather than just entering the vein. The bevel facing upward allows the blood to enter the needle with minimal trauma.
22. The needle needs to be inserted quickly, with one smooth gentle motion. As the insertion is accomplished, follow the direction of the vein that was previously identified; if the vein is running at an angle across the arm or hand, this is how the needle should be directed into the vein. Approximately a third of the needle is usually below the surface of the skin when the insertion is complete.	Smooth insertion minimizes the trauma to the patient. It is important to follow the direction of the vein as the needle is inserted; this allows a better opportunity for the blood to enter the needle without obstruction. The needle needs to be inserted far enough to enter the vein, but not so far that it punctures both sides of the vein. 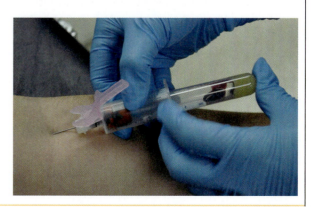

Continued

Procedure 8-1: Venipuncture Using the Evacuated Tube System—cont'd

Procedure	Rationale
23. While keeping the needle firmly seated in the vein, push the first tube into the needle holder, with the label facing downward. Use the index and middle fingers of the nondominant hand by placing them on either side of the flared edge at the bottom of the evacuated tube holder. Place the thumb of the nondominant hand on the bottom of the tube, and squeeze or pull the thumb toward the fingers, pushing the tube into the holder. If the needle is placed appropriately in the vein, blood should start to enter the tube as soon as the needle has pierced the stopper.	The hand used to hold the evacuated tube holder should rest firmly against the arm to keep the needle in place. If the label on the tube is facing upward, it is difficult to see the blood as it enters the tube. 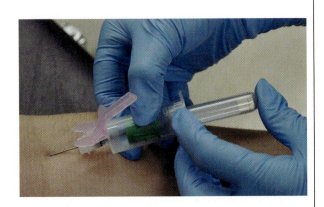
24. If only one tube is necessary for the tests ordered, release the tourniquet once the blood has started to enter the tube. If there is more than one tube necessary, the tourniquet may stay in place until the last tube has been inserted, as long as the length of time has not exceeded 1 minute since the tourniquet was applied.	The tourniquet must not stay on longer than 1 minute. It is always necessary to release the tourniquet before the needle is removed from the arm to avoid bleeding from the venipuncture site and introduction of air into the last vacuum tube used.
25. If it is necessary to use more than one tube for the blood draw, push against the flanges to remove the tube from the holder. Be careful not to disturb the needle placement as the tube is removed. Insert the next tube needed for the tests ordered, following the appropriate order of draw.	It is important to keep applying gentle pressure on the arm of the patient with the back of the fingers that are supporting the evacuated tube holder while removing and inserting tubes to keep the needle in place within the vein. It may be necessary to change tubes more than once when there are multiple tubes necessary for the tests ordered.
26. As each tube with additive is removed from the holder, invert the tube gently at least one or two times. This may be accomplished while the next tube is filling.	Tubes with anticoagulant added must be inverted sufficiently to mix the sample with the additive or the blood will clot and the specimen will need to be redrawn.
27. As the last tube is filling, ask the patient to relax the fist. Verify that the tourniquet has been released, and remove the last tube from the holder.	This is important to avoid a potential bruise or hematoma at the draw site, and also to avoid introduction of excess air into this last tube.

Procedure	Rationale
28. As the needle is removed from the skin, place gauze over the site without applying initial pressure. The needle is to be removed quickly, and at the same angle as the insertion. Do not apply pressure to the site with the gauze until the needle has been removed completely from the skin, as this will cause pain for the patient.	The gauze placed over the site will minimize bleeding as the needle is removed. 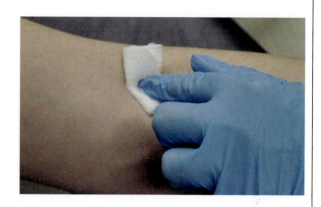
29. Ask the patient to apply pressure to the site for 3 to 5 minutes. Do not allow the patient to bend his or her arm.	The pressure should be adequate to stop any bleeding before the patient leaves the drawing area. Bending the arm increases the risk for bleeding and bruise formation.
30. Once the needle has been removed from the arm, immediately activate the needle safety device and discard the entire setup in the biohazardous sharps container. Do not remove the needle from the evacuated tube holder before disposal. *Never recap contaminated needles.*	The evacuated tube setup is designed to be used one time and discarded without removing the needle before disposal. Recapping contaminated needles increases the risk of needlestick accidents and potential exposure to bloodborne pathogens. 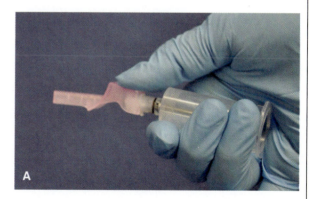

Continued

Procedure 8-1: Venipuncture Using the Evacuated Tube System—cont'd

Procedure	Rationale
	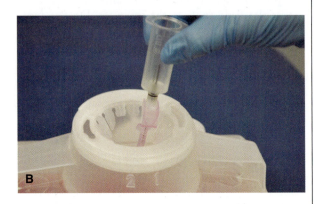
31. As the patient is applying pressure to the draw site, gently invert the blood specimens containing anticoagulant 5 to 10 times.	Insufficient mixing of the anticoagulant with the specimen will result in clotted blood and a sample that must be discarded.
32. Label the tubes, including the full name of the patient, birth date (or other unique identifier assigned by the health-care provider), the date and time of collection, and the initials of the person who drew the sample.	All samples must be labeled using at least two unique identifiers. The date and time provide additional information that may be necessary for interpretation of the results.
	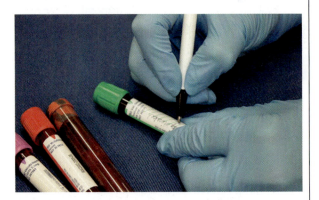
	Identification of the phlebotomist may be helpful if there are questions about the procedure or the specimens collected.
33. Use the requisition form or the labels to verify that all the necessary tubes were drawn for the specimens ordered.	Verifying the details of the blood draw once more in the presence of the patient allows for a redraw to be performed immediately if something is missing.

Procedure	Rationale
34. Observe any special handling instructions for the specimens.	Some types of specimens must remain at room temperature, whereas others may need to be put on ice immediately. This should be information that is ascertained before the procedure starts.
35. Monitor the patient for any signs of distress from the procedure.	These may include pallor, perspiration (especially on the upper lip or forehead), increased anxiety, or light-headedness. If the patient is exhibiting any of these symptoms, it is best to have him or her lie down if possible. This may be easily accomplished if the patient is in a chair that can recline. If not, a cold compress on the forehead and/or the back of the neck may help. Continue to converse with the patient and move the blood out of sight. Ask for assistance if you feel that your patient is feeling faint. If the patient loses consciousness, it may be necessary to lower him or her to the floor from the phlebotomy chair.
36. Once the tubes have been labeled, check the draw site for bleeding. If it has not stopped bleeding, apply pressure for another few minutes, and if the bleeding is still present, contact a physician.	It is important to look under the gauze for 2 or 3 seconds before applying the adhesive bandage to be certain that the site has actually stopped bleeding.
37. If the bleeding has subsided, apply an adhesive bandage, but leave the gauze in place to allow for additional pressure.	Self-adhesive bandages (such as Coban) may be wrapped around the site rather than applying an adhesive to the skin directly. Self-adhesive bandages may be especially effective for those patients who are on anticoagulant therapy.
38. Advise the patient to avoid heavy lifting or excessive exercise of the arm used for venipuncture for at least 1 hour.	Heavy lifting or exercise could cause the site to resume bleeding.
39. Assist the patient to stand (if necessary) and thank him or her for being cooperative.	Patients may be a bit light-headed, and assistance may be needed when he or she first stands up.
40. Discard all trash, and place the tubes in an appropriate vessel for processing. Never touch full tubes of blood without wearing gloves.	Touching the tubes of blood without wearing gloves offers potential opportunities for exposure to bloodborne pathogens.
41. Remove gloves and sanitize hands.	Hands must always be sanitized after removing gloves.

Continued

Procedure 8-1: Venipuncture Using the Evacuated Tube System—cont'd

Procedure	Rationale
42. Document the procedure in the patient's chart as well as on the requisition form. Include the date and time of collection, what was collected, and if there were any circumstances that were out of the ordinary. Also document where the vein was accessed (such as right arm, left hand, etc.). The documentation should include the type (color) of tubes drawn, as well as the identity of the person who collected the sample.	All patient interactions must be carefully documented. The site used for vein access should always be written in the chart or on the requisition form so that if there are any negative outcomes associated with the procedure, the site has been noted.

Date	
1/18/2020:	*Phlebotomy performed in right antecubital area for CMP and CBC. Tiger top and lavender top tube drawn.*
1100 a.m.	*Connie Lieseke, CMA (AAMA)*

Procedure 8-2: Venipuncture Using a Syringe

A syringe and needle may be used for venipuncture in situations in which the available veins are prone to move during the blood draw, or when the vein may not be capable of supporting the vacuum exerted from an evacuated tube. This may be the case if the vein is small, or if it lacks "bounce" when palpated. Syringe draws are an excellent choice in the antecubital area when the veins are not quite suitable for a blood draw using an evacuated tube system setup.

TASK

Successfully perform a venipuncture using a syringe. After the blood has been obtained, transfer it successfully into the necessary tubes for analysis. The process must be completed within 5 minutes.

CONDITIONS

- Hand-washing supplies and/or alcohol-based hand sanitizer
- Disposable gloves
- Tourniquet
- 70% isopropyl alcohol
- Syringe (5- to 15-mL capacity)
- 21- to 23-gauge safety enabled needle
- Transfer device

- Laboratory requisition form or labels with specified test
- Evacuated tubes
- 2 x 2 gauze pads
- Adhesive bandage or wrap
- Test tube rack
- Biohazardous sharps container
- Biohazardous disposal bag

CAAHEP/ABHES STANDARDS

 CAAHEP Standards

I.P.I.2: Perform Venipuncture **I.A.I.1:** Apply critical thinking skills in performing patient assessment and care **III.P.III.3:** Select appropriate barrier/personal protective equipment (PPE) for potentially infectious situations

 ABHES Standards

- Medical Office Laboratory Procedures: Collect, label and process specimens: Perform venipuncture
- Medical Office Clinical Procedures: Apply principles of aseptic techniques and infection control
- Medical Office Clinical Procedures: Use Standard Precautions

Procedure	Rationale
1. Gather the requisition form and/or labels for the blood draw, and greet the patient. Identify yourself appropriately.	The requisition or labels are necessary to collect the correct type of specimen. It is always correct practice to identify yourself to the patient.
2. Wash hands (if they are visibly soiled) or apply hand sanitizer. Allow hands to dry completely.	Clean hands stop the spread of infection. Hands should be completely dry before attempting to apply gloves, or it will be difficult to put the gloves on the wet hands.
3. Verify the identification of the patient by asking for his or her name and at least one other unique identifier (such as the patient's birth date). Compare this information to the requisition form or labels.	Patient identification must always be verified using at least two unique factors.
4. Verify whether diet restrictions were followed, and time of last medication dose, if needed.	Many laboratory tests require fasting specimens or other dietary restrictions. Drug dosage times are especially important for appropriate interpretation of the laboratory results.
5. Have the patient sit in the phlebotomy chair with appropriate arm support, and extend his or her arm to expose the antecubital area.	The arm should be supported for the venipuncture process, and the antecubital area will be the first area that is considered for the blood draw.
6. Apply gloves.	Gloves are required for procedures in which there is reasonable anticipation of exposure to blood or other potentially infectious materials.
7. Apply the tourniquet approximately 3 in. above the antecubital area (or above the wrist if a hand draw is necessary) and select an appropriate draw site using palpation. Use the tips of the ring finger and middle finger in a gentle probing motion as the antecubital area is examined. An appropriate vein will feel flexible and firm. Do not allow the tourniquet to remain on the arm for more than 1 minute.	The tourniquet needs to be placed high enough that it will not block the venipuncture site. Only blood vessels that can be palpated should be used for venipuncture; just looking at them is not sufficient. The thumb should never be used to feel for a vein, as there may be a pulse felt from the thumb that can be misleading. The thumb is also not as sensitive as the fingers.
8. While palpating, have the patient make a fist, but *do not* allow the patient to pump his or her hand.	Pumping the hand can cause erroneous results because of hemoconcentration.
9. If an appropriate site is not identified on the first arm, examine the other arm. If the antecubital area is not appropriate on either arm, examine the back of the hands for other opportunities.	It is important to choose the best site before inserting the needle. If the first arm examined doesn't provide a vein that is appropriate, check the other arm. If necessary, the back of the hands may be considered as a blood draw site.
10. Once an appropriate site is selected, determine the direction of the vein; is it running straight up and down or at an angle across the arm? Establish a visible landmark (a mole or dimple in the skin, etc.) for reference.	The needle must be inserted in such a way that it follows the direction of the vein for the best chance of success. A landmark is helpful so that the chosen venipuncture site can be identified after cleaning the area.

Continued

Procedure 8-2: Venipuncture Using a Syringe—cont'd

Procedure	Rationale
11. Have the patient open the hand to relax the fist until the tourniquet is reapplied.	Relaxing the hand will help the blood to flow normally as the site is prepared.
12. Remove the tourniquet.	A tourniquet may not stay on the arm for more than 1 minute, or hemoconcentration may result.
13. Apply 70% isopropyl alcohol to the area in a circular motion with the draw site at the center of the circle. Allow the site to air-dry.	70% isopropyl alcohol will kill most of the bacterial contaminants on the surface of the skin. Never blow or fan the site to speed up the drying process, as this recontaminates the clean area.
14. As the alcohol is drying, assemble the necessary supplies.	Supplies need to be close by for ease of use and patient safety.
a. Open the sterile package holding the syringe	Syringes should remain sterile until the time of use.
b. Pull back and push forward the plunger of the syringe several times to verify whether it moves smoothly. Be certain that the plunger is pushed forward as far as it goes before continuing with the process.	"Exercising" the plunger in this way allows for smooth movement when pulling back the plunger to allow blood to enter the syringe. If the plunger does not move smoothly or is too loose within the barrel of the syringe, it should be discarded.
c. Remove the needle from the sterile wrapper. Do not take off the cap covering the end of the needle until just before insertion into the patient's arm.	The needle must remain sterile until just prior to insertion. It cannot touch other surfaces before piercing the skin of the patient.
d. Attach the needle to the syringe tip.	Verify that this is a secure connection so that blood will not leak out around the needle during the venipuncture process.
e. Place gauze pads and adhesive bandage within reach of the nondominant hand for use at the end of the venipuncture.	Supplies to be used during the venipuncture process should be within easy reach of the nondominant hand to avoid reaching over the site where the needle is inserted in the arm.
f. Organize tubes needed for analysis and unwrap transfer device. Place within easy reach.	When the venipuncture procedure is finished, it is necessary to transfer the blood into the tubes quickly to avoid clot formation in the sample. Organization of supplies before the process is critical.
g. Verify that the tubes are not expired and that the anticoagulant is placed away from the rubber stopper within the tube. (You may need to shake the tube lightly to get the anticoagulant to move away from the stopper.) Check for any obvious defects in the tubes.	Use of an expired tube may result in a loss of vacuum and an unsuccessful blood draw. Potential crossover of anticoagulant from one tube to another should be minimized as much as possible. Defective (such as cracked or chipped tubes) should be discarded immediately.
15. Once the alcohol is dry and the supplies are assembled, reapply the tourniquet. Do not repalpate the venipuncture site, or if absolutely necessary, clean the end of the gloved finger with alcohol before touching the site.	If the site is touched after cleansing, it will need to be cleaned again before the venipuncture can begin.

Procedure	Rationale
16. Have the patient make a fist.	Forming a fist may help with the visualization of the veins once the tourniquet is reapplied.
17. Remove the cap to expose the end of the needle to be inserted into the arm. Do not allow this needle to touch anything before piercing the skin.	Touching this needle to any surface before it pierces the skin will cause contamination and possible introduction of bacteria into the vein.
18. Stabilize the chosen vein by anchoring it with the thumb of the nondominant hand about 2 in. below the draw site, and/or off to the side. Make sure that the skin is pulled taut over the vein.	It is important to stabilize the vein, but if the thumb is placed too close to the draw site, it will be in the way of the needle insertion and could cause interference with the angle used for the process and result in an unsuccessful blood draw.
19. As you prepare to pierce the skin with the needle, it is good practice to warn the patient by saying something like, "Here we go; you will feel a stick."	If the patient is not expecting the skin to be pierced, he or she may be startled and move the arm or hand, causing an unsuccessful venipuncture.
20. Insert the needle at an angle of approximately 15 degrees, with the bevel up. The actual insertion site is approximately $1/4$ to $1/2$ inch below the identified draw site so that the needle is actually inserted into the vein at the chosen site.	If the angle is significantly less or more than 15 degrees, it may slide just above the vein or puncture through both sides of the vein rather than just entering the vein. The bevel facing upward allows the blood to enter the needle with minimal trauma.
21. The needle needs to be inserted quickly, with one smooth gentle motion. As the insertion is accomplished, follow the direction of the vein that was previously identified; if the vein is running at an angle across the arm or hand, this is how the needle should be directed into the vein. Approximately a third of the needle is usually below the surface of the skin when the insertion is complete.	Smooth insertion minimizes the trauma to the patient. It is important to follow the direction of the vein as the needle is inserted; this allows a better opportunity for the blood to enter the needle without obstruction. The needle needs to be inserted far enough to enter the vein, but not so far that it punctures both sides of the vein. 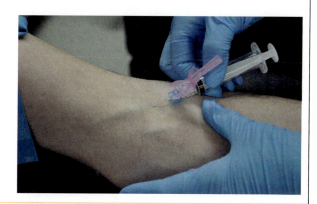

Continued

Procedure 8-2: Venipuncture Using a Syringe—cont'd

Procedure	Rationale
22. When using the syringe technique, there may be a "flash" of blood visible in the hub of the needle as soon as it is inserted in the vein. Gently pull back on the plunger of the syringe to create a vacuum and pull the blood into the syringe.	It is important to pull back relatively slowly because if the plunger is pulled back too fast, it can cause hemolysis. It is also possible that if the vein is small, it will collapse with the pressure applied by pulling the plunger back too quickly.
23. Continue to pull back slowly on the plunger and monitor the volume of blood entering the syringe. Keep gentle pressure on the arm of the patient with the back of the fingers holding the syringe. 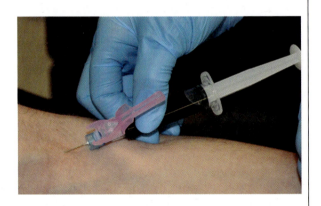	The medical assistant must continue to pull back on the plunger so that the blood will continue to enter the syringe. To keep the needle from moving during the process, pressure should be applied with the back of the fingers holding the syringe.
24. When the required amount of blood has almost been obtained, release the tourniquet and have the patient open his or her fist.	The tourniquet must not stay on longer than 1 minute. It is always necessary to release the tourniquet and have the patient open the fist before the needle is removed from the arm to avoid bleeding from the venipuncture site.
25. As the needle is removed from the skin, place gauze over the site, without applying initial pressure. The needle is to be removed quickly, and at the same angle as the insertion. Do not apply pressure to the site with the gauze until the needle has been removed completely from the skin, as this will cause pain for the patient.	The gauze placed over the site will minimize bleeding as the needle is removed.
26. Ask the patient to apply pressure to the site for 3 to 5 minutes. Do not allow the patient to bend his or her arm.	The pressure should be adequate to stop any bleeding before the patient leaves the drawing area. Bending the arm increases the risk for bleeding and bruise formation.

Procedure	Rationale
27. Once the needle has been removed from the arm, immediately activate the needle safety device. Grasp the needle at its base, and remove it from the syringe. Discard the needle in the biohazardous sharps container. *Never recap contaminated needles.*	The needle must be removed from the syringe so that the transfer device can be applied. Recapping contaminated needles increases the risk of needlestick accidents and potential exposure to bloodborne pathogens.
28. Screw the transfer device onto the end of the syringe filled with blood.	Make sure this is a secure seal so that the blood will flow adequately.
29. While holding the syringe upright, insert each evacuated tube into the open end of the transfer device. Follow the recommended order of draw.	Holding the syringe upright will minimize the opportunity for anticoagulant crossover as the transfer device is used.

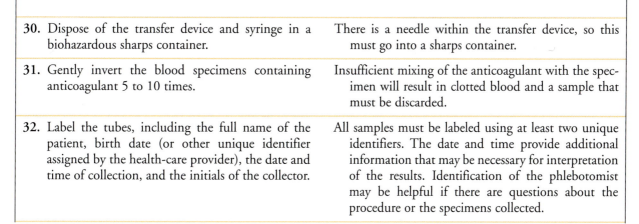

Procedure	Rationale
30. Dispose of the transfer device and syringe in a biohazardous sharps container.	There is a needle within the transfer device, so this must go into a sharps container.
31. Gently invert the blood specimens containing anticoagulant 5 to 10 times.	Insufficient mixing of the anticoagulant with the specimen will result in clotted blood and a sample that must be discarded.
32. Label the tubes, including the full name of the patient, birth date (or other unique identifier assigned by the health-care provider), the date and time of collection, and the initials of the collector.	All samples must be labeled using at least two unique identifiers. The date and time provide additional information that may be necessary for interpretation of the results. Identification of the phlebotomist may be helpful if there are questions about the procedure or the specimens collected.

Continued

Procedure 8-2: Venipuncture Using a Syringe—cont'd

Procedure	Rationale
33. Use the requisition form or the labels to verify that all the necessary tubes were drawn for the specimens ordered.	Verifying the details of the blood draw once more in the presence of the patient allows for a redraw to be performed immediately if something is missing.
34. Observe any special handling instructions for the specimens.	Some types of specimens must remain at room temperature, whereas others may need to be put on ice immediately. This should be information that is ascertained before the procedure starts.
35. Monitor the patient for any signs of distress from the procedure.	These may include pallor, perspiration (especially on the upper lip or forehead), increased anxiety, or light-headedness. If the patient is exhibiting any of these symptoms, it is best to have him or her lie down if possible. This may be easily accomplished if the patient is in a chair that can recline. If not, a cold compress on the forehead and/or the back of the neck may help. Continue to converse with the patient and move the blood out of sight. Ask for assistance if you feel that your patient is feeling faint. If the patient loses consciousness, it may be necessary to lower him or her to the floor from the phlebotomy chair.
36. Once the tubes have been labeled, check the draw site for bleeding. If it has not stopped bleeding, apply pressure for another few minutes, and if the bleeding is still present, contact a physician.	It is important to look under the gauze for 2 or 3 seconds before applying the adhesive bandage to be certain that the site has actually stopped bleeding.
37. If the bleeding has subsided, apply an adhesive bandage, but leave the gauze in place to allow for additional pressure.	Self-adhesive bandages (such as Coban) may be wrapped around the site rather than applying an adhesive to the skin directly. Self-adhesive bandages may be especially effective for those patients who are on anticoagulant therapy.
38. Advise the patient to avoid heavy lifting or excessive exercise of the arm used for venipuncture for at least 1 hour.	Heavy lifting or exercise could cause the site to resume bleeding.
39. Assist the patient to stand (if necessary) and thank them for their cooperation.	Patients may be a bit light-headed and assistance may be needed when he or she first stands up.
40. Discard all trash, and place the tubes in an appropriate vessel for processing. Never touch full tubes of blood without wearing gloves.	Touching the tubes of blood without wearing gloves offers potential opportunities for exposure to bloodborne pathogens.
41. Remove gloves and sanitize hands.	Hands must always be sanitized after removing gloves.

Procedure	Rationale
42. Document the procedure in the patient's chart as well as on the requisition form. Include the date and time of collection, what was collected, and if there were any circumstances that were out of the ordinary. Also document where the vein was accessed (such as right arm, left hand, etc.). The documentation should include the type (color) of tubes drawn, as well as the identity of the person who collected the sample.	All patient interactions must be carefully documented. The site used for vein access should always be written in the chart or on the requisition form so that if there are any negative outcomes associated with the procedure, the site has been noted.

Date	
1/18/2020:	*Phlebotomy performed in left antecubital area for H&H. Lavender top tube drawn.*
1100 a.m.	*Connie Lieseke, CMA (AAMA)*

Procedure 8-3: Venipuncture Using the Butterfly (Winged Infusion) System

The butterfly system is often used for obtaining blood from patients with small, fragile veins. It is the system of choice when performing blood draws from the hand of patients. When utilized for venipuncture, 23-gauge needles are usually used.

TASK

Successfully perform a venipuncture using a butterfly (winged infusion) system. The process must be completed within 5 minutes.

CONDITIONS

- Hand-washing supplies and/or alcohol-based hand sanitizer
- Disposable gloves
- Tourniquet
- 70% isopropyl alcohol
- Butterfly needle (winged infusion set)
- Evacuated tube holder and luer adapter, or syringe and transfer device
- Laboratory requisition or labels with specified test
- Evacuated tubes
- 2 x 2 gauze pads
- Adhesive bandage or wrap
- Test tube rack
- Biohazardous sharps container
- Biohazardous disposal bag

CAAHEP/ABHES STANDARDS

CAAHEP Standards

I.P.I.2: Perform Venipuncture **I.A.I.1:** Apply critical thinking skills in performing patient assessment and care **III.P.III.3:** Select appropriate barrier/personal protective equipment (PPE) for potentially infectious situations

ABHES Standards

- Medical Office Laboratory Procedures: Collect, label and process specimens: Perform venipuncture
- Medical Office Clinical Procedures: Apply principles of aseptic techniques and infection control
- Medical Office Clinical Procedures: Use Standard Precautions

Continued

Procedure 8-3: Venipuncture Using the Butterfly (Winged Infusion) System—cont'd

Procedure	Rationale
1. Gather the requisition and/or labels for the blood draw, and greet the patient. Identify yourself appropriately.	The requisition or labels are necessary to collect the correct type of specimen. It is always correct practice to identify yourself to the patient.
2. Wash hands (if they are visibly soiled) or apply hand sanitizer. Allow hands to dry completely.	Clean hands stop the spread of infection. Hands should be completely dry before attempting to apply gloves, or it will be difficult to put the gloves on the wet hands.
3. Verify the identification of the patient by asking for his or her name and at least one other unique identifier (such as the patient's birth date). Compare this information to the requisition or labels.	Patient identification must always be verified using at least two unique factors.
4. Verify whether dietary restrictions were followed, and time of last medication dose, if needed.	Many laboratory tests require fasting specimens or other dietary restrictions. Drug dosage times are especially important for appropriate interpretation of the laboratory results.
5. Have the patient sit in the phlebotomy chair with appropriate arm support, and extend his or her arm to expose the antecubital area.	The arm should be supported for the venipuncture process, and the antecubital area will be the first area that is considered for the blood draw.
6. Apply gloves.	Gloves are required for procedures in which there is reasonable anticipation of exposure to blood or other potentially infectious materials.
7. Apply the tourniquet approximately 3 in. above the antecubital area (or above the wrist if a hand draw is necessary) and select an appropriate draw site using palpation. Use the tips of the ring finger and middle finger in a gentle probing motion as the antecubital area is examined. An appropriate vein will feel flexible and firm. Do not allow the tourniquet to remain on the arm for more than 1 minute.	The tourniquet needs to be placed high enough that it will not block the venipuncture site. Only blood vessels that can be palpated should be used for venipuncture; just looking at them is not sufficient. The thumb should never be used to feel for a vein, as there may be a pulse felt from the thumb that can be misleading. The thumb is also not as sensitive as the fingers.
8. While palpating, have the patient make a fist, but *do not* allow them to pump his or her hand.	Pumping the hand can cause erroneous results because of hemoconcentration.
9. If an appropriate site is not identified on the first arm, examine the other arm. If the antecubital area is not appropriate on either arm, examine the back of the hands for other opportunities.	It is important to choose the best site before inserting the needle. If the first arm examined doesn't provide a vein that is appropriate, check the other arm. If necessary, the back of the hands may be considered.

Procedure	Rationale
10. Once an appropriate site is selected, determine the direction of the vein; is it running straight up and down or at an angle across the arm? Establish a visible landmark (a mole or dimple in the skin, etc.) for reference.	The needle must be inserted in such a way that it follows the direction of the vein for the best chance of success. A landmark is helpful so that the chosen venipuncture site can be identified after cleaning the area.
11. Have the patient open the hand to relax the fist until the tourniquet is reapplied.	Relaxing the hand will help the blood to flow normally as the site is prepared.
12. Remove the tourniquet.	A tourniquet may not stay on the arm for more than 1 minute, or hemoconcentration may result.
13. Apply 70% isopropyl alcohol to the area in a circular motion with the draw site at the center of the circle. Allow the site to air-dry.	70% isopropyl alcohol will kill most of the bacterial contaminants on the surface of the skin. Never blow or fan the site to speed up the drying process, as this recontaminates the clean area.
14. As the alcohol is drying, assemble the necessary supplies. Start by opening the sterile package holding the butterfly setup and uncurling the tubing by gently stretching it.	Supplies need to be close by for ease of use and patient safety. The butterfly system should remain sterile until just before use. If the tubing stays tightly curled, it is difficult to use it effectively.
Option 1. Butterfly System With a Syringe	
a. Open the sterile package holding the syringe b. Pull back and push forward the plunger of the syringe several times to verify whether it moves smoothly.	Syringes should remain sterile until the time of use. "Exercising" the plunger in this way allows for smooth movement when pulling back the plunger to allow blood to enter the syringe. If the plunger does not move smoothly or is too loose within the syringe, it should be discarded.
c. Attach the end of the butterfly tubing to the syringe. d. Open a transfer device and place within reach.	This tubing needs to be attached securely to allow the blood to enter the syringe. There is a limited amount of time allowed to transfer the blood from the syringe to the tubes before it clots, so it is important to have the transfer device ready.
Option 2. Butterfly System With Evacuated Tube Holder	
a. Verify that the butterfly system has a luer adapter to be used with the evacuated tube holder. b. Screw the butterfly tubing with the adapter attached into the evacuated tube holder.	The luer adapter has a needle covered with a rubber sleeve that pierces the tubes when using the evacuated tube holder. The tubing and the holder must be securely attached to one another to allow the blood to flow appropriately into the tubes.

Continued

Procedure 8-3: Venipuncture Using the Butterfly (Winged Infusion) System—cont'd

Procedure	Rationale
15. Place gauze pads and adhesive bandage within reach of the nondominant hand for use at the end of the venipuncture.	Supplies to be used during the venipuncture process should be within easy reach of the nondominant hand to avoid reaching over the site where the needle is inserted in the arm.
16. Organize tubes needed for analysis and place within easy reach.	To allow for the blood collection process to proceed smoothly, it is necessary organize the supplies before getting started.
17. Verify that the tubes are not expired and that the anticoagulant is placed away from the rubber stopper within the tube. (You may need to shake the tube lightly to get the anticoagulant to move away from the stopper.) Check for any obvious defects in the tubes.	Use of an expired tube may result in a loss of vacuum and an unsuccessful blood draw. Potential crossover of anticoagulant from one tube to another should be minimized as much as possible. Defective (such as cracked or chipped tubes) should be discarded immediately.
18. Once the alcohol is dry and the supplies are assembled, reapply the tourniquet. Do not repalpate the venipuncture site, or if absolutely necessary, clean the end of the gloved finger with alcohol before touching the site.	If the site is touched after cleansing, it will need to be cleaned again before the venipuncture can begin.
19. Have the patient make a fist.	Forming a fist may help with the visualization of the veins once the tourniquet is reapplied.
20. Remove the cap to expose the end of the needle to be inserted into the arm. Do not allow this needle to touch anything before piercing the skin.	Touching this needle to any surface before it pierces the skin will cause contamination and possible introduction of bacteria into the vein.
21. Stabilize the chosen vein by anchoring it with the thumb of the nondominant hand about 2 in. below the draw site, and/or off to the side. Make sure that the skin is pulled taut over the vein.	It is important to stabilize the vein, but if the thumb is placed too close to the draw site, it will be in the way of the needle insertion and could cause interference with the angle used for the process and result in an unsuccessful blood draw.
22. As you prepare to pierce the skin with the needle, it is good practice to warn the patient by saying something like, "Here we go; you will feel a stick."	If the patient is not expecting the skin to be pierced, he or she may be startled and move the arm or hand, causing an unsuccessful venipuncture.
23. Grasp the butterfly needle with the wings on either side. The textured area of the plastic wings is designed to be against the fingers; this allows the bevel of the needle to face upward.	If the needle is not grasped appropriately, the bevel will point downward and could affect the success of the blood draw.

Procedure	Rationale
24. Insert the needle at an angle of 5 to 10 degrees, with the bevel up. The actual insertion site is approximately $1/4$ to $1/2$ inch below the identified draw site so that the needle is actually inserted into the vein at the chosen site.	If the angle is significantly less or more than 5 to 10 degrees, it may slide just above the vein or puncture through both sides of the vein rather than just entering the vein. The bevel facing upward allows the blood to enter the needle with minimal trauma. 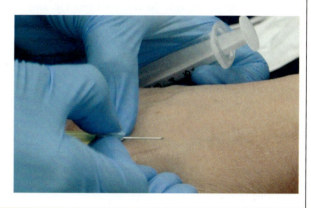
25. The needle needs to be inserted quickly, with one smooth gentle motion. As the insertion is accomplished, follow the direction of the vein that was previously identified; if the vein is running at an angle across the arm or hand, this is how the needle should be directed into the vein. Approximately a third of the needle is usually below the surface of the skin when the insertion is complete.	Smooth insertion minimizes the trauma to the patient. It is important to follow the direction of the vein as the needle is inserted; this allows a better opportunity for the blood to enter the needle without obstruction. The needle needs to be inserted far enough to enter the vein, but not so far that it punctures both sides of the vein.
26. When the needle pierces the vein, the blood will immediately be present in the tubing. As soon as there is blood present, begin to pull the plunger of the syringe back slowly, if using a syringe. If the evacuated tube holder is used, push on the first tube to be drawn so that the vacuum pulls the blood through the tubing.	The blood will not flow into the tubing adequately without the vacuum of the plunger or the evacuated tube. Do not pull back quickly, or it may cause hemolysis or collapse the vein.
27. If using the syringe system, continue to pull back slowly on the plunger and monitor the volume of blood entering the syringe. Change the evacuated tubes as needed if using these directly to draw the blood. Keep gentle pressure on the arm of the patient with the back of the fingers holding the butterfly setup.	The medical assistant must continue to pull back on the plunger so that the blood will continue to enter the syringe. To keep the needle from moving during the process, pressure should be applied with the back of the fingers holding the syringe.
28. When the required amount of blood has almost been obtained, release the tourniquet and have the patient open the fist.	The tourniquet must not stay on longer than 1 minute. It is always necessary to release the tourniquet and have the patient open the fist before the needle is removed from the arm to avoid bleeding from the venipuncture site.

Continued

Procedure 8-3: Venipuncture Using the Butterfly (Winged Infusion) System—cont'd

Procedure	Rationale
29. As the needle is removed from the skin, place gauze over the site, without applying initial pressure. The needle is to be removed quickly, and at the same angle as the insertion. Do not apply pressure to the site with the gauze until the needle has been removed completely from the skin, as this will cause pain for the patient.	The gauze placed over the site will minimize bleeding as the needle is removed.
30. Ask the patient to apply pressure to the site for 3 to 5 minutes. Do not allow the patient to bend his or her arm if the draw was performed in the antecubital space.	The pressure should be adequate to stop any bleeding before the patient leaves the drawing area. Bending the arm increases the risk for bleeding and bruise formation.
31. Once the needle has been removed from the arm, immediately activate the needle safety device.	The safety device may be a push-button device that is activated while the needle is still in the skin, or it may be activated right after removal. It is imperative that the medical assistant keeps his or her fingers behind the needle while activating the safety device.
32. If a syringe was used for the procedure, remove the tubing from the end of the syringe and discard the butterfly unit into a biohazardous sharps container. If an evacuated tube system was used, discard the evacuated tube holder with the butterfly setup.	The tubing must be removed so that the transfer device can be applied to put the blood into the tubes.
33. Screw the transfer device onto the end of the syringe filled with blood.	Make sure this is a secure seal so that the blood will flow adequately.
34. While holding the syringe upright, insert each evacuated tube into the open end of the transfer device. Follow the recommended order of draw.	Holding the syringe upright will minimize the opportunity for anticoagulant crossover as the transfer device is used.
35. Dispose of the transfer device and syringe in a biohazardous sharps container.	There is a needle within the transfer device, so this must go into a sharps container.

Procedure	Rationale
36. Gently invert the blood specimens containing anticoagulant 5 to 10 times.	Insufficient mixing of the anticoagulant with the specimen will result in clotted blood and a sample that must be discarded.
37. Label the tubes, including the full name of the patient, birth date (or other unique identifier assigned by the health-care provider), the date and time of collection, and the initials of the collector.	All samples must be labeled using at least two unique identifiers. The date and time provides additional information that may be necessary for interpretation of the results. Identification of the phlebotomist may be helpful if there are questions about the procedure or the specimens collected.
38. Use the requisition form or the labels to verify that all the necessary tubes were drawn for the specimens ordered.	Verifying the details of the blood draw once more in the presence of the patient allows for a redraw to be performed immediately if something is missing.
39. Observe any special handling instructions for the specimens.	Some types of specimens must remain at room temperature, whereas others may need to be put on ice immediately. This should be information that is ascertained before the procedure starts.
40. Monitor the patient for any signs of distress from the procedure.	These may include pallor, perspiration (especially on the upper lip or forehead), increased anxiety, or light-headedness. If the patient is exhibiting any of these symptoms, it is best to have him or her lie down if possible. This may be easily accomplished if the patient is in a chair that can recline. If not, a cold compress on the forehead and/or the back of the neck may help. Continue to converse with the patient and move the blood out of sight. Ask for assistance if you feel that your patient is feeling faint. If the patient loses consciousness, it may be necessary to lower him or her to the floor from the phlebotomy chair.
41. Once the tubes have been labeled, check the draw site for bleeding. If it has not stopped bleeding, apply pressure for another few minutes, and if the bleeding is still present, contact a physician.	It is important to look under the gauze for 2 or 3 seconds before applying the adhesive bandage to be certain that the site has actually stopped bleeding.
42. If the bleeding has subsided, apply an adhesive bandage, but leave the gauze in place to allow for additional pressure.	Self-adhesive bandages (such as Coban) may be wrapped around the site rather than applying an adhesive to the skin directly. Self-adhesive bandages may be especially effective for those patients who are on anticoagulant therapy.
43. Advise the patient to avoid heavy lifting or excessive exercise of the arm used for venipuncture for at least 1 hour.	Heavy lifting or exercise could cause the site to resume bleeding.

Continued

Procedure 8-3: Venipuncture Using the Butterfly (Winged Infusion) System—cont'd

Procedure	Rationale
44. Assist the patient to stand (if necessary) and thank him or her for being cooperative.	Patients may be a bit light-headed and assistance may be needed when he or she first stands up.
45. Discard all trash, and place the tubes in an appropriate vessel for processing. Never touch full tubes of blood without wearing gloves.	Touching the tubes of blood without wearing gloves offers potential opportunities for exposure to blood-borne pathogens.
46. Remove gloves and sanitize hands.	Hands must always be sanitized after removing gloves.
47. Document the procedure in the patient's chart as well as on the requisition form. Include the date and time of collection, what was collected, and if there were any circumstances that were out of the ordinary. Also document where the vein was accessed (such as right arm, left hand, etc.). The documentation should include the type (color) of tubes drawn, as well as the identity of the person who collected the sample.	All patient interactions must be carefully documented. The site used for vein access should always be written in the chart or on the requisition form so that if there are any negative outcomes associated with the procedure, the site has been noted.

Date	
1/18/2020:	*Phlebotomy performed in right hand for BMP and Hematocrit level. Lavender top tube drawn.*
1100 a.m.	*Connie Lieseke, CMA (AAMA)*

Procedure 8-4: Blood Collection From a Capillary Puncture

Capillary punctures are performed frequently to obtain blood for CLIA-waived tests, as well as to draw blood for testing on children and infants. Blood obtained by capillary puncture is the preferred specimen type in these situations. In some situations in which it has been difficult to perform a successful venipuncture for adults, a capillary puncture specimen may also be obtained for testing.

TASK

Successfully perform a capillary puncture and obtain blood necessary for the tests ordered. The process must be completed within 5 minutes.

CONDITIONS

- Hand-washing supplies and/or alcohol-based hand sanitizer
- Disposable gloves
- 70% isopropyl alcohol
- Disposable safety equipped lancet
- Laboratory requisition form or labels with specified test
- Microcollection tubes
- 2 x 2 gauze pads
- Hand warmer (if necessary)
- Adhesive bandage or wrap
- Biohazardous sharps container
- Biohazardous disposal bag

CAAHEP/ABHES STANDARDS

 CAAHEP Standards

I.P.I.3: Perform Capillary Puncture   **I.A.I.1:** Apply critical thinking skills in performing patient assessment and care **III.P.III.3:** Select appropriate barrier/personal protective equipment (PPE) for potentially infectious situations

 ABHES Standards

• Medical Office Laboratory Procedures: Collect, label and process specimens: Perform capillary puncture
• Medical Office Clinical Procedures: Apply principles of aseptic techniques and infection control
• Medical Office Clinical Procedures: Use Standard Precautions

Procedure	Rationale
1. Gather the requisition form and/or labels for the blood draw, and greet the patient. Identify yourself appropriately.	The requisition or labels are necessary to collect the correct type of specimen. It is always correct practice to identify yourself to the patient.
2. Wash hands (if they are visibly soiled) or apply hand sanitizer. Allow hands to dry completely.	Clean hands stop the spread of infection. Hands should be completely dry before attempting to apply gloves, or it will be difficult to put the gloves on the wet hands.
3. Verify the identification of the patient by asking for his or her name and at least one other unique identifier (such as the patient's birth date). Compare this information to the requisition or labels.	Patient identification must always be verified using at least two unique factors.
4. Verify whether dietary restrictions were followed, and time of last medication dose, if needed.	Many laboratory tests require fasting specimens or other dietary restrictions. Drug dosage times are especially important for appropriate interpretation of the laboratory results.
5. Have the patient sit in the phlebotomy chair with appropriate arm support, and extend his or her arm so that the hand may be accessed easily. Massage the fingertips if necessary for warmth, or apply a commercial warming device, hand warmer, or warm towel.	The patient should be secure and comfortable for the capillary puncture process. The fingers must be warm for a successful capillary blood draw; warming the site and massaging will allow much better blood flow. A commercial warming device works well, or immersing the finger or heel in warm water will also help. The temperature of the warming device or water should not exceed 42°C (108°F). Three to five minutes is generally sufficient to warm the site.
6. Assemble necessary equipment within reach. This includes the necessary tubes for the tests ordered, gauze, alcohol, and an adhesive bandage.	Once the incision is made, the process will go quickly, so it is important to have all supplies within reach.
7. Apply gloves.	Gloves are required for procedures in which there is reasonable anticipation of exposure to blood or other potentially infectious materials.

Continued

Procedure 8-4: Blood Collection From a Capillary Puncture—cont'd

Procedure	Rationale
8. Choose the appropriate finger for the blood draw, and disinfect the fingertip with an alcohol swab. Allow the alcohol to dry completely before performing the skin puncture. Do not fan or blow on the site to dry the alcohol.	For both adults and children, the ring finger or middle finger should be used. The index finger is more sensitive and more callused, and the little finger does not have enough flesh to protect the bone from puncture. The thumb should never be used as a capillary puncture site. The alcohol may contaminate the specimen if not allowed to dry completely before performing the puncture. Blowing or fanning the site may recontaminate the skin after cleansing.
9. Choose the correct lancet for the age of the patient and the site selected. The number of tubes to be drawn must also be taken into consideration when choosing a device to use for the incision.	Lancets come with different depths and widths. There are recommendations for ages and uses provided by the manufacturers. Lancet devices designed for home use that produce only a drop of blood do not provide enough blood to be used for microcollection tubes.
10. Remove the cap from the lancet device. Do not allow the surface to be placed against the patient's skin or to touch anything else before it is utilized.	This part of the device must remain sterile until use.
11. Perform the dermal puncture by holding the lancet device firmly against the skin and activating the device. Use the lateral side of the ring or middle fingertip, perpendicular (opposite) to the lines of the fingerprint. Immediately discard the lancet into a biohazardous sharps container.	The lateral sides of the fingers need to be used to avoid potential damage to the bone. The incision needs to be perpendicular to the lines of the fingerprint to keep the blood from following the fingerprint and flowing away from the incision site.
12. Wipe away the first drop of blood, then gently massage the finger to achieve blood flow.	The first drop of blood is contaminated with tissue fluid, and must be discarded. The finger should be continuously massaged from the proximal to the distal end of the fingertip. Do not squeeze right at the collection site as this can contaminate the specimen with tissue fluid and cause erroneous results.
13. Fill the required tubes in the correct order of draw. If anticoagulant is used in the tubes, tap them against the countertop to mix the specimen as the tube is filled. Do not touch the collection device against the incision while collecting the specimen. Instead, touch it to the drop of blood as it forms at the collection site.	The capillary order of draw must be followed to avoid cross-contamination. The tubes must be mixed well during the collection process to avoid clotting. The collection device is to be used only to collect blood that is free flowing; scraping or touching the incision site can cause infection and/or irritation.
14. If a microhematocrit tube is to be filled, hold it horizontal to the site to avoid introduction of air bubbles to the specimen.	Capillary tubes that are held at a slant allow air to enter the microhematocrit tube. The capillary tube will fill with capillary action if held horizontal to the incision site. Plug the end of the capillary tube when filled appropriately.

Procedure	Rationale
15. When the desired tubes have been collected, apply gauze to the puncture site and instruct the patient to apply direct pressure, if he or she is capable.	Direct pressure helps the bleeding to stop.
16. Tightly cap and invert any microcollection tubes containing anticoagulant 8 to 10 times.	Tubes must be thoroughly mixed to avoid clotting.
17. Label the tubes with the patient's name, birth date (or other unique identification number), your initials, the date and the time of the blood draw.	For microcollection tubes, it may be necessary to write this information on a label to be attached to the tube. The microcollection tubes may also be placed inside larger tubes that are labeled appropriately. Capillary tubes may also be labeled in this way, as it is very difficult to label the actual collection container.
18. Use the requisition form or the labels to verify that all the necessary tubes were drawn for the specimens ordered.	Verifying the details of the blood draw once more in the presence of the patient allows for a redraw to be performed immediately if something is missing.
19. Observe any special handling instructions for the specimens.	Some types of specimens must remain at room temperature, whereas others may need to be put on ice immediately. This should be information that is ascertained before the procedure starts.
20. Monitor the patient for any signs of distress from the procedure.	These may include pallor, perspiration (especially on the upper lip or forehead), increased anxiety, or light-headedness. If the patient is exhibiting any of these symptoms, it is best to have him or her lie down if possible. This may be easily accomplished if the patient is in a chair that can recline. If not, a cold compress on the forehead and/or the back of the neck may help. Continue to converse with the patient and move the blood out of sight. Ask for assistance if you feel that your patient is feeling faint. If the patient loses consciousness, it may be necessary to lower him or her to the floor from the phlebotomy chair.
21. Once the tubes have been labeled, check the draw site for bleeding. If it has not stopped bleeding, apply pressure for another few minutes, and if the bleeding is still present after 5 minutes, contact a physician.	It is important to look under the gauze for 2 or 3 seconds before applying the adhesive bandage to be certain that the site has actually stopped bleeding.
22. If the bleeding has subsided, apply an adhesive bandage, but leave the gauze in place to allow for additional pressure.	Adhesive bandages should not be applied for capillary punctures on small children as they may pose a choking hazard. Newborns may have adhesive bandages applied if they are not able to remove them. Self-adhesive bandages (such as Coban) may be wrapped around the site rather than applying an adhesive directly to the skin. Self-adhesive bandages may be especially effective for those patients who are on anticoagulant therapy.

Continued

Procedure 8-4: Blood Collection From a Capillary Puncture—cont'd

Procedure	Rationale
23. Assist the patient to stand (if necessary) and thank them for their cooperation.	Patients may be a bit light-headed, and assistance may be needed when they first stand up.
24. Discard all trash, and place the tubes in an appropriate vessel for processing. Never touch full tubes of blood without wearing gloves.	Touching the tubes of blood without wearing gloves offers potential opportunities for exposure to bloodborne pathogens.
25. Remove gloves and sanitize hands.	Hands must always be sanitized after removing gloves.
26. Document the procedure in the patient's chart as well as on the requisition form. Include the date and time of collection, what was collected, and if there were any circumstances that were out of the ordinary. Also document where the specimen was obtained (such as right middle finger, left hand, etc.). The documentation should include the type (color) of tubes drawn, as well as the identity of the person who collected the sample.	All patient interactions must be carefully documented. The site where the specimen was obtained should always be written in the chart or on the requisition form so that if there are any negative outcomes associated with the procedure, the site has been noted.

Date	
1/18/2020:	*Capillary puncture performed in right ring finger for CBC. Lavender top microcollection tube drawn.*
1100 a.m.	*Connie Lieseke, CMA (AAMA)*

the analysis. It is the job of the medical assistant to process the specimen properly so that it can be tested.

Obtaining Serum for Testing

When blood is allowed to clot and is then spun down in a centrifuge, the liquid portion is called **serum.** Serum is plasma that no longer has the clotting factors included, as they have been used up in the blood clot that formed in the tube. Analytes such as glucose, lipids, cholesterol, electrolytes, hormones, enzymes, and antibodies may be dissolved in serum. To isolate this liquid so that the tests can be performed, it is necessary to separate it from the rest of the blood specimen. Whenever drawing blood for serum or plasma, it is necessary to collect approximately 2.5 times as much blood as the volume needed for the testing procedure. For instance, if there is 1 mL of serum required for an electrolyte test, the medical assistant drawing the blood should obtain at least 2.5 mL of blood.

Tubes without anticoagulants are used to collect samples for serum testing. These include red top tubes, as well as those that contain thixotropic gel and clot activators. The blood must be allowed to stand for at least 30 to 45 minutes at room temperature to clot thoroughly before the specimen can be further processed. If the specimen is spun in the centrifuge before there is a chance for a solid clot to form, the clotting factors will not be mixed in with the cells at the bottom of the tube when centrifuged; instead, they will form a large fibrin clot in the serum layer. A *fibrin clot* is a soft, sticky mass that makes it very difficult to separate out serum for testing. Although the tube must be allowed to clot completely before centrifuging, it should not be more than an hour after the blood draw is performed before the tube is spun, as prolonged contact with the cells in the tube may allow chemical changes to take place in the serum, which will affect the test results. Potential changes may include a decreased serum glucose level, an increased serum iron level, and elevated serum potassium levels, among others.

To fully separate the serum from the cells, the specimen should be centrifuged for at least 10 minutes. The serum may then be removed from the specimen and placed in a transfer tube. There are various methods that may be used to remove the liquid portion of the blood; remember that regardless of the method used for separation, adequate personal protective equipment should be worn at all times, including a face shield or plastic-mounted barrier shield, gloves and a laboratory coat. (See Fig. 8-15.) The methods that may be used for separation include the following:

- **SST or PST tubes:** These tubes contain a thixotropic gel that forms a barrier between the cells and the serum (or plasma with PST tubes) so that the liquid can remain in the tube, but be separated from the cells. If it is necessary to remove the serum and put it in a transfer tube, it can be poured out because the gel forms a solid barrier to the cells in the bottom of the tube.
- **Transfer pipette:** A pipette may be used to aspirate the liquid out of the tube and transfer it into another tube. Care must be taken not to aspirate out any of the cells that are present in the bottom of the tube; if the serum appears a hazy red color while aspiration is taking place, it should be spun again to remove any cells that may have been accidentally aspirated into the specimen. If the serum still appears to be red after recentrifugation, it is hemolyzed and the specimen will, in most circumstances, have to be redrawn. If the serum is no longer red, separate the serum again from the cells that have settled to the bottom of the tube.
- **Plunger-type separators:** These are devices that have a filter on one end of a plastic tube, with an opening

at the other end. After the specimen has been centrifuged, the rubber stopper is removed from the top of the tube and the filter end of the separator is carefully inserted into the specimen tube and pushed down through the serum or plasma. Proper protective equipment must be used when performing this procedure to keep from potentially splashing the liquid into the eyes or mucous membranes. Also, once the separator has been place in the tube, it is important to pull it back up a bit to provide an air barrier between the serum and the cells. This keeps the blood cells in the bottom of the tube from being in contact with the serum, causing chemical changes as they metabolize nutrients in the liquid.

Test Your Knowledge 8-16

How are specimens processed if serum is to be separated from the cells?   (Outcome 8-17)

Specimen storage instructions for most chemistry tests will advise that the serum and/or plasma be refrigerated within a few hours after processing to protect the various analytes from changing in concentration. Follow the directions provided in the laboratory directory for handling the serum specimen after it has been separated. Also, if a transfer tube is used, the labeling on the tube is critical. Not only does the patient information need to be included, but there also has to be a notation of the

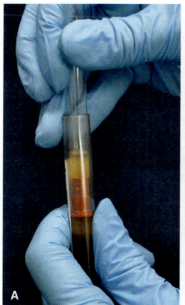 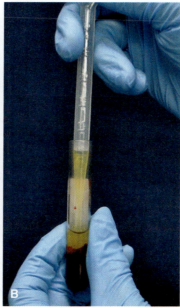

Figure 8-15. A and B.   (A) Serum tube after centrifugation and (B) various devices used for separation of serum.

type of specimen (serum or plasma) and the type of anticoagulant present in the tube, because many body fluids are similar in appearance. Transfer tubes are available that are color coded to match the color tube originally used for the specimen collection, which may help eliminate confusion.

Obtaining Plasma for Testing

The liquid portion of the blood in our bodies is **plasma.** Plasma is made up of approximately 90% water, with dissolved substances making up the remaining portion. Plasma may be analyzed for levels of chemicals involved in the clotting process such as fibrinogen and prothrombin. Other common tests performed on plasma specimens include levels of electrolytes, calcium, glucose, and creatinine.

Because plasma is the liquid portion of the blood that contains factors that contribute to clotting, a specimen that is to be used for plasma testing must not be allowed to clot. A tube that contains an anticoagulant (such as heparin) must be used for the collection. The medical assistant should consult the laboratory directory to see what type of anticoagulant is to be used for specimen collection before the venipuncture is performed. It may be possible to use a PST tube, which contains anticoagulant and a thixotropic gel that will separate the plasma from the blood cells in the specimen after centrifugation. As in the case of serum, it is necessary to collect a blood specimen that is approximately 2.5 times the required volume for the test ordered. Appropriate labeling of the transfer tube is essential; remember to include a notation that the fluid is plasma in addition to the patient's name and other necessary information.

Unlike the process for obtaining a serum sample, plasma samples should be well mixed, then centrifuged as soon as possible. There is no need to allow the specimen to sit for an extended period of time before centrifuging, as the blood is not going to clot in the tube. This makes plasma samples the specimen of choice for most STAT chemistry tests, because the samples can be processed and the test performed quickly after collection.

After centrifugation, a sample that has had anticoagulant added will separate into three layers. This will include a layer containing the red blood cells, topped by a very small layer that contains the white cells and platelets (sometimes called the buffy coat), with the liquid plasma present as the top layer in the tube. The tube in Figure 8-16 is an example of the appearance of a tube to be used for plasma separation after centrifugation.

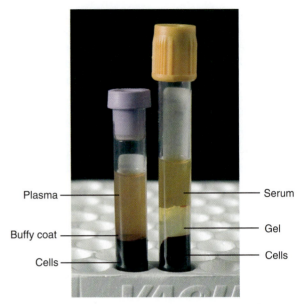

Plasma —
Buffy coat —
Cells —
— Serum
— Gel
— Cells

Figure 8-16   The tube on the left shows plasma after centrifugation. Note the cells, buffy coat, and plasma. The tube on the right shows serum separated from the clotted cell by gel. *Reprinted with permission from Eagle S, Brassington C, Dailey C, and Goretti C:* The Professional Medical Assistant: An Integrative, Teamwork-Based Approach. *Philadelphia: FA Davis, 2009.*

The actual separation methods for plasma are the same as those used for serum, including the use of a PST tube, the transfer pipette, or the plunger-type separators. Remember, whenever separating the liquid portion of the blood from the cells, it is imperative that the appropriate personal protective equipment is used to protect the employee from potential exposure. Removal of the rubberized stoppers may create an aerosol that could get into the mouth or eyes, so face shields must be worn in addition to gloves and a protective laboratory coat. Also, all supplies must be disposed of appropriately; the stoppers and any other specimen containers must be disposed of as biohazardous materials.

Test Your Knowledge 8-17
Describe one way that serum and plasma are different.
(Outcome 8-18)

Whole Blood Specimens

Tests that count or examine the cells present in the blood require a whole blood specimen. These tests are often performed in the hematology department, and include complete blood counts, platelet counts, and hemoglobin and hematocrit tests. For tests requiring whole blood specimens, the blood is drawn into tubes that contain anticoagulants so that the cells are not involved in clot formation, which would make it very difficult to count the cells or examine their appearance. Potassium EDTA is the anticoagulant that is usually preferred; this is present in the lavender top evacuated tubes.

Whole blood specimens are to be well mixed at the time of the initial blood draw, and again just prior to analysis. The specimens used for whole blood testing are not to be centrifuged, as the analysis is performed on the formed elements within the sample. In some small physician office laboratories, the medical assistant may place the whole blood specimens directly on a "rocker" that keeps the specimen mixed until the analysis can be performed. Remember that the mixing and inversion of these samples must be a gentle motion to avoid damaging the cells. Eight inversions of the tube immediately after drawing the blood should provide appropriate mixing of the specimen.

Test Your Knowledge 8-18

True or False: Tests that utilize whole blood specimens require that the specimen be centrifuged before testing.

(Outcome 8-17)

Unaccepable Specimen Types

In certain situations, the specimen collected and processed will be rejected for the test ordered. There are numerous reasons for specimen rejection, including the following:

- **Hemolyzed specimens:** *Hemolysis* means that the red blood cells in the specimen have been damaged and broken. It may be a result of a traumatic venipuncture in which the cells were damaged as they entered the needle, or hemolysis may be the result of mishandling the tube after the blood draw. Hemolysis is evident in the specimen after centrifuging by the presence of a pink to red tint in the plasma or serum. (Fig. 8-17 is an example of a hemolyzed specimen.) Potassium, magnesium, and iron levels are examples of tests for which a hemolyzed specimen is unacceptable. To avoid hemolysis, be sure that the tubes used for the blood draw are kept at room temperature, and be sure to use the appropriate sized needle for the draw. Also, if using a syringe, do not pull back on the plunger with a great deal of force, as this may damage the cells. Use good technique when performing venipunctures, and *gently* invert all tubes when mixing.

- **Lipemic specimens: Lipemia** is the presence of excess lipids (fatty molecules) in the blood. Plasma or serum in a lipemic specimen will appear cloudy or milk-like after centrifugation. These lipid molecules interfere with the testing methods for many analytes. Some laboratories are capable of clearing the specimen with a special type of centrifuge, whereas others will reject the lipemic specimens (Fig. 8-17).

- **Quantity not sufficient:** When the medical assistant does not draw enough blood to perform the tests ordered, the specimen may be rejected as **quality not sufficient (QNS)** because the amount drawn is not enough for the tests to be performed on it. In almost all situations, these samples will need to be redrawn so that there is enough specimen to complete the tests ordered.

- **Clotted specimens:** When a whole blood specimen is necessary for the test ordered, a clotted specimen is unacceptable. The clotting process draws in the cells in the specimen to be involved in the clot. This means that even if the clot is small, the cell count in the tube will be inaccurate, because it is impossible to know how many cells are involved in the clot and how many are floating freely in the specimen. To avoid clotted specimens, be sure to invert the specimens thoroughly during the collection process.

- **Incorrect anticoagulant use:** Each anticoagulant uses a different principle to keep the blood from clotting. Some bind up the calcium in the specimen, as it is necessary for the clotting process to proceed. Others make the platelets in the specimen nonadhesive so that they cannot cling to one another. Tests are designed to be performed using a specific anticoagulant, and if the incorrect one is used, it may alter the test results. For instance, potassium EDTA may cause false elevation of the potassium levels if a lavender top tube was used

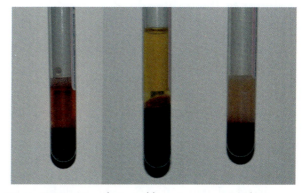

Figure 8-17 Hemolysis and lipemia present in plasma tubes on left and right.

for the plasma sample. Sodium citrate is an anticoagulant that binds up the calcium in the specimen so that it cannot participate in the clotting process. This means that calcium levels performed on plasma from these light blue top tubes would be very low, as the calcium is not in solution in a way that it can be tested.

- **Fibrin clots:** Tubes without added anticoagulant must be allowed to clot properly before centrifugation, or it may be impossible to obtain enough serum from the specimen to perform the tests ordered. This may result in a request for a specimen to be recollected. It may be possible to physically remove the fibrin clot and recentrifuge the specimen, but this may lead to damaged red cells and hemolysis.

Test Your Knowledge 8-19

Examples of inappropriate specimens may include:
  a. Hemolyzed and lipemic specimens
  b. Partially filled specimen tubes for multiple tests
  c. Blood collected in tubes with the wrong anticoagulant
  d. All of the above   (Outcome 8-19)

POTENTIAL NEGATIVE OUTCOMES OF VENIPUNCTURE AND CAPILLARY PUNCTURE

Regardless of the skill level exhibited by the medical assistant, sometimes the person who is attempting a venipuncture may be unsuccessful. In addition, even when the person drawing the blood is successful, there may be physical patient complications resulting from the blood draw. It is important to realize that these negative outcomes are sometimes unavoidable, and to know what action should be taken if they occur.

Inability to Draw Blood

Veins are not solid objects that are incapable of movement. Sometimes even when the vein is anchored tightly, it will move just a bit as the needle is inserted. Or, the health-care worker who is drawing the blood may not insert the needle far enough or go in just a bit too far so that the blood does not enter the needle. It is never acceptable to "probe" when drawing blood. However, recommendations from the Clinical and Laboratory Standards Institute do allow the phlebotomist to move the needle a bit further into the vein or a bit further out of the vein to see if the blood will start to flow. Sometimes a slight change in the location or angle of the needle is all that is necessary for the blood to enter the needle. The needle should never be moved from side to side after insertion into the arm, as this will cause damage to the tissues and pain for the patient. If the slight movements (small increments in or out) are not enough to allow blood to enter the needle, discontinue the draw, and try again. Be sure to check for alternative sites before using the same area for a second attempt. If the person drawing the blood is still unsuccessful after two attempts, he or she should seek assistance from another qualified employee.

Fainting Patients

Some patients experience light-headedness, dizziness, or fainting during or immediately after a blood draw. This may be due to **vasovagal syncope**, which is the body's exaggerated reaction to the sight of blood. Some of these patients may have had negative experiences in the past, whereas others cannot identify a specific reason for their reaction. Each person who experiences vasovagal syncope has his or her own triggers, which may include emotional distress, the sight of blood, and/or pain. The trigger causes a response in the body that includes a drop in blood pressure and a decreased heart rate. Young patients, thin patients, nervous individuals, and those who are very quiet (or sometimes *very* talkative) are more prone to fainting. Also, hunger, fatigue, and environmental factors such as excessive heat or strong smells may make the situation worse. There are usually some symptoms that occur prior to the actual fainting episode such as nausea, yawning, dizziness, weakness, perspiring, pallor, and a flushed feeling of warmth. If the patient communicates any of these symptoms, the blood draw should be discontinued. The medical assistant should help the patient to put the head down between the legs if he or she is still conscious. This may help to keep the patient from fainting. If the patient shares a history of fainting, he or she should be drawn in the supine position, and the medical assistant should make additional efforts to talk to the patient during the procedure to monitor the level of consciousness. If a patient does faint when sitting up in a phlebotomy chair, the primary focus should be safety for the patient and the medical assistant. Discontinue the draw, remove the tourniquet and the needle, activate the safety device on the needle, and bandage the draw site. Call for assistance from a coworker. If the patient is still unconscious, it may be necessary to lower him or her to the floor from the chair, with special care taken to protect the head from hitting anything during the process. The patient's legs should be elevated to help the blood flow return to the heart and brain, and a health-care provider should be notified of the situation.

Rolling Veins

The median cubital vein is usually quite stable, which makes it an excellent choice for venipuncture. If this vein cannot be used for phlebotomy procedures, the other veins in the antecubital area may be considered. However, these are not as well anchored, and have a tendency to "roll" or move away when the venipuncture is attempted. Special care must be taken to anchor these veins very well to avoid this problem.

Hematoma Formation

A hematoma is the result of blood leaking into the tissues from a vein. It can occur in routine venipunctures, but is more common when the process did not go smoothly. If the initial insertion of the needle is too deep, the needle may puncture and go through the vein, which allows excessive blood to leak from the punctures in the vein. Conversely, if the needle does not go far enough into the vein, the bevel may not be totally within the vessel, and blood may leak out around the slant at the end of the needle. (See Fig. 8-18 for examples.) Hematomas can also be the result of too little pressure applied after the venipuncture procedure, with subsequent bleeding around the puncture site. When a hematoma forms, there is a sudden swelling (and sometimes a discoloration) around the site where the needle is inserted. If this occurs, the tourniquet and then the needle need to be removed and pressure should be applied immediately. The medical assistant should be sure to keep pressure on the site for at least 5 minutes, and also should be sure to document the situation. The patient may experience pain and more swelling in the area. The healthcare provider may suggest ice application and anti-inflammatories to help with the discomfort.

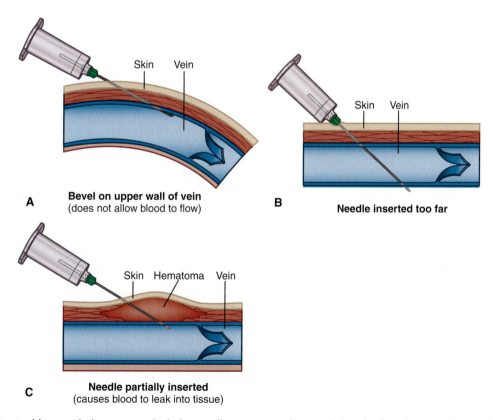

A **Bevel on upper wall of vein**
(does not allow blood to flow)

B **Needle inserted too far**

C **Needle partially inserted**
(causes blood to leak into tissue)

Figure 8-18 Problems with the way in which the needle is entering the vessel. (A) The first drawing shows what occurs if the angle of insertion is too shallow and the needle goes above the vein. (B) The second drawing shows what occurs if the angle of insertion is too high, and the needle goes through the vein. (C) The third shows what can happen if the needle is not inserted far enough into the vein. *Reprinted with permission from Strasinger S, and Di Lorenzo M: Phlebotomy Textbook, ed. 3. Philadelphia: FA Davis, 2011.*

Collapsing Veins

Fragile veins may collapse with the amount of pressure used to withdraw blood during a venipuncture procedure. Small veins or veins that have been damaged with IV therapy or medication treatment are more prone to collapse. If the medical assistant recognizes that the vein is small or appears fragile, the evacuated tube system should not be used for the venipuncture, as this will increase the likelihood of venous collapse. A syringe and needle or a butterfly system should be used instead.

Nerve Damage

Venipuncture procedures performed in the median cubital vein rarely cause irritation to the nerves in the arm, as this vein is not usually in close proximity to the medial nerve. When drawing from the antecubital area, blood draws performed from the basilic vein are the most likely to cause nerve irritation or damage due to the close proximity to the nerve. If a patient complains of excessive pain during a blood draw (especially if hc or she describes it as shooting pain that goes up or down the arm), the procedure should be discontinued immediately. Never attempt a venipuncture from the underside of the wrist, as there are numerous opportunities to cause nerve irritation or damage in this area.

Infection

Infection or excessive irritation at the site of a venipuncture is not common, but can occur. To minimize the risk, the medical assistant should always clean the site thoroughly before the procedure, and also allow the alcohol used to disinfect the site to dry completely before the needle is inserted. If the alcohol has not been allowed to dry, it can cause irritation to the skin in the area, which makes the site more prone to infection. Using good judgment when choosing a site for venipuncture will also help to minimize the chances of inflammation and infection.

> **Test Your Knowledge 8-20**
> True or False: The angle at which the needle is inserted for venipuncture has no impact on whether the procedure has a negative outcome.   (Outcome 8-20)

OTHER PROCESSING PROCEDURES

Processing a blood specimen may include centrifugation, separation of plasma or serum from the cells, and appropriate storage of the specimen until testing occurs. In addition, the medical assistant may be asked to create and stain a smear from a whole blood specimen so that the healthcare provider or other qualified professional may view it.

PREPARATION OF A PERIPHERAL BLOOD SMEAR FOR STAINING

When it is necessary to view the red blood cell **morphology** (appearance and size), identify the types and percentages of various types of white blood cells, and quantitate the number of platelets present in the circulation, a peripheral blood smear may be utilized. Automation has replaced the need to perform a manual examination of the slide for most hematology testing procedures, but there is still a need to examine the slide manually in many

Procedure 8-5: Creation of Peripheral Blood Smear

A peripheral blood smear may be requested at the time of the initial blood draw, or it can be created using blood from a lavender top tube containing EDTA anticoagulant. This procedure will explain how to create a smear using the lavender top tube. If creating a smear at the time of the blood draw, the procedure only differs with the initial application of the sample to the slide.

TASK

Successfully create a peripheral blood smear to be stained and used for a manual differential count or pathologist examination. The process must be completed within 5 minutes.

CONDITIONS

- Hand-washing supplies and/or alcohol-based hand sanitizer
- Disposable gloves
- Clean glass slides
- DIFF-SAFE device
- Lavender top (EDTA) tube filled with blood
- Biohazardous sharps container
- Biohazardous disposal bag

CAAHEP/ABHES STANDARDS

 CAAHEP Standards

III.P.2: Practice Standard Precautions

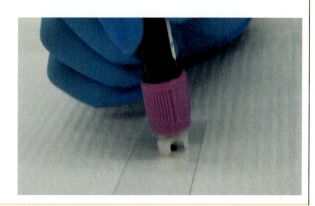 **ABHES Standards**

None

Procedure	Rationale
1. Sanitize hands (allow them to dry) and apply gloves.	Gloves must be worn for any procedures in which exposure to blood or other potentially infectious materials is anticipated.
2. Invert the blood tube 8 to 10 times to mix the sample.	The specimen must be well mixed or it will provide erroneous results when the blood smear is examined.
3. Insert DIFF-SAFE device into the top of the lavender top tube.	The device has a blunt metal cannula that is inserted through the rubber stopper on top of the tube. This is performed while the tube is in an upright position.
4. Turn the tube upside down and push the DIFF-SAFE device to the slide until a drop of blood is released.	Pushing down on the tube with the DIFF-SAFE device against the slide will release a drop of blood onto the slide.

Continued

Procedure 8-5: Creation of Peripheral Blood Smear—cont'd

Procedure	Rationale
5. Pull the second slide back into the drop of blood at an approximate 30-degree angle, allowing the blood to flow along the edge of the slide.	This process must occur quickly. The angle allows for correct application of the blood across the slide. 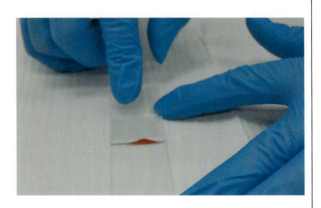
6. Once the blood has flowed to cover approximately three-quarters of the width of the slide, push the second slide forward to spread the blood across the original slide.	Push the spreader slide forward smoothly with a rapid motion. Do not apply weight or additional pressure during this step, or the slide will not move smoothly across the surface. The entire process must occur in less than 15 seconds or the drop of blood will begin to dry and the distribution of the cells will be uneven across the slide. Smears should have a "feathered" edge, with visible edges on the heaviest part of the smear. Ideally there will be no holes or ridges in the blood pattern. If the cell distribution is too thick, it will be difficult to see the morphology of the red blood cells clearly, and it may be difficult to visualize the white blood cells as well. The completed smear should have an appearance that is similar to a thumbprint, with a heavy distribution at the beginning of the smear and a gradual decrease in the thickness across the slide. 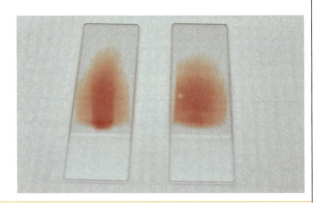

Procedure	Rationale
7. Allow the slide to air-dry.	The slide must be completely dry before it is stained or the appearance of the cells will be altered during the staining process.
8. Remove the DIFF-SAFE device from the top of the tube and discard the device in a biohazardous sharps container. Also discard the second slide used for spreading in the biohazardous sharps container. Store the tube as directed by the laboratory.	The device and the slide are contaminated with blood and are considered to be a sharp.
9. Label the slide with a pencil or a grease pen with the name of the patient and other identification as required by the laboratory.	All slides need to be properly labeled before staining.
10. Transfer the slide to the appropriate area of the laboratory for drying and staining.	The medical assistant should not touch the slide without gloves on, so the transport should occur before the gloves are removed.
11. Remove gloves and sanitize the hands.	Hands must always be sanitized after removing gloves.
12. Document the procedure in the patient's chart if it is available.	In a physician office laboratory, this procedure should be documented in the patient's chart. If the medical assistant is working in a laboratory setting where the chart is not available, this step is not necessary.

Date	
1/18/2020:	Blood smear prepared from lavender top tube. ∿∿∿∿∿∿∿∿∿∿∿∿∿∿∿
1100 a.m.	∿∿∿∿∿∿∿∿∿∿∿∿∿∿ Connie Lieseke, CMA (AAMA)

instances. A lavender top EDTA tube may be used or, in some cases, a drop of blood may be taken directly from a capillary puncture and applied to the slide. The safest method of applying the drop of blood to the slide from the tube is to use a DIFF-SAFE device (Alpha Scientific Corporation, Malvern, Pennsylvania), which eliminates the need to open the tube to gain access to the blood.

WRIGHT'S STAIN PROCEDURE

Once the peripheral blood smear has been prepared, it must be stained so that it can be examined. There are various products available for this staining process,

including Diff-Quik stain by Dade Behring. Wright's stain is another common stain often used in the physician office laboratory as well as in larger laboratories. It is a hematology stain that is used for staining smears made from blood and bone marrow samples. Wright's stain allows for visualization of the red blood cells and platelets in the sample, as well as differentiation of the various types of white cells that are present. The stain contains methanol, which acts as a fixative for the cells, as well as an acidic red dye and a blue dye that is alkaline in pH. These stains are absorbed differently by the formed elements in the blood to allow for them to be examined and counted.

Procedure 8-6: Quick Stain of Peripheral Smear Using Camco Quik Stain II

The Camco Quik Stain procedure allows for the cells to be stained appropriately so that they can be identified by an individual who is qualified to perform this microscopic evaluation. This may be performed for a differential examination, in which a technician or technologist will count the various types of white cells present and report a percentage of each type. The stain solution may be poured into small vessels for dipping the slides, or it may be applied with a pipette to a slide on a rack that is suspended over a sink or other receptacle.

TASK

Stain a peripheral blood smear using Camco Quik Stain II.

CONDITIONS

- Air-dried blood smear
- Camco Quik Stain II solution
- Distilled water with a pH of 6 or 7
- Laboratory wipes
- Sink or other receptacle for excess stain

CAAHEP/ABHES STANDARDS

None

Procedure	Rationale
1. Sanitize hands, and allow them to dry completely. Apply gloves.	Gloves must be worn for any procedures in which exposure to blood or other potentially infectious materials is anticipated. In addition, the stain will discolor the fingers if gloves are not utilized.
2. Dip the blood smear in the stain solution for 10 seconds. Alternatively, the smear may be placed on a rack and stain may be added until the slide is covered with the stain for 10 seconds.	The 10 seconds is a minimum staining time. If the smear is thick, additional staining time may be necessary.
3. Allow excess stain to drain from the slide. Apply or dip in distilled water for 20 seconds.	It is necessary to allow at least 20 seconds for the process to be complete.
4. Wipe away any excess stain that may be present on the back of the slide with a laboratory wipe.	Excess stain on the back of the slide will obscure the view when examining the smear under the microscope.
5. Allow the slide to air-dry. Make sure that there is no excess water standing on the slide.	This type of smear does not need to be heat fixed. Excess water may change the staining characteristics or increase the time necessary for the slide to dry.
6. Dispose of the laboratory wipe in the trash and put away supplies.	All work areas should remain clean and organized.
7. Remove gloves and sanitize hands.	Gloves should be removed before proceeding to the next task. Hands must always be sanitized after removing gloves.

SUMMARY

Blood collection is the most common and most important part of the preanalytical process for laboratory testing. To perform quality venipuncture and capillary puncture, it is imperative that the medical assistant or phlebotomist understands the basics of the anatomy and physiology of the cardiovascular system as well as areas and situations to avoid when collecting blood. Following recommended procedures during the collection process is critical, which includes knowledge of how to safely use the various collection devices.

Patient identification and appropriate preparation are of utmost importance. Knowledge of the various tube types to be used is very important in collecting the sample correctly. Order of draw is critical to avoid crossover contamination. Finally, processing the samples appropriately is the final preparatory step before testing the sample. This may include centrifugation and separation of the plasma or serum, or it may include preparation and staining of slides.

TIME TO REVIEW

1. The bevel of a needle is:　　　　Outcome 8-1
   a. The interior hollow space of the needle
   b. The slanted tip at the end of the needle
   c. The diameter of the needle
   d. None of the above

2. The flanges of an evacuated tube holder:　Outcome 8-1
   a. Allow for the needle to be screwed on the holder
   b. Provide a space for the tube to be inserted
   c. May be used to provide leverage when inserting and/or removing tubes
   d. Are decorative only

3. True or False: Interstitial fluid　　Outcome 8-1
   is the fluid located between the cells of the tissues.

4. True or False: Venules are larger　　Outcome 8-1
   in diameter than are veins.

5. Identify all the ways that veins　　Outcome 8-3
   and arteries are the same:
   a. Transport blood
   b. Connect to capillaries
   c. May be punctured to withdraw blood for testing

   d. Have multiple layers of cells in the walls of the vessels
   e. Have a distinct pulse that can be felt with palpation
   f. Have valves that prevent backflow
   g. Are varied in size throughout the body

6. Mark the veins below in　　　　Outcome 8-5
   order of preference for venipuncture procedures by numbering them 1, 2, and 3:

   _____ Cephalic vein
   _____ Basilic vein
   _____ Median cubital vein

7. True or False: Capillary punctures　　Outcome 8-6
   on infants may be performed on the great toe.

8. An example of an area to avoid　　Outcome 8-7
   when choosing a site for venipuncture is:
   a. Scarred skin
   b. Varicose veins
   c. Veins on the back of the hand
   d. None of the above
   e. a and b

9. How is a butterfly (or winged　　Outcome 8-8
   infusion set) different from the needle used for evacuated tube draws or syringe draws?

10. Using the following order of　　Outcome 8-9
    draw, create a mnemonic that will help you to remember the order the tubes are to be drawn with an evacuated tube system or a syringe draw.

    Yellow, light blue, red, green, lavender, gray

11. Describe one way that a medical　　Outcome 8-12
    assistant might put a child at ease before a blood collection is to be performed.

12. Why is it important to verify　　Outcome 8-14
    whether a patient has properly prepared for a test before the medical assistant performs the blood draw?

13. Why would a peripheral smear be used?　Outcome 8-16
    a. To test for certain hormones
    b. To scan for bacteria
    c. To identify various types of white blood cells
    d. To perform ABO blood typing

14. What is one practice that can   Outcome 8-15
help to protect patients and employees during invasive procedures?

15. Capillary specimens may be preferred: Outcome 8-13
    a. When performing CLIA-waived tests that use whole blood
    b. When the patient's medical condition warrants it
    c. For infants
    d. All of the above

16. Which part of the hand is used   Outcome 8-15
to hold the evacuated tube holder when the medical assistant performs a venipuncture?

17. Do all capillary puncture devices   Outcome 8-15
provide incisions that are the same depth?

Case Study 8-1: How long was this sitting here?

A blood specimen for a glucose level and electrolyte analysis was drawn on Mr. Dee at 9:30 a.m. Shortly after the blood draw, Shannon, the medical assistant who was covering the laboratory area of the office, was asked to fill in for another employee who became ill at work. At 2 p.m., after lunch, Shannon went back into the laboratory and processed the specimens that she had drawn that morning so that they were ready to be picked up by the laboratory courier at 2:30.

Just before closing, Shannon received a call from the laboratory alerting the health-care provider that the potassium was elevated above the reference range for Mr. Dee, and the glucose levels were well below the reference range. The laboratory suggested that the specimen needed to be redrawn before the health-care provider acted on these results.

1. What event of the day may have affected these blood levels?
2. Do you agree that the specimen should be redrawn before the physician acts on the results obtained from the original specimen?

Case Study 8-2: Clumps

John George is performing a blood draw for a CBC, differential, and platelet count on Mrs. Charrone. As he completes the blood draw, he notices that she is looking really pale and is no longer conversing with him. He removes the tourniquet and the needle with the evacuated tube holder and lavender top tube from her arm just as she loses consciousness. He gently lowers her to the floor as she slides out of the phlebotomy chair, and elevates her feet as he calls for help. Within a few minutes she regains consciousness and after monitoring her for a few minutes, the health-care provider states that she is ready to leave the office. John helps her out to the waiting room to meet her husband, after which he returns to the blood draw area to process the specimen. He labels the specimen appropriately and places it on the blood rocker for the laboratory technician working in the testing area to access it for the CBC, differential, and platelet count.

In about an hour, the laboratory technician comes to find John and asks him if he remembers anything unusual about this blood draw. The laboratory technician said that the platelet count is extremely low with the initial analysis and that the hematology instrument flagged the sample with an error. The laboratory technician is going to recheck the specimen and create a blood smear to look at the sample more thoroughly.

1. How do you think the events of this blood draw may have affected the platelet count?
2. What do you think the technician may find when she looks at the blood smear?

RESOURCES AND SUGGESTED READINGS

"DIFF-SAFE Blood Dispenser: Directions for Use"
Provides step-by-step instructions on how to use a DIFF-SAFE Blood Dispenser http://www.alpha-scientific.com/Diff-safe2.html

"NCCLS simplifies the order of draw."
 by Ernst D, Calam R. Medical Laboratory Observer, May 2004
 National Committee for Clinical Laboratory Standards. Procedures for the Collection of Diagnostic Blood Specimens by Venipuncture. Approved Standard, H3-A5, Wayne, PA; 2003.

"Preanalytical Errors in the Emergency Department."
 from BD Company, LabNotes. 17, no. 1, 2007 http:// www.bd.com/vacutainer/labnotes/Volume17Number1/

"Preparation of Peripheral Blood Smear Staining With Wright's Stain
 Directions on how to stain a peripheral blood smear using Wright's Stain http://www.scribd.com/doc/8801750/ Preparation-of-Peripheral-Blood-Smear-Staining-With-Wrights-Stain

"Staining the Cells."
 How to stain a blood smear; instructions on how to stain a peripheral blood smear http://www.tpub.com/content/ medical/14295/css/14295_286.htm

"Venipuncture Technique Using the Multisample Vacutainer System"
 Description of the use of the Vacutainer© system with details http://www.phlebotomycert.com/multi_vtainer_systm.htm

"Newborn Screening"
 Washington State Department of Health. In-depth information about the various disorders that may be detected by newborn screening. Includes links to more detailed information about the collection process and specimen handling. http://www.doh.wa.gov/ehsphl/phl/newborn/ disorders.htm#msud

Chapter 9

Collection and Processing of Urine Samples

Constance L. Lieseke, CMA (AAMA), MLT, PBT(ASCP)

CHAPTER OUTLINE

Learning Outcomes

After reading this chapter, the successful student will be able to:

9-1 Define the key terms.

9-2 Explain the necessity of obtaining different types of urine samples for laboratory testing.

9-3 Compare and contrast various urine specimen types.

9-4 Describe how urine specimens are to be processed after collection.

9-5 Describe changes that may occur in urine specimens if they are left at room temperature after collection.

9-6 Analyze the details for proper labeling of the various types of urine specimens presented in the text.

9-7 Examine the necessary patient education for collection of samples to be used for specialized urine testing procedures.

9-8 Instruct a patient on the proper collection procedure for a clean-catch midstream urine specimen.

9-9 Instruct a patient on the proper collection procedure for a 24-hour urine specimen.

CAAHEP/ABHES STANDARDS

 CAAHEP Standards

I.P.I.6: Anatomy and Physiology: Perform patient screening using established protocols
I.A.I.2: Anatomy and Physiology: Use language/verbal skills that enable patients' understanding

 ABHES Standards

• Medical Laboratory Procedures: e. Patient Instructions (collection of urine and feces); Instruct patients in the collection of a clean-catch mid-stream urine specimen.

KEY TERMS

Aliquot	Indwelling catheter	24-hour urine collection
Distal urethra	Intermittent (straight) catheter	2-hour postprandial specimen
Diurnal variation	Prostatitis	Urinalysis
Fasting urine specimen	Prostatitis specimen collection process	Urinary meatus
First morning void		Urine culture
Formed elements	Random	
Glucose tolerance urine specimen	Suprapubic aspiration	

TYPES OF URINE SPECIMENS

Urine analysis is one of the most common tests performed in the clinical laboratory. The collection process for urine specimens is noninvasive, and is relatively easy to accomplish because the production of urine by the body is an ongoing process. It is important to remember, however, that proper collection and processing procedures are essential for the urine laboratory results to be accurate and meaningful. (Table 9-1 summarizes the various types of urine specimens.)

Specimen collection procedures may vary based on the length of time for the collection, dietary limitations, specimen volume requirements, and the method of collection. Many urine specimens are collected to diagnose potential urinary tract infections, in which case they are usually **random** collections; they could be collected at any time of the day, as long as the collection procedures

---

TABLE 9-1

Types of Urine Specimens

Specimen Type	Time of Collection	Uses
Clean-catch midstream urine specimen	Random	Urinalysis, culture, random chemistry testing, urine pregnancy testing
Intermittent (straight) catheter specimen	Random	Urinalysis, culture, random chemistry testing, urine pregnancy testing
Indwelling catheter specimen	Not appropriate for urinalysis, culture, or chemistry testing	Not appropriate for urinalysis, culture, or chemistry testing
Suprapubic aspiration specimen	Random	Urinalysis, culture, random chemistry testing, urine pregnancy testing, urine cytology
Prostatitis specimen	Random as part of procedure	To check for bacterial prostatitis
First morning void specimen	Upon rising	Urine pregnancy testing, specific chemistry tests; urinalysis, culture
24-hour urine specimen	24 hours of collection	Chemistry testing
2-hour postprandial specimen	2 hours after a 100-g carbohydrate meal	Glucose and ketones
Glucose tolerance testing	As part of a glucose tolerance testing procedure	Glucose and ketones
Infant urine specimens	Random	Urinalysis

are followed appropriately. Other urine specimens are collected for chemical analysis to aid in the diagnosis of specific problems with the kidneys or other organ systems. These chemicals often change in concentration throughout the day, which is known as **diurnal variation.** To provide accurate results, specimen collection in these circumstances is carried out over a specific period of time at a certain time of the day. Procedures for collection may also include dietary restrictions for some tests to limit potential erroneous results because of a diet rich in a particular substance.

The guidelines that should be followed whenever a urine specimen is to be collected include the following:

- All specimen containers must be correctly labeled. In the case of urine collection, this should occur immediately after the patient returns the specimen container to the laboratory or health-care facility. All labels should include the patient's name, birth date or other unique identifier, and the date and time of the collection. Labels must be placed on the container itself, not just on the lid. It is also a good idea to document the type of specimen (e.g., urine) in the container; many body fluids have a similar appearance when received in the laboratory.
- The required specimen volume must be verified before instructing the patient on collection requirements.
- Any medication the patient is taking that may potentially interfere with the test results needs to be documented on the requisition form.
- For timed specimens, the start and finish time (and dates if appropriate) must be documented on the container.
- Dietary restrictions must be communicated to the patient before collection, both verbally and in writing.
- Collection of urine for analysis during the menstrual cycle should be avoided if possible; the presence of red blood cells may interfere with the testing procedures for some analytes. If it is not possible to delay the collection, care must be taken to instruct the patient on proper cleaning techniques to avoid gross contamination, and a notation should be placed on the laboratory requisition form (and/or in the patient chart if available) that the patient is menstruating.
- Specimen containers that have preservatives added need to be clearly marked, and in these situations, there should be an additional container provided for the patient to use during collection to avoid urinating directly into the specimen container with the preservative.
- Patients should *always* be provided with a specimen container, so that they are not using a jar or other container from home. Although these may appear "clean,"

they may contain chemicals or other substances that can affect the urine test results.
- Any instructions for collection must be given to the patient verbally and in writing. These include storage instructions for the specimen until it is returned for analysis.

Test Your Knowledge 9-1

Please provide two reasons that a urine specimen may be ordered for testing. (Outcome 9-2)

Test Your Knowledge 9-2

List one item that is the same for all urine collection procedures. (Outcome 9-2)

POINT OF INTEREST 9-1
Urine drug screens

Many health-care providers and laboratories are now involved in preemployment physicals. These may include urine drug screens for drugs of abuse. This type of urine collection has very specific procedural parameters designed to prove that the specimen collected was not tampered with prior to the completion of testing. There are guidelines that dictate the steps involved in the collection procedures, as well as guidelines that outline the security of the specimen during transportation and processing. A series of documentation on a standardized form is necessary; this process establishes the *chain of custody* for the specimen. Federal regulations require preemployment, postaccident, and random drug screening for some jobs, whereas other large nonfederal employers choose to ensure a drug-free environment by requiring their employees to undergo testing. The following is a summary of the steps involved in a urine drug specimen collection procedure:

1. Collectors must be appropriately trained for the process.
2. The collector verifies that there is a bluing agent (some sort of dye) added to the toilet before the donor process begins.
3. The donor is greeted and must provide photo identification. In some situations, alternative forms of identification are acceptable from an employer representative.

Continued

4. The collector fills out the first step of the chain of custody form, and the donor signs to verify the accuracy of this information.

5. The donor leaves all purses, coats, and so on outside of the restroom to eliminate the possibility of smuggling in concealed substances to contaminate the urine.

6. The donor washes and dries his or her hands.

7. The collector must tape the toilet lid and the faucet handles with tamper-proof tape so that there is no access to other water sources.

8. The collector remains in the restroom (if there is a private stall) or outside the restroom door if there is no private stall during the collection process. Sometimes a witnessed collection is requested, in which case the donor must be watched by the collector during the collection.

9. The donor is not allowed to wash his or her hands until the specimen is handed to the collector and the follow-up quality control measures and documentation have been completed. The urine specimen must remain within the site of the donor and the collector during this process.

10. The collector verifies the volume received, the appearance of the urine, and records the temperature of the specimen. If there is a problem with the temperature or the appearance of the urine specimen, the collection process is void.

11. As the donor observes, tamper-proof collection labels are placed over the top of the collection container and the donor initials these labels. The date and time are also added to these labels.

12. These steps are documented on the chain of custody form.

13. From this point forward, every individual involved in transportation, processing, or testing of the specimen must document their actions and the purpose of their actions on the chain of custody form.

Clean-Catch Midstream Urine Specimen Collection

When a urinalysis or urine culture is ordered for a patient, it is important the specimen be as contaminant free as possible. A **urinalysis** includes physical observations and chemical analysis of the urine specimen, and may also include a microscopic examination of the urine sediment. A **urine culture** is designed to test for bacterial growth in the urine specimen. In both these situations, it is imperative that the specimen received for testing is representative of the urine in the urinary bladder and urethra, rather than contaminants that might be present on the outside of the body. A clean-catch midstream urine specimen collection technique is the best noninvasive method to obtain a urine specimen for these tests. This procedure involves cleaning the external opening of the urinary tract and obtaining a midstream urine specimen.

The clean-catch midstream urine collection technique offers an opportunity to obtain a specimen that has less contamination with epithelial cells and bacteria from the distal urethra and urinary meatus than a specimen obtained without proper cleansing and technique. The **distal urethra** is the area of the urethra that is closest to the outside of the body. The **urinary meatus** is the exterior opening of the urinary tract. Because these are both near the outside of the body, they are naturally potential sources of exterior contamination. Even though all urine specimens must pass through this area of the urinary tract as they exit the body, the goal is to obtain a specimen that contains the bacteria and other microscopic structures that are clinically significant, (those that are present in the bladder) and minimize those that are essentially contaminants. This is critical for patients to be properly diagnosed and treated for urinary tract infections.

Test Your Knowledge 9-3

Why is the cleansing process for a clean-catch midstream urine specimen so important?   (Outcome 9-2)

Test Your Knowledge 9-4

Should a urine collection container be labeled before or after it is given to the patient for collection?

(Outcome 9-6)

Catheterized Specimens

Another way to avoid potential specimen contamination is to use a catheter to obtain the specimen. Only a licensed health-care professional may insert a catheter. This process may also be used when the patient is not capable of following the directions or performing the procedures necessary for a clean-catch urine collection procedure, such as those who are very young or those who may have physical limitations. Catheters may be

(Text continues on page 203)

Procedure 9-1: Instructing a Patient for Collection of a Clean-Catch Midstream Urine Specimen for Urinalysis and/or Culture

Clean-catch midstream urine specimens are required by most laboratories for performance of urinalysis and cultures. By cleansing appropriately and providing a midstream specimen that comes from the bladder and upper urethra, most extraneous microorganisms will be eliminated from the specimen.

TASK

The student will demonstrate the ability to properly instruct a male or female patient how to collect a clean-catch midstream urine specimen.

CONDITIONS

- Appropriately labeled sterile urine collection container
- Three moist antiseptic towelettes
- Hand-washing facilities
- Paper towels

CAAHEP/ABHES STANDARDS

 CAAHEP Standards

I.P.I.6: Anatomy and Physiology: Perform patient screening using established protocols
I.A.I.2: Anatomy and Physiology: Use language/verbal skills that enable patients' understanding

 ABHES Standards

Medical Laboratory Procedures: e. Patient Instructions (collection of urine and feces); Instruct patients in the collection of a clean-catch mid-stream urine specimen.

Procedure	Rationale
1. Wash hands and gather necessary supplies for the patient.	Hand washing breaks the chain of infection.
2. Greet and identify the patient. Verify the test orders and the labeling on the container.	The patient identity should always be verified for every procedure. Verification of test orders and labeling reduces the potential for error.
3. Provide the patient with a sterile container and three antiseptic towelettes.	The patient will need to refer to these items as the procedure is explained. The towelettes will be used for cleansing around the urinary opening area. Strong antiseptics should not be used because of the potential irritation to the external urinary structures.

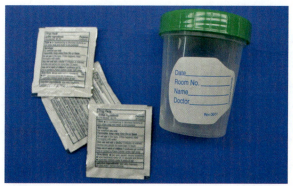

Continued

Procedure 9-1: Instructing a Patient for Collection of a Clean-Catch Midstream Urine Specimen for Urinalysis and/or Culture—cont'd

Procedure	Rationale
Instructions for Male Patients	

a. Instruct the patient to wash and dry his hands, and once in the restroom, remove his underwear.

Hand washing breaks the cycle of infection, and removing the undergarments allows for better access during the cleaning process.

b. The patient should carefully remove the lid of the specimen container and place it with the inside up on the counter near the toilet where the container can easily be accessed for the collection process. Emphasize the importance of keeping the interior of the container sterile.

Placing the lid with the inside up prevents contamination from microorganisms that may be present on the countertop.

c. Male patients who are uncircumcised must pull back the foreskin, and keep it withdrawn during the cleaning and collection process.

Pathogenic microorganisms may be present under the foreskin.

d. The tip of the penis must be cleansed three times:

Thorough cleansing eliminates potential contaminating substances. Once the cleaning process has started, the patient should keep holding the penis until the specimen has been obtained to eliminate the possibility of recontamination.

- Wipe with the first wipe from front to back on one side of the tip of the penis.
- Wipe with the second wipe from front to back on the other side of the tip of the penis.
- Use the third wipe over the urinary opening (the meatus) from front to back. Note: A new antiseptic towelette must be used to clean each side of the penis and an additional towelette used to clean the tip of the penis. (A total of three towelettes are to be used for the cleansing process.)
- Some laboratories may provide a fourth towelette to clean the outside of the container after the collection.

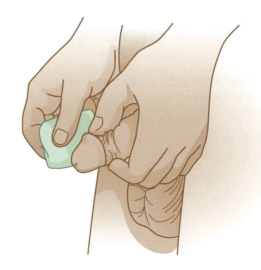

Procedure	Rationale
e. Instruct the patient to pick up the specimen container so that he is ready when for the collection. Begin to urinate into the toilet. Stop the urine stream, move the specimen container into a position where it will intersect the urine stream, and urinate into the container until it is at least half full. Stop the urine stream again and move the container out of the way. Remind the patient not to touch the inside of the container.	This process flushes out microorganisms that may be present near the opening of the urethra and allows collection of a specimen that represents the urine that was present in the bladder and upper urethra.
f. Instruct the patient to finish urinating into the toilet.	The specimen must be *midstream*; the first and last part of the urine void should not be included in the specimen submitted to the laboratory.
g. The patient must carefully replace the lid on the container without contaminating the interior of the cup or lid. If urine is present on the outside of the cup, dry it off with toilet tissue or a paper towel, and discard the waste.	Contamination must be avoided on the inside of the container so that the specimen represents the urine as it is inside the body.
h. Instruct the patient to wash and dry his hands.	Clean hands prevent the spread of microorganisms.
i. Instruct the patient to place the urine in the designated area of the laboratory if the specimen is collected in the office. If it is a home collection, instruct the patient to refrigerate the specimen until it can be transported to the testing location.	The specimen will need to be refrigerated or tested in a timely manner to preserve the integrity of the test results.

Instructions for Female Patients

Procedure	Rationale
a. Instruct the patient to wash and dry her hands, and once in the restroom, remove her underwear.	Hand washing breaks the cycle of infection, and removing the undergarments allows for better access during the cleaning process.
b. The patient should carefully remove the lid of the specimen container and place it with the inside up on the counter near the toilet where the container can easily be accessed for the collection process. Emphasize the importance of keeping the interior of the container sterile.	Placing the lid facing up prevents contamination with microorganisms that may be present on the countertop.
c. Instruct the patient to move her knees apart until she can easily reach her labia. (These are the structures that cover the urinary opening in females.)	It is important that the patient has full access to the labia to clean the area properly.

Continued

Procedure 9-1: Instructing a Patient for Collection of a Clean-Catch Midstream Urine Specimen for Urinalysis and/or Culture—cont'd

Procedure	Rationale
d. Instruct the patient to spread apart the labia with one hand to expose the urinary opening (the urinary meatus). The labia will need to remain spread apart until the cleaning and collection process is complete.	The labia must remain apart after the area is cleaned to eliminate the potential for recontamination of the site.

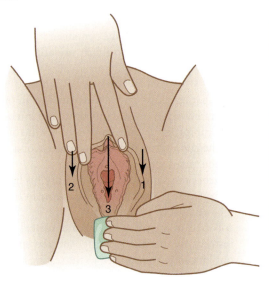

e. The patient needs to clean the area three times, using a clean antiseptic towelette each time. • The first towelette should be used to clean from front to back on one side of the urinary opening. • Use the second towelette to wipe front to back on the other side of the urinary opening. • The third towelette is to be used to wipe front to back across the urinary opening for the final cleansing step. • Some laboratories may provide a fourth towelette to clean the outside of the container after the collection.	Cleansing in this manner avoids potential contamination from the anal area (front to back) and provides an opportunity to thoroughly clean away potential pathogenic microorganisms that could enter the specimen while urinating.
f. Instruct the patient to pick up the urine specimen container in the hand that is not holding the labia apart.	The specimen container must be in hand before the patient starts to urinate.
g. The patient should begin to urinate into the toilet. After a small amount has entered the toilet, stop the urinary stream and place the specimen container under the urinary opening.	This initial urine stream flushes out potential contaminants that may have been around the urinary meatus.

Procedure	Rationale
h. Instruct the patient to urinate directly into the specimen container, filling it at least half full. Tell the patient to stop urinating and move the specimen container out of the way. Remind the patient to avoid contamination of the interior of the specimen container.	This is a *midstream* specimen that includes urine from the bladder and the upper part of the urethra.
i. Instruct the patient to finish urinating into the toilet.	The first and last part of the urine specimen should not be submitted to the laboratory.
j. The patient must carefully replace the lid on the container without contaminating the interior of the cup or lid. If urine is present on the outside of the cup, dry it off with toilet tissue or a paper towel.	Contamination must be avoided on the inside of the container so that the urine is representative of the conditions on the inside of the body.
k. Instruct the patient to wash and dry her hands.	Hand washing stops the spread of microorganisms.
l. Instruct the patient to place the urine in the designated area of the laboratory if the specimen is collected in the office. If it is a home collection, instruct the patient to refrigerate the specimen until it can be transported to the testing location.	The specimen will need to be refrigerated or tested in a timely manner to preserve the integrity of the test results.
4. Verify whether the patient understood the instructions as given, and check if he or she has any additional questions. Supply contact information for future questions.	This is a critical step for the appropriate collection of the specimen.
5. Provide the patient with a written copy of the instructions.	A written copy will allow patients to refresh their memory when the collection is performed.

Date	
10/24/2016:	*Patient provided supplies and written and verbal instructions for a clean-catch midstream urine collection procedure.*
11:58 a.m.	*Connie Lieseke, CMA (AAMA)*

used in various ways (listed below), and it is imperative that the requisition form and the patient chart include documentation of the type of collection performed.

- **Intermittent (straight) catheter:** There may be times that it is necessary to empty the bladder for a patient who is unable to do so. If this is a temporary situation, an **intermittent (straight) catheter** may be used for the process. This catheterization procedure involves a small, stiff, plastic tube that is placed through the urethra into the bladder to allow the bladder to be drained. This procedure may also be used to obtain a specimen for urinalysis and culture, as the potential for contamination is greatly reduced. Catheterization, however, does include risks of bacterial infection because the lining of the urethra may be damaged as the catheter is inserted or removed.

- **Indwelling catheter: Indwelling catheters** are designed for long-term use. They may be inserted in surgery patients for a few days after surgery, or they may be inserted in patients who have permanently lost the ability to control urination. These catheters are larger in diameter than the straight catheters, and have a small "balloon" that is pumped up to keep them in place within the bladder once they have been inserted. Indwelling catheters continuously drain the urine from the bladder into a collection bag. This bag is emptied periodically. Indwelling catheters are *not* recommended as a source of urine for urinalysis or urine cultures, as the catheters are kept in place for extended periods of time and become contaminated with bacteria. If a patient with an indwelling catheter needs to have a urinalysis, it is best for the catheter to be removed and for the health-care professional to use a straight catheter to obtain the specimen for analysis.

Test Your Knowledge 9-5

Which type of catheterization procedure is used to obtain a urine specimen for a routine culture?

(Outcome 6-3)

Suprapubic Aspiration

There are times, especially with young children, when it is imperative that a urine specimen be collected quickly, without contamination. Skilled health-care professionals (such as physicians or nurse practitioners) may choose to perform a **suprapubic aspiration** to obtain a specimen for urinalysis and culture. A needle is placed externally through the abdomen directly into the bladder, and a urine specimen is withdrawn. This procedure may also be used to collect urine for *cytology* examination, a procedure in which the cells present in the specimen are examined by a pathologist or cytologist for abnormalities in their appearance.

Prostatitis Specimen Collection

Prostatitis (inflammation of the prostate) may be caused by various factors. Prostate enlargement and/or use of urinary catheters are often linked to this condition. The tissue of the prostate may be inflamed, or there may be an infection with pathogenic microorganisms. In order to plan the correct course of action, it may be necessary to collect a urine specimen utilizing a special procedure. In a **prostatitis specimen collection** process, there are three specimens collected in close progression. The patient is provided with three antiseptic towelettes and three sterile specimen collection containers, numbered sequentially 1, 2, and 3. The patient cleansing process is the same as that required for the clean-catch midstream collection procedure. However, rather than urinating into the toilet at the beginning of the process, the first small amount of urine passed goes into collection cup 1. Next, the midstream specimen goes collected in cup 2. After this collection is completed into cup 2, the health-care provider will massage the patient's prostate to allow prostatic secretions to enter the urethra for collection. After the prostate has been massaged, the patient will immediately urinate into the third cup. Cultures are performed on all three specimens. If the second specimen has a high concentration of bacteria present, the third specimen is considered to be invalid, because of contamination by the bacteria already present in the urethra. Generally, if there is an infection of the prostate, the bacterial count of the third specimen will be much higher than that of the first two specimens.

Timed Urine Specimen Collections

Most urine specimens collected in the office setting are random collections, because the time of day is not significant for the desired results. The clean-catch midstream urine collections used for urinalysis and culture are usually random specimens. Remember, however, that the time of collection still must be recorded accurately. A random collection is not always desirable for all urine specimens. There are situations in which the *time* of collection is critical:

- **First morning void specimen:** A specimen that is collected when the patient first rises from sleep is known as a **first morning void** specimen. This specimen is concentrated (ideally it should be approximately 8 hours since the patient last voided)

POINT OF INTEREST 9-2
Proper documentation for urine collection procedure education

This chapter includes a lot of information about different types of urine collection procedures. The key component in all these processes is patient education. The patient should be provided with the appropriate collection supplies in all situations, as well as verbal and written instructions for the collection process. Every laboratory should develop its own literature to distribute to patients so that there is standardization of information provided for collection and storage of the specimens. Government regulations require that the instructions for patients are to be provided in their native language whenever possible. In addition, it is very important to remember that whenever instructions are provided for the patient, doing so must be documented properly in the patient chart.

because it has been in the bladder during the night while the patient slept. The first morning void specimen is recommended for urine pregnancy tests (especially if it is very early in the potential pregnancy) and for detection of the presence of protein or albumin in the urine. It may also be used for routine urinalysis and culture, but the clean-catch midstream collection procedure should still be followed. There will be more dissolved substances present in this specimen than in those found later in the day, and it may also contain more microscopic structures.

- **24-hour urine collection:** Routine urinalysis testing reports the presence or absence of numerous chemicals in the urine specimen and provides a rough quantitative estimate of the amount present for that chemical. For some chemical components, however, it is necessary to have an exact measurement of the amount of that chemical present in the urine. These analytes are not present in the same concentration at all times; they may vary with the time of the day (diurnal variation), or their concentration may be changed with exertion or the hydration status of the individual. To account for these variables, it is often desirable to collect all the urine produced by a patient over the period of an entire day. This is called a **24-hour urine collection.** This collection process is used to test for various substances; among the most common are the following:
  - Urea nitrogen: Urea nitrogen is a by-product of protein metabolism, and is used as an indicator of kidney function.
  - Urine electrolytes: Urine electrolyte tests include those that check for the level of calcium, chloride, potassium, and sodium in the urine. These tests may be ordered together or individually. They are often part of a clinical workup for suspected endocrine disorders or hormonal imbalances or kidney dysfunction. Urine calcium levels are sometimes ordered for patients with recurring kidney stone formation. Situations that cause electrolyte imbalances in the bloodstream may also result in abnormal urine electrolyte levels.
  - Catecholamines: Catecholamines are substances that are created by nerve tissue and by the adrenal glands of the body. They include norepinephrine, dopamine, and epinephrine. Urine specimens do not contain the intact catecholamine molecules; instead, we test for the breakdown products of these compounds. The breakdown products include homovanillic acid (HVA), vanillymandelic

acid (VMA), normetanephrine, and metanephrine. Urine catecholamines may be ordered as a group or individually. This test may be used when an adrenal gland tumor is suspected (pheochromocytoma), and it may also be ordered for patients with symptomatic hypertension.
  - 17-Hydroxysteroids: This test is often performed when there is suspicion of Addison's disease, which is a type of adrenal insufficiency.
  - Urine total protein: The level of total protein in the urine may be an indicator of kidney damage.
  - 5-Hydroxyindoleacetic acid: More commonly known as 5-HIAA, this test may be performed to detect a specific type of tumor, the carcinoid tumor, of the digestive tract. 5-HIAA is a metabolite of serotonin in the urine, and these intestinal tumors secrete unusually high amounts of serotonin.
  - Urine creatinine: Creatinine is a breakdown product of creatine, present in muscle tissue throughout the body. Creatinine is cleared from the body exclusively by the kidneys, and the test is ordered to screen for possible kidney dysfunction.

In some situations, blood is also drawn and tested for the same analyte as the urine specimen at the end of the 24-hour interval. For example, when urine creatinine is ordered, there is often a blood draw performed for creatinine as well, so that both results can be used to reach a diagnosis.

Urine specimens collected over a 24-hour period may have dietary or fluid restrictions; this is to limit potential erroneous results because of a diet rich in a particular substance. Patient education concerning these restrictions is *critical* for a meaningful urine test result. The patient must be given the instructions verbally and in writing, and documentation of the education should be added to the patient's chart.

It may also be necessary to deliver (or even ship) these urine specimens directly to a laboratory for processing, rather than returning them to the health-care provider's office. These instructions should be explained clearly before the collection process is started. The patient should be provided with all shipping materials and written instructions so that the specimen is delivered successfully.

When refrigeration is not possible (especially when the specimen must be transported over long distances) chemical preservatives may be utilized to keep the 24-hour urine specimen from undergoing changes upon standing. Chemical preservatives (such as boric acid or dilute hydrochloric acid) are often added to 24-hour urine specimen containers to keep chemical changes from occurring before the specimen is tested. These additives for 24-hour urine specimen collection are listed in Table 9-2.

Test Your Knowledge 9-6

When providing instructions to a patient for a 24-hour specimen collection, what should the patient be told about urinating directly into the container that contains hydrochloric acid as a preservative? (Outcome 9-7)

There are additional handling procedures that are required by 24-hour urine specimens once they arrive at the laboratory. These procedures include proper documentation of the total specimen volume upon arrival at the laboratory, and verification of the times included in the collection. The specimen must also be well mixed and an **aliquot,** which is a small sample, must be poured off for further chemical testing. Figure 9-1 shows a 24-hour urine collection container.

Procedure 9-2 details the instructions for collection of a 24-hour urine specimen.

Glucose Testing Specimens

Glucose is not usually present in the urine at levels high enough to be measured. However, in patients with diabetes mellitus, blood glucose concentrations may reach levels that are high enough to cause glucose to "spill" into the urine. There are several urine collection procedures that may assist with the diagnosis or monitoring of those with diabetes mellitus or gestational diabetes. These include the following:

- **2-hour postprandial specimen:** For a **2-hour postprandial specimen,** the patient is instructed to empty the bladder before a meal that contains approximately 100 g of carbohydrates. Two hours after meal completion, the patient is to collect a urine specimen. Ideally, the patient will also have a blood sample drawn 2 hours after eating so that both results can be used to evaluate the patient's condition. Because there will not be a culture or complete urinalysis performed on the specimen, 2-hour postprandial urine specimens do not need to be collected using the clean-catch midstream urine collection procedures, The specimen is tested only for the presence of glucose. (Additional

TABLE 9-2	
Additives used for 24-hour urine specimens	
Test Ordered	**Preservative Added**
Aldosterone	1 g boric acid per 100 mL urine
Amylase	Add NaOH; adjust pH to 6 or above
Urine calcium	Add HCl to adjust pH 1.5–2.0
Catecholamines	Add HCl to adjust pH to 2–3 or add 25 mL 6N HCl
Cyclic AMP (adenosine monophosphate)	10 mL 6M HCl
17-Hydroxy-corticosteroids	Boric acid to adjust pH 5–7
Urine phosphorus	HCl to adjust pH to 1.5–2
Testosterone	1 g Boric acid per 100 mL
Uric acid	NaOH to adjust pH to 8 or above
Dopamine	Glass container with 25 mL HCl
Homovanillic acid (HVA)	Glass container with 25 mL HCl
Iodine	Glass container with 25 mL acetic acid
Vanillymandelic acid (VMA)	Glass container with 25 mL 6N HCl
Urea nitrogen	25 mL 6N HCl
5-Hydroxy-indoleacetic acid (5-HIAA)	25 mL 6N HCl

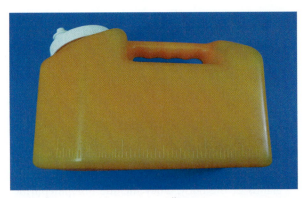

Figure 9-1 A 24-hour urine collection container. Notice the large-volume capacity, the measurements along the side of the container, and the amber color, which blocks light exposure, as some chemical concentrations are decreased with exposure to light. This 24-hour urine collection container includes a special closure adaptation to make it easy to pour the specimen when it arrives at the laboratory.

information about this procedure is included in Chapter 17.)

- **Glucose tolerance urine specimen:** Glucose tolerance urine specimen tests are used for diagnosis of gestational diabetes or diabetes mellitus. Urine and blood specimens are collected at specific intervals after a fasting patient is given a high glucose substance to drink. The first urine specimen collected should ideally be a "fasting" specimen, meaning that it is the second morning void, not the first. The first morning void contains the breakdown products from the food ingested the night before the test; the second morning void should be representative of the body in a state of fasting. After the patient has been given the high glucose substance to drink, a blood and urine collection is performed at least three more times at hourly intervals for 3 more hours. Additional samples may be collected depending on the policy for that particular laboratory. It is not necessary to use the clean-catch midstream collection procedures for this test, as the specimens collected are not used for cultures or complete urinalysis procedures.

Procedure 9-2: Instructing a Patient for Collection of a 24-Hour Urine Specimen

This process collects all urine that is produced by the body over a 24-hour period. It is noninvasive, and provides a great deal of information about the patient's renal function. Remember, urine contains many chemical substances such as sodium, potassium, and creatinine that are dissolved in water. Because the concentration of these chemicals may vary throughout the day, it is important to collect all the urine produced over a 24-hour period for an accurate assessment.

TASK

Provide the necessary supplies and education for a patient to successfully complete a 24-hour urine specimen collection.

CONDITIONS

- An appropriately labeled 24-hour urine collection container (or more than one container if a high volume of urine is anticipated)

- Warning sticker if preservative is added to the specimen container
- An additional smaller container (such as a urinal device) for urine collection
- Written patient instructions, including any dietary restrictions for the collection period

CAAHEP/ABHES STANDARDS

 CAAHEP Standards

I.P.I.6: Anatomy and Physiology: Perform patient screening using established protocols
I.A.I.2: Anatomy and Physiology: Use language/verbal skills that enable patients' understanding

 ABHES Standards

None

Procedure	Rationale
1. Wash hands and gather necessary supplies for the patient. Verify any dietary restrictions and/or preservative requirements for the test ordered by checking the laboratory reference guide. Check to see if the instructions for the analyte ordered include a blood draw.	Hand washing breaks the chain of infection. It is imperative that the medical assistant verify all restrictions and special instructions before meeting with the patient. There should be a written copy of all instructions (including dietary restrictions) available so that they can be provided to the patient.

Continued

Procedure 9-2: Instructing a Patient for Collection of a 24-Hour Urine Specimen—cont'd

Procedure	Rationale
2. Add preservative to the collection container if necessary, using appropriate safety precautions. Apply warning label if acid was added to the container.	Warning labels must be added to the container if there has been preservative added (e.g., hydrochloric acid) that could harm the patient. If there is a harmful preservative added to the container, the patient must be told that he or she cannot urinate directly into the container or splash the specimen on bare skin. **Danger Acid**
3. Greet and identify the patient. Verify the test order once more.	The patient identity must always be verified for every procedure. Verification of test orders and labeling reduces the potential for error. Some laboratories have labels that include the dietary restrictions that are also attached to the container.
4. Provide the patient with the 24-hour urine collection container and an additional smaller, wide-mouth container for urine collection.	The 24-hour urine collection container will be amber or dark in color. It will hold approximately 3 liters of urine. The dark color protects some of the urine chemicals from decomposing with exposure to light. The smaller container is used to collect the specimen during urination, after which it will be added to the large container.
5. Instruct the patient that the 24-hour specimen must remain refrigerated during the collection process. Also emphasize that *all* urine collected during the 24-hour period must be collected in the container provided.	For accurate results the patient must understand that *all* the urine in the 24-hour period must be collected and preserved appropriately. For convenience, the patient may want to choose a day for collection when he or she will be home most of the time.
6. Instruct the patient that upon arising on the first day of the 24-hour period he or she is to empty the bladder by urinating into the toilet. This is the start time of the collection period, so the patient is to note this time on the collection container and on any paperwork that may have been provided for the process.	For accurate results, this part of the process should be emphasized; it is a bit difficult to understand without a thorough explanation.

Procedure	Rationale
7. Explain to the patient that all the urine for the next 24 hours (after that initial void) must be saved in the large container. Instruct the patient that he or she may use the smaller collection container during the urination process, but this urine must all be added immediately to the larger container.	It must be stressed that all the urine must be collected during the 24-hour period for the test results to be valid.
8. Explain to the patient that if for any reason all the urine is not put in the container, the collection process must be started over.	The reference ranges for the tests are dependent on 24-hour specimens; any urine not added to the specimen container may potentially affect the results.
9. Explain to the patient that the 24-hour collection period ends the following day at the same time that the process was started. This urine (from the following morning at the same time) is to be added to the collection container to complete the process. Document this time on the collection container and on any additional paperwork as required.	Emphasize that the 24-hour period starts and ends with an empty bladder.
10. Tell the patient to transport the filled container to the laboratory as directed. It may be necessary to collect blood when the specimen is returned to the laboratory.	The patient should be notified before the collection process begins if there is a blood draw necessary so that he or she is anticipating this.
11. Verify whether the patient understood the instructions as given, and check if there are any additional questions. Supply contact information for future questions.	This is a critical step for the appropriate collection of the specimen.
12. Provide the patient with a written copy of the instructions.	A written copy will allow the patient to refresh his or her memory when the collection is performed.

Date	
10/24/2013:	*Patient provided supplies and written and verbal instructions for a 24-hour urine collection procedure.*
11:58 a.m.	*Connie Lieseke, CMA (AAMA)*

Test Your Knowledge 9-7

How is a first morning void specimen different from a 24-hour urine specimen?   (Outcome 9-3)

Urine Collection Procedures for Infants and Pediatric Patients

It can be very difficult to collect a urine specimen from an infant or young child using noninvasive procedures. A routine specimen may be obtained by using a special type of collection bag designed to be attached to the skin surrounding the urinary opening of a young child or infant. The area around the urinary meatus must be carefully cleaned to reduce contamination, and care must be used to attach the device securely so that the urine does not leak out around the adhesive. It is also important to inform the parents of the patient (if the collection is to be completed at home) to check for the presence of urine in the bag often so that it can be transferred to an appropriate sterile collection cup and refrigerated. Figure 9-2 shows a pediatric urine collection

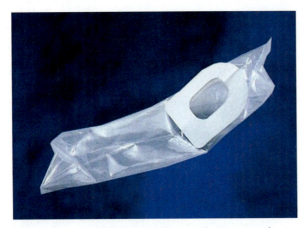

Figure 9-2 Pediatric urine collection device. Note the adhesive surrounding the opening of the bag. The adhesive surface will be applied to the child's cleansed skin surrounding the urinary opening. *Courtesy of Zask, Inc.*

bag. A suprapubic aspiration or straight catheterization procedure may be performed by the physician (or other qualified health-care professional) for young children and infants if a sterile specimen is necessary for proper diagnosis.

Test Your Knowledge 9-8

Why is a special collection device necessary to collect a urine specimen from an infant?   (Outcome 9-3)

URINE SPECIMEN PROCESSING

Because urine can be collected relatively easily without invasive procedures, it is often taken for granted. A urine specimen may have drastic changes occur while standing at room temperature, so care must be taken to handle the specimen correctly after collection until the testing process is complete. Urine that is not processed correctly can lead to misdiagnosis and incorrect treatment for the patient.

Although urine is not considered to be capable of transmitting HIV, hepatitis B, or hepatitis C, it is important that the processor uses gloves and a protective laboratory coat when handling urine samples. Other pathogenic microorganisms may be present in the urine specimen, and employees need to be certain to protect themselves appropriately. Protective eyewear may also be considered if there is a potential for splashing the specimen. This may be particularly critical when handling specimens that have acid added as

---

POINT OF INTEREST 9-3
What now?

Once the specimen has been collected and returned to the laboratory or physician's office, it is up to the medical assistant to process and store it correctly. Here are a few basic guidelines:

- While still in the presence of the patient, verify that the specimen is correctly labeled with name, birth date, and other identifying information.
- Verify and, if necessary, document the date and time of collection on the appropriate paperwork.
- Review the collection process with the patient; ask specifically whether there were any problems with the specimen collection or storage. If the collection or storage of the specimen was incorrect, the specimen should be discarded at this time, and the patient should be provided with materials to perform a recollection.
- Some facilities will have the medical assistant immediately document the color, appearance, and specific gravity of the specimen before it is refrigerated, as these can change once the specimen temperature decreases.
- Specimens for urinalysis, culture, and most other procedures are to be tested or refrigerated as soon as possible, and always within 1 hour of arrival at the laboratory.
- Twenty-four-hour urine collections may need to be mixed well and an aliquot may need to be poured off. This aliquot would then be forwarded to the main laboratory for analysis. (This step will be dependent on the policy of the laboratory performing the 24-hour urine collection container.)

---

preservative, or those that may have a lot of blood present in the urine.

Test Your Knowledge 9-9

Why are gloves worn when handling urine specimens in the laboratory?   (Outcome 9-4)

Refrigeration and Preservation

Urine specimens should be refrigerated (at 2° to 8°Celsius) immediately after collection if they cannot be analyzed within 1 hour of collection. If the specimen is collected in a patient's home, instructions about refrigeration are especially critical. The sample should stay cool until delivered to the laboratory; if a patient has numerous errands to run, or if the patient is going to work, it is important that the patient use a cooler to keep the urine refrigerated until it is delivered to the laboratory.

There are numerous changes that may occur as the urine is left standing at room temperature, but the most dramatic is the change in the bacterial count. The bacteria present in urine specimens are capable of multiplying very rapidly; the bacterial count of the specimen may double within 2 hours at room temperature. This means that the patient may initially be treated for a urinary tract infection based on a high bacterial count reported as part of the urinalysis, when there were actually very few bacteria present in the specimen at the time of collection. Refrigeration halts most of the changes that may occur in the urine specimen, and reduced temperatures are especially effective at limiting the replication process of bacteria. The potential changes to a urine specimen with extended room temperature storage are listed in Table 9-3.

Test Your Knowledge! 9-10

What change in the urine specimen is most dramatic if the specimen is left out at room temperature for more than an hour?

(Outcome 9-5)

TABLE 9-3

Changes in urine specimen when left at room temperature for more than 1 hour

Changes in Urine Specimen	Details and/or Clinical Significance
Decreased clarity and slight color change	Crystallization of solutes; may also cause color interpretation to change as these form
pH increases	Bacteria in specimen convert urea to ammonia and CO_2 is lost
Ketones decrease	Ketones decrease with time at room temperature
Bilirubin and urobilinogen decrease	Exposure to light causes these chemicals to degrade in the specimen
Cells and casts dissolve	Microscopic examination is inconclusive as identification of microscopic features is inaccurate
Bacterial count increases	Bacteria continue to multiply exponentially
Glucose decreases	Glucose is used by bacteria and other cellular components as an energy source

Although it is necessary to preserve urine specimens at reduced temperatures to stabilize some of the analytes, it is important to remember that these reduced temperatures may also affect the specimen. Refrigeration may increase the *specific gravity* of the specimen, and cause some diffuse microscopic crystallization within the urine specimen as well. The specific gravity is a measurement of the amount of dissolved substances in the urine specimen. (More information about specific gravity is covered in Chapter 20.) Urine that has been refrigerated may also change in color and appearance, and these parameters are recorded as part of a routine urinalysis in many situations. In order to counteract the effects of refrigeration on these testing parameters, the urine specimens should be allowed to return to room temperature before routine urinalysis testing is performed. This reverses most of the changes. Also remember the urine specimens must be well mixed with gentle inversion or swirling of the specimen container before testing.

Additives (preservatives) may also be used for specimens that are to be tested for common urinalysis tests and/or set up for urine cultures. Many manufacturers produce tubes with additives for this purpose. An example is BD Vacutainer Plus Plastic Conical urinalysis preservative tubes, which contain chlorhexidine, ethyl paraben, and sodium propionate for preservation of urine specimens for urinalysis. Some of these additive tubes cannot be used for certain types of test procedures; it is imperative that the medical assistant check the package insert to verify whether a specific type of collection container with an additive may be used for the procedure ordered. These special additive tubes are not usually given to the patient for transfer at home; the urine specimen is added to the tube once it arrives at the laboratory or physician office. Because microscopic examinations of the specimens are performed, it is also important that the **formed elements** (substances in the urine specimen such as cells and microorganisms) are preserved so that they can be documented as part of the examination. Additives may assist with the preservation of these substances as well as the chemical components present in the specimen.

Proper Disposal of Urine and Supplies

After testing, laboratories may immediately discard urine samples, or keep them refrigerated for a few days for potential follow-up testing and troubleshooting of test results. When the urine is no longer needed, it may be flushed down the sink, and the specimen containers may be disposed of as regular (nonbiohazardous) trash.

Urine is not considered a biohazard in the same way that blood and other body fluids are. Sinks used for disposal of urine should be disinfected daily with a concentration of 10% bleach or another approved laboratory disinfectant.

SUMMARY

Urine testing is a common method of screening for disorders of metabolism, pregnancy, and potential infection within the body. Proper patient preparation and education are essential to ensure a quality specimen that will yield meaningful results. Collection methods, required volume, and the need for preservatives will vary, depending on the test ordered. Also, once the urine specimen arrives at the laboratory, it is imperative that the specimen is appropriately processed and preserved in a timely manner to prevent overgrowth of microorganisms and potential erroneous results.

TIME TO REVIEW

1. How is a suprapubic aspiration   Outcome 9-3
   different from a catheterization?
   a. The urine is collected from a different part of the urinary system
   b. The collection device used is different for each procedure
   c. The amount of urine collected is not the same for the two types of procedures
   d. All of the above

2. True or False: The urine collected   Outcome 9-3
   using the clean-catch midstream collection procedure may be collected at any time of the day.

3. Which of these statements is not   Outcome 9-4
   true of indwelling catheters?
   a. Indwelling catheters are inserted and used continuously for an extended period of time
   b. Indwelling catheters are often colonized with bacteria
   c. Indwelling catheters may be used to collect a urine specimen after they have been in place for a few days
   d. Indwelling catheters may be used for patients who have problems with incontinence

4. Which of these measurements   Outcome 9-5
   may change when urine is left at room temperature for longer than 1 hour? (Circle all that apply.)
   a. Color
   b. Glucose concentration
   c. Bacterial count
   d. Appearance of microscopic elements
   e. pH
   f. Specific gravity

5. True or False: It is not necessary to   Outcome 9-6
   provide two unique identifiers (such as patient name and birth date) on a urine specimen container.

6. True or False: Labels for urine   Outcome 9-6
   specimen containers may be placed on the lid only; it is not necessary to label the container.

7. Which of these urine specimen types   Outcome 9-3
   may be collected at random times? (Circle all that apply.)
   a. Clean-catch midstream urine specimens
   b. Specimens to check for prostatitis
   c. Specimens used to check for the presence of glucose as part of a glucose tolerance test
   d. Suprapubic aspiration specimens
   e. Urine pregnancy test specimens
   f. Culture specimens

8. The urinary meatus is: Outcome 9-1
   a. Part of the bladder
   b. The excess skin removed during the process of circumcision
   c. The external opening of the urethra
   d. Part of the prostate gland

9. True or False: Different collection   Outcome 9-2
   techniques for urine specimens are necessary because chemicals are not present in urine in the same concentration at the same time each day.

10. Diurnal variation means: Outcome 9-1
    a. Fluctuations in the value of an analyte that occur during each day.
    b. Concentration of urine in the morning void specimen.
    c. Changes in urinary pH when urine is left at room temperature
    d. None of the above

11. True or False: An aliquot of a urine   Outcome 9-1
    specimen refers to a small portion (or fraction) of the whole.

Case Study 9-1: Postoperative pain

Mr. Johnson has had pain in his perineal area for more than a week, and he has noticed that he is urinating quite frequently. Mr. Johnson decides that he should call the physician for an appointment, because he now has a fever and doesn't feel as if he can go to work. He recently had abdominal surgery, and was catheterized with an indwelling catheter for several days before he was mobile.

1. What are two possible explanations for his discomfort and frequent urination?
2. How could the physician decide on the correct diagnosis? What procedures might be utilized?

Case Study 9-2: Specimen dropoff

Mrs. Brown brings her 24-hour urine specimen container to the office. The medical assistant who is working at the front desk receives the specimen from Mrs. Brown.

1. What does the medical assistant need to do before Mrs. Brown leaves the office?

RESOURCES AND SUGGESTED READINGS

"Prostatitis"
Neal Chamberlain, computerized teaching materials for the Infectious Disease Course at Kirksville College of Osteopathic Medicine http://www.atsu.edu/faculty/chamberlain/Website/lectures/lecture/prostate.htm

"Acute Bacterial Prostatitis"
Overview of prostatitis, with specific information about diagnosis and treatment http://www.drrajmd.com/conditions/prostate/prostatitis/acute_bacterial_prostatitis.htm

"Care Gram 24-Hour Urine and Food Drug Restrictions"
Information about dietary and medication restrictions for 24-hour urine collections from Licking Memorial Health Systems http://www.lmhealth.org/pdf/CareGrams/Lab%20Tests/24%20Hour%20Urine%20&%20Food%20Drug%20Restrictions%201616-0550.pdf

"CAP Today: Cloudy or Clear? Best Forecasts for Urine Cultures," CAP today online newsletter, November 2006
Details for a study about preanalytical errors with urine specimen collection for cultures http://www.cap.org/apps/portlets/contentViewer/show.do?printFriendly=true&contentReference=cap_today%2Ffeature_stories%2F1106Urine.html

"24-Hour Urine Collection"
Southwestern University Health Library selection about 24-hour urine collection; includes clinical significance and details about the collection process http://www.utsouthwestern.edu/patientcare/healthlibrary/healthtopics/0,,P08955,00.html

"Best Practice: Tips for Urinalysis"
Becton, Dickinson online newsletter, LabNotes, 13, no. 2, 2003
Details about urine processing for urinalysis and urine cultures, including information about preservative tubes that are available http://www.bd.com/vacutainer/labnotes/2003spring/best_practice.asp

"Sample Meal for a 2-Hour Postprandial Glucose Test"
Patient instructions for 2-hour postprandial glucose testing procedure from the Delaware Valley Institute of Fertility and Genetics http://www.startfertility.com/patient_fld/form_pdfs/Sample_Meal-2-hr_PP_glucose_test.pdf

"Laws, Regulations, Standards and Guidelines"
A publication of the New Jersey Hospital Association with a summary of laws, regulations, standards, and guidelines that pertain to language assistance for diverse populations in the health-care setting that may not have English as their native language http://www.njha.com/publications/pdf/Laws_Regulations_Standards_and_Guidelines.pdf

Chapter 10

Collection and Processing of Samples for Microbial Studies

Constance L. Lieseke, CMA (AAMA), MLT, PBT(ASCP)

CHAPTER OUTLINE

Learning Outcomes

After reading this chapter, the successful student will be able to:

10-1 Define the key terms.

10-2 Demonstrate understanding of the general guidelines to be followed when collecting for microbiology testing.

10-3 List various types of media used for bacterial and viral specimen setup.

10-4 Describe how the collection processes and supplies for bacterial, viral, and fungal specimens may differ.

10-5 Compare and contrast sample collection of throat swabs for streptococcal screens and cultures.

10-6 Explain the collection procedure for sputum samples.

10-7 Differentiate the types of urine specimens that may be used for cultures.

10-8 Describe the procedure for collecting a specimen for a blood culture.

10-9   Describe how a cerebrospinal fluid (CSF) sample is collected, and explain how the sample should be processed after collection.

10-10   Explain how genital screening samples are processed.

10-11   Demonstrate an understanding of the various types of wound cultures and how their processing differs.

10-12   Compare and contrast collection and processing of stool samples as compared to other common microbiology specimen types.

10-13   State when a nasopharyngeal specimen may be necessary, and describe the collection technique used.

10-14   Describe the technique used for eye and ear culture sample collection procedures.

10-15   Classify the various types of fungal infections, and describe the techniques used to collect fungal culture samples.

10-16   Differentiate the requirements and use of a KOH prep and a wet mount specimen preparation.

10-17   Explain how a stool sample is collected and preserved for an examination for the presence of ova and parasites.

10-18   Summarize the sample collection process used for detecting a pinworm infection.

10-19   Explain the steps involved in performance of a Gram stain, as well as the differential appearance of the stained organisms.

10-20   Explain how a microbiological sample is plated for growth.

10-21   Describe how sensitivity testing is performed and explain the clinical significance of the process.

10-22   Translate a microbiology laboratory report, and explain the clinical significance of the values.

CAAHEP/ABHES STANDARDS

 CAAHEP Standards

I.A.I.2. Use language/verbal skills that enable patients' understanding
III.C.III.3. Discuss infection control procedures
III.C.III.5 List major types of infectious agents
III.C.III.7. Match types and uses of personal protective equipment (PPE)
III.C.III.9. Discuss quality control issues related to handling microbiological specimens
III.P.III.2. Practice Standard Precautions
III.P.III.3. Select appropriate barrier/personal protective equipment (PPE) for potentially infectious situations
III.P.III.7. Obtain specimens for microbiological testing
III.A.III.1. Display sensitivity to patient rights and feelings in collecting specimens
III.A.III.2. Explain the rationale for performance of a procedure to a patient
III.A.III.3. Show awareness of patients' concerns regarding their perceptions related to the procedure being performed

 ABHES Standards

- Apply principles of aseptic techniques and infection control
- Use standard precautions
- Practice quality control
- Perform selected CLIA-waived tests that assist with diagnosis and treatment, #5: Microbiology testing
- Dispose of biohazardous materials
- Collect, label and process specimens, #3: Perform wound collection procedures, #4: Obtain throat specimen for microbiology testing
- Instruct patients in the collection of a fecal specimen

KEY TERMS

Aerobes

Agar

Anaerobes

Antibiotic sensitivity testing

Broth

Candle jar

Cerebrospinal fluid (CSF) samples

Colonies

Cover slip

Culture

Culture and sensitivity (C&S) report

Disk-diffusion method

Ectoparasites

Endoparasites

Eustachian tube

Exudate

Gram stain

Hanging drop slide

Hemolytic uremic syndrome

Inoculation

Kirby-Bauer method

KOH (potassium hydroxide)

Lumbar puncture

Medium (pl., media)

Methicillin-resistant *Staphylococcus aureus* (MRSA)

Minimum inhibitory concentration (MIC) method

Motility

Mycoses

Nasopharyngeal collection technique

Nasopharynx

Normal flora

Otitis

Otitis externa

Otitis media

Ova and parasite examination (O&P)

Parasites

Pathogen

Petri dish

Pinworm

Resistant

Scabies

Sensitive

Septicemia

Sequela

Slant

Sputum

Strep screens

Trichomoniasis

Wet mount

Wood's lamp

Zone of inhibition

Microbiology is the study of organisms that require magnification to be seen by the human eye. As introduced in Chapter 3, microorganisms are everywhere! These tiny creatures have been the objects of study since the early 1700s, when Antony Leeuwenhoek first recorded observations of bacteria he watched with his homemade microscopes. These "animalcules" (as Leeuwenhoek called them) were described in great detail, and Leeuwenhoek hired an illustrator to provide pictures of the living creatures that he observed. However, the idea that microorganisms were capable of spreading disease was understood much later. In 1847, Ignaz Semmelweis was working in a maternity hospital in Siena, Italy, when he realized that some sort of "invisible agent" seemed to spread from the mothers who died of puerperal fever after childbirth to the other mothers in the ward. He insisted that the physicians working in the ward begin to wash their hands between

patients, and also had the practitioners change their laboratory coats after performing autopsies before they worked with expectant mothers. These small changes resulted in a dramatic drop in the mortality rates in the maternity ward of the hospital. Unfortunately, Semmelweis was ridiculed for his strict enforcement of the rules, and was subsequently fired.

It would still be almost 100 years before observations such as the ones made by Semmelweis began to change the way that the world viewed microorganisms and their relationship to disease. Louis Pasteur and Robert Koch were responsible for many of the theories that we use in microbiology today. In the late 1800s, they conducted a series of experiments to suggest that bacteria cause disease, and these scientists went even further to prove that bacteria did not spontaneously generate, but instead replicated at a very fast pace when introduced to an environment that supported their growth. It was also proved during this time that bacteria could be kept from contaminating a certain area if the appropriate precautions were taken. These were revolutionary ideas that continue to shape the way we view microorganisms today.

When working with microbiological samples, it is important to keep these core concepts in mind, as our goal is to avoid extraneous contamination of the specimens, to provide appropriate samples for testing to allow for proper patient diagnosis and treatment, and to nurture the growth of microscopic organisms so that they can be identified. We now know that the microscopic "animalcules" that can cause harm do not include only bacteria. Microbiology testing may also focus on viruses, fungi, and parasites. Because of this variety, collection methods and testing procedures vary, depending on the type of specimen collected and the organism that is thought to be present. The laboratory may process these samples in the general microbiology department, or there may be subdivisions for bacteriology, virology, mycology, and/or parasitology. This chapter presents collection and handling procedures for the most common types of microbiological tests ordered.

MICROBIOLOGY SAMPLE COLLECTION GUIDELINES

In order to provide appropriate treatment, health-care providers need to know which type of pathogen is causing the symptoms exhibited by the patient. A **pathogen** is a microorganism that is capable of causing disease in the body. Most infectious diseases are caused by viruses or bacteria. Treatment choices vary dramatically based on the causative organism present in the specimen collected for testing. Variables for treatment may be based on the type of pathogen present (such as viruses, bacteria, fungi, or parasites), the amount of the microscopic organism isolated, as well as sensitivity testing for antimicrobials suitable for treatment. The microorganism that causes a disease is a pathogen, so health-care providers must always remember which organisms may be present as part of the **normal flora** (resident bacteria present in certain areas of the body) as these may contaminate the specimen, and their presence may be misleading.

Test Your Knowledge 10-1

What is the term used to describe a microorganism that causes disease?.   (Outcome 10-1)

To assure quality processes and valid results, specific guidelines should be followed whenever collecting or processing samples for microbiology testing. These include the following:

Specimen collection

- Collect the sample from the area of infection, and avoid contamination from surrounding areas if at all possible. This is especially critical when collecting samples for wound cultures.
- Ideally, bacterial culture specimens should be collected before antibiotics are introduced. If the antibiotics have already been administered, the causative organism may not be present in high enough numbers to identify it appropriately.
- Use the correct collection and transportation methods. Research what type of swab or container is to be used, and how the sample is to be handled after collection until it reaches the laboratory. Package inserts should be consulted for specific collection techniques. Some samples are to be refrigerated immediately, whereas others are to remain at room temperature until they are transported to the laboratory for processing.
- Always collect a sufficient quantity of sample for testing.
- Be certain that the sample is appropriately labeled, including the source (be as specific as possible), the patient's name, the identification of the individual performing the specimen collection, and the date and time of the collection. Document this information on the requisition form appropriately as well.
- Verify and adhere to any sample restrictions for transport time. Also verify whether the sample needs to be protected from light after collection.
- Use sterile supplies, and be careful to maintain sterility while performing sample collection procedures.
- Store all laboratory specimens in a refrigerator or other container dedicated for that use.

Personnel

- All personnel participating in the collection, processing, or testing of microbiological specimens must be appropriately trained in all procedures.
- Personnel should participate regularly in competency testing to assure quality of collection, processing and testing of specimens.
- Wear appropriate personal protective equipment (PPE) when performing specimen collection or specimen processing. This may include items such as gloves, a laboratory coat, face shield, or special respiratory equipment such as that needed for processing samples that may contain tuberculosis.

Media

- A medium provides nutrition for microorganisms when grown in the laboratory environment. There is an expiration date associated with all media to ensure appropriate performance. Media should be discarded when outdated.
- For a medium to function as designed, it cannot be allowed to dry out or become contaminated. In addition, there are specific storage requirements for each type of medium, and these must be followed carefully.
- Verify that the correct medium is used for each type of specimen collection, as this can have a profound effect on the results.
- Medium performance should be verified on a regular basis by inoculating the medium with a known microorganism to observe growth.

Stains

- All products used for staining microorganisms have expiration dates provided by the manufacturer, after which the stains must be discarded. Stain performance should be verified on a regular basis by staining microorganisms with predictable staining characteristics to observe staining patterns.

Test Your Knowledge 10-2

What must be documented on the sample after the collection of a microbiology specimen?   (Outcome 10-2)

Test Your Knowledge 10-3

Should bacterial culture specimens be collected before or after antibiotic therapy has been started?

(Outcome 10-2)

Types of Media

The growth of any microorganism in the laboratory is dependent on the presence of an appropriate nutrition source and other chemicals necessary for survival. These are provided in a culture **medium** (plural, **media**). The medium may be in the form of a liquid nutrient broth, a semi-solid gel, or a solid gel. **Agar** is a thickening agent added to the medium that allows the gel to solidify so that the microorganisms will grow on the surface. A medium may be provided in tubes, or it may be provided in a small shallow container, known as a **Petri dish.** Figure 10-1 shows various types of media used in a microbiology setting. Some laboratories create their own media, but most purchase commercially prepared media, which provide a longer shelf life, fewer impurities, and more consistent appearance and performance. All types of media contain nutrients and additives that support the growth of microorganisms. Ingredients may include blood, vitamins, dyes, sugar mixtures, and organic sources of nutrition such as vegetable extracts.

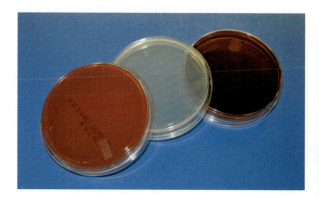
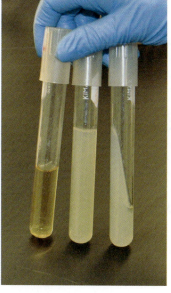

Figure 10-1 Types of media. Note the presence of the agar plate, the slant, and the broth.

Culture media is classified into categories based on whether the medium enriches the growth of all bacteria or selectively inhibits growth of certain bacteria.

- *Selective media* have additives that prevent the growth of certain types of bacteria while promoting the growth of other select species. One example is Thayer Martin agar, used for specimens when a gonorrhea infection is suspected. It has lysed red blood cells, which provide an easy source of hemoglobin to promote the growth of the *Neisseria gonorrhoeae* organism, but the medium also contains vancomycin, colistin, and nystatin. These are antibiotics that prohibit the growth of other common nonpathogenic microorganisms often found concurrently with gonorrhea.
- *Differential media* allow for different types of bacteria to be identified based on an indicator. A common differential medium used in the laboratory is MacConkey agar, which has a special dye additive. If the organisms growing on the agar ferment lactose (the indicator), their growth will appear pink on the medium plate. This colored growth allows the microbiologists to make a preliminary identification of the pathogenic microorganisms based on their ability to ferment lactose.
- *Enriched media* include nutrients that allow for a wide variety of organisms to grow. Blood agar is an example of an enriched medium that is designed to support growth of microorganisms that flourish in the human body, including both pathogens and nonpathogens.

Solid gel is provided in a tube (called a **slant**) or in a Petri dish. Liquid medium (usually called nutrient **broth**) comes in a tightly sealed tube. It is important to keep all forms of media from drying out or becoming contaminated after receipt at the laboratory or physician office. The media should be refrigerated for storage, but must be brought to room temperature before use. All forms of media have a limited shelf life, so it is important to be aware of their expiration date.

Test Your Knowledge 10-4

What are two ways that culture media may differ?

(Outcome 10-3)

Microbiology Terms

A **culture** is a group of microorganisms grown in a laboratory environment using prepared media. The word *culture* is used whether the sample is bacterial, viral, or fungal. A culture is created when a medium source has a specimen added for potential growth. The culture is the most

common test performed in the microbiology laboratory. The process of adding the specimen to a medium source is known as **inoculation.** Inoculation may occur in the physician office immediately after specimen collection, or it may be performed once the specimen arrives at the laboratory. The visible growth that occurs once the specimen has been added to the medium may be seen as **colonies** (or clumps) of growth, especially with bacterial cultures. The unique appearance of the colonies present on the culture may allow for preliminary identification of the microorganism. To accelerate bacterial growth, the specimen is usually placed in an incubator that is kept near body temperature (37°Celsius) for 24 to 48 hours. Some organisms must be placed in an environment with little to no oxygen present for growth (**anaerobes**), whereas others like an oxygen-rich environment (**aerobes**). There are incubators or other devices that are specifically designed to provide these parameters for culture growth.

Preliminary laboratory results for bacterial cultures are often available within 24 to 48 hours after the specimen has been submitted to the laboratory. Each laboratory establishes a definitive time frame before which they will not report a negative result for a bacterial culture. This means that the laboratory gives the sample a chance to grow for at least a few days before posting a negative result. Most pathogenic bacteria are relatively easy to grow in the laboratory, and identification techniques have been established for most of these microorganisms.

Viral cultures require a longer time for growth and identification, and require use of different types of media than those required for bacterial cultures. Because viruses are parasitic intracellular organisms, viral cultures require living tissue and cells to support growth and replication. It is imperative that the person collecting a viral specimen for culture pay scrupulous attention to specimen collection protocol, the technique of collection, and transportation requirements. Viral culture specimens should be collected, in general, within 72 hours of symptom onset. Collection swabs made of calcium alginate should not be used for collection of viral culture specimens, and cotton-tipped swabs with wooden shafts must also be avoided. Generally, viral specimens are refrigerated to preserve their integrity if there will be a delay in transportation. Because it is a complicated process, viral culture processing is usually performed only in large reference laboratories. It may be 7 to 10 days before a viral culture result is confirmed. For this reason, if a viral infection is suspected and the patient's symptoms warrant it, the health-care provider may administer antiviral medication to the patient without a culture result or identification of the organism.

Fungal cultures are even slower to grow than viral cultures. The fungal elements in a specimen may be difficult to isolate because of the faster-growing organisms present in or on the specimen, such as bacteria. A selective media is used, including nutrition sources such as brain and/or heart extract, blood, dextrose, and natural nutrition sources such as potatoes. Antibiotics may be added to retard the growth of the bacteria in the specimen so that the fungal elements can be identified. The exact type of media used will be dictated by the specific source of the specimen within the body, as, for example, the types of fungus growing on the skin may be very different from those growing in the lungs. A fungal culture may take up to 4 weeks to report results; it is generally a minimum of 21 days before a negative result can be released.

Test Your Knowledge 10-5

Which type of culture (viral, bacterial, or fungal) is quickest to grow? (Outcome 10-4)

POINT OF INTEREST 10-1
Bioterrorism

Prior to September 11, 2001, the threat of widespread bioterrorism was a rare topic in most casual conversations. However, the climate changed with the events of that day and the weeks that followed. The Centers for Disease Control and Prevention (CDC) strongly recommends that all laboratories (even those in physician offices) continue to monitor their procedures and remain aware of those that could create aerosols. An aerosol is a suspension of fine particles (such as bacteria or viruses) in the air. For those facilities in which the risk of aerosol formation is heightened because of the types of procedures performed and the patient population served, a biosafety hood is recommended. The procedures would be performed within the hood workspace, and any microorganisms released into the air would be vented out of the room.

Health-care facilities also must remain educated about what to do in case of an exposure within their facility; fast, appropriate action can save lives. The agents may be bacterial or viral in nature. Most, but not all, agents that could be used for bioterrorism would be spread through the aerosol form. It is difficult to predict which agents may be used for a biological attack, but the following are some that are considered to be most probable:

- **Anthrax:** In the 1800s, Louis Pasteur documented work that he performed with this bacterium, and there are reports of soldiers using anthrax in World War I to deliberately infect animals that were to be eaten by the enemy. In October and November 2001, there were 22 cases of deliberate infection with the anthrax bacterium in the United States. Anthrax is caused by *Bacillus anthracis* and is a gram-positive, spore-forming bacillus. In nature, the spores may be present in the soil, and they are either ingested or picked up on the skin and hair of animals when they are feeding. Humans usually become infected only when they come in contact with animals or products that are contaminated, and infection is rare. There are three routes of infection for anthrax:

  - *Cutaneous:* The most common natural route is cutaneous, or via the skin; humans may be infected when handling contaminated wool, or occasionally from the spores in the soil. The cutaneous infection causes a papule that progresses with time into a necrotic ulcer. If the ulcer penetrates deep enough into the skin, the patient's bloodstream may become infected, which can lead to more serious consequences.

  - *Inhalation:* The route that is used most often for deliberate infection is via inhalation. The exposed patient has flu-like symptoms. Within days, the patient suffers from hypoxia and has difficulty breathing, as pulmonary edema and further damages within the lungs progress. Approximately 50% of those who are infected via the inhalation develop meningitis, and the morbidity rate is quite high. Prior to 2001, there had been only 20 cases of anthrax infection via inhalation reported in the United States.

  - *Gastrointestinal:* The ingestion of poorly cooked, contaminated meat allows anthrax entrance via the gastrointestinal route. The patient may have abdominal discomfort, bloody diarrhea, and vomiting, and may have visible ulcerations in the oropharynx when examined. Essentially, the necrotic lesions that are visible with cutaneous exposure form within the GI tract and impair the patient's ability to digest food properly.

  All forms of anthrax exposure can be treated with antibiotics if caught early. Once the more serious symptoms have developed, it may be difficult treat successfully. Ciprofloxacin or doxycycline is often used successfully for early treatment. Anthrax is not passed from person to person.

- **Brucellosis:** Brucellosis is a disease that is common in cattle, sheep, goats, and pigs in many areas of the world. It may also affect domestic animals such as dogs. Humans may be infected by direct exposure to an animal host. There are very few human infections in the United States because of a rigid vaccination program, but the disease is much more frequent in other areas of the world. Infection causes flu-like symptoms in most humans, but can lead to much more serious CNS problems, as well as heart damage. Brucellosis forms an aerosol very easily, so to avoid potential inhalation in the workplace, it is important to remember not to "sniff" cultures in the microbiology area. This practice may be very dangerous.

- **Botulism:** The symptoms associated with botulism are related to the toxin produced by the spore-forming bacterium *Clostridium botulinum*. This toxin is one of the most lethal natural substances known to humans. The toxin paralyzes the muscles of those infected, which eventually leads to paralysis of the lungs, and death. The toxin is not used as an aerosol as much as some of the other microorganisms considered as threats for bioterrorism use, but the bacteria could be very lethal if added to a common food source or used in a contained area. *C. botulinum* may also be introduced into the body through a wound; there is evidence that armies in the past added it to their swords to enhance the damage done during hand-to-hand combat. For those infected, the most important consideration is the treatment of symptoms, as the damage caused by the toxin spreads quickly throughout the body.

- **Plague:** Everyone who has studied world history has heard of the plague in medieval Europe. The plague is caused by the bacteria *Yersinia pestis* and may infect humans through two different routes. One is the bubonic plague, which is usually caused by the bite of a flea or tick carried on a host rodent. The other is through inhalation. This is the method that causes concern for potential use of this bacterium as a bioterrorist weapon. The pneumonic plague may be spread from person to person via droplets in the air after the initial infection, and is relatively easy to isolate and grow in large amounts. Thus, initial infection could lead to wider and wider mortality. Infection may easily cause respiratory failure and death. The bacterium is treatable with tetracycline and/or fluoroquinolone for at least 7 days if given orally, or IV streptomycin or gentamycin, but the infection must be caught early.

- **Smallpox:** Smallpox is different from the other microorganisms that are considered bioterrorist threats because it is a virus instead of a type of bacterium. The last natural case of smallpox in the United States occurred in 1949, and the causative agent (the variola virus) is considered to have been eradicated by a long-term, aggressive, and worldwide vaccination campaign that has been carried out since 1980. There is no specific treatment for the smallpox virus infection except for supportive care of the symptoms. The variola virus appears to infect only humans, and it may be passed from person to person through infected body fluids and contaminated bedding. It is very rarely passed through the aerosol route, and is not naturally present in nature, so use of the virus as a bioterrorist tool would require more effort than some of the other agents discussed here.

- **Hemorrhagic fever viruses:** These viruses are carried by a host or vector, usually a rodent (such as a rat or mouse) or a tick, flea, or mosquito. For some of the viruses (Ebola and Marburg, for instance) the host is still unknown. Once a human has been infected, it is possible to spread the virus from person to person through contaminated body fluids. Outbreaks are sporadic around the world, and usually remain limited to the area where the vector or host is located, but this has the potential to change. Because of the ease of travel today, coupled with the fact that rats and mice can "stow away" on ships and planes, it is possible for these diseases to become widespread within a relatively short period of time. Those who are infected have flu-like symptoms early in the disease process. Then as the disease progresses, there may be evidence of hemorrhaging under the skin, and bleeding from all orifices of the body. Multiple organs are affected by the virus, and it usually is the organ failure that causes fatalities, not the loss of blood. There are no vaccines or cures for these infections at this time; infected individuals are quarantined and treated symptomatically.

- **Tularemia:** Tularemia is caused by the bacterium *Francisella tularensis* and is carried often by rodents, rabbits, or wild hares. It is *very* infectious; only a small number of the bacteria entering the body will cause disease. It is easy to spread this bacterium as an airborne weapon, so it would be a likely choice for bioterrorist activities. It causes a severe respiratory illness and life-threatening pneumonia, and is not difficult to find in nature. It is treatable with early intervention and aggressive antibiotic treatment.

DETAILED MICROBIOLOGY SAMPLE COLLECTION PROCEDURES

Procedures and supplies may vary for the different microbiology collection processes, but there are common techniques shared by all the systems. Specimens may be collected in a sterile cup or tube or, more commonly, on a swab to be transported to the laboratory. These collection swabs are commercially prepared and supplied in a sterile pull-apart package. The package includes a sterile swab (often made of Dacron) and a transport medium designed to keep the swab from drying out before it reaches the laboratory. Culturette (manufactured by Becton, Dickinson) is an example of a system used for transport. Figure 10-2 includes some of the common sample collection devices available. The following are some techniques to be used for all culture collections:

- Be certain that a laboratory request form has been completed for the patient. The specific source of the specimen must be documented.
- Verify the collection technique necessary for the test ordered, as well as how the specimen is to be handled after collection: refrigeration, room temperature storage, frozen. Most bacterial culture specimens are to be kept at room temperature until transported.
- Always sanitize your hands, and wear appropriate personal protective equipment (PPE). In some situations, this may be a face shield or a disposable gown that covers your scrubs. In patients who have a wound that is positive for methicillin-resistant *Staphylococcus aureus* (MRSA), for example, it is often necessary to take extra precautions and to dispose of all the PPE used in collection before leaving the presence of the patient.
- If using a swab, check the package for signs of potential contamination (e.g., water stains, torn outer packaging) and verify that the expiration date has not passed. If using a different type of collection container, ensure that the package is sterile by examining the outer wrapper or safety seal.
- For swab packages, carefully peel apart the plastic outer envelope, using aseptic technique. Put this

down on a flat surface. Pick up the swab by the lid that is attached to the end of the "stick" end of the swab. (The lid is permanently attached to the swab in most cases.) It is very important that the swab does not touch any other surfaces before the specimen is collected, or extraneous organisms may be added to the culture specimen.

- Collect the specimen appropriately, avoiding any other areas of the body except those needed for the collection.
- Without setting down the inoculated swab, remove the cap from the collection tube (still sitting inside the sterile plastic package) and insert the inoculated swab fully into the collection tube until the lid clicks closed. It may be necessary to activate the transport medium present in the tube by breaking an ampule at the bottom of the tube; this will depend on the type of collection device used.
- Remove gloves and other PPE that was used in the collection process, and sanitize the hands.
- Label the specimen carefully, documenting the specimen source, patient's name, the date, the time, the source (be specific), and your initials or identification. Chart the procedure in the patient's chart if it is available to you.
- If the specimen is to be transported via courier to a laboratory for workup, place it in a biohazardous specimen bag. The requisition form goes into the outer pocket of the bag. If the bag has an area for documentation for handling and storing the specimen, mark this appropriately (e.g., room temperature, refrigerated).
- Place the specimen in the pickup area for the courier to transport to the laboratory.

> ### Test Your Knowledge 10-6
> When using a swab to collect a culture specimen, is it acceptable to set it down on a countertop while getting the patient situated for the collection procedure?
>
> (Outcome 10-2)

Throat Sample Collections for Culture or Strep Screens

Samples may be taken from the throat of patients for group A strep screens for general cultures, or sometimes both types of specimens at the same time. For both a strep screen sample and a culture sample the collection procedure is identical, but the materials used for the collection may differ. Before beginning the collection, it is

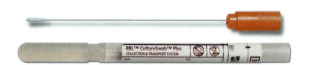

Figure 10-2   Swab collection devices. *Courtesy of BD, Inc.*

important to verify whether the physician wants a culture to be performed, a strep screen, or both. Once the strep screen is performed, it is not possible to use the sample for the culture setup. If both a culture and a strep screen are ordered, the culture plate may be inoculated before the strep screen is performed, but not afterward. It is also possible to use two swabs (these are packaged as a double swab) at the same time to collect the sample so that one can be used for each procedure. Be careful about the type of collection swab used; strep screens recommend the use of rayon collection swabs. Cotton swabs or wooden tipped swabs are not to be used for strep screens. Some of the CLIA-waived procedures don't recommend the use of liquid or gel transport media after collection.

Throat samples are used most commonly to test for streptococcal infections with a **group A strep screen** rapid test completed in the physician office. Group A streptococcus (a subtype of *Streptococcus pyogenes)* is the most common cause of streptococcal throat infection. Those who are positive for streptococcal infection of the throat should be treated immediately to avoid sequela that can develop as a result of the initial strep infection. A **sequela** is a serious secondary complication or infection that follows as a result of the primary bacterial infection. For a group A streptococcal infection, these complications may include heart damage and kidney damage from glomerulonephritis. Throat specimen collections are performed using a sterile swab, often made of Dacron, rayon, or a cotton mixture. For a throat culture, the sterile swab is part of a packaged culture collection kit, with transport media usually present in the transport tube. The throat culture specimen is transported to the laboratory for processing, whereas a strep screen sample is usually processed immediately after collection by performing a CLIA-waived strep screen test. A sterile swab provided with the strep screen kit is used for the collection, and there is no transport medium present. Remember to verify whether the physician wants both a strep screen and a culture to be performed, as the medical assistant needs to know this information before performing the strep screen.

> ### Test Your Knowledge 10-7
> What is one way that a collection for a throat culture and a rapid strep screen are similar?   (Outcome 10-5)

Strep screens are one of the most common CLIA-waived tests performed in all types of laboratories. The test is simple to perform, and requires only a sample taken from the back of the throat, a tongue depressor, personal protective equipment, and the supplies in the kit. The entire process takes approximately 10 minutes from the time the order is received to the time the result may be reported. This fast turnaround time and the ease with which the test can be performed allow the patient to be treated immediately if the screen is positive for the streptococcus A antigen. The CLIA-waived group A strep screen procedure is presented in Chapter 24.

> ### Test Your Knowledge 10-8
> Is it acceptable to collect only one swab if a strep screen *and* a throat culture are ordered?   (Outcome 10-5)

> ### Test Your Knowledge 10-9
> Are the samples for a strep screen and for a throat culture collected from different areas of the throat?
> (Outcome 10-5)

Sputum Samples

When patients are diagnosed with a lower respiratory infection, such as pneumonia, it is important to identify the causative organism if possible. This allows the health-care provider to plan the best course of action for treatment. Sputum samples are necessary for culture and organism identification in these situations. **Sputum** is the substance produced from a deep cough or from aspiration caused by inserting a tube down the patient's throat. Aspiration of sputum is primarily performed on patients who are intubated in an inpatient setting, but sputum cultures may be collected by patients at home without aspiration.

The medical assistant is not usually involved with the actual collection process for a sputum sample if employed in a physician office, but it is important that the procedure is explained thoroughly to the patient so that he or she may produce a quality sample. Sputum samples are collected into a sterile container (such as a urine cup or a centrifuge tube) and transported immediately to the laboratory for processing. Ideally, a sputum collection system will protect the sample from UV light. The system should also prevent the health-care employees processing the specimen from being exposed to the sputum. Becton, Dickinson offers a sputum collection system that does both, composed of a large centrifuge tube enclosed in an amber "funnel" tube with a lid on the top (Fig. 10-3). The amber outer container is important, as *Mycobacterium tuberculosis,* the causative

Procedure 10-1: Collection of a Throat Specimen for Culture or Strep Screen

Throat culture collections are very common procedures in physician offices. It is important to perform the collection process correctly to ensure meaningful results. Remember to communicate appropriately with the patient to assist with the collection process.

TASK

Collect an appropriate specimen from the throat for a culture or strep screen. Complete the procedure within 5 minutes.

CONDITIONS

- Hand sanitization equipment
- Gloves
- Tongue depressor
- Safety shield
- Sterile culture swab or swab provided with strep screen kit
- Label
- Laboratory requisition form
- Biohazardous waste container
- Biohazardous transport bag

CAAHEP/ABHES STANDARDS

 CAAHEP Standards

I.A.I.2. Use language/verbal skills that enable patients' understanding, **III.C.III.3:** Discuss infection control procedures, **III.C.III.9:** Discuss quality control issues related to handling microbiological specimens. **III.P.III.2:** Practice Standard Precautions, **III.P.III.3:** Select appropriate barrier/personal protective equipment (PPE) for potentially infectious situations, **III.P.III.7:** Obtain specimens for microbiological testing, **III.A.III.1:** Display sensitivity to patient rights and feelings in collecting specimens, **III.A.III.2:** Explain the rationale for performance of a procedure to the patient.

 ABHES Standards

- Apply principles of aseptic techniques and infection control
- Use standard precautions
- Practice quality control
- Perform selected CLIA-waived tests that assist with diagnosis and treatment, #5: Microbiology testing
- Dispose of biohazardous materials
- Collect, label and process specimens, #3: Perform wound collection procedures, #4: Obtain throat specimen for microbiology testing

Procedure	Rationale
1. Greet and properly identify the patient, using at least two unique identifiers. Introduce yourself.	It is imperative that the identity of the patient is verified before the specimen is collected. The medical assistant should always identify him- or herself with any patient interaction.
2. Explain the procedure to the patient. Answer any questions that the patient may have about the collection process.	Explaining the procedure will help the patient know what to expect and will facilitate cooperation. Answering questions allows the medical assistant to display sensitivity to patient rights and feelings in collecting specimens.
3. Sanitize hands (allow them to dry) and apply gloves.	Gloves must be worn for any procedures in which exposure to blood or other potentially infectious materials is anticipated.

Continued

Procedure 10-1:   Collection of a Throat Specimen for Culture or Strep Screen—cont'd

Procedure	Rationale
4. Gather necessary supplies within reach. If a strep screen is ordered, be certain to use the swab supplied with the kit. If a throat culture is requested, use a sterile swab packaged with the transport media.	Organization of supplies is important so that the collection procedure may continue without interruption.
5. Position the patient in an upright position. If necessary, adjust available lighting so that the back of the throat is well lit.	The back of the throat must be well lit and accessible for the collection to be successful.
6. Put on face safety shield.	Because this procedure may initiate coughing or gagging in some individuals, it is important that the medical assistant protect against potential exposure.
7. While holding the tongue depressor in one hand and the collection swab in the other, instruct the patient to open his or her mouth wide.	The mouth must be opened wide to gain full access to the collection area.
8. Push down on the tongue lightly with the tongue depressor, and insert the swab into mouth. Be certain to avoid touching the tongue, cheeks, gums, or teeth with the collection swab.	Introduction of extraneous microorganisms may result in inaccurate culture results.
9. Gently brush the swab against the tonsillar area and the back of the throat. A gentle rotating motion works best. Be sure to touch any white or inflamed patches present with the collection swab.	Adequate sample must be obtained for the accuracy of the culture results. White areas may represent clusters of bacteria, so it is important that these are included in the sample.
10. After removing the swab from the mouth, place it in the sterile container. If only a throat culture is requested, slide the swab into the container and activate the preservative or coat the swab. If a strep screen was ordered, only rayon swabs may be used for the collection, and liquid preservative is not recommended in the swab container.	It is important that the swab be processed appropriately so that the results are representative of the bacteria present in the throat. CLIA-waived strep screen package inserts will specify whether liquid preservatives (such as Amies or Stuart media) can be used. Rayon swabs with dry transport are recommended for strep screen specimen collection and transport.
11. Dispose of the tongue depressor in the biohazard garbage.	Proper disposal is necessary for quality control purposes.
12. Label the specimen appropriately and place the labeled specimen in a biohazardous transport bag to go the laboratory.	The specimen should always be labeled in the presence of the patient.
13. Remove gloves and safety shield.	Gloves should be removed when no longer necessary.

Procedure	Rationale
14. Wash hands, and thank the patient for being cooperative. Add documentation to the laboratory requisition form if needed.	Hands must be washed whenever gloves are removed. The requisition form must be completed with the date and time of collection as well as the source of the culture.
15. Chart the procedure appropriately.	All patient interactions should be recorded on the chart.

Date	
1/18/2014	*Throat culture specimen collected.* ～～～～～～～～～～～～～～ *Connie Lieseke, CMA (AAMA)*
11:10 a.m.	～～～～～～～～～～～～～～～～～～～～～～～～～～～～～

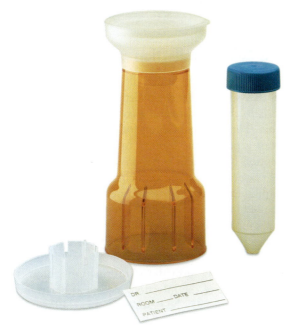

Figure 10-3   BD sputum collection container. The inner tube may be removed from the bottom of the container with minimum exposure potential for the employee. *Courtesy of BD, Inc.*

agent of tuberculosis infection, does not live long when exposed to light. The specimen must remain protected from light until it is processed in the laboratory, or this pathogenic microorganism may not be isolated from the culture even though it is present. Once the specimen arrives at the laboratory, the technician will remove the inner "tube" that contains the sputum and process the specimen according to protocol to set up the culture.

Patients collecting sputum samples must be instructed that a deep cough is absolutely necessary to produce an acceptable specimen. If saliva rather than sputum is submitted for testing, the specimen will most likely contain only normal flora for upper respiratory system, and the culture results will be inconclusive. It is recommended that the sample be obtained first thing in the morning, after the patient brushes his or her teeth and rinses the mouth, but before ingesting food or drink. Because the pathogenic microorganisms responsible for many lower respiratory infections are spread by droplets in the air, it is necessary that the patient perform collection in a private area, preferably at home. Do not allow a patient to attempt to produce a sputum culture specimen in the waiting room of the physician office, as this will potentially expose the other patients to the pathogenic microorganisms distributed as aerosol when the patient coughs. The sample must be delivered to the laboratory as soon as possible after collection, preferably within 2 hours. The specimen should not be refrigerated, nor exposed to extreme heat.

> **Test Your Knowledge 10-10**
>
> Why should a sputum specimen *not* be collected in the waiting room of a physician office?   (Outcome 10-6)

Once the specimen arrives at the laboratory, the technician (or sometimes, in an inpatient setting, a respiratory specialist) will decide whether the specimen is acceptable for culture. The technician also documents the volume and appearance of the specimen. A sputum sample that has too many epithelial cells present and is too "watery" in appearance is often a saliva sample; it was not the result of a deep cough and is not suitable for culture setup. Sputum color and thickness are not indicators of any specific illness, and this information should never be interpreted in this way.

Urine Samples for Culture

Urine specimens used for culture must be collected in a manner that reduces potential contamination by non-pathogenic microorganisms. This may be accomplished by utilizing the clean-catch midstream collection method (see Chapter 9), or alternatively, urine may be collected for culture with a straight catheter or suprapubic aspirate taken directly from the bladder. Urine samples for culture should never be taken from an indwelling catheter, as the potential for extraneous contamination is very high. The medical assistant must be sure to document on the requisition form whether the specimen was obtained from a catheter or via the clean-catch midstream urine method, as the amount of urine applied to the agar plate and the interpretation of the results are different for each type of specimen. Figure 10-4 shows an example of the different sizes of inoculation loops used for urine specimens.

Patients must be provided with a sterile cup for the urine collection, and given instructions in how to perform

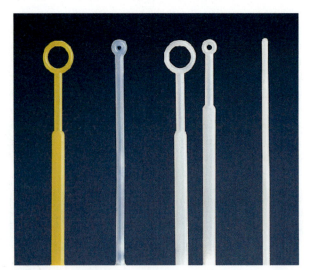

Figure 10-4   Urine loops for culture. The larger loop is used to apply urine collected via catheterization and the smaller loop is used for inoculation of urine collected via the clean-catch method. *Courtesy of Fisher HealthCare, Inc.*

the collection to provide a satisfactory culture sample. It is also imperative that within 1 hour of collection the specimen is set up for culture, refrigerated, or preserved in some way to keep the bacterial count stable. Urine tubes with preservative are available for this purpose. The bacteria present in the culture specimen will multiply at a very high rate if the urine is left at room temperature for more than an hour, so the culture results may appear to be erroneously abnormal.

> ### Test Your Knowledge 10-11
> Which of these urine specimen types may not be used for cultures?
> a. Specimens taken from indwelling catheters
> b. Specimens obtained using a straight catheter
> c. Specimens collected via the clean-catch midstream collection technique
> d. None of the above   (Outcome 10-7)

Blood Culture Collection

Health-care providers order blood culture collections when they suspect that the patient may have pathogenic bacteria in the bloodstream, a condition known as **septicemia.** The National Center for Injury Prevention and Control is part of the Centers for Disease Control and Prevention (CDC) and is responsible for compiling statistics about injuries and reducing their consequences. According to its statistics, septicemia was the 10th leading cause of death in the United States in 2006, responsible for more than 30,000 deaths. Septicemia is often a complication of urinary tract infections, pneumonia, and infected wounds. Blood cultures assist the health-care provider by providing information about the causative agent of the infection, as well as determining which antibiotics will be best to use for treatment. It is common for blood cultures to be ordered just before or just after a fever has spiked, and they are often ordered as STAT blood draws. Ideally, blood cultures will be drawn before antibiotics have been administered.

Special bottles that contain nutrients capable of supporting all bacterial growth are used for blood cultures, one that includes special nutrition and a unique atmosphere to encourage growth of microorganisms that need oxygen to grow (**aerobes**) and one that is specially designed to support growth of microorganisms that do not do well in the presence of oxygen (anaerobes). There may be special instructions with the order for the timing of the blood draws; some practitioners ask that they are drawn 30 minutes apart, whereas others will have them done serially, which means that they are drawn at regular intervals over a set period of time. The order may also be to draw two blood cultures, which means that they are to be drawn one after the other in two different sites.

Test Your Knowledge 10-12
Why are multiple bottles inoculated when collecting blood cultures?   (Outcome 10-8)

Because bacteria are not usually present in the bloodstream, the presence of any growth in the blood culture is considered to be abnormal. It is imperative that a detailed, controlled aseptic process is followed to clean and disinfect the skin as thoroughly as possible before the specimens are drawn to avoid contamination with normal skin flora. Contamination of the specimen may lead to thousands of dollars worth of treatment that otherwise would have been unnecessary and additional hospitalization days.

Each laboratory will have established protocol for the blood cultures drawn and processed within its facility. The majority of methods will include the use of a combination of 1% to 2% tincture of iodine provided in applicator sticks or cleaning pads, or 10% povidone provided in cleaning packets. Alcohol pads may also be used for a two-step cleaning process. The blood culture collection supplies may be purchased as a kit; Figure 10-5 shows an example. Surgical asepsis must be followed carefully to keep from contaminating the sample, so the site must not be repalpated after cleaning unless sterile gloves have been applied.

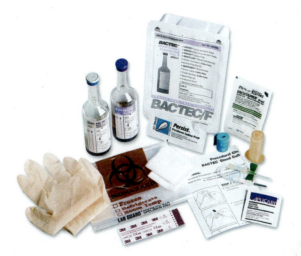

Figure 10-5 Blood culture collection kit containing two bottles, an iodine-based scrub and brush, and alcohol pads. *Courtesy of BD, Inc.*

A syringe with a safety needle may be used to obtain the specimen for the blood cultures (at least a 20-mL syringe for adults; at least a 10-mL syringe for children) or a butterfly setup may be used. The firm bioMérieux has created BacT/ALERT, a blood culture system that includes a butterfly adapter that can be used to fill the blood culture bottles directly during the venipuncture, eliminating the need to transfer the blood from the syringe to the bottles. The BacT/ALERT setup also includes an adapter that allows blood to be drawn directly into other blood tubes if there are additional samples ordered at the same time as the blood culture specimens. This helps to minimize the invasive procedures performed for that patient.

Adult specimens should have approximately 10 mL of blood added to each bottle. The vacuum will automatically pull the blood into the bottle from the syringe or from the vein if a butterfly setup and adapter are used. Monitor the flow carefully, as the vacuum does not always stop when the correct amount of blood has been added, and it is possible to overfill the blood culture bottles. Depending on the manufacturer's recommendations, pediatric draws will most likely call for 2 to 5 mL of blood per bottle.

There are special blood culture bottles available for patients who have already started on antibiotic therapy. These include substances that neutralize or remove the antibiotics from the blood so that they cannot interfere with the growth of the microorganisms. Examples are the Antimicrobial Removal Device (ARD), produced by Becton, Dickinson, or a Fastidious Antimicrobial Neutralization bottle, made by bioMérieux.

Test Your Knowledge 10-13
How many times is the draw site cleaned/disinfected prior to blood culture collections?
  a. One time
  b. Two times
  c. Three times
  d. Four times   (Outcome 10-8)

Cerebrospinal Fluid Samples

Cerebrospinal fluid (CSF) samples are used to help diagnose various diseases of the central nervous system. These diseases include meningitis and encephalitis caused by bacterial, viral, fungal, or parasitic infections. CSF samples are collected only by a qualified health-care provider by means of a **lumbar puncture,** in which a needle is placed between the lower lumbar vertebrae into

(Text continues on page 234)

Procedure 10-2: Blood Culture Collection Procedure

Blood cultures are ordered when the health-care provider suspects an infection of the bloodstream with a pathogenic microorganism. The collection process is similar to that of a typical blood draw, but there are specific procedures for disinfection of the puncture site and inoculation of the blood culture media that must be followed carefully. Blood cultures that are contaminated with normal skin flora may result in improper treatment and prolonged hospital stays.

TASK

Perform a venous blood culture collection.

CONDITIONS

- Laboratory requisition form
- Hand sanitization equipment
- Gloves
- Blood culture bottles
- 10% Povidone iodine swab stick or other antiseptic scrub kit
- Alcohol prep pads
- 22- or 23-gauge, 1-in. needle and 20-mL syringe **or** 22- or 23-gauge butterfly setup with luer adapter and special bottle cap for inoculation of blood culture bottles
- Biohazardous sharps container
- Biohazardous waste container

CAAHEP/ABHES STANDARDS

 CAAHEP Standards

I.A.I.2: Use language/verbal skills that enable patients' understanding, **III.C.III.3:** Discuss infection control procedures, **III.C.III.5:** List major types of infectious agents, **III.C.III.8:** Differentiate between medical and surgical asepsis used in ambulatory care settings, identifying when each is appropriate, **III.C.III.9:** Discuss quality control issues related to handling microbiological specimens. **III.P.III.2:** Practice Standard Precautions, **III.P.III.3:** Select appropriate barrier/personal protective equipment (PPE) for potentially infectious situations, **III.P.III.7:** Obtain specimens for microbiological testing, **III.A.III.1:** Display sensitivity to patient rights and feelings in collecting specimens, **III.A.III.2:** Explain the rationale for performance of a procedure to the patient.

 ABHES Standards

- Apply principles of aseptic techniques and infection control
- Use standard precautions
- Practice quality control
- Dispose of biohazardous materials
- Collect, label and process specimens

Procedure	Rationale
1. Verify the test ordered on the requisition form. Pay special attention to the time and/or frequency of the blood culture specimen collection. Note the age of the patient.	The test and identification on the specimen label should be verified every time to avoid erroneous results. Blood cultures may be ordered as STAT draws, which must be performed immediately, or they may be ordered at specific frequencies, such as 1 hour apart. The patient's age may be significant, as there are often special blood culture bottles or differences in the required blood volume for pediatric patients.
2. Gather necessary supplies. Verify the expiration date on the blood culture bottles and antiseptic solution.	Expired bottles and antiseptics may not be used.
3. Wash hands (if they are visibly soiled) or apply hand sanitizer. Allow hands to dry completely.	Clean hands stop the spread of infection. Hands should be completely dry before attempting to apply gloves, or it will be difficult to put the gloves on the wet hands.

Procedure	Rationale
4. Apply tourniquet to the desired site and select an appropriate venipuncture site. Release tourniquet.	It is important to establish a visual landmark for the venipuncture site chosen, as it will not be possible to repalpate the site before insertion of the needle. The tourniquet must be removed because appropriate skin cleansing techniques for blood culture collection take more than 1 minute.
5. Cleanse the venipuncture site.	The cleansing process will vary with laboratory policies. Some sites prefer a two-step process, in which the site is vigorously cleansed with alcohol for 30 seconds, followed by use of a povidone or iodine swab stick. If a povidone/iodine swab stick or cleaning pad is used, the solution must be applied using a concentric circle motion, beginning at the chosen venipuncture site and moving outward without going over any area more than once. If an alcohol/chlorhexidine cleansing kit is used, the site must be scrubbed vigorously for at least 30 to 60 seconds. This is the recommended method for cleaning the site for infants older than 2 months of age or for those with iodine sensitivity. Regardless of the cleansing method, the site must be allowed to dry completely before insertion of the needle into the skin.
6. Prepare the setup for the blood draw. This may be a needle and syringe (at least 20 mL) or a butterfly setup with a luer adapter attached to a special cap that goes over the blood culture bottles and allows the blood to be introduced directly into the bottles.	The choice of needle setup is based on the size and condition of the veins. The ideal ratio of blood to the medium in the bottles is 1:10. This means that each bottle should have 10 mL of blood added for optimal results.
7. Mark the blood culture bottles on the side with the minimum and maximum volumes.	Blood culture bottles do have a vacuum that functions to pull in the blood specimen from a syringe or butterfly. However, the vacuum in these bottles is not controlled as carefully as that in the evacuated tubes, so care must be used to monitor the amount of blood added to the bottle. It is possible to overfill the blood culture bottles. It is important to make a mark on the bottle so that the phlebotomist can estimate when the appropriate amount of blood has been added.
8. Prepare the blood culture bottles. Flip off the removable bottle cap and clean the rubber stopper with an alcohol prep pad. Discard this pad and cover the rubber stopper with a clean alcohol prep pad. Leave this pad in place until the blood is added to the bottle.	Asepsis is critical for blood culture collections. Every precaution must be followed to eliminate an opportunity for bacterial contamination of the specimen.

Continued

Procedure 10-2: Blood Culture Collection Procedure—cont'd

Procedure	Rationale
9. Reapply the tourniquet and withdraw the necessary volume of blood; 20 mL is the desirable volume for most blood culture procedures. Draw the blood using a butterfly setup or a syringe with a needle attached.	20 mL of blood will provide 10 mL per bottle, which is the desired volume for best detection and identification of infective microorganisms.

Option 1: Blood Collection Using a Butterfly Setup

a. Assemble the butterfly setup with a luer adapter attached to the end of the tubing. Screw the other end of the luer adapter into the special adapter cap designed for the blood culture bottles to be used, or an evacuated tube holder if this works for the bottles.	By using the luer adapter and the special cap, the blood can be added directly into the blood culture bottles without need of additional transfer procedures. 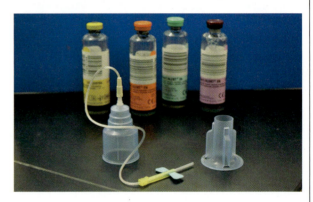
b. Using appropriate venipuncture technique, insert the butterfly needle into the vein. Continue to hold the butterfly device or tape in place.	It is important to secure the needle to avoid damage to the vein and to ensure a successful blood draw.
c. Remove the alcohol pad from the top of the bottle and push down the adapter to pierce the septum of the blood culture bottle. Blood should be added to the aerobic bottle first.	The vacuum in the blood culture bottle will pull the blood from the vein.
d. Monitor the bottle volume and pull up the adapter to remove the needle from the stopper when the desired amount of blood has been added to the bottle.	It is possible to overfill the bottles, so this is an important step to follow.
e. Follow the same procedure to add blood to the anaerobic bottle. Monitor the volume as necessary and pull up the adapter when the desired volume has been reached.	Anaerobic bottles should be filled after the aerobic bottles.

Procedure	Rationale
Option 2: Blood Collection Using a Syringe and Needle	
a. Open the sterile package holding the syringe.	Syringes should remain sterile until the time of use.
b. Pull back and push forward the plunger of the syringe several times to verify whether it moves smoothly.	"Exercising" the plunger in this manner allows for smooth movement when pulling back the plunger to allow blood to enter the syringe. If the plunger does not move smoothly or is too loose within the syringe, it should be discarded.
c. Remove the needle from the sterile wrapper. Do not take off the cap covering the end of the needle until just before insertion into the patient's arm.	The needle must remain sterile until just prior to insertion. It cannot touch other surfaces before piercing the skin of the patient.
d. Attach the needle to the syringe tip.	Verify that this is a secure connection so that blood will not leak out around the needle during the venipuncture process.
e. Reapply the tourniquet, taking care not to touch the venipuncture site. Using appropriate technique, withdraw 20 mL of blood into the syringe, and have the patient place pressure over the venipuncture site.	Special care must be utilized to keep the disinfected site without contamination; 20 mL of blood is optimal for the blood culture procedures.
f. If the bottle is designed to fit a transfer device, activate the safety device on the needle, remove it from the syringe, and discard it in a biohazardous sharps container. Attach the transfer device to the syringe. Remove the alcohol pad from the top of the bottle and push down the transfer device to pierce the septum of the blood culture bottle. Blood should be added to the aerobic bottle first.	The blood culture bottles may come with a very small neck that is designed for use with a standard transfer device such as that in an evacuated tube system.
g. If the bottle is not designed for a transfer device to fit over the top of the bottle, it will be necessary to add the blood to the bottle with the needle on the syringe. Verify that the blood culture bottle is on a stable, flat surface. Remove the alcohol prep pad from the top of the bottle, and puncture the septum with the needle on the syringe, puncturing the aerobic bottle first.	Do not hold the blood culture bottle with your hand while puncturing the septum, as this will increase the chance of an accidental needlestick. Place the bottle on the counter or tabletop.
h. Monitor the volume in the blood culture bottle as the blood is introduced and remove the needle when 10 mL have been added.	Do not overfill the blood culture bottle.
i. Repeat the process to add 10 mL to the anaerobic bottle. Discard the syringe/needle setup in a biohazardous sharps container.	Avoid contamination of the septum on the anaerobic bottle.

Continued

Procedure 10-2: Blood Culture Collection Procedure—cont'd

Procedure	Rationale
10. Label both bottles and the requisition form with the date, time and site of the blood draw, as well as the birth date or other patient ID and the initials of the collector. Transport to the laboratory as soon as possible for processing.	Accurate labeling and documentation are always necessary.
11. Clean the iodine solution off the patient's arm using an alcohol swab. Clean up the work area and chart the procedure.	The iodine solution may become irritating to the skin if left on the patient's arm after the procedure.

Date	
3/12/2014:	Blood culture collection X2 from right and left arm. ～～～～～～～ Connie Lieseke, CMA (AAMA)
4:40 p.m.	～～～～～～～～～～～～～～～～～～～～～～～～～～～～～～～

the subarachnoid space, and a sample of cerebrospinal fluid is withdrawn for analysis. This procedure may also be known as a spinal tap. Generally, four tubes are used for the collection, with 1 to 8 mL of fluid placed in each tube. The tubes are numbered in order of collection, which is a very important part of the procedure. In most situations, the first tube collected during the lumbar puncture is used for chemical analysis, including protein and glucose levels. The second tube is used for culture and other microbiology testing, and the last tube collected is used to perform a cell count to look for presence of red and/or white blood cells.

Medical assistants may aid in the collection procedure for CSF samples, and they may also process the samples to be delivered to the laboratory. All CSF analysis must be conducted on a STAT basis, as the integrity of the cells present in the specimen may deteriorate rapidly once the spinal fluid leaves the body. Some tubes used for CSF collection are already labeled with numerals that are raised on the side of the tube, but if not, the numbering of the tubes as the fluid is added is *critical*, as is the assurance that sterile technique is maintained when handling the specimen. The tubes must be closed securely after the fluid is added and labeled appropriately with all patient demographic information and the date and time of the collection. Ideally, if the medical assistant knows that a lumbar puncture is to be performed in the office, he or she may contact the laboratory to request a STAT courier pickup before the procedure is

started, so that the courier will arrive very shortly after the process has been completed. Do not refrigerate or freeze CSF samples after collection before the routine testing can be performed.

> **Test Your Knowledge 10-14**
>
> What is the additional information required on the CSF collection tubes that is not required for other types of microbiology samples?   (Outcome 10-9)

Genital Samples

Genital cultures use several types of media to identify microorganisms that cause common genital infections such as cervicitis (inflammation of the cervix), urethritis (inflammation of the urethra), or pelvic inflammatory disease. Not all organisms that cause genital infections can be easily cultured, but common infective agents isolated and identified with culture procedures include yeast infections caused by *Candida albicans*, and bacterial infections (vaginosis) caused by *Gardnerella vaginalis, Neisseria meningitides,* or *Haemophilus ducreyi.* Another common infection of the genitals is **trichomoniasis,** which is a sexually transmitted disease caused by the parasite *Trichomonas vaginalis.* This parasite is identified through microscopic examination of vaginal smears and other testing methods, but not cultures.

Many sexually transmitted diseases, such as chlamydia, herpes, human papillomavirus infection, and syphilis, are not typically identified through culture, because the causative microorganisms are difficult to grow in the laboratory. More often, these diseases are identified through serological tests that check for the presence of antigens or antibodies. If a culture order is received for these microorganisms, the order should be verified before proceeding with collection. If the health-care provider really wants a culture to be performed, the medical assistant should carefully investigate the collection and processing procedures so that the culture is viable and the results are meaningful.

Cultures from the genitals of patients are usually ordered if the patient complains of itching, discharge, or burning, or if the patient has visible lesions on or near the external genitalia. Remember to use standard precautions at all times when assisting with the collection or processing of these specimens. The specimens may be collected via aspiration (as in the case of abscesses), or more commonly swabs are used to obtain a specimen from open lesions or discharge. When collecting a urethral swab from a male patient, a small swab on a wire may be inserted into urethra to obtain the culture specimen. It may also be necessary to collect specimens from the rectum if the sexual history of the patient makes this a probable site for infection.

Vaginal and rectal culture specimens may also be collected from pregnant women to test for the presence of group B streptococci. This is an important procedure to avoid newborn infection with these bacteria, which can cause pneumonia or sepsis. Women infected with group B streptococci are usually asymptomatic, so this screening process is necessary as part of a routine prenatal checkup. A swab is used for the collection, and the specimen is handled following general bacterial culture guidelines.

If a cervical culture is requested (as in the case of suspected gonorrhea), the specimen collection will require the use of a speculum to widen the vaginal opening and provide access to the cervix. Excess mucus and drainage are to be wiped away from the opening of the cervix, after which a collection swab is inserted into the opening of the cervix and rotated several times to obtain the specimen. Cervical specimens are often collected at the same time that a specimen is collected for a Pap procedure. Specimens collected for gonococci cultures may be transported in a tube that contains charcoal mixed in the transport medium. The charcoal is designed to absorb any interfering substances in the specimen that might decrease the growth rate of the gonococci bacteria.

> **Test Your Knowledge 10-15**
> What type of collection device is used for most genital sample collections?
> a. An aspirate using a needle and syringe
> b. Skin scrapings
> c. Swabs
> d. Urine samples   (Outcome 10-10)

A medical assistant may be asked to inoculate the agar plates used to support bacterial growth from genital culture specimens in the physician office at the time of collection. It may be necessary to inoculate more than one type of agar to isolate the causative organism. Chocolate agar, which contains lysed (broken) red blood cells, is commonly inoculated with the specimen, as it supports the growth of most pathogenic bacteria that may be present in the genital area. Chocolate agar is shown in Figure 10-6. Pathogens commonly present in the genital area need growth factors that are present inside the red cells, so the red blood cells are lysed when preparing the nutrient agar. However, if the health-care provider wants to determine whether the patient may be infected with *Neisseria gonorrhoeae* (the causative agent of gonorrhea), he or she will also want to inoculate a Petri dish that contains Thayer Martin agar. Thayer Martin agar contains lysed red cells just as the chocolate agar. In addition, Thayer Martin agar contains

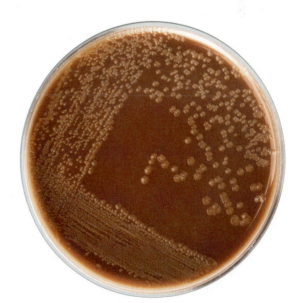

Figure 10-6 Chocolate agar. *Courtesy of Fisher HealthCare, Inc.*

antibiotics (vancomycin, colistin, and nystatin), which inhibit the growth of other bacteria on the agar plate. This allows for the gonococci to grow without competing with other normal flora from the vaginal area. The gonococci also like to grow in an environment with a low oxygen concentration. A special CO_2 tablet may be added to the bag that contains the agar plate after it has been inoculated to enhance the growing environment, or the inoculated agar plate may be placed in a **candle jar,** a special enclosed container in which the medical assistant places the specimen. After the specimen is added, the medical assistant lights a candle and inserts it into the container until the flame goes out. This process removes oxygen from the environment inside the container and enhances the growth of *N. gonorrhoeae* if present.

POINT OF INTEREST 10-2
Pap smears and human papillomavirus

A Pap smear, or Pap test, is performed on a sample of cells collected from a woman's cervix during a pelvic examination. The Pap test does not detect the presence of infection with sexually transmitted pathogenic microorganisms, but it does detect changes in the cells of the cervix that may develop into cancer. It also detects malignant cervical cells that may already be present. A genital culture may be obtained at the same time that a Pap sample is collected, and this may be tested for the presence of the genital human papillomavirus (HPV), or other suspected infectious agents. A special kit is used for collection of the sample for the Pap smear, which may include a brush-like device, a swab, and/or a wooden spatula. Once the sample has been collected by the health-care provider, it is placed into a solution for preservation and transport to the laboratory. Medical assistants may be responsible for processing the sample appropriately after collection. Once the specimen arrives at the laboratory, a cytotechnologist examines the sample under a microscope to look for evidence of abnormal cervical cells.

Certain strains of the genital HPV may cause genital warts in males and females. Other strains of HPV may cause changes in the cells of the cervix that lead to cervical cancer. The cellular changes are detected with the Pap smear, but the presence of HPV and verification of the type of HPV infection must be accomplished with a separate sample collection. Vaccines are available for protection against many of the most common strains of HPV. Cervarix and Gardasil vaccinations are available for women. If necessary, these vaccinations may begin at 9 years of age, but the recommended age range is 11 to 26 years. Gardasil protects against the strains of HPV linked to cervical cancer, and also protects against most genital warts. Cervarix is specific for the HPV strains that cause cervical cancer. Males may also be vaccinated with Gardasil for protection. These vaccinations are recommended for boys and young men ages 9 to 26 years.

Wound Cultures

A wound is any break in the skin. A wound may be a deep break, an abrasion on the surface of the skin, a surgical incision, or a scratch. Even an ingrown toenail with signs of infection may be processed as a wound. Wound cultures may be ordered when a patient has redness, swelling, drainage, or heat in or around a wound. Cultures collected from breaks in the skin are the most varied in collection techniques, processing procedures, and results. The most important aspects of wound culture collection to remember are the following:

- Only culture the wound; not the area around it. Contamination from extraneous bacteria will complicate the culture process, and may cause inaccurate results and incorrect treatment.
- It is best to collect a culture from a clean wound; the process washes away transient bacteria present in the area that are not involved in the actual infection.
- Deep wounds and aspirates are usually collected and processed as anaerobic culture specimens, as the bacteria growing in this environment do not prefer exposure to environmental oxygen because they are growing well in the deep tissues of the body. Anaerobic culture specimens are collected using special culture kits that protect the specimen from oxygen exposure while providing moisture to keep the specimen viable.
- It is very important that the source is documented thoroughly when working with wound cultures. Details of the culture source will dictate how the culture is set up and which types of pathogens the microbiologist is expecting to identify from the wound. Normal flora may be pathogenic if present as an overgrowth (very high in numbers) within a certain area of the body, or if present in an area that is usually considered to be sterile, such as the eye. Documentation of the patient's name, the date and time of collection, and the source of the sample should be affixed to the collection container as well as added to the requisition form and the patient chart. The source

information includes details about the side of the body (for instance, wound left hand thumb) for the wound.

- If **exudate** (fluid from the blood vessels in the area of the infection) or pus is present, the health-care provider may culture this drainage. However, in the case of abscesses, sometimes the culture is not performed, as the most important aspect is to clear the area of all the abscess material, not find out what caused the abscess.

- Results obtained from someone with a chronic wound may be very different from those of a patient with a wound that has just become infected. Sometimes the quantitative results (number of colonies or bacteria present in the culture specimen) may indicate whether current treatment is working for a specific wound.

- A **Gram stain** is often performed from the original collection swab at the same time the culture is set up. Gram stains provide information about the shape and staining characteristics of the pathogen. Observation of the slide after performing a Gram stain can provide preliminary information to guide how the culture is to be started, based on the types of bacteria present. For instance, gram-positive cocci often grow better on certain media than do gram-negative rods.

- Swabs are usually used to collect wound culture specimens. Be sure to keep the swab sterile until the specimen is collected. If an aspirate is taken using a needle and syringe, the needle must be removed from the syringe before transporting the specimen. In this situation the aspirate is often transferred into a sterile tube for transport. Identification of the transfer tube is essential; the laboratory will not know what type of fluid is submitted without the documentation, as many body fluids are very similar in appearance. Wound culture specimens should be delivered to the laboratory as soon as possible, and should not be refrigerated or frozen before the culture medium is inoculated.

Test Your Knowledge 10-16

True or False: It is not advisable to wash a wound before collecting a culture specimen.   (Outcome 10-11)

Stool Specimens

Cultures for stool specimens differ from many of the other cultures that we have discussed because of the copious amount of normal flora that is present in the digestive tract. The culture medium used to process stool samples is very selective; it has been designed to encourage the growth of known gastrointestinal pathogens, while discouraging the growth of the normal flora of the area. Only pathogenic microorganisms are processed further for identification and treatment. Sometimes the physician may also ask for a specimen to be collected to check for the presence of parasites in the gastrointestinal (GI) tract. This is known as an **ova and parasite examination (O&P)**, during which the microbiologist will be looking for the presence of parasites or their ova (eggs). Stool cultures may be ordered when a patient has diarrhea that lasts more than a few days, or when there is mucus or blood visible in the stool. A patient may be exposed to pathogenic bacteria from eating food or drinking water that has been contaminated. Common sources include water from a contaminated well, lake, or stream, or undercooked eggs, poultry, or beef. Unpasteurized milk is another potential source. When patients travel outside the country, there may be exposure to bacteria that have become part of the normal flora for the occupants of that area, but that will make visitors sick who are not habituated to them.

Stool specimens for bacterial cultures are collected in a sterile cup. The stool specimen must be fresh for culture setup. The specimen should be delivered to the laboratory within 2 hours of collection, and the specimen must be protected from extremes in heat during transport. The sample cannot be taken from the water in the toilet bowl, and the sample cannot contain urine. Toilet tissue also should not be mixed in with the sample. To successfully collect a stool culture specimen, it is recommended that the patient spread plastic wrap across the back half of the toilet seat so that the stool can be collected on this plastic wrap when eliminated. It is important that urine is not introduced to the plastic wrap. For patients who are wearing diapers, it may be necessary to line the diaper with plastic wrap for successful collection.

Test Your Knowledge 10-17

Why is it important for the medium used for stool cultures to be so selective?   (Outcome 10-12)

Common pathogens isolated from stool specimens include the following:

- *Clostridium difficile:* Infection with this bacteria often follows use of broad-spectrum antibiotics, which disrupt the balance of normal flora in the body and allow this opportunistic bacteria to flourish. *C. difficile* is a spore-forming bacterium that may live on surfaces (hospital beds, walls, etc.) for extended periods of time. The bacteria are shed in the stool of infected individuals, and the infection may be life threatening if not treated appropriately. Patients may form a pseudomembrane, or artificial lining in the intestinal tract that impairs absorption of nutrients from the food they ingest. *C. difficile* is difficult to grow as a culture (hence the name *difficile,* "difficult"), but a toxin is secreted by the bacteria that may be detected in the stool specimen or in blood from an infected individual.

- *Salmonella:* This name actually describes a group of bacteria of the *Salmonella* genus. *Salmonella* species live in the intestines of many animals, such as baby chickens, cattle, or pigs. They may also be present in the feces of turtles and domestic animals. Food that has been contaminated with animal feces is the most common means of transmission. The bacteria are transmitted via the fecal-oral route, and usually cause abdominal cramping and severe diarrhea within 1 to 2 days of infection. Most of the time the infection is resolved without antibiotic treatment within a week, but occasionally the *Salmonella* bacteria may enter the bloodstream and cause more serious illness. To avoid infection with this organism, patients should always wash and cook food thoroughly, keep eggs refrigerated, and wash their hands using soap and clean water after working with or petting animals.

- *Shigella:* This name describes a genus of bacteria that causes diarrhea, including *Shigella sonnei* and *Shigella flexneri.* These two types cause almost all cases of *Shigella* infection in the United States. *Shigella dysenteriae* type 1 can cause deadly epidemics, but is very rarely seen in the United States. *Shigella* is transmitted through fecal material from one person to another. Common methods for transmission include food handlers who do not wash their hands after using the restroom, and small children who share wading pools. Infected patients will continue to shed the bacteria in their stools, which often appear bloody, for several weeks after the symptoms have subsided.

- *Campylobacter:* This spiral-shaped organism causes diarrhea, abdominal cramps, nausea, and fever in infected patients. The most common species of the *Campylobacter* genus to cause disease is *Campylobacter jejuni.* Most cases are spread by the feces of birds or the ingestion of birds, as they are able to carry the bacteria without being ill with it themselves. Infection may occur from exposure to raw or undercooked poultry, but occasionally a dog or cat may be infected and the owner may become infected from them. *Campylobacter* can cause disease with very little exposure, so cross-contamination can occur between, for example, cutting boards in a food

preparation area and a preparer's unwashed hands, leading to illness. *Campylobacter* infection is the most common bacterial infection causing diarrhea in the United States. Usually it resolves without antibiotic treatment, but there are many documented cases of infected patients who developed the neurological disorder Guillain-Barré syndrome. The *Campylobacter* infection acts as a "trigger" to cause an autoimmune response in which the body attacks the nervous system, causing paralysis.

- *Escherichia coli:* This family of bacteria is present in our environment, and is part of our normal flora. However, there are certain strains of *E. coli* that can cause illness, especially when they are introduced into areas of our body where *E. coli* is not normally found. Some of the *E. coli* families, also known as enterohemorrhagic or verocytotoxic types of *E. coli,* produce the Shiga toxin. The most common one to cause disease in the United States is *E. coli* O157:H7. When a patient has become infected with this type of *E. coli,* the toxins produced by the bacteria cause the illness. Those who are infected usually start to feel ill within a few days of ingesting the bacteria. Symptoms include severe abdominal cramps, vomiting, and diarrhea, which may be bloody. In most patients the infection resolves within a week. However, approximately 5% to 10% of those who are infected with *E. coli* O157:H7 develop **hemolytic uremic syndrome,** which can be life threatening. Hemolytic uremic syndrome occurs when the toxins produced by the bacteria begin to destroy the red blood cells and platelets of the infected patient. The torn or broken red cells begin to block the small capillaries in the kidneys, which can lead to total renal failure.

Nasopharyngeal Specimens

When an upper respiratory infection is suspected, it may be necessary to collect a specimen using a **nasopharyngeal collection technique,** commonly used when collecting samples to test for presence of viral microorganisms. The **nasopharynx** is the area of the pharynx (throat) that runs from the back of the nasal cavity down to the back of the throat that is visible through the mouth. Nasopharyngeal specimens are usually collected by entering the pharynx through the nose, but they may also be collected by going through the mouth and "sweeping" the area of the pharynx that is above the uvula. Some key points are the following:

- Generally, nasopharyngeal swab specimens will be collected 3 to 7 days after the symptoms have started, and before antibiotics or antiviral medications have been administered.

- Always verify the order before collecting the sample. Verify whether a viral culture or a bacterial culture is requested, and have the correct supplies on hand to handle the specimen appropriately after collection. Copan Diagnostics makes several types of "flocked" swabs designed for maximum specimen collection potential. Nasopharyngeal swabs traditionally have a flexible shaft, which may be made of wire or flexible thin plastic. Only Dacron or rayon swabs should be used for viral samples.

- To collect the sample on the nasopharyngeal swab, it is necessary first to measure how far the swab needs to be inserted for the collection. The depth of insertion is approximately half the length from the earlobe to the base of the nose (nostril) of the patient. This should be measured and marked on the nasopharyngeal swab shaft so that it is visible during the collection. The swab is inserted into the nose parallel to the roof of the mouth. Continue to insert the swab until the depth of insertion has been reached and slight resistance is felt, indicating that the nasopharynx has been reached. The swab should be rotated several times, and left in place for a few seconds to absorb any mucus that is present. Remove the swab in the same way that it was inserted. It may be necessary to insert the swab in the other nostril and repeat the process. The swab is then placed immediately into the viral transport media (or bacterial transport media if ordered) and processed according to the directions provided by the testing laboratory.

Eye Cultures

Samples from the eye may be taken from the *conjunctiva,* the mucous membrane that covers the inner area of the eyelid and extends to cover the exposed surface of the eye. The conjunctiva can be accessed just under the upper and lower eyelids. Eye cultures less commonly are obtained as corneal scrapings or an aspirate from the eyeball. In the outpatient setting, conjunctival samples will be the most commonly collected. When assisting with this procedure, it is important to remember that the microbiology laboratory will prefer a sample from each eye, even if the infection is suspected in only one eye. This allows the laboratory to compare any normal flora that may be present, and assists with identification of potential pathogens. Also, the collection swabs should be moistened with sterile saline or nutrient broth before use to minimize discomfort when the collection swab is rubbed across the delicate surfaces of the eye.

Common pathogens present in the eye may be isolated by inoculation of the specimens on 5% sheep's blood agar, chocolate agar, and mannitol salt agar. The pathogens often include *Streptococcus* genus, as well as *Haemophilus* genus, and occasionally *Gonorrhoeae* bacteria may be evident, especially in a newborn infant whose mother had minimal prenatal care.

> **Test Your Knowledge 10-18**
>
> Why is the swab used for eye culture samples usually moistened prior to use?   (Outcome 10-13)

Ear Cultures

The human ear is separated into three sections: the outer ear, the middle ear (located right behind the tympanic membrane), and the inner ear. The middle ear is connected to the back of the throat by a small structure known as the **eustachian tube**. Inflammation (with or without infection) of the ear is called **otitis** and is further specified by adding the location to the name. **Otitis media** describes inflammation or infection of the middle ear, and **otitis externa** describes inflammation and/or infection of the outer ear canal.

Otitis media is the most common type of ear infection, and usually develops as a result of blockage of the eustachian tube. When this tube is blocked, fluid builds up in the middle ear, and if there are bacteria or viruses present (such as those causing a sore throat or the common cold), these may be introduced to the fluid within the ear by the eustachian tube. (The middle ear is usually a sterile environment.) This is a common disorder in children, as their eustachian tubes are shorter and straighter than those of adults. If the pressure builds up too much within the middle ear, the tympanic membrane may rupture, and the health-care provider will take a culture specimen of the drainage with a sterile swab. Sometimes it may be necessary to take a culture specimen of the fluid behind the tympanic membrane when it has not ruptured. A procedure called *tympanocentesis* may be performed, in which the health-care provider inserts a needle through the tympanic membrane and aspirates a sample of the fluid that is built up in the middle ear. Another procedure that may allow access to the fluid is a *myringotomy,* in which a tiny incision is made into the eardrum to allow for drainage of the infected fluid. In this situation, a sterile syringe may be used to aspirate some of the sample for a culture, or a sterile swab can be used to obtain the sample as it drains out of the eardrum.

Otitis externa is a condition that is often known as swimmer's ear. When moisture is introduced into the external ear canal, it can create a perfect environment for bacterial or fungal growth to occur. Otitis externa may also be caused by excess moisture or a break in or irritation to the skin of this area. The introduction of foreign objects (such as cotton-tipped swabs) or chemicals (such as those present in hair-care products or dyes) may contribute to the development of otitis externa. The outer ear usually itches, and there is often discharge and pain in the area as well. If a culture is needed to identify the infective microorganism, a sterile swab is used to swipe the lesions and/or obtain a sample of the discharge. The outer ear canal does contain normal flora, such as *Staphylococcus epidermis, Staphylococcus aureus,* and *Corynebacterium* genus.

Test Your Knowledge 10-19

Which type of otitis is often linked to excessive moisture in the ear?
  a. Otitis externa
  b. Otitis media   (Outcome 10-14)

SPECIAL SAMPLE COLLECTION AND PROCESSING PROCEDURES

The role of a medical assistant does not end with the collection and labeling of the specimens. Sometimes there are special procedures that must be completed after the collection so that specimens can be examined, or unique collection requirements for certain specimens that require prior setup.

Fungal Sample and Culture Collection Procedures

As was presented earlier in this chapter, specimen collection procedures performed to detect the presence of fungal elements may be different from those procedures used for bacterial or viral organisms. Successful isolation and identification of fungal elements are dependent on very specific collection methods, rapid transport, and use of the correct growth medium once the sample arrives at the laboratory. Fungi may be isolated from wounds, abscesses, hair follicles, or lesions on the skin. *Tinea pedis* (athlete's foot) and *Tinea unguium* (a fungal infection of the nails) are frequently seen in the physician office. Fungal infections are referred to as **mycoses** and are further identified by the area of infection and/or the causative organisms. Common classifications of fungal infections include the following:

- **Superficial or cutaneous mycoses:** These infect the outermost (dead) layers of the skin and hair, as well as the epidermis, hair follicles and deeper layers of the visible skin. *Tinea corporis* (ringworm) is an example of this type of infection.
- **Subcutaneous mycoses:** These fungal infections occur in the dermis and subcutaneous layers of the skin, and may affect the muscles and tissue layers beneath the skin. Often these are chronic infections that resulted from an initial wound when the fungus was introduced into the body.
- **Systemic mycoses:** Systemic fungal infections may be present in multiple organs and/or areas of the body. They are often introduced to the body through the respiratory tract. Systemic fungal infections may be caused by opportunistic fungal organisms in patients who have suppressed or inactive immune systems (such as HIV-positive patients), or they may be caused by a pathogen that is introduced to the body.

Sample collection procedures will differ according to the site of infection. It is important that the medical assistant and health-care provider verify which type of specimen is necessary for the infection before the collection process begins. Sometimes the health-care provider will utilize a **Wood's lamp,** which shines a fluorescent light over the infected area. Certain types of fungi will fluoresce when exposed to this light, and the physician may use this information without the need of an actual specimen collection to prescribe treatment. Table 10-1 summarizes the type of specimen needed and the collection method used to identify the fungal elements in various areas of the body. Sample types include scrapings of skin lesions for superficial infections, nailbed samples, aspirates from abscesses, or swabs used to sample vaginal drainage.

Test Your Knowledge 10-20

Are all fungal infections superficial?   (Outcome 10-15)

Potassium Hydroxide Preparation

Many times it is not necessary to identify the specific *type* of fungus responsible for an infection; the most important information is whether a fungal element is the causative agent. Patient treatment is based on the presence of the fungi without further identification. An examination of the sample under the microscope with a drop or two of 10% to 20% potassium hydroxide (**KOH)** solution is

TABLE 10-1		
Information needed for collection of samples for fungal cultures*		
Type of Infection	**Specimen Required**	**Collection Method**
Skin lesions	Skin scrapings	Use the dull edge of a scalpel or a glass slide; scrape across the lesion. If there are not enough loose pieces created with this action, adhesive tape may be used to pick up a sample. Transport dry in sterile container.
Fungal infection of the hair	Pieces of hair with roots attached	Pluck out the hair (including root material) with sterile forceps. Transport dry in sterile container.
Nail infection	Pieces of nail and debris from underneath the nail	Samples from discolored or misshapen parts of the nail preferable; may use microdrill method to provide samples from the more proximal parts of the nail for better capture of the fungi. Samples scraped from underneath the nail may also provide fungal elements. Transport dry in sterile container.
Abscesses and other subcutaneous infections	Aspirate taken with a needle and syringe, or a sterile swab moistened with saline brushed over the surface from deepest area of infection possible	Sample only the actively infected areas for best results. Be certain that the sample amounts are adequate for culture.
Deep tissue infections	Samples of tissue	Tissue to be excised; will be minced, then cultured for fungal elements.
*For all cultures, specimen ideally will be processed within 2 hours of collections.		

performed immediately after collection to search for the presence of fungi. The KOH dissolves other organic elements in the specimen such as hair, mucus, skin cells, and bacteria, but it does not dissolve the fungus that may be present. This allows the health-care provider to visualize the fungus and decide on a plan of treatment without waiting for a culture result. Some fungal species do not show up with the KOH treatment, so the health-care provider may order a culture in addition to the microscopic examination if a fungal infection is suspected upon examination. It is important to remember that results from a fungal culture may not be available until weeks after the sample is submitted, so alternative methods of detection are very important to avoid delay in treatment.

Wet Mount Procedure

A **wet mount** is a means by which living organisms may be observed under the microscope. *Trichomonas vaginalis* is a common sexually transmitted parasitic microorganism that needs to be visualized as it is alive and active via a wet mount examination. A wet mount is prepared by adding a few drops of saline to a sample (usually a swab with secretions on it) then placing a drop of saline/sample mixture onto a microscopic slide. A **cover slip** (a small piece of plastic or glass) is applied over the solution on the slide, and the health-care provider examines the sample. Diagnosis is made by examining the structural characteristics and movement of the microorganism. Wet mount examinations (as well as KOH preps) are performed in physician offices only by health-care providers or trained laboratory professionals, but not by medical assistants. The medical assistant may set up the sample appropriately and bring it into focus on the microscope for examination, but the health-care provider or other appropriately trained personnel will be responsible for performance of the examination.

A **hanging drop slide** is another way that a sample, especially those exhibiting a lot of movement, may be examined for live microorganisms. In this case, a special depression slide is used. These slides have a "scoop" out of the center of the slide, which forms a depression. A cover slip is also used and petroleum jelly is applied with an applicator to the four corners of the cover slip. A drop of the sample (often an inoculated swab that has been agitated in saline) is placed on the center of the cover slip.

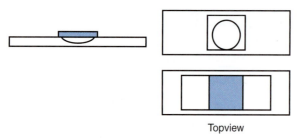

Topview

Figure 10-7 A depression slide. Note how the "scoop" is taken from the middle of the slide. This is covered with a cover slip. The sample is actually placed on the cover slip with the depression set over this area and the slide flipped for viewing under the microscope.

The depression slide is placed over the cover slip, where the petroleum jelly seals the edges. The setup is inverted so that the specimen drop is "hanging" from the cover slip over the depression. This allows an excellent opportunity to examine the sample for anatomy and **motility** (movement) of the microorganisms that are present. An example of a hanging drop slide can be seen in Figure 10-7.

Test Your Knowledge 10-21

How are KOH preps and wet mounts similar? How are they different?   (Outcome 10-16)

Sample Collection Procedures for Detection of Parasites

Organisms that live on or in a host and use their host for nourishment are known as **parasites.** Pathogenic microorganisms that use the human body for nourishment include **ectoparasites,** which live on the outside of the body, and **endoparasites,** which live within the human body. These parasites feed off the human host, at the expense of the health of the human that they occupy.

Common ectoparasites that use humans as hosts include lice, mites, fleas, and ticks. Diagnosis of these infections usually occurs with the visual examination of the site. For instance, the health-care professional may take a scraping from the skin of the infected individual and examine it under the microscope to see if there are mites present. **Scabies** is a parasitic infection with *Sarcoptes scabiei,* and this may be diagnosed with a skin scraping. The Burrow ink test is another method sometimes used for verification of scabies infections, performed by rubbing the site with an ink pen, then wiping away the ink with an alcohol pad. If there is a parasitic scabies infection then the burrow holes left from where

the microorganisms entered the skin will be evident. When a lice infection is suspected, the diagnosis is usually made with careful examination of the hair for the adult lice or the nits that are present near the scalp. Most infections with ectoparasites do not cause the host to become ill; however, secondary infections from the scratching and breaks in the skin may be problematic.

The most common internal parasitic infection in the United States is caused by *Giardia lamblia.* This single-cell parasitic microorganism is passed in the feces of animals. Untreated water in ponds and mountain streams are contaminated with feces from indigenous animals in the area such as beaver, muskrat, elk, and deer. The human host then ingests the parasite by drinking this contaminated water. The presence of the *Giardia* in the water cannot be detected without the use of a microscope, as it does not change the water's color, smell, or taste. Infection by other internal parasites such as roundworms, tapeworms, and hookworms may also occur, but this is not as common in the United States as it is in other areas of the world. Endoparasites can damage their hosts by causing cellular destruction, chewing damage to the gastrointestinal tract, anemia, blood vessel damage, bloody diarrhea, and failure to absorb nutrients.

Ova and Parasite Examination

For most endoparasites, the ova and parasite examination (O&P) is used to make a visual identification of the presence of adult parasites or eggs in the stool. Most parasites have adult forms and produce ova (eggs) or cysts with sexual or asexual reproduction. When the gastrointestinal tract is infected with parasites, the adult parasites or their eggs are shed into the stool of the infected host. The O&P test is performed by placing thin smears of stool (fresh or preserved) onto slides and examining and/or staining them for examination. The sample may need to be spun in a centrifuge for concentration before the slide is prepared to allow for easier detection of any parasites or ova present. The microbiologist will be able to detect the presence or absence of adult parasites or the eggs (ovum), and based on the anatomical structures observed, an identification of the species may also be performed.

When a patient is to be tested for the presence of ova and parasites, he or she is provided with a collection kit that includes a container for the stool specimen, as well as one or two small bottles of preservative solution (Fig. 10-8). The bottles must be appropriately labeled to warn the patient that they contain strong chemicals that could be harmful if swallowed or allowed to remain on bare skin for extended periods of time. The bottles may have a "scoop" built into the cap for the patient to add

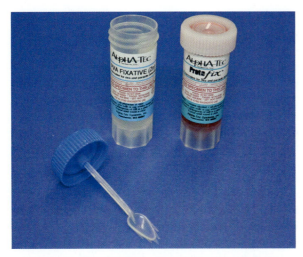

Figure 10-8 Ova and parasite collection kit. There are two different types of preservatives provided, and each bottle has a scoop in the lid that is used to add the stool specimen to the preservative.

the stool specimen to the preservative in the bottle. Common preservatives are 10% buffered formalin and polyvinyl alcohol (PVA). The formalin allows for extended preservation of the parasites and eggs, but the stool sample may be used only for wet mount observation; it cannot be stained for a more permanent record of the examination. PVA does preserve the sample for a reasonable amount of time, but it also allows for staining of the slide for further study. Some laboratories will provide two bottles with different fixatives. The patient should be advised to collect the stool sample into the larger container (provided) or use some other method to collect the sample without contamination of urine or water. Then, the patient should use the scoop or a provided applicator to put a small part of the sample into the provided preservative bottles and return it to the laboratory or physician office.

Sometimes a stool culture is ordered at the same time as the sample for the ova and parasite examination, so it is important that the medical assistant give appropriate instructions for the time intervals before the specimen arrives back at the office. Some laboratories will also prefer a fresh stool sample, in which case it needs to be delivered to the laboratory within 1 hour of collection to preserve the anatomical features of the parasitic microorganisms for identification. It is also common for health-care providers to order multiple sample collections, as the parasites and/or eggs may be shed at random times in the stool. Identification of the specimen collection date and time is very important.

Test Your Knowledge 10-22

How does a collection procedure for an ova and parasite examination differ from a stool culture collection procedure?

a. The O&P collection procedures include containers with preservative solution, but stool culture sample procedures do not

b. Stool specimens for cultures can be kept at room temperature for extended periods of time, whereas specimens for O&P cannot be stored at room temperature

c. The procedures are exactly the same for both types of collections

d. None of the above   (Outcome 10-17)

Pinworm Collection Procedures

Pinworm infections, caused by the parasite *Enterobius vermicularis,* are the most common type of worm infections in the United States. The pinworm is a small white worm that can infect the colon and rectum of humans. School-age children and those who are institutionalized are at highest risk for this type of infection, as well as those who care for this population. The adult pinworms are large enough that they can sometimes be seen around the rectum without magnification. The adult female pinworm leaves the rectum at night and lays her eggs around the opening. Within a couple of hours these eggs are infectious, and may be shed into the underwear and bedclothes. This infection often causes intensive anal itching.

Testing for pinworm infection must occur first thing in the morning, before the individual has had a bowel movement or bathed, as these actions may remove the eggs from the rectal area. A piece of clear adhesive tape (sticky side down) may be pressed against the perianal area, and any eggs in the area will stick to the tape. This process may need to be repeated for several days before eggs are identified. The eggs can then be viewed under the microscope when placed on a slide. A "pinworm paddle" may also be used for the collection. Becton, Dickinson produces a tool called the FALCON SWUBE Pinworm Paddle, which is a clear plastic paddle with one adhesive side at the wide end. This sticky side is placed against the perianal area, and then the paddle is placed within a tube to keep it secure until it is examined. The actual paddle can be used as a slide under the microscope, as it is transparent. Figure 10-9 shows the FALCON SWUBE Pinworm Paddle.

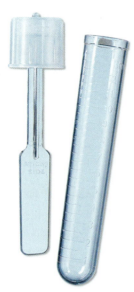

Figure 10-9   The FALCON SWUBE Pinworm Paddle for pinworm collection. The end of the collection device is pressed against the anus to collect the sample. The sample is transported in the outer tube to the laboratory where the actual collection device may be placed on the microscope for examination. *Courtesy of BD, Inc.*

Test Your Knowledge 10-23
What role does adhesive tape play in the collection of the samples for pinworm detection?   (Outcome 10-18)

PROCESSING MICROBIOLOGY SAMPLES

This chapter has explained the collection process and immediate handling for many different types of microbiology samples. In a physician office, the medical assistant is often responsible for one more step; the processing of the sample to prepare it for growth of the culture. This may include inoculation of the growth medium, slide preparation, and Gram staining, or even initiating the process for antibiotic sensitivity testing.

Slide Preparation and Gram-Staining Procedure

Developed in 1884, the **Gram stain** is a technique that quickly and inexpensively provides information about the bacteria that are present in a sample. Identification of the microorganisms is based on the fact that almost all bacteria will preferentially absorb different colors of stains, based on characteristics of their cell walls.

When the slide is viewed using the microscope, those bacteria that retain the crystal violet dye will appear purple and be identified as gram positive. Gram-negative organisms will have retained the safranin counterstain, and will appear pink when examined. Figure 10-10 shows gram-positive and gram-negative bacteria after staining. Gram-stained slides also allow the appearance and shape (e.g., cocci, bacilli) microorganisms to be viewed. Complete identification (such as genus and species) cannot be ascertained with a Gram stain, but the microorganism's characteristics that can be determined will assist the physician in making appropriate initial treatment decisions. If the Gram stain is performed at a laboratory outside of the physician office, the preliminary results are often called in to the physician office. The medical assistant must be very careful to document all information and report it to the physician in a timely manner.

Test Your Knowledge 10-24
Why are two different types of stains used for the Gram-staining procedure?   (Outcome 10-19)

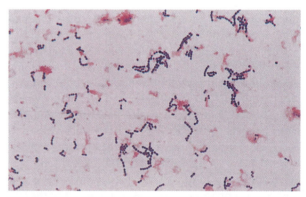
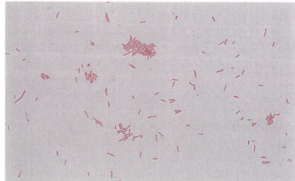

Figure 10-10   Gram-negative and gram-positive bacteria. The purple bacteria *(top)* are gram positive, and the pink bacteria *(bottom)* are gram negative.

Procedure 10-3: Gram-Staining Procedure

The Gram stain is one of the most common procedures performed in the microbiology department. It is a differential stain that allows bacteria to be classified into one of two groups depending on the way that the cell wall reacts with the dyes used in the staining process. The cell walls of the gram-positive bacteria have a greater affinity for the crystal violet stain than the bacteria classified as gram negative. When viewed under the microscope, the gram-positive bacteria will appear purple in color as a result of the crystal violet stain, and the gram-negative bacteria will appear pink in color as a result of the safranin counterstain.

TASK

Perform a Gram stain on a bacterial smear.

CONDITIONS

- Heat-fixed glass slide with bacterial smear
- Gram stain supplies (crystal violet, Gram's iodine, 95% ethyl alcohol, and safranin)
- Gloves
- Forceps
- Water
- Laboratory wipes

CAAHEP/ABHES STANDARDS

 CAAHEP Standards

III.C.III.9: Discuss quality control issues related to handling microbiological specimens. **III.P.III.2:** Practice Standard Precautions, **III.P.III.3:** Select appropriate barrier/personal protective equipment (PPE) for potentially infectious situations, **III.A.III.** Applied Microbiology/Infection Control

 ABHES Standards

- Apply principles of aseptic techniques and infection control
- Use standard precautions
- Practice quality control
- Perform selected CLIA-waived tests that assist with diagnosis and treatment, #5: Microbiology testing

Procedure	Rationale
1. Sanitize hands and apply gloves.	The gloves will protect the hands from becoming stained by the materials used in this procedure.
2. Grasp the slide in the forceps. Hold it over the sink or other waste container. Flood the slide with the crystal violet stain and allow it to be covered for 1 minute.	The slide should be held over the sink to allow excess stain to drain. It is important to keep the stain in contact with the slide for 1 full minute.
3. Pour off stain from slide and flush gently with water. Blot against laboratory wipes to remove excess water.	The slide should be flushed until the liquid stain is removed from the slide. It may be necessary to rub the underside of the slide with a laboratory wipe to remove excess stain if it drips onto the back of the slide.
4. Apply Gram's iodine to the slide for one minute.	The Gram's iodine forms a complex to keep the crystal violet attached to the gram-positive bacteria.

Continued

Procedure 10-3: Gram-Staining Procedure—cont'd

Procedure	Rationale
5. Pour off the Gram's iodine and flush the slide with alcohol. Allow the alcohol to run over the slide until the alcohol runs clear. This may take 20 to 30 seconds, and depends on the thickness of the smear.	The alcohol is a decolorizing agent, and it is imperative that the slide is flushed with this until it runs clear.
6. Rinse the alcohol from the slide with gentle running water. Blot off any excess water by tapping the slide against a laboratory wipe. Clean the underside of the slide with a laboratory wipe if necessary to remove excess stain.	Rinsing the water stops the decolorization process.
7. Cover the slide with safranin stain. Allow the slide to be covered for 20 seconds.	The safranin is the counterstain, which gives color to the gram-negative organisms that did not absorb the crystal violet stain. Without it, they would appear colorless on the slide when viewed under the microscope.
8. Rinse the slide once more with water. If necessary, use alcohol on the underside of the slide to remove any residual stain. Blot the stained slide with a laboratory wipe to absorb excess water.	This is the final stage of the process. It is important to make sure that the residual stain is removed so that the light will not be obscured when the slide is viewed under the microscope.
9. Put away supplies and clean the work area.	The laboratory area must remain clean and tidy.

POINT OF INTEREST 10-3
Tuberculosis and other acid-fast bacilli

Certain types of bacteria resist colorization during the Gram-staining procedure. These bacteria have a higher concentration of lipids in their cell walls, so they do not retain the crystal violet or the safranin stain. At the end of the Gram-staining procedure they remain essentially colorless. In order to identify these bacteria, the Ziehl Neelsen stain is often used to identify these bacteria, known as acid-fast bacilli. The most common group of bacteria that reacts in this way is from the genus *Mycobacterium*. Many species are harmless to humans, but there are a few notable exceptions. *Mycobacterium tuberculosis* is the causative agent of tuberculosis, *Mycobacterium avium* is a bacterium that is capable of causing lung disease, and *Mycobacterium leprae* causes leprosy.

Tuberculosis (TB) is a disease that has been around for a very long time. Active infection is on the rise, and it is imperative that the health-care community remain aware and educated about how to identify and treat this infection. *M. tuberculosis* is most often thought of causing a lung infection, but the bacterium may infect any area of the body. Other common infection sites include the kidneys and the central nervous system. The bacteria are spread through the air when an infective individual coughs, speaks, sneezes, or sings. There are two types of tuberculosis infection:

1. **Latent infection:** A patient has latent tuberculosis infection when he or she has become infected with the bacteria, but does not become actively ill. In the case of latent infection, the patient's immune system has "walled off" or isolated the bacterium to the extent that it does not cause immediate harm. The TB infection may spread at a later date, especially if the patient develops other conditions that lower natural immunity, such as HIV infection. The patients with latent infection will show a positive reaction on the tuberculosis skin test, and they need to be treated to kill the bacteria in their bodies before they cause active infection.

2. **Tuberculosis disease:** A patient with tuberculosis disease has the *M. tuberculosis* bacteria in the body, but the immune system has not rendered it inactive. The bacterium has caused active illness. Symptoms may include severe coughing for an extended period of time, spitting or coughing up blood, fatigue, anorexia, chills, fever, and night sweats. Patients with tuberculosis disease are infectious, and may infect those around them in their home or workplace. They may also infect the health-care professionals who care for them.

To aid in controlling tuberculosis disease, certain high-risk groups should be tested for latent infection, as well those who show symptoms of the active disease. These groups include those who have been exposed to a TB-positive person, patients who have a compromised immune system, those who have lived in or traveled to a country where TB is widespread in the population, those who are incarcerated, and those who are health-care professionals. The tuberculin skin test is the most common way to screen for latent infection, and this test is offered at local health departments as well as many physician offices. Those who immigrated to the United States from another country may have received the bacille Calmette-Guerin (BCG) vaccine against tuberculosis, which is given in countries outside of the United States. However, the BCG vaccine is not considered to offer lifetime immunity. Individuals who have received the BCG vaccine should still receive the tuberculosis skin test. They may show a false-positive result; if that is the case, patients will require follow-up chest x-rays and a physical examination to determine TB status. There is also a blood test now available for tuberculosis infection, called an interferon-gamma release assay. It does not check for the presence of the TB bacilli; rather, it tests for the body's immune response to the bacteria. It is relatively expensive to perform, and not yet in widespread use. An example of this test is the Quantiferon-GOLD test. Those who have had the BCG vaccine have less of a chance of a false positive with the blood test than they do the skin test.

Fortunately, tuberculosis infection, whether the infection is latent or active, is treatable. Those who test positive with the skin test or the blood test are treated with a regime that may last 6 to 12 months, and includes several medications at once. *M. tuberculosis* has become problematic in recent years, with development of several antibiotic resistant strains. Treatment with more than one medication at once seems to reduce the chance of developing resistance. Common medications include isoniazid, rifampin, ethambutol, and pyrazinamide. Patients with active infection are required to take their medication; if there is a high risk of noncompliance, they may even be placed in a directly observed therapy program in which a local health nurse will monitor their dosages daily. Incarceration is also an option; if the local health authority feels that a patient poses a high risk to other individuals and if that patient is noncompliant, jail time may be required.

Plating and Inoculation of Media

In some situations, laboratories may request that the physician office laboratory inoculate the media at the time of collection. A nutrient broth or slant may sometimes be innoculated. These types of media encourage growth of microorganisms but do not allow for isolation of specific colonies for further growth and identification. To accomplish separation of the growth into definitive colonies, an agar plate is used with a specific pattern of inoculation to create isolated colonies of the organism to be further identified and tested. The pattern of inoculation may be different depending on the type of agar plate or type of specimen. A common method used to add a sample to an agar plate is the quadrant method, in which the agar plate is divided into four parts, either mentally or with a grease pencil if necessary. The sample is applied to one quadrant of the plate fairly heavily with a swab that is twirled for full exposure. Successive quadrants are "streaked" with the sample by passing through the previous quadrant one time to pick up specimen, then continuing with numerous streaks that are close together. The goal is to provide an opportunity for growth of isolated colonies so that these can be further tested for identification and possibly sensitivity tested. Figure 10-11 illustrates the quadrant streaking method.

Test Your Knowledge 10-25

Which of these may be used for inoculation?
   a. Agar plates
   b. Slants
   c. Liquid nutrient broth
   d. All of the above   (Outcome 10-20)

Procedure 10-4: Quadrant Streaking Inoculation Procedure

To isolate microorganisms from pure culture or to isolate specific colonies from agar plates that contain mixed flora, it is necessary to set up a streak plate. The most common method used for this procedure is the quadrant streaking method. The plate is divided into four sections, and the sample is streaked across each area, with every quarter slightly overlapping the previous area.

TASK

Prepare a streak plate using the quadrant streaking method.

CONDITIONS

- Agar plate
- Inoculation loops or sterilization equipment
- Gloves
- Culture specimen on swab

CAAHEP/ABHES STANDARDS

 CAAHEP Standards

III.C.III.3: Discuss infection control procedures, **III.C.III.9:** Discuss quality control issues related to handling microbiological specimens. **III.P.III.2:** Practice Standard Precautions, **III.P.III.3:** Select appropriate barrier/personal protective equipment (PPE) for potentially infectious situations,

 ABHES Standards

- Apply principles of aseptic techniques and infection control
- Use standard precautions
- Practice quality control
- Dispose of biohazardous materials
- Collect, label and process specimens

Procedure	Rationale
1. Remove the lid of the agar plate and place face down on the countertop.	The lid should be placed so that it does not become contaminated.
2. Sanitize hands and apply gloves.	Gloves protect the hands from the microorganisms in the culture.
3. Mentally divide the agar plate into four quadrants. This may also be accomplished physically by drawing a four-part diagram on the bottom of the agar plate.	The quadrant method requires that the plate be divided into four sections.
4. Use the culture swab to inoculate the first quadrant on the agar plate. Gently roll the swab across this area for complete coverage.	The first quadrant must have an adequate amount of specimen present for the rest of the procedure to proceed correctly.
5. Turn the agar plate so that the second quadrant is at the top. Use the inoculation loop to apply sample into the next quadrant by passing it into the original application two times, then spreading it across the second quadrant without entering the first quadrant again.	The sample becomes less concentrated as it is spread across the second quadrant.
6. Using a new sterile inoculation loop (or sterilize and cool a reusable loop) repeat the procedure with the subsequent quadrants.	Each quadrant will be inoculated in the same way with a very small amount pulled from the previous quadrant and spread out.
7. Label the plate and incubate as directed.	Appropriate incubation will be necessary to allow for specimen growth.
8. Put away supplies and clean the work area.	The laboratory area must remain clean and tidy.

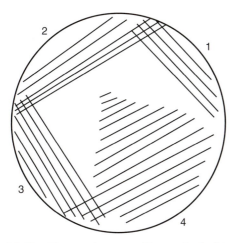

Figure 10-11   The quadrant streaking method of inoculation. The culture swab or a loop of a liquid sample is placed across quadrant 1. A sterile inoculating loop is used for the second quadrant; the streaks overlap quadrant 1 three times, then the swipes continue to fill the quadrant. Another sterile inoculating loop is used for the third quadrant, and the same procedure is used. This process is repeated once more for the fourth quadrant.

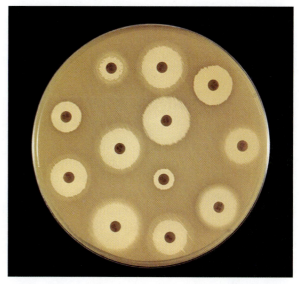

Figure 10-12   Antibiotic sensitivity plate showing the disk-diffusion method. Note the zones of inhibition around some of the antibiotic disks. *From CDC/Gilda L. Jones.*

Antibiotic Sensitivity Testing

Antibiotic sensitivity testing is performed to determine how effective antimicrobial therapy is against a certain type of bacteria. There are numerous methods available for this procedure; instruments such as the VITEK 2 (produced by the firm bioMérieux) are capable of performing antibiotic sensitivities in a fully automated fashion. These automated methods use the **minimum inhibitory concentration (MIC) method** to determine which antimicrobial agent is best to use for a specific pathogenic bacteria. However, many laboratories use an older, more laborious method of testing known as the **disk-diffusion method** (also known as the **Kirby-Bauer method**) for antibiotic sensitivity testing.

To set up the disk-diffusion (Kirby-Bauer) procedure, a solution of the diluted specimen is applied to cover an entire Mueller Hinton agar plate. Absorbent paper discs that have been impregnated with various antibiotics are applied directly to the specimen on the plate (Fig. 10-12). The antibiotics are absorbed into the specimen and the agar as the plate is incubated for a period of 18 to 24 hours. If an organism is **sensitive** to a specific antibiotic, it will have a **zone of inhibition** around the disc for that specific medication, meaning that the antibiotic is able to stop the growth of that particular microorganism so that no growth occurs near the disc on the agar plate. If bacterial growth is present right up to the disc and there is no visible zone of inhibition, this bacteria is

resistant. A resistant bacteria is not susceptible to the action of a particular antibiotic, so a patient should not be treated with this medication. The zone of inhibition is measured for each type of bacteria, and reported in the laboratory report so that the health-care provider will have the knowledge needed to treat the patient appropriately using antibiotics that will inhibit the growth of the specific pathogen. The Clinical and Laboratory Standards Institute (CLSI) outlines the reporting methods for disk-diffusion antibiotic testing. The technician reading the results in the microbiology laboratory will measure each zone of inhibition for the antibiotics used. He or she will then use the NCCLS to report the antibiotic susceptibility as sensitive, moderately susceptible, or resistant.

The minimum inhibitory concentration testing procedure is usually performed using an automated instrument. A plastic panel with rows of small wells that are filled with a specific concentration of antibiotic is used. The microbiology technician will inoculate each well with a dilution of the culture specimen. (This may also be performed automatically.) After incubating for approximately 24 hours, the wells are checked for evidence of bacterial growth, which presents as a cloudy appearance. The well that has the lowest concentration of a specific antibiotic that does not show evidence of growth is reported as the minimum inhibitory concentration of that specific antibiotic. The laboratory report will include the list of antibiotics tested and the MIC for each of them. It will also interpret these data further to state whether that bacteria is susceptible, moderately susceptible, or resistant to the antibiotic.

Test Your Knowledge 10-26

Why are antibiotic discs used when performing
sensitivities?   (Outcome 10-21)

POINT OF INTEREST 10-4
Antibiotic resistance

The discovery and further development of antibiotics
has been an incredible asset to public health. Millions
of lives have been saved, and our life expectancy has increased as a result of the positive steps we have taken to
battle infectious diseases. Unfortunately, these steps are
not without complications. As we develop more and
more complex drugs, the microorganisms in our environment are beginning to develop resistance to our antibiotics. This is especially evident in the drug classifications that are considered first line of defense: the drugs
that are cheapest and easiest to use. This resistance is
most recognizable in the types of infections that are
most prevalent: those that cause diarrhea, sexually
transmitted diseases, diseases of the upper and lower
respiratory tract, and especially those that are nosocomial (acquired as a result of hospitalization). Some of
the most serious problems include the following:

- Vancomycin-resistant *Enterococcus* (VRE): *Enterococcus* is a genus of bacteria that normally is found
  in the gastrointestinal system. However, when the
  bacteria are introduced into other areas of the body
  (the urinary tract, for instance) they are considered
  to be pathogenic, and cause serious infections.
  Many strains have developed a resistance to vancomycin, which was commonly used to treat this
  type of infection.
- **Methicillin-resistant *Staphylococcus aureus*
  (MRSA):** Staph is a common bacterium found as
  normal flora in various areas of our bodies. However, when introduced into a wound or into the
  bloodstream, it can be a virulent pathogen. Methicillin is a classification of antibiotic that has historically worked well against staph infections, but the
  levels of resistance are rising dramatically to this
  drug. MRSA is an aggressive pathogen, and may be
  difficult to treat effectively because of its virulence.
  It is estimated that up to 20% of our population
  may be colonized with MRSA at this point.
- Multiresistant *Mycobacterium tuberculosis*: As the
  number of cases of TB rises around the world,
  more and more show resistance to one or more of
  the drugs used for treatment. The regime used for

those who have active or latent TB infection now
includes more than one drug, as this seems to slow
the development of resistant strains, and accelerate
the elimination of the pathogen.

Scientists believe that there are multiple factors that
contribute to antibiotic resistance: the widespread use
of antibiotics in our food sources, historical prescribing patterns of health-care providers worldwide, and
patient compliance issues. Whenever an antibiotic is
prescribed as treatment for a bacterial infection, the
microorganisms either will be eliminated from the patient or they will not. Those bacteria that are not eliminated have now been exposed to the antibiotic, and
many have developed a way to "resist" the effects of
that particular medication. As these bacteria multiply,
their offspring will also have this natural resistance.

Medical assistants can help with educating patients
about the importance of this issue. Encourage patients
to keep the following issues in mind with antibiotic use:

Always take antibiotics as prescribed. This includes the frequency of the prescription (e.g., take
one pill two times per day) as well as the length of
time for the dosage. Many patients are tempted to
stop taking the medication as soon as they feel better;
this allows the bacteria that are still present in their
bodies to survive and develop resistance to the antibiotic that they were taking. Patients need to take the
prescription as it was written.

Do not take prescriptions that belong to other people. These medications were not prescribed for the
specific type of infection that the patient may be exhibiting. Even if two people have the same infection,
the required dosage for a medication may be different
for each. Self-medicating in this way is a dangerous
practice, and contributes to antimicrobial resistance.

Do not insist on antibiotics when the health-care
provider feels that the infection is viral in nature. Antibiotics are not effective against viral infections, and
taking them when they are not necessary only exposes
the body to these medications when they are not
needed.

Do not insist on a "higher grade" antibiotic when
the more common drug may be just as effective.
Many patients feel that penicillin, tetracycline, and
similar first-line drugs could not be the best thing for
them, as they are convinced that the newest drug developed must be better. Follow the guidance of your
health-care provider and your pharmacist; they are
more familiar with the specific dosage recommendations for these drugs.

MICROBIOLOGY TEST RESULTS

It can be difficult to interpret the results for microbiology testing by identifying the information that is clinically significant. Both the culture report and the sensitivity result may be present on the same document. This may be ordered or reported as a **culture and sensitivity (C&S) report**. Each laboratory has a unique system that it uses for reporting, but there are a few similarities common to all reports. The report will provide information about the microorganisms that are isolated from the culture, as well as relative amounts of these different microorganisms. When the report is final, there may also be antibiotic sensitivity data provided for bacterial cultures so that the health-care provider will be able to suggest treatment with the best medication available. This may be reported in several ways, so it is important for the medical assistant to gain an understanding of the report format used by his or her laboratory in order recognize abnormal values and bring them to the attention of the health-care provider. Figure 10-13 provides an example of a microbiology laboratory report.

Test Your Knowledge 10-27

What is a C&S report used to document?

(Outcome 10-22)

LZ labs

Laboratory Services
P.O. Box 44444
Seattle, WA 98124-1944

Patient: Thompson, Casandra   (MR#: 123456)
DOB: 01/25/1930, (81Y)   Sex: F
PCP: Grant, D.

Status: FINAL
Collected: 02/02/2012 15:20
Resulted: 02/06/2012 09:12
Printed: 02/09/2012 10:33
LabID: 18081424

Culture, Urine
SPECIMEN DESCRIPTION — Urine. 81yo female with catheter related UTI.
SPECIAL REQUESTS — Report principal pathogen only.
RESULT — Providencia rettgeri
REPORT STATUS — Final 02/08/2012

SUSCEPTIBILITY
ORGANISM — Providencia rettgeri
METHOD — MIC
Ampicillin — 16 Intermediate
Amoxicillin/Clavulanic Acid — 32 Resistant
Cefazolin — Resistant
Ceftriaxone — <=8 Susceptible
Gentamicin — <=4 Susceptible
Nitrofurantoin — >128 Resistant
Trimeth-sulfamethoxazole — >4 Resistant
Aztreonam — <=2 Susceptible
**SUSCEPTIBILITY COMMENT — See below:
Enterobacter, Citrobacter and Serratia species may develop resistance during prolonged therapy with third-generation cephalosporons. Repeat testing of these organisms is recommended after 4 days of therapy.
Cefepime — <=2 Susceptible
Ciprofloxacin — 1 Susceptible
Amikacin — <=4 Susceptible
Imipenem — <=1 Susceptible
Meropenem — <=1 Susceptible
Pip/tazobactam — <=8 Susceptible
Tobramycin — Resistant

Performing Laboratory
LZ Laboratory,   Lincoln George, M.D.
42600 1st Ave, Seattle, WA 98168 206-983-4456

Figure 10-13 Microbiology laboratory report.

SUMMARY

One of the most diverse areas of the laboratory is the microbiology department. Specimen requirements, processing procedures, and culture techniques are very specific and varied. Basic aseptic procedures and labeling techniques are common for all specimen types. As part of their role in quality microbiology testing, medical assistants need to remain knowledgeable about the type of test ordered, the specimen required for each kind of test, and the processing requirements. It is also very important that medical assistants know how to read the microbiology reports used by the laboratory so that clinically significant results are recognized and handled appropriately.

TIME TO REVIEW

1. Inoculation is the: Outcome 10-1
   a. Addition of a specimen to a culture medium for growth
   b. Addition of antibiotics to a culture medium
   c. Separation of colonies on a culture plate
   d. Gram staining of a specimen

2. True or False: Mycoses are the   Outcome 10-1
   various types of fungal infections that may be present on or in humans.

3. Hemolytic uremic syndrome   Outcome 10-1
   is a severe consequence of which type of infection?
   a. *Shigella*
   b. *Salmonella*
   c. *E. coli* O157:H7
   d. *Yersenia*

4. A nasopharyngeal culture   Outcome 10-13
   specimen is obtained by access through the:
   a. Mouth
   b. Nose
   c. Eye
   d. Pharynx

5. Which of these is not a type   Outcome 10-3
   of culture media?
   a. Slant
   b. Broth
   c. Agar
   d. Aerobe

6. True or False: Sample collection   Outcome 10-4
   supplies and transport media for bacterial, viral, and fungal cultures are all different.

7. Why should sputum samples   Outcome 10-6
   be protected from light?

8. Which of these statements is   Outcome 10-8
   false concerning the collection procedures for blood cultures?
   a. Blood cultures are rarely collected
   b. Aseptic technique is essential to avoid contamination of the specimen and misdiagnosis of the patient
   c. Blood is usually added to more than one bottle after collection
   d. Physicians may order blood cultures to be drawn serially at set time intervals

9. Genital samples may be used   Outcome 10-10
   to detect infections with:
   a. *Candida albicans*
   b. *Trichomonas vaginalis*
   c. *Neisseria meningitides*
   d. All of the above

10. Preservatives are used for   Outcome 10-17
    transport of specimens to be examined for presence of ova and parasites because:
    a. The preservatives provide nutrition for the parasites in the sample
    b. The appearance of the parasites and their eggs are kept near those of their natural state in the body
    c. The preservatives keep the parasites alive so that they can grow in the laboratory
    d. All of the above

11. What time of day should a   Outcome 10-18
    pinworm sample collection occur?
    a. Just before bedtime
    b. Randomly; the time of day is not important
    c. First thing in the morning
    d. Right after bathing in the morning

12. Gram-positive microorganisms   Outcome 10-19
    will appear _____ after the Gram-staining procedure is complete.
    a. pink
    b. purple
    c. blue
    d. black

13. The quadrant method describes: Outcome 10-20
    a. A technique used to inoculate an agar plate
    b. A technique used for Gram stains
    c. A technique used for collection of wound culture specimens
    d. A calculation used for antibiotic sensitivity reporting

14. When reading a microbiology   Outcome 10-22
    laboratory report, why is it important for the healthcare provider to be familiar with the normal flora commonly present in the area of the body where the specimen was collected?

Case Study 10-1: How long is too long?

Marti is a certified medical assistant working in a busy internal medicine practice. There is a new receptionist who is working at the front counter this week, and Marti has found that the receptionist is a bit overwhelmed by the volume of patients the practice is seeing today. The morning appears to be uneventful, but at 2 p.m., the new receptionist brings a urine specimen back to Marti. The receptionist tells Marti that it was dropped off that morning before lunch, but that she forgot to do anything with it until now. Marti sees that the physician has ordered a culture on the urine specimen, and that the urine is in a specimen cup without preservative.

1. What should Marti do?

Case Study 10-2: A sticky situation

Mrs. Oliver brings in her 3-year-old who is complaining of intense anal itching. Lanette, the medical assistant, is asked to collect a sample for examination of potential pinworm infection. This is a procedure she has not performed often, and Lanette is a bit nervous. She decides that the best approach is to speak very little to Mrs. Oliver and the child so that process goes quickly.

1. For this procedure, is this the best approach?
2. If you were Lanette, how would you explain the process to Mrs. Oliver and her child?

RESOURCES

"Antimicrobial Resistance"
World Health Organization
Excellent overview about the progressing issues with antibiotic resistance around the world http://www.who.int/mediacentre/factsheets/fs194/en/

"Antony van Leeuwenhoek (1632–1723)"
History of Leeuwenhoek and the early discoveries of bacteriology http://www.ucmp.berkeley.edu/history/leeuwenhoek.html

BacT/ALERT blood culture collection procedure
An overview of the supplies provided with the culture collection kit and their use. http://www.biomerieux-usa.com/upload/Worksafe-Blood-Culture-Collection-Procedure-1.pdf

"Lumbar Puncture and Spinal Fluid" by John E. Greenlee, MD.
Information about how a spinal fluid specimen is obtained, and how it is processed umed.med.utah.edu/neuronet/pda/2002/HO%20LP%20Spinal%20Fluid%20Greenlee%202002.doc

"Cerebrospinal Fluid Analysis," in Encyclopedia of Surgery: A Guide for Patients and Caregivers
Great article on the clinical indications of a need for CSF collection, the laboratory test results, and potential poor outcomes of the procedure. http://www.surgery-encyclopedia.com/Ce-Fi/Cerebrospinal-Fluid-CSF-Analysis.html

"Disease Listing: Campylobacter General Information"
CDC Division of Foodborne, Bacterial and Mycotic Disease. http://www.cdc.gov/nczved/dfbmd/disease_listing/campylobacter_gi.html

"Disease Listing: Salmonella General Information"
CDC Division of Foodborne, Bacterial and Mycotic Disease, http://www.cdc.gov/nczved/dfbmd/disease_listing/salmonellosis_gi.html

"Disease Listing: Shigella General Information"
CDC Division of Foodborne, Bacterial and Mycotic Disease, http://www.cdc.gov/nczved/dfbmd/disease_listing/shigellosis_gi.html

"Pinworm Fact Sheet"
CDC Division of Parasitic Diseases
Great information about pinworm infestation http://www.cdc.gov/ncidod/dpd/parasites/pinworm/factsht_pinworm.htm

"Educational Commentary on the Preservation of Fecal Specimens for Ova and Parasite Examination"
Excellent information about pros and cons of different preservatives used for O&P examinations; sponsored by the American Society of Clinical Pathology http://www.api-pt.com/pdfs/2002Amicro.pdf

"Training Material Facilitates Proper Nasopharyngeal Swab Collection"
Training module for nasopharyngeal swab collection http://www.rapidmicrobiology.com/news/2023h4.php

"UV Light Cuts Spread of Tuberculosis," Science Daily, March 19, 2009
Information about studies performed for new methods of controlling the spread of tuberculosis within healthcare facilities http://www.sciencedaily.com/releases/2009/03/090316201505.htm

Specimen Collection and Processing
What Does it All Mean?

As this section clearly points out, proper specimen collection and processing is paramount to obtain accurate and reliable laboratory results. Our Case in Point for this section demonstrates the importance of proper specimen collection and processing.

Case in Point

As you may recall, Wilma F. is a 70-year-old female who presented to the doctor's office where you work complaining of burning and painful urination. She felt hot to the touch as confirmed by her temperature that was 101.5°F. The doctor asked you to collect blood and urine samples for laboratory testing.

Based on the patient's symptoms and the fact that Wilma has a history of urinary tract infections (UTIs), it is likely that she once again has an infection. If she only has a UTI, the urine collected for culture will reveal significant microorganism growth but the bloodstream will be free of microorganisms and the corresponding blood culture results will be reported as "negative." If however, microorganisms establish residence in Wilma's bloodstream, her blood culture results will be considered "positive." It is common for patients to start out with a UTI and then progress into a bloodstream infection. In these cases, the same microorganisms often are found in both the blood and urine culture specimens.

In Wilma's case, she has symptoms of both a blood and urine infection. Wilma's high temperature suggests a possible blood infection whereas her problems with urination indicate a urine infection. The question now is: What microorganisms are causing these problems for Wilma? With the appropriate collection and handling of Wilma's urine and blood samples, the chances of getting reliable and accurate laboratory results is excellent. While the doctor is waiting for the results to come back, he will likely begin Wilma on a suitable treatment known to treat a variety of microorganisms, often referred to a broad-spectrum treatment. He will then adjust treatment if necessary after the microorganisms have been identified and the laboratory results are obtained.

On the Horizon

The study of blood and blood-forming tissues is known as *hematology*. *Coagulation* refers to the clotting of blood. Because these two concepts interconnect, corresponding testing is often conducted in the same area of the clinical laboratory. The results generated by performing hematology and coagulation testing are of monumental importance in the diagnosis and monitoring of a number of diseases and conditions.

Relevance for the Medical Assistant

Medical assistants may be called upon to collect samples and in some instances perform CLIA-waived tests that fall into the hematology and coagulation category. An understanding of this area of laboratory testing is essential to recognize the clinical significance of test results and to anticipate the needs of the health-care provider when dealing with the patients. In addition, medical assistants need to have a full understanding of their role in the preanalytical process while preparing patients and specimens for testing

Continued on page 258.

Hematology and Coagulation On the Horizon

The fundamental concepts associated with hematology and coagulation are covered in six chapters that make up this section of the text, as outlined below.

Chapter 11: Overview of Hematology introduces the reader to the formation, description, and analysis of the three key types of cells in the circulating blood: red blood cells (RBCs), white blood cells (WBCs), and platelets.

Chapter 12: Complete Blood Count With Differential explores the key components of the most commonly ordered battery of hematology tests, known as a complete blood count (CBC).

Chapter 13: Hemoglobin and Hematocrit examines the description, theory, and testing (with emphasis on CLIA-waived procedures) of these two important hematology tests: hemoglobin (Hgb) and Hematocrit (Hct). An independent examination of each test as well as an investigation of the relationship between them are made, because of their importance in the diagnosis and monitoring of hemoglobinopathies, anemia, and polycythemia.

Chapter 14: Erythrocyte Sedimentation Rate covers the description, theory, and testing (with emphasis on CLIA-waived tests) of the erythrocyte sedimentation rate (ESR) test. This test, often in combination with other laboratory tests, is of importance in instances of inflammation changes and in monitoring pregnancies.

Chapter 15: Coagulation Studies introduces the reader to the purpose of coagulation studies, the mechanism of blood clotting, disorders associated with abnormal coagulation test results, and commonly performed coagulation tests. Select coagulation laboratory tests that are useful in the diagnosis of disorders and monitoring of anticoagulant therapy as well as specimen requirements for testing are covered.

Continued from page 256.

Case in Point

You are the primary medical assistant working at Midtown Medical. In the midst of a very busy Monday, Margie, the receptionist, informs you that a new patient, M.J., has been worked into the schedule and is here now to be evaluated. After greeting M.J. and recording his weight and height, you take him into the examination room. While preparing to take his blood pressure and pulse, you ask M.J. what brings him in to see the doctor today. You find out that up until a few weeks ago, this 38-year-old male had been in the best of health. The symptoms he has been experiencing consist of an overall feeling of being tired and weak, and every time he brushes his teeth his gums bleed. After questioning M.J. further, you find out that he was recently hospitalized after a tractor accident and had received a blood transfusion at that time. You notice while talking to him that he looks very pale. The doctor orders blood to be drawn for a complete blood count (CBC), and coagulation studies (PT and APTT). The following results are obtained:

LABORATORY REPORT
PATIENT: M.J.

Complete Blood Count (CBC)

Test	Patient Result	Reference Range for Adult Males
WBC count	10.0	4,000–11,000/mm^3
RBC count	3.0	5.5–6.5 × 10^6/mm
Hgb	9.0	14–18 g/dL
Hct	30	42%–54%
RBC Indices	>>>>>>>>>	>>>>>>>>>
MCV	86	80–96 femoliters
MCH	31	27–33 picograms
MCHC	35	33–38 g/dL
Platelet count	28	140–400 × 10^3/mm^3
Differential	>>>>>>>>>	>>>>>>>>>
Neutrophils	65	50%–70%
Bands	5	3%–5%
Lymphocytes	23	23%–30%
Monocytes	6	3%–7%
Eosinophils	1	1%–3%
Basophils	0	0%–1%
Cell morphology	Few schistocytes present	

Coagulation Studies

Test	Patient Result	Reference Range
Prothrombin time (PT)	18 seconds	10–14 seconds
Activated partial thromboplastin time (APTT)	47 seconds	20–35 seconds

Questions for Consideration:

- What type and color of blood-drawing tube should be used for this patient so that the laboratory can perform the complete blood count (CBC) test?
- What type/color of blood-drawing tube should be used for this patient so that the laboratory can perform the coagulation studies?
- Examine the patient's laboratory results. Which of these results is/are considered as "abnormal" (that is, out of the reference range)?
- What laboratory results obtained most likely account for the patient's being pale?
- What is the purpose of the coagulation studies tests (PT & APTT)?

Chapter 11

Overview of Hematology

Nikki A. Marhefka, EdM, MT(ASCP), CMA (AAMA)

CHAPTER OUTLINE

Hematopoiesis—Blood Cell Formation
Types of Blood Cells in the Circulating Blood
    Erythrocytes—Red Blood Cells
    Leukocytes—White Blood Cells
        Granular White Blood Cells
        Agranular White Blood Cells
    Thrombocytes—Platelets

Analysis of the Formed Elements
Summary
Time to Review
Case Studies
Resources and Suggested Readings

Learning Outcomes   *After reading this chapter, the successful student will be able to:*

11-1 Define the key terms.

11-2 Summarize the process of blood cell formation.

11-3 State the three types of formed elements in the circulating blood and the function of each cellular element.

11-4 Describe the appearance of a reticulocyte and provide examples of situations in which there are increased numbers of reticulocytes in the circulating blood.

11-5 Differentiate the appearance and function of the five types of leukocytes normally present in the circulating blood.

11-6 Describe the appearance of a band cell, and explain when there may be an increased number of band cells in the circulating blood.

11-7 Describe the appearance and function of platelets.

11-8 List three CLIA–waived hematology testing procedures that may be performed in a physician office.

CAAHEP AND ABHES STANDARDS

 CAAHEP Standards met:

I.C.I.2. Identify Body Systems
I.C.I.4. List major organs in each body system
I.C.I.5. Describe the normal function of each body system
I.C.I.6. Identify normal pathology related to each body system

 ABHES Standards met:

None

KEY TERMS

Agranular	Granlocyte-macrophage colony-stimulating factor (GM-CSF)	Monocyte
Band cell		Myeloid
Basophil	Hematocrit	Neutrophil
Bilobed	Hematology	Phagocytosis (phagocytic, phagocytize)
Blast cells	Hematopoiesis	
Complete blood count (CBC)	Hemoglobin	Platelet
	Hemostasis	Pluripotent
Diapedesis	Heparin	Polychromatic stain
Eosinophil	Histamine	Polymorphonuclear
Erythrocyte	Interleukin	Red blood cell (RBC)
Erythrocyte sedimentation rate (ESR)	Intrinsic factor	Reticulocyte
Erythroid	Leukocyte	Reticulum
Erythropoietin	Lobulated	Stem cells
Formed element	Lymphocyte	Thrombocyte
Granular	Lymphoid	Thrombopoietin
Granulocyte	Megakaryocyte	Thrombus
		White blood cell (WBC)

Blood is a specialized connective tissue that consists of **formed elements** suspended in liquid plasma. Approximately 38% to 48% of the total blood volume is made up of these formed elements, including **red blood cells (RBCs; erythrocytes), white blood cells (WBCs; leukocytes),** and **platelets (thrombocytes).** The cells function in important ways to keep the human body healthy and safe. The primary function of the erythrocytes is to carry oxygen to the tissues of the body, whereas the leukocytes help to fight off infection within the body. The thrombocytes are present to assist with blood clotting and repair of blood vessel damage. Each of the cell types may be identified by characteristics of its nucleus and cytoplasm.

Hematology is defined as the study of blood and blood-forming tissues. However, more specifically, it is the word used to describe the study of the formed elements in the blood. This chapter explores the process involved with the formation of cellular elements in the bone marrow, and discusses identification and functions of erythrocytes, leukocytes, and thrombocytes.

> **Test Your Knowledge 11-1**
>
> List the three formed elements present in the circulating blood.   (Outcome 11-3)

HEMATOPOIESIS—BLOOD CELL FORMATION

Blood cell formation, a process known as **hematopoiesis** (Fig. 11-1), occurs primarily in the red bone marrow. In children, most bones contain red marrow. In the adult (individuals greater than age 20), red marrow is found in the flat bones (vertebrae, ribs, iliac crest, and sternum). **Stem cells** are the precursors of all blood cells and are present in the bone marrow. They are pluripotent, which means that they have the ability to differentiate into several types of specialized cells. These stem cells may divide into precursor stem cells classified as **myeloid** or **lymphoid.** Erythrocytes and most of the white blood cells are capable of arising from myeloid precursor cells. Specialty white blood cells responsible for the majority of the body's immune protection, known as **lymphocytes,** arise from the lymphoid precursor

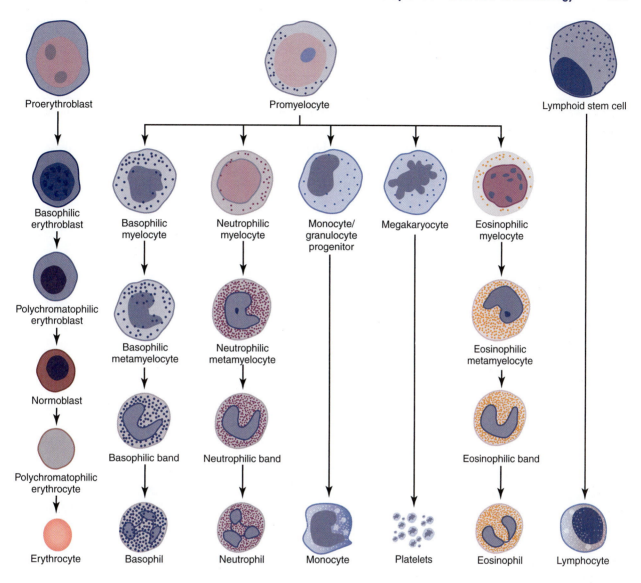

Figure 11-1   Hematopoiesis. The production and maturation of the blood cells and fragments.

stem cells. It is important to note that lymphocytes are also produced and processed in the thymus gland and secondary lymph organs, in addition to their production in the bone marrow. Descriptions of the formed elements in the blood are summarized in Table 11-1.

Myeloid and lymphoid stem cells, once developed, differentiate to produce **blast cells,** which are the first identifiable immature cell stages of what eventually become erythrocytes (RBCs), leukocytes (WBCs), and thrombocytes. Blast cells mature and go through a number of stages before they are transformed into mature cells. Numerous functions of the spleen are associated

with the development, storage, breakdown, and removal of specific blood cells, as noted in Box 11-1.

Under normal circumstances, only the mature blood cells will enter the circulating blood. Immature forms of the blood cells may be present in the circulating blood in disease states. For example, immature red blood cells may be evident in the circulating blood with anemia, and immature white blood cells may be present with leukemia. The cellular components of the bone marrow can be studied by making slides of the marrow, staining it, and studying it under the microscope. The sample for evaluation is obtained from the marrow cavity of the flat bones.

TABLE 11-1

Formed Elements of the Circulating Blood

Blood Cell	Size	Description	Function
		Leukocytes	
Neutrophil	9–15 microns	Multilobed nucleus, grayish purple granules	Phagocytic, increases in bacterial infection
Band cell	9–15 microns	C-shaped nucleus, grayish purple granules	An immature neutrophil, increases in bacterial infection
Eosinophil	10–16 microns	Bilobed nucleus, large red-orange granules	Phagocytic, detoxifying
Basophil	10–14 microns	Bilobed nucleus, large blue-black granules	Release histamine and heparin
Lymphocyte	7–18 microns	Large dark nucleus, little light blue cytoplasm (There are larger ones with larger less dense nuclei and more cytoplasm.)	Produce antibodies, involved in cell-mediated immunity
Monocyte	12–20 microns	Large foamy convoluted nucleus, little or no granules in cytoplasm	Travel to tissue to become macrophage, phagocytic
Erythrocytes	6–8 microns	No nucleus, biconcave discs	Carry oxygen in blood to the tissues
Thrombocytes	0.5–3 microns	Small cytoplasmic fragments	Blood clotting

---

BOX 11-1   Functions of the spleen associated with blood cells

- Site of red blood cell formation in the fetus
- Site of worn out red blood cell and platelet removal
- Site of old red blood cell breakdown
- Site of hemoglobin (from the worn-out red cells) decomposition
- Stores some iron from hemoglobin decomposition
- Contains red blood cell and platelet pools for use when needed
- Areas of lymphocyte proliferation and immune surveillance and response

A number of factors are produced by the body to stimulate the production of blood cells. **Intrinsic factor** helps with B_{12} absorption in the digestive tract, and B_{12} is critical for red blood cell formation. **Thrombopoietin** from the liver stimulates production of platelets, and **granulocyte-macrophage colony-stimulating factor (GM-CSF)** increases the formation of leukocytes. **Interleukins** influence the growth and activation of the lymphocytes. **Erythropoietin** stimulates the bone marrow to produce more red blood cells when needed in the body. When the oxygen level is low in the tissues, the kidneys produce more erythropoietin to stimulate the differentiation and growth of the **erythroid** (pertaining to erythrocyte) cells in the bone marrow to increase the number of circulating red blood cells. Blood loss, such as from a bleeding ulcer, anemia, or low oxygen levels in the lungs due to high altitude or lung disease cause an increase in erythropoietin.

POINT OF INTEREST 11-1
Bone marrow aspiration

In some clinical situations, medical practitioners need to visualize what is occurring in the bone marrow to make an accurate diagnosis. A bone marrow biopsy is not a procedure that is performed casually because the process may be painful and is very invasive. A sample of the red marrow may be obtained to look for the cell distribution, iron stores, or cell maturity. The information gained from the sample may provide valuable clues needed for a differential diagnosis, and therefore, may be very valuable.

Red bone marrow is found in the ribs, sternum, ilium, vertebrae, and the epiphyses of the long bones of adults. In children, it is found in the shafts of the long bones as well. The red marrow is generally the same in each of these areas, so a sample may be taken from any location. The site for the biopsy and aspiration is usually the posterior iliac crest. The sternum and the broad end of the tibia are other sites that may be utilized, although not as frequently as the iliac crest.

A sample of the bone marrow can be obtained using a special hollow needle with a stylus insert. The aspiration is completed using sterile technique to prevent infection and/or inflammation of the bone, which is called osteomyelitis. The patient is usually in a prone position so that the iliac crest is fully exposed and supported. The skin, subcutaneous tissues, and the periosteum are anesthetized with a local anesthetic to reduce discomfort to the patient. A special hollow aspirate, needle is used to penetrate through the layers of tissue and into the bone. A twisting motion is necessary for the needle to reach the destination. Once the marrow cavity has been entered, the stylus part of the needle device is removed, and a syringe is attached to the end of the hollow needle that is exposed. Fluid is aspirated, and some of the marrow material is obtained. The medical assistant or laboratory technologist that is assisting with the procedure must verify whether the sample is valid by observing its appearance.

The aspirated sample is placed on a clean glass slide. The liquid sample from the marrow may be spread across the slide using a similar procedure as that used when preparing a blood smear. There will also be solid components of the bone marrow obtained; these are called spicules, and they are slowly rotated across a slide to make impressions for examination. These solid components are then placed in preservative for further studies if necessary. The slides are stained and the preparations are assessed under the microscope by a pathologist or hematologist.

After the procedure has been completed, the medical assistant will prepare the slides, clean up the supplies and assist with the application of a pressure bandage to the puncture site.

Test Your Knowledge 11-2

Define *hematopoiesis*.   (Outcome 11-2)

Test Your Knowledge 11-3

Stem cells are described as pluripotent. What does this mean?   (Outcome 11-2)

TYPES OF BLOOD CELLS IN THE CIRCULATING BLOOD

As was introduced earlier in this chapter, there are three categories of cells circulating in blood: erythrocytes, leukocytes, and thrombocytes. A description and function of the primary members in each category are detailed in the following sections.

Erythrocytes—Red Blood Cells

Erythrocytes, also known as red blood cells (RBCs), are the most numerous formed element in the blood. The number of red blood cells in the body varies with the gender and age of the patient, but there are approximately 4.2 to 6.5 million in a milliliter of blood. Normal red blood cells measure 6 to 8 microns in diameter. The red blood cells are smaller than the white blood cells in the body, but larger than the platelets. Red blood cells perform their duties within the blood vessels and do not enter the tissues normally.

The primary function of red blood cells is to carry oxygen to all tissues of the body. Each red blood cell contains an iron pigment responsible for oxygen transport known as **hemoglobin.** Oxygen enters the capillaries that surround the alveoli of the lungs and moves to each red blood cell, where it attaches to the hemoglobin. Hemoglobin is a protein composed of an iron-containing pigment and globulin (a type of protein). Hemoglobin gives red blood cells their characteristic reddish color. Blood is a brighter red color in the arteries as more oxygen is attached and is darker red in the venous blood because of less oxygenation. It is interesting to note that some carbon dioxide is carried through the blood via hemoglobin in the red blood cells to be released in the lungs.

Circulating red blood cells have no nuclei and are biconcave (the center is thinner than the thicker edges) in shape. Their unique shape and the lack of a nucleus allow red blood cells to increase their surface area for gas diffusion (oxygen transport) and allow the cells to contain more hemoglobin than a cell with a nucleus. The biconcave shape of the erythrocyte also eases the cells' passage through the capillaries to bring oxygen to the tissues.

Each red blood cell has a life span of approximately 120 days. Mature red blood cells have no organelles and therefore a limited metabolism. Erythrocytes are not capable of producing proteins or enzymes. Red cells undergo much stress as they traverse the blood vessels in the body and they have no repair mechanisms. The red cells are continuously monitored and the old, worn-out ones are recognized and engulfed by the macrophages or the reticuloendothelial system of the liver, spleen, and bone marrow. The functions of the spleen are presented in Box 11-1.

Immature red blood cells, called **reticulocytes,** may also be found in the circulating blood. Reticulocytes exhibit a blue network when stained with a special stain because the cells have not fully matured and still have residual structures present in the cell cytoplasm. The reticulocytes will also appear as large bluish red blood cells when viewed with the standard stains used for peripheral blood smears. The blue network is remnant RNA (ribonucleic acid) left in the cell when the nucleus is expelled near the end of the red blood cell maturation. With use of special staining procedures, the remnant RNA is visualized as fine, thread-like strands known as **reticulum.** These immature reticulocytes should remain in the bone marrow until maturity. However, when the demands of the body are increased for red blood cells (as in the event of hemorrhage or massive blood cell destruction), reticulocytes enter the circulating blood. Normally, less than 5% of the circulating red blood cells are reticulocytes. Both erythrocytes and reticulocytes are pictured for comparison in Figure 11-2.

Test Your Knowledge 11-4

Do mature erythrocytes contain a nucleus?

(Outcome 11-3)

Test Your Knowledge 11-5

What type of immature red blood cell may increase if a patient has hemorrhaged due to an injury?

(Outcome 11-4)

Leukocytes—White Blood Cells

Leukocytes are specialized cells that play an essential role in the immune response of the body. White blood cells are the largest blood cells and vary in size from 7 to 20 microns. The total number of white blood cells is 4,300 to 10,800 per cubic millimeter in normal circulating blood. The white blood cells spend most of their life span in the tissues of the body, but the vascular circulation allows white blood cells a mode of transportation throughout the body so that they can respond where necessary. Some WBCs only live a few hours, whereas others live for months or years. Many of them die when they have completed destroying foreign invaders. There are five mature types of white blood cells that are generally found in circulating blood: *neutrophils, lymphocytes, monocytes, eosinophils,* and *basophils* (Fig. 11-3). These cells may be categorized in various ways based on their appearance. One such method is to define them as **granular** or **agranular.**

Granular White Blood Cells

White blood cells that have names ending in –phil (neutrophil, eosinophil, and basophil) have distinct granules visible in their cytoplasm and are known as **granulocytes.** These granules contain digestive enzymes that are designed to destroy or damage foreign cells or microorganisms, or

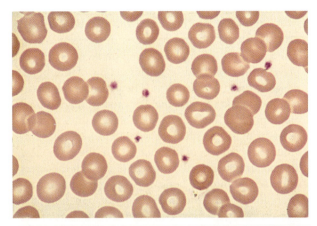

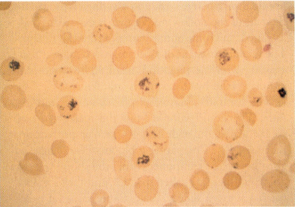

Figure 11-2   Top: Erythrocytes in the circulating blood. Bottom: Reticulocytes The endoplasmic reticulum is visible with new methylene blue stain. *From Harmening, DM: Clinical Hematology and Fundamentals of Hemostasis, ed 5.* FA Davis, Philadelphia, 2009, *with permission.*

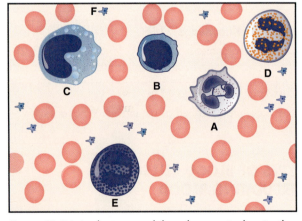

Figure 11-3   Leukocytes and thrombocytes in the circulating blood. A. neutrophil. B. lymphocyte. C. monocyte. D. eosinophil. E. basophil. F. platelet.

chemicals that assist with the process of destroying invaders. The nuclei of granular cells are arranged in lobes or sections. This appearance of the nucleus is described as **lobulated.** White cells are distinguished by the staining of their nucleus and granules when using a **polychromatic stain** (a stain having many colors, such as Wright's stain). The granular cells live only a few days and dissolve as they age, or are destroyed when they have participated in bacterial destruction.

Neutrophils make up the majority of circulating granular cells, and provide much of the body's protection against infection. A typical neutrophil measures 9 to 15 microns in diameter, has a nucleus with 3 to 5 lobes, and has gray/pale purple granules in its cytoplasm. A neutrophil may also be called a **polymorphonuclear** (PMN) leukocyte, or "poly," because of the multiple lobes of its nucleus. Some laboratories may also describe a neutrophil as a "seg," referring to the segmented appearance of the nucleus in these cells.

The primary function of neutrophils is **phagocytosis,** which is the act of engulfing and destroying foreign invaders. The majority of the circulating white blood cells of adults are usually neutrophils. The number of neutrophils often increases when a bacterial infection is present in the body. A mature neutrophil lives for 10 to 24 hours in the circulating blood. Typically, it takes about 30 minutes for the neutrophil to engulf bacteria. This process destroys the cell, and we often see these dead white cells accumulated as pus.

A **band cell,** as seen in Figure 11-4, is an immature form of the neutrophil that may appear in the circulating blood when there is a high demand for neutrophils by the body. Neutrophils are the first to respond to infection or injury, so the need is increased for an acute infection. The nucleus of a band cell is C shaped as the nucleus has not

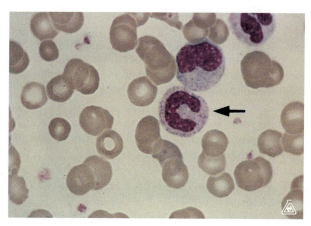

Figure 11-4 A band cell has a C-shaped nucleus and the same granules as the neutrophil.

had a chance to mature into lobes or sections. The cytoplasm of a band cell is the same as that of a mature cell. Normal circulating blood may have some band cells, but they usually make up less than 10% of the total. Band cells may also appear in the circulating blood of patients suffering from disease states that result in overproduction of neutrophils in the bone marrow.

Eosinophils are 10 to 16 microns in diameter, have **bilobed** nuclei (that is, each nucleus has two lobes or sections), and have large orange/red granules in the cytoplasm. These cells phagocytize invaders attached to antibodies (antigen-antibody complexes) and detoxify foreign substances. (Additional information on these concepts is located in Chapter 24.) An increase in the number of eosinophils is often seen in allergic reactions, myocardial disease, or with parasitic infection. Eosinophils enter the tissues from the blood capillaries and live there for about 6 days.

> **Test Your Knowledge 11-6**
>
> What is the type of white blood cell that will increase in production when a patient has a bacterial infection?
>
> (Outcome 11-5)

> **Test Your Knowledge 11-7**
>
> What is the name of the white blood cell that may be increased in number in an allergic reaction? How can this cell be differentiated from the other types of white blood cells?
>
> (Outcome 11-5)

Basophils are 10 to 14 micron in diameter, have bilobed nuclei, and large dark blue granules in the cytoplasm. The nucleus is often hard to see, as the granules are so large and dark that they obscure it from view. The granules found in the cytoplasm of basophils contain **heparin** and **histamine.** Heparin helps to prevent blood from clotting, whereas histamine makes blood vessel walls more permeable so that white cells can get into tissues to phagocytize foreign cells and invaders. An increase in basophils is often seen in the presence of chronic infection, when there is healing of infection, in allergic asthma, or in contact allergies. Basophils have a life span of about 6 days.

Agranular White Blood Cells

Lymphocytes and monocytes are considered agranular, as they have few visible cytoplasmic granules. **Monocytes** are the largest of the white blood cells with a diameter of 12 to 20 microns and have a large, convoluted, less densely stained nucleus. The cytoplasm often has a "ground-glass" appearance and a pale blue or light gray color. In addition, the cytoplasm of monocytes often contains vacuoles (holes) when viewed under the microscope. Monocytes travel through the vessel walls and out of the circulatory system into the tissues as needed in a process called **diapedesis.** Monocytes are phagocytic in function as they destroy and remove dead cells from tissue. They defend the body against microorganisms and malignant cells. Monocytes live in the circulating blood for 8 to 24 hours and then as macrophages in the tissue for several months. The macrophages assist with removal of all types of old, damaged, or nonfunctional blood cells.

Lymphocytes are the smallest of the white blood cells, with dark, dense nuclei that often take up most of the cell. Lymphocytes traditionally have a small amount of light blue cytoplasm. Lymphocytes may vary in size from 7 to 19 microns in diameter. Lymphocytes appear slightly larger than red blood cells when viewed on a stained slide. Lymphocytes mature into B cells, T cells, and natural killer cells. B lymphocytes become plasma cells and form antibodies. T cells and natural killer cells are active in cell-mediated immunity. (More information about the body's defense system may be found in Chapter 24.) Lymphocytes are usually the most predominant white blood cell in the circulating blood of children until about age 10 years, but they are the second most prevalent type of white blood cell in adults. An increase in number may be seen in viral infections at all ages. The life span of the T cells is months to years and the B cells live only a few days.

Test Your Knowledge 11-8

What type of white blood cell has forms that make antibodies and are active in cell-mediated immunity?

(Outcome 11-5)

Thrombocytes—Platelets

Thrombocytes, or platelets, are spherical or ovoid cell fragments which are 0.5 to 3 microns in diameter (Fig. 11-3). There are normally 150,000 to 450,000 platelets per millimeter of blood. Platelets are cytoplasmic fragments of large bone marrow cells called **megakaryocytes.** Two-thirds of the platelets are in the circulating blood at any given time, whereas the other third is stored in a pool in the spleen. The typical platelet life span is 8 to 10 days.

Platelets actively participate in **hemostasis** (the stoppage of bleeding or of circulation). Platelets prevent blood loss and have three functions that begin the clotting process (for more information on hemostasis see Chapter 15). When a capillary is damaged, platelets stick together and adhere to the sides of the cut to form a plug that fills the opening. While forming the plug, platelets secrete a chemical known as serotonin designed to help constrict the blood vessels. Platelets also activate the complex chemical process of coagulation to enhance the platelet plug. Younger platelets are larger and more metabolically active and are more effective in hemostasis.

Platelets sometimes clot within the blood vessels when there is no vessel wall damage. This may result in a **thrombus** (blood clot), which adheres to the wall of a vessel or organ. These clots can occlude (block) the vessels and potentially stop the flow of blood. When the body's tissue does not receive oxygen from the blood, body cells will die. A thrombus may be the cause of a heart attack or a stroke.

Test Your Knowledge 11-9

What are the three hemostatic functions of platelets that prevent blood loss?   (Outcome 11-7)

ANALYSIS OF THE FORMED ELEMENTS

In reference and hospital laboratories erythrocytes, leukocytes, and platelets may be identified and counted by automated analyzers capable of processing large volumes of specimens. The cells that make up the formed elements in the blood are typically identified by size, appearance, and other specific characteristics. A **complete blood count (CBC)** is the most commonly ordered hematology test. As the test name implies, this comprehensive test provides practitioners with important information about all three formed elements in the circulating blood. The process of cell formation (hematopoiesis) may be studied by collecting and microscopically examining bone marrow samples in large laboratories. Types of hemoglobin can be identified by the technique of hemoglobin electrophoresis. (More information about these tests is presented in Chapters 12 and 13.)

In the physician office and at the bedside in hospitals, CLIA-waived hematology testing is often performed. The hemoglobin concentration of the blood cells is often measured using a CLIA-waived procedure. The **erythrocyte sedimentation rate** and the **hematocrit** value are other common CLIA-waived tests performed in physician office laboratories. The hematocrit is the percentage of red blood cells in a given volume of blood, and the erythrocyte sedimentation rate is a screening test for inflammation that measures the speed at which erythrocytes settle out of anticoagulated blood. Medical assistants or phlebotomists often perform these tests in the physician office laboratory.

Test Your Knowledge 11-10

Name three CLIA-waived hematology tests.

(Outcome 11-8)

SUMMARY

Hematology is the study of the cellular (or formed) elements in the blood. The cells of the circulating blood are predominantly formed in the bone marrow by the process of hematopoiesis. Each type of cell matures from the same pluripotent stem cell. The stem cell differentiates into blast cells for each kind of blood cell and then continues to mature into the functioning cells that are released into the circulating blood. These functioning cells include erythrocytes, leukocytes, and thrombocytes. Erythrocytes carry oxygen, leukocytes are part of the immune system, and platelets participate in blood clotting.

Erythrocytes contain hemoglobin, which enables them to transport oxygen throughout the body. An increase of a more immature form of the erythrocyte, the reticulocyte, in the circulating blood can show that the bone marrow is trying to provide sufficient red blood cells at times of crisis. This may mean that the body has increased its demands for oxygen, or that there is a need to replace lost blood cells.

There are five types of leukocytes normally seen in the circulating blood. These white blood cells are neutrophils, eosinophils, basophils, lymphocytes, and monocytes. Each cell is identified by the properties of its nucleus and cytoplasm and has a specific function in the immune process. Thrombocytes are small round cell fragments that are involved in the clotting process.

Blood cells and platelets can be counted and tested for their ability to function. Large analyzers in the reference and hospital laboratories can perform many tests on a large number of specimens or highly specialized testing. The medical assistant can perform the CLIA–waived testing of hemoglobin, hematocrit, and the erythrocyte sedimentation rate. An abnormal number of the formed elements or an abnormal test result can be indicative of a disease process. Testing procedures and clinical significance of the formed elements in the blood are discussed in the following chapters.

TIME TO REVIEW

1. What is the difference between   Outcome 11-1
   erythropoietin and thrombopoietin?

   a. Erythropoietin stimulates red blood cell formation and thrombopoietin stimulates white blood cell formation
   b. Erythropoietin stimulates platelet production and thrombopoietin stimulates white blood cell production
   c. Erythropoietin stimulates red blood cell formation and thrombopoietin stimulates platelet production
   d. Erythropoietin stimulates platelet production and thrombopoietin stimulates red blood cell production

2. True or False: During hematopoiesis   Outcome 11-2
   all blood cells are derived from stem cells.

3. Which of these statements does not   Outcome 11-3
   describe the appearance or function of erythrocytes?

   a. Erythrocytes are biconcave in shape
   b. Erythrocytes assist in blood clot formation
   c. Erythrocytes carry oxygen throughout the body
   d. Erythrocytes are the most numerous found elements in the bloodstream

4. What is the substance in the   Outcome 11-1
   red blood cells to which oxygen attaches?

   a. Nuclei
   b. Vacuoles
   c. Reticulum
   d. Hemoglobin

5. Immature red blood cells that still   Outcome 11-5
   contain some endoplasmic reticulum which may be visualized in the circulating blood in periods of high demand are called:

   a. Granulocytes
   b. Reticulocytes
   c. Band cells
   d. Lymphocytes

6. The number of white blood cells in   Outcome 11-3
   the circulating blood is 4,300 to 10,800 per milliliter and their main function is in:

   a. Participation in the immune response of the body
   b. Carrying oxygen to the cells of the body
   c. Blood clotting
   d. Liver function

7. The cytoplasm of these cells   Outcome 11-6
   have large dark granules that contain heparin and
   histamine:

   a. Neutrophils
   b. Eosinophils
   c. Basophils
   d. Monocytes

8. The type of white blood cells that   Outcome 11-6
   are most prevalent in adults and that phagocytize
   foreign invaders are called:

   a. Neutrophils
   b. Eosinophils
   c. Basophils
   d. Monocytes

9. The function of these cells is   Outcome 11-6
   to remove dead cells from tissue. They are called
   macrophages when they have traveled into the tissues:

   a. Neutrophils
   b. Eosinophils
   c. Basophils
   d. Monocytes

10. An immature neutrophil that may be   Outcome 11-7
    visualized in the circulating blood in a severe infec-
    tion is called a:

    a. Granulocyte
    b. Reticulocyte
    c. Band cell
    d. Lymphocyte

11. Which of the formed   Outcome 11-3, Outcome 11-8
    elements are involved in hemostasis and prevent
    blood loss?

    a. Reticulocytes
    b. Thrombocytes
    c. Erythrocytes
    d. Leukocytes

Case Study 11-1: Meaning of abnormal results

Dr. Stewart has ordered a CBC to be collected on Mr. Marcus. Lily, the medical assistant, draws the blood sample and sends it to the local reference laboratory with the courier that afternoon. The next day, the results are available and Lily reviews them before placing them on the chart for Dr. Stewart to read. The leukocyte count and the neutrophil count are both flagged as elevated above the normal range.

1. What do you think these two elevated results may mean?

RESOURCES AND SUGGESTED READINGS

"Fun Science Gallery: Let's Observe the Blood Cells" Contains pictures and descriptions of the various blood cells. http://www.funsci.com/fun3_en/blood/blood.htm

Chapter 12

Complete Blood Count With Differential

Nikki A. Marhefka, EdM, MT(ASCP), CMA (AAMA)

Learning Outcomes

After reading this chapter, the successful student will be able to:

12-1 Define the key terms.

12-2 Identify the component tests of a complete blood count (CBC).

12-3 Recognize the normal reference ranges for each CBC component.

12-4 Identify examples of disorders that are characterized by an increased red blood cell, white blood cell, or platelet count.

12-5 Identify situations where the white blood cell count may be decreased.

12-6 State the clinical significance of the erythrocyte indices included in a CBC.

12-7 For the five types of normal white blood cells identified on a differential, state the normal reference range in the form of percentages.

12-8 Identify examples of diseases characterized by an abnormal white blood cell differential.

12-9 Differentiate terms used to describe normal and abnormal red blood cell morphology using appropriate medical terminology.

12-10 Describe the appearance of platelets when viewed under the microscope.

12-11 Summarize the general principle of electrical impedance as it relates to automated CBC testing.

CAAHEP AND ABHES STANDARDS

 CAAHEP 2008 Standards

 ABHES 2010 Standards

I.C.1.6. Identify common pathology related to each body system

I.A.I.1. Apply critical thinking skills in performing patient assessment and care

None

KEY TERMS

Anemia	Leukocytosis	Ovalocyte
Anisocytosis	Leukopenia	Poikilocytosis
Blast	Lysed	Polychromatic stain
Complete blood count (CBC)	Macrocyte	Polycythemia
Differential	Mean corpuscular hemoglobin (MCH)	Red blood cell index
Electrical impedance		Sickle cell
Hematocrit (Hct)	Mean corpuscular hemoglobin concentration (MCHC)	Spectrophotometrically
Hemoglobin (Hgb)	Mean corpuscular volume (MCV)	Spherocyte
Hemocytometer	Microcyte	Target cell
Histogram	Morphology	Thrombocythemia
Hyperchromic	Normochromic	Thrombocytopenia
Hypochromic	Normocytic	Thrombocytosis
Leukemia		

A complete blood count (CBC) provides physicians and other health-care professionals with an overview of cells and cell fragments in the circulating blood. The amounts of different types of cells in the specimen as well as physical characteristics of these cells are included in the CBC results. Used alone or along with other diagnostic and laboratory tests, the CBC helps the physician diagnose disorders, follow the course of treatment, and determine prognoses. This chapter introduces the reader to each of the major CBC components as well as presents an overview of automated analyzers used in CBC testing.

COMPLETE BLOOD COUNT

The **complete blood count (CBC)** comprises a series of tests, each with its own reference range, as listed in Table 12-1. The tests are usually performed using an automated hematology analyzer, but some of them may also be performed using manual methods. Components of a CBC include the following:

- *A white blood cell (WBC) count,* providing the number of white blood cells present in the sample.
- A *red blood cell (RBC) count,* which provides the total number of red blood cells present in the specimen.
- **Hemoglobin** concentration, which is the concentration of the iron-containing pigment in red blood cells which binds to oxygen.
- **Hematocrit,** which is the percentage of red blood cells in a given volume of blood.
- Three **red blood cell indices,** defined as numerical descriptions of the RBCs present.
- A *platelet count,* which provides a quantitative measurement of the platelets present in the specimen
- The *white blood cell differential,* which provides quantitative information about the types of white blood cells present in the specimen.

TABLE 12-1

Suggested Reference Ranges for Component Tests of the Complete Blood Count

White blood cell count	4,300 to 10,800/mm³
Red blood cell count	Adult female: 4.2–5.9 × 10⁶/mm³
	Adult male: 4.6– 6.2 × 10⁶/mm
Hemoglobin concentration	Adult female: 12 to 16 g/dL
	Adult male: 13 to 18 g/dL
Hematocrit	Adult female: 37%–48%
	Adult male: 45%–52%
Red blood cell indices	MCV 80–100 femtoliters
	MCH 27–31 picograms/cell
	MCHC 32–36 g/dL
Platelet count	150 to 450 × 10³/mm³
Differential	
Neutrophils	54%–65%
Lymphocyte	25%–40%
Monocyte	2%–8%
Eosinophil	1%–4%
Basophil	0%–1%

The hemoglobin and hematocrit tests included in the CBC are CLIA-waived test procedures. However, the other tests included in the complete blood count are categorized as moderately or highly complex by CLIA. Medical assistants may perform moderately complex automated hematology testing with appropriate documented training and supervision. Medical assistants can also perform a normal manual differential from a stained blood smear if they are specially trained and appropriately supervised for this moderately complex procedure.

For the CLIA moderately complex tests, the following additional steps must be taken for appropriate documentation, training, and quality control:

1. All laboratories that perform tests of moderate complexity must be registered with the Centers for Medicare & Medicaid Services (CMS) as a moderately complex laboratory. The Certificate of Waiver that is used for CLIA-waived testing procedures will not be valid if the tests of higher complexity are also performed in the laboratory.
2. The requirements for quality control increase with the higher level of test complexity. This includes the documentation of daily calibration and maintenance, the testing of two levels of quality control performed routinely, and participation in a proficiency testing program.
3. Those employees who perform these tests must also have documentation of all training, and regular documented updates when the process changes.

> **Test Your Knowledge 12-1**
> What tests are components of the CBC? (Outcome 12-2)

Complete Blood Count Specimen Requirements

Blood samples for the complete blood count can be collected by venipuncture or capillary collection. The CBC requires a well-mixed lavender top tube containing EDTA as an anticoagulant. There is an emphasis on the mixing of the sample for CBC analysis because the whole blood tested must represent the circulating blood in the body. If the sample is not inverted five to ten times immediately after collection, small clots may form, leading to inaccurate results.

A lavender Microtainer tube will be used in the capillary collection process for a CBC. As in the case of the tube used for venipuncture, the specimen in the Microtainer tube must be mixed during and immediately following the collection process. A steady, consistent blood flow is necessary so that small clots do not form during the blood collection. CLIA-waived analyzers have special collection chambers that can be filled directly with blood from a capillary puncture, eliminating the need for a Microtainer tube. These collection chambers are placed in the instrument for testing.

White Blood Cell Count

The total number of WBCs in the circulating blood (known as a white blood cell count) is another component of a CBC. There is no distinction between types of white blood cells in this total white blood cell count. Since there are so many blood cells, a method known as *scientific notation* is used to express the values for the white blood cell count and the red blood cell count. Scientific notation is used when numbers are too large to be written in the common decimal format, in which the numbers are reported as a number $\times 10^6$. The normal reference range for the WBC count is approximately 4.3 to 10.8 $\times 10^3/mm^3$ (4,300 to 10,800 cells per cubic mm).

Leukocytosis is the term used when the white blood cell count exceeds the normal range. The most frequent cause for an elevation of leukocytes is infection. Increased WBC counts may also be associated with stress, intense exercise, trauma, inflammation, and pain. Smoking may also cause slight leukocytosis.

In addition, white blood cell counts are usually elevated well above the normal range in the presence of leukemia. In cases of leukemia, white blood cell counts may range from 30,000 to 200,000 per cubic millimeter of blood. Leukemia is a cancer of the bone marrow in which a large number of immature white blood cells are being produced or disease states in which mature forms live an exceptionally long time. These white blood cell clones are not capable of performing their roles as part of the immune system. Leukemias are classified according to the predominant cell type present, and whether the disease is acute or chronic in nature. Table 12-2 provides more information about the various types of leukemia.

Leukopenia refers to a WBC count that is below the normal range (values below 4,000 per cubic millimeter). The number of white blood cells may be decreased in a chronic viral infection. Exposure to lead, mercury, some chemotherapy agents, and radiation may also cause the white blood cell count to be diminished.

> **Test Your Knowledge 12-2**
>
> What is the reference (normal) range of the red blood cell count for an adult?   (Outcome 12-3)

Red Blood Cell Count

Red blood cells are the most prevalent formed element in circulating blood. Because there are so many red blood cells, scientific notation is used as it is for the white blood cell count to express these values. There are millions of red blood cells present in each specimen, so these are reported as 10^6. The reference (normal) ranges for red blood cell measurements will vary based on the age and gender of the patient. For instance, adult males normally

TABLE 12-2		
Types of leukemias		
Type	**Abbreviation**	**Description**
Chronic myelogenous (granulocytic) leukemia	CML	A large number of all types of white blood cells and platelets; subtyped according to the type of predominant cell
Acute myelogenous (granulocytic) leukemia	AML	The bone marrow produces a large number of granulocytic blast cells; predominantly an adult leukemia
Chronic lymphocytic leukemia	CLL	Accumulation of lymphocytes that live a long time; predominately identified in older adults
Acute lymphocytic (lymphoblastic) leukemia	ALL	Abnormal growth and development of lymphocytes; diagnosed most frequently in children
Hairy cell leukemia	HC or HCL	Excess B lymphocytes are produced; these lymph have projections that make them look "hairy"; generally affects middle-aged and older adults

have more red blood cells present in their bodies than do adult females. Red blood cell counts are performed using an automated hematology analyzer. The reference ranges will vary from 4.2 to 6.2×10^6 cells per microliter.

Red blood cell counts that exceed the normal range may be present in various diseases, including **polycythemia** (a condition that results in an excess of RBCs). Those results below the normal range suggest a reduction in the oxygen-carrying capacity of the blood known as **anemia.** The various types of anemia are further described in Chapter 13.

Test Your Knowledge 12-3

List two disorders that are characterized by an increased white blood cell count.   (Outcome 12-4)

Hemoglobin and Hematocrit

Hemoglobin (Hgb) is an iron-containing pigment present in all red blood cells and is responsible for oxygen transport. The Hgb concentration is typically measured in grams per deciliter (g/dL). For this test, RBCs are **lysed** (broken open) and the free hemoglobin enclosed in the cell is then measured **spectrophotometrically.** Spectrophotometric measurements measure color changes produced by the hemoglobin present in a sample using a specific wavelength of light. The reference ranges for hemoglobin also vary by gender and age. The hemoglobin normal range for adults is 12 to 18 g/dL.

The **hematocrit (Hct)** is the amount of space occupied by the red blood cells in a whole blood sample as compared to the total sample volume. A hematocrit can be measured directly utilizing hematocrit tubes after centrifugation, or the hematocrit result may be calculated using the hemoglobin and one of the red blood cell indices, called the mean corpuscular volume (MCV). This red blood cell index represents the average volume of the individual red blood cells in a sample. The hematocrit is always reported as a percentage, and the reference ranges vary with gender and age of the patient. Adult normal ranges include values from 38% to 52%. More details of hemoglobin and hematocrit testing and further evaluation of their clinical significance are provided in Chapter 13.

Red Blood Cell (Erythrocyte) Indices

A typical CBC includes three calculated values that help classify RBCs in terms of size and hemoglobin concentration. The calculations use the word *corpuscular* in referring to the red blood cells. These calculations are known as **red blood cell indices:**

1. **Mean corpuscular volume (MCV),** defined as the average volume of a red blood cell in a sample
2. The average weight of hemoglobin in the red blood cells in a sample, known as **mean corpuscular hemoglobin (MCH)**
3. **Mean corpuscular hemoglobin concentration (MCHC),** the average weight of hemoglobin in a given volume of packed blood cells

These values are calculated from the hemoglobin concentration, the hematocrit value, and the red blood cell count. The indices are most often used to classify various types of anemias. Table 12-3 includes more information about each of the indices, including a brief description, the

---

TABLE 12-3

Red Blood Cell (Erythrocyte) Indices

Red Blood Cell Index Units	Description	Formula	Suggested Reference (normal range)
MCV: Mean corpuscular volume Femtoliters	The average volume of red blood cells in the specimen	$\dfrac{\text{Hematocrit (\%)} \times 10}{\text{RBC count (millions)}}$	80–100 fL
MCH: Mean corpuscular hemoglobin Picograms per cell	Content or weight of hemoglobin in the average red blood cell	$\dfrac{\text{Hemoglobin (g/dL)} \times 100}{\text{red blood cell count (million)}}$	27–31 pg/cell
MCHC: Mean corpuscular hemoglobin concentration g/dL	The average concentration of hemoglobin in a volume of packed cells	$\dfrac{\text{Hemoglobin (g/dL)} \times 100}{\text{hematocrit (\%)}}$	32–26 g/dL

fL is the abbreviation for femtoliters, and pg is the abbreviation for picograms.

formula used for calculation, and a suggested reference range. These indices provide clinicians with valuable information about the size and condition of the red blood cells in the sample as well as more details about the amount of hemoglobin present. The calculated indices may be compared with the appearance of the corresponding red blood cells as noted on a stained blood smear to verify their clinical significance and the accuracy of the values.

Test Your Knowledge 12-4

What information is provided by the red blood cell indices?

(Outcome 12-6)

Platelet Count

As was introduced in Chapter 11, platelets are small cell fragments that interact with chemicals in the bloodstream to assist in the clotting process. The reference ranges for platelet counts may vary with the blood sample collection technique employed. Capillary collection values are lower than those in venous blood because some of the platelets in the area are immediately involved with the formation of the plug for the injury of the skin puncture. The venous reference range for the platelet count is 150×10^3 to $450 \times 10^3/mm^3$ (150,000 to 450,000 per cubic millimeter).

Thrombocytopenia means a decreased platelet count. Platelets may be decreased with some types of infection and in situations where the individual has been exposed to certain medications or toxic substances. **Thrombocytosis** refers to an increased platelet count in the circulation, and may be associated with a variety of diseases. If the platelet count is increased in response to a specific "trigger," it is known as *reactive thrombocytosis.* When the elevated platelet count becomes pronounced over an extended period of time and the bone marrow begins to produce excessive amounts of abnormally functioning platelets, the condition is known as **thrombocythemia.** Thrombocythemia is considered to be a serious condition, as these excess platelets can cause small clots to form intravascularly, or the platelets may not function properly to stop bleeding when needed.

Leukocyte Differential Count

A **differential** is a process by which the percentage of the five normal types of white blood cells in the circulating blood is calculated. These cell types include the following:

1. **Neutrophils:** First responders to foreign invasion of the body

2. **Eosinophils:** Assist with allergic reactions, parasitic infections, and chronic inflammation
3. **Basophils:** Play a key role in the inflammatory process
4. **Lymphocytes:** Ingest and kill microorganisms and play a key role in the immune response with antibody formation
5. **Monocytes:** Attack and eliminate foreign substances; monocytes function as macrophages in the tissues of the body

As introduced in Chapter 11, immature neutrophils, known as *band cells*, are also identified and reported separately when a leukocyte differential is performed. The band cells may be increased in number during a bacterial infection because the bone marrow is attempting to produce an increased amount of white blood cells (especially neutrophils) to meet the body's need. Immature cells that are earlier in the developmental stage than band cells are not normally present in the bloodstream, and their presence indicates a serious infection or other blood disorder. The immature forms of other white blood cell types may occasionally be present and must be identified, as their presence may assist with a diagnosis or prognoses.

When reporting the leukocyte differential, each type of white blood cell is reported as a percentage (%). This procedure is completed utilizing automated methods or performed manually with visualization of a stained blood smear by a properly trained clinical laboratory professional. In blood samples for most adults, neutrophils are typically seen in the greatest numbers (between 54% and 65%). Lymphocytes are next in frequency; 24% to 40% would be the normal range. Monocytes make up approximately 2% to 8% of the white blood cell count. The rest of the white blood cells are made up of eosinophils, which total 1% to 4%, and the basophils, which make up 1% or less of the circulating white blood cells. The immature neutrophils (band cells) may total up to 5% of the normal differential as well. The cells are identified on a stained slide by their size, shape, color, and the structures within the cell. Automated instruments may also report these parameters. Table 12-4 provides a summary of information about the various types of white blood cells.

The results of the differential can be used for initial diagnosis or to monitor treatment. An increase in neutrophils often indicates a bacterial infection. With acute infections, there usually will be an increase in the number of the immature band cells as well as an overall increase in neutrophils. Eosinophils may increase in number with allergies and parasitic infections. Lymphocytes often

The order of frequency for the presence of the five types of white blood cells may be remembered by using this simple sentence: **N**ever **L**et **M**onkeys **E**at **B**ananas! Starting with the most prevalent to the least, the five types of white blood cells identified in the circulating blood are **N**eutrophils, **L**ymphocytes, **M**onocytes, **E**osinophils, and **B**asophils.

exceed the normal range in viral infections. In immediate hypersensitivity reactions (such as asthma) basophils are often increased. An increase of monocytes may suggest a chronic infection (tuberculosis is an example) or the presence of a malignancy.

Lymphocytes may be elevated with infectious mononucleosis. In addition to the increase in the percentage of lymphocytes, many of the lymphocytes may be larger than normal. *"Reactive" lymphocytes* are also identified with mononucleosis; these are larger than the typical lymphocyte, and when visualized under the microscope, they have a nucleus that is less dense than a typical lymphocyte. An increase of regular, larger, and reactive lymphocytes accompanied by other physical signs and symptoms and a positive mono screening test will be used to diagnose infectious mononucleosis.

The white blood cell differential is significant for patients with leukemia because the various types of leukemia are categorized by the type of predominant white blood cell present in the bone marrow and bloodstream. Leukemia classification is also based on whether the disease process is acute or chronic in nature. The acute leukemias primarily present with immature white blood cells in the form of **blasts** (the earliest form of the white blood cell that is identifiable), while the chronic types of leukemia are characterized by dramatically increased numbers of dysfunctional mature cells. In acute lymphoblastic leukemia, the differential would have many immature lymphocytes, referred to as *lymphoblasts*. The blood smear of a patient with chronic myelogenous leukemia typically has an increased number of the granulocytic white blood cells, (neutrophils, eosinophils and basophils). The granulocytic white blood cells have granules present in their cytoplasm.

Test Your Knowledge 12-5
Describe the appearance of a normal red blood cell on a stained blood smear.   (Outcome 12-9)

Clinical Facts

- Viral infection caused by the Epstein-Barr virus
- Virus enters through the oropharynx, transmitted in saliva; called "the kissing disease"
- Most prevalent in adolescents and young adults
- Virus infects the B-cell lymphocytes

Clinical Symptoms

- Fatigue
- Fever
- Sore throat
- Swollen lymph glands

Hematological Features

- Slight elevation in the white blood cell count (12,000 to 25,000)
- Increased percentage of lymphocytes (60% to 90%)
- Presence of reactive (atypical) lymphocytes
  - Larger T cells than normally visualized
  - Larger; nuclei with more open chromatin and deep indentations
  - Cytoplasm with basophilia, azurophilic granules, and vacuoles

Immunology Features

- Positive rapid-screen mono test
- Increased heterophile antibody titer

Treatment

- Rest
- NSAIDs, such as ibuprofen
- No lifting or contact sports if the spleen is enlarged

Peripheral Blood Smear

A peripheral blood smear may be used for a manual white blood cell differential as well as visualization of other formed elements in the blood. A blood smear consists of a slide with a drop of blood spread across it. The blood sample may be created directly from a capillary puncture or from an EDTA-anticoagulated venous blood sample that is less than 2 hours old. The smear is then dried, stained, and viewed under the microscope. White blood cells, red blood cells, and platelets are observed. Examination of cell **morphology** (appearance

TABLE 12-4

White Blood Cell Types in the Circulating Blood and Reference Ranges for the Leukocyte Differential

White Blood Cell	Image of Cell	Description of Morphology	Percentage Normally Present (suggested reference range)
Neutrophil	(From Harmening, DM: Clinical Hematology and Fundamentals of Hemostasis, ed. 5. FA Davis, Philadelphia, 2009, with permission.)	Multilobed nucleus; lavender gray granules in cytoplasm	54%–65%
Lymphocyte	(From Harmening, DM: Clinical Hematology and Fundamentals of Hemostasis, ed. 5. FA Davis, Philadelphia, 2009, with permission.)	Large, dense, dark blue nucleus; small amount of pale blue cytoplasm	25%–40%
Monocyte	(From Harmening, DM: Clinical Hematology and Fundamentals of Hemostasis, ed. 5. FA Davis, Philadelphia, 2009, with permission.)	Foamy, convoluted nucleus; ground glass–looking cytoplasm	2%–8%
Eosinophil	(From Harmening, DM: Clinical Hematology and Fundamentals of Hemostasis, ed. 5. FA Davis, Philadelphia, 2009, with permission.)	Bilobed nucleus; large orange-red granules in cytoplasm	1%–4%

TABLE 12-4—cont'd

White Blood Cell Types in the Circulating Blood and Reference Ranges for the Leukocyte Differential

White Blood Cell	Image of Cell	Description of Morphology	Percentage Normally Present (suggested reference range)
Basophil	(From Harmening, DM: Clinical Hematology and Fundamentals of Hemostasis, ed. 5. FA Davis, Philadelphia, 2009, with permission.)	Bilobed nucleus (difficult to see clearly); large dark blue granules in cytoplasm	0%–1%
Band cell (immature neutrophil)	(From Harmening, DM: Clinical Hematology and Fundamentals of Hemostasis, ed. 5. FA Davis, Philadelphia, 2009, with permission.)	C-shaped nucleus; lavender-gray granules in cytoplasm	0%–5%

of the red blood cells including their size, color, and shape) and determination of size are used to identify each type of blood cell. The leukocyte differential, the red blood cell morphology, and a platelet estimate are reported as part of the results. Examination of the blood smear is necessary when the automated results indicate that there is a need to double-check the differential count or cell morphology of the specimen, or when the method used for the CBC does not allow for an automated white blood cell differential.

Test Your Knowledge 12-6

What characteristics of the white blood cells are used to differentiate the different types?   (Outcome 12-7)

Blood smears are stained with a **polychromatic stain,** which consists of a combination of an alkaline and acidic component that allows for cells to appear in a variety of colors. Wright's stain is a popular polychromatic stain used for blood smears. Different structures will absorb more of one color or the other, as they will naturally be attracted to the alkaline or acidic components of the stain. The resulting colors and cell structural appearance are used to differentiate the cells. Nuclei are stained blue by the basophilic (alkaline) part of the stain; other structures are stained red orange by the eosinophilic (acid) stain component. Some structures pick up both stain components.

Manual Leukocyte Differential

For performance of a manual differential, the stained blood smear is placed on the stage of microscope and the immersion oil objective (100X) is used to magnify the blood smear. An area where cells appear in a single layer and are not overlapped is located while looking at the slide. The viewing field is moved from side to side across the width of the smear. Typically 100 consecutive white blood cells are observed and accounted for by type. The size of the cell and the structures of the nucleus and the cytoplasm are used to identify each white blood cell type. An electronic or a manual tabulator keeps count. When 100 cells are counted, the percentage of each type is the total number observed.

> **Test Your Knowledge 12-7**
>
> List the five white blood cell types in order from those of the greatest number to those of the least.
>
> (Outcome 12-7)

Red Blood Cell Morphology

As well as counting the different types of WBCs on a differential, it is important to observe the RBCs and pay careful attention to their size and shape. As introduced in Chapter 11, normal red blood cells are circular biconcave disks with pale centers. They are 6 to 8 microns in diameter. They are a soft red color and have no nuclei. Red blood cells are smaller than white blood cells and larger than platelets. The red blood cells on the stained slide should all be similar in size, with natural slight differences in the sizes and shapes. These normal red blood cells are called **normocytic** and **normochromic**. The suffix –cytic refers to the size and shape of the red blood cells and the suffix –chromic refers to the color of the cells when viewed under the microscope.

Normocytic red blood cells are the normal size of 6 to 8 microns. Normochromic red blood cells have a center that is paler than the surrounding cell, which means that they contain a sufficient concentration of hemoglobin. In hematological disorders, the red blood cells may vary in the amount of hemoglobin, the size and shape of the cells, the staining characteristics (pale or dark red) and the structures present within the cells.

> **Test Your Knowledge 12-8**
>
> What is the term used to describe a red blood cell visualized on a stained smear that is paler or lighter in color than a normal erythrocyte?   (Outcome 12-9)

Red blood cells that have too little hemoglobin will have larger, paler central areas than normal cells. These cells are described as **hypochromic. Spherocytes** are RBCs that assume a spherical shape and are said to be **hyperchromic,** because they have excess hemoglobin concentration and thus no central pallor. **Polychromatic** (a multicolored appearance achieved using a mixture of varied colored stains) red blood cells appear a little more bluish in hue as they contain RNA that attracts the alkaline component of the stain. **Anisocytosis** is a condition in which there is a variety of sizes of red blood cells present. Cells larger than normal size are considered **macrocytes** and those smaller than normal are **microcytes**.

> **Test Your Knowledge 12-9**
>
> What is the term used when the red blood cells on a smear are varied in shape more than usual?
>
> (Outcome 12-9)

Poikilocytosis describes red blood cells that are present on the slide in a variety of different shapes. Some types of cells are named for their descriptive shape. Examples of these include teardrops, helmet cells, **sickle cells** (arch-shaped cells that result from low oxygen tension and that contain an abnormal substance known as hemoglobin S, and elliptical-shaped cells known as **ovalocytes.** Cells that have a reduced hemoglobin concentration (known as **target cells)** have so little hemoglobin that there is only a slight ring of color at the edges. These target cells have a spot of trapped hemoglobin in the center (the bull's eye of the target). Figure 12-1 includes examples of normal and abnormal red blood cell morphology.

Immature nucleated red blood cells may be present on the slide when there has been an event that puts an extreme demand on the bone marrow for production of new blood cells. These nucleated red blood cells (NRBCs) will have a blue staining nucleus. NRBCs are not normally present in the circulating blood of an adult but they may be seen in fetal blood or that of young infants. If NRBCs are present, it is important to report this as part of the CBC result, as their presence may be clinically significant.

Platelet Morphology and Estimated Count

Platelets are small, oval-shaped, and purple cellular fragments when visualized on the stained blood smear. A platelet estimate may be calculated by counting the number of platelets on a stained blood smear in fields viewed under the microscope where cells are not overlapped and red blood cell morphology is easily visualized. Ten fields are counted, and the average number of platelets per field is multiplied by 20,000 to achieve a platelet estimate. In a normal platelet count, there are 8 to 20 platelets on an oil immersion field.

Manual Blood Cell Counts

Red blood cells, white blood cells, and platelets may be counted manually by a qualified laboratory professional. This is not a CLIA-waived procedure, so in most circumstances it is not a procedure that will be

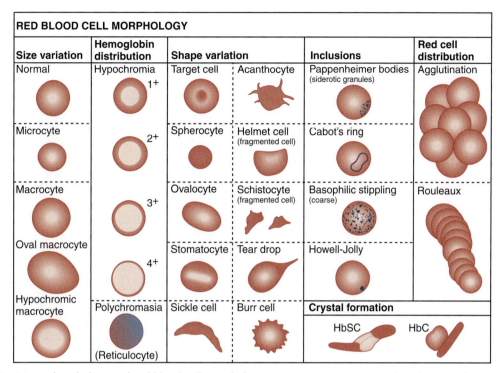

Figure 12-1 Normal and abnormal red blood cell morphology. *From Harmening, DM: Clinical Hematology and Fundamentals of Hemostasis, ed. 5. FA Davis, Philadelphia, 2009, with permission.*

performed by a medical assistant. A manual cell count may be necessary when the automated system is non-functional or in situations in which the cell counts are too low to be measured by the instrument commonly used. For a manual count, blood samples are mixed with a specified amount of diluent (Fig. 12-2A) and added to a **hemocytometer.** The hemocytometer is a chamber of specific dimension and depth that has a grid marked for counting the cells under the microscope (Fig. 12-2B). The cells are counted using the magnification of the microscope. Because of the standardized dilution ratio and dimensions of the hemocytometer, a mathematical calculation is used to determine the number of cells in a milliliter of blood.

AUTOMATED ANALYZERS FOR COMPLETE BLOOD COUNT TESTING

Blood cell analyzers have come into use with advances in technology. In hospitals and reference laboratories, these analyzers allow for large volumes of tests to be performed in a short period of time. Automated instruments in the physician office laboratory have added greater accuracy and precision to the results. Most of these test procedures

use **electrical impedance** (a process for counting blood cells that depends on their resistance to the flow of an electrical current) and light-scattering principles to count and differentiate blood cells. Beckman-Coulter, Abbott, ABX, and Bayer-Technicon are companies that produce these automated analyzers for large-scale, time-efficient hematology testing.

In electrical impedance analyzers, the cells pass through an opening with an electrical current flowing through it. The changes of electrical resistance due to the formed elements in the sample are monitored and they are counted as voltage pulses. These pulses are proportional in height to the volume of the cells, which allows them to be identified as white blood cells, red blood cells, or platelets.

Some instruments may also use a beam of light to measure the number and size of the cells in the sample, a process called light scattering. A light-sensitive detector measures the light scattered as the sample is introduced into a chamber and the beam of light is interrupted. The size of the pulse detected is proportional to the size of the cellular element. Many of the analyzers use a combination of these two techniques to count the formed elements in the blood sample. A

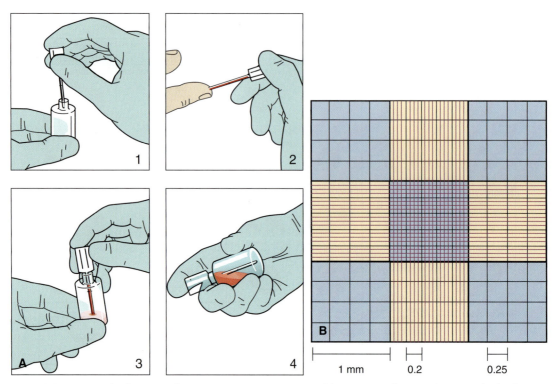

Figure 12-2   (A) Steps involved in using the Unopette system. *From Wedding, ME, and Toenjes, SA: Medical Laboratory Procedures. FA Davis, Philadelphia, 1998, with permission. (B) Hemocytometer counting chamber. From Ciesla, B: Hematology in Practice, ed. 2, FA Davis, Philadelphia, 2012, with permission.*

graph of the distribution of cell sizes made during cell counting on an automated analyzer, known as a **histogram,** may also be reported. An example of the results of an automated CBC is shown in Figure 12-3.

The automated white blood cell differential is performed by a combination of techniques. The information gathered using these techniques is combined to classify the type of white blood cell. The cell volume can be determined by electrical impedance, electromagnetic procedures define nuclear characteristics and granular composition, and light-scattering techniques can analyze cell surface and morphological and granular qualities to determine the type of white blood cell. The automated analyzers work well for the vast majority of specimens, but they do have their limitations. Certain samples with abnormal results must have a manual differential performed for accurate results.

The QBC STAR Centrifugal Hematology System (QBC Diagnostics) is an example of an automated instrument that tests one sample at a time (Fig. 12-4). It

may be used in the physician office laboratory where automation is desired, but specimen-testing volumes are not high. The QBC STAR system is a CLIA test of moderate complexity, so those performing the testing will participate in proper training of specified quality assurance procedures. The analysis tube used for testing within the instrument may be filled with EDTA-anticoagulated blood or directly from a capillary puncture. The analysis tube contains a dye and a special "float" that is used for the testing process. The tube is filled with blood and placed directly into the analyzer. The testing process involves centrifugation within the instrument and use of the "float" to measure different parameters of the specimen. This instrument is desirable for some office settings because there are no liquid reagents to work with, and the calibration of the instrument is done internally. The analysis tubes contain all the reagents necessary for the procedure. The QBC Star is capable of measuring most of the components of a typical CBC, with the exception of a red blood cell count and some of the indices.

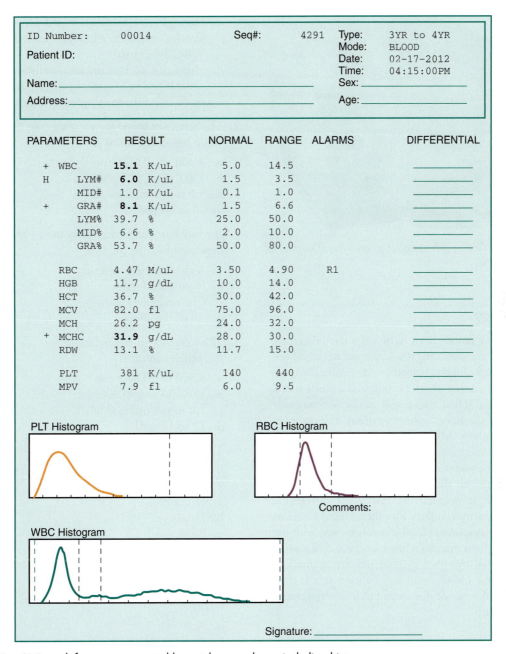

ID Number:	00014		Seq#:	4291	Type:	3YR to 4YR
Patient ID:					Mode:	BLOOD
					Date:	02-17-2012
					Time:	04:15:00PM
Name:					Sex:	
Address:					Age:	

PARAMETERS		RESULT		NORMAL	RANGE	ALARMS	DIFFERENTIAL
+	WBC	**15.1**	K/uL	5.0	14.5		_____
H	LYM#	**6.0**	K/uL	1.5	3.5		_____
	MID#	1.0	K/uL	0.1	1.0		_____
+	GRA#	**8.1**	K/uL	1.5	6.6		_____
	LYM%	39.7	%	25.0	50.0		_____
	MID%	6.6	%	2.0	10.0		_____
	GRA%	53.7	%	50.0	80.0		_____
	RBC	4.47	M/uL	3.50	4.90	R1	_____
	HGB	11.7	g/dL	10.0	14.0		_____
	HCT	36.7	%	30.0	42.0		_____
	MCV	82.0	fl	75.0	96.0		_____
	MCH	26.2	pg	24.0	32.0		_____
+	MCHC	**31.9**	g/dL	28.0	30.0		_____
	RDW	13.1	%	11.7	15.0		_____
	PLT	381	K/uL	140	440		_____
	MPV	7.9	fl	6.0	9.5		_____

PLT Histogram

RBC Histogram

Comments:

WBC Histogram

Signature: _____

Figure 12-3   CBC result from an automated hematology analyzer, including histograms.

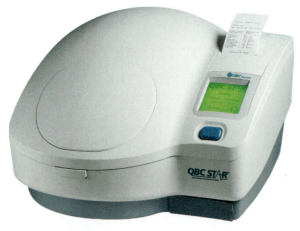

Figure 12-4   QBC STAR hematology analyzer. *Courtesy of QBC Diagnostics.*

SUMMARY

The complete blood count (CBC) is a comprehensive hematology test consisting of a white and red blood cell count, hemoglobin and hematocrit determinations, red blood cell indices, a platelet count, and a white blood cell differential. These tests may be performed manually or by use of automated instrumentation. The three red blood cell indices (MCV, MCH, MCHC) are calculations that numerically describe the size of the red blood cells and the amount of hemoglobin that they contain.

There may be times in which examination of a blood smear is necessary to clarify the differential results or view morphology for other cellular elements in a sample. A stained blood smear is viewed with the microscope for a manual white blood cell differential, red blood cell morphology, and platelet estimation. The complete blood count can be used as a tool to diagnose and monitor disease and to follow the course of treatments.

TIME TO REVIEW

1. Choose the correct list of   Outcome 12-2
   components of a complete blood count.

   a. Hemoglobin, hematocrit, red blood cell count, white blood cell count, erythrocyte sedimentation rate, WBC differential
   b. Hemoglobin, hematocrit, red blood cell count, white blood cell count, red blood cell indices, platelet count, WBC differential

c. Hemoglobin, hematocrit, red blood cell count, platelet count, erythrocyte sedimentation rate, WBC differential
   d. Hemoglobin, hematocrit, red blood cell count, white blood cell count, hemoglobin electrophoresis, WBC differential, platelet count

2. The reference range for an adult   Outcome 12-3
   white blood cell count is:

   a. 4,300 to 10,800/mm^3
   b. 140,000 to 400,000/mm^3
   c. 5.0 to 6.5 million/mm^3
   d. 12 to 14 g/dL

3. A white blood cell count may be   Outcome 12-5
   decreased because of:

   a. A chronic viral infection
   b. Exposure to toxins
   c. Chemotherapy use
   d. All of the above

4. The reference or normal range for   Outcome 12-3
   the platelet count is:

   a. 4,300 to 10,800/mm^3
   b. 150,000 to 450,000/mm^3
   c. 5.0 to 6.5 million/mm^3
   d. 12 to 14 g/dL

5. This type of white blood cell is the   Outcome 12-7
   most numerous in a healthy adult and makes up about 60% of the white blood cells:

   a. Eosinophil
   b. Monocyte
   c. Neutrophil
   d. Lymphocyte

6. This is the term used to describe   Outcome 12-9
   a variety of sizes of red blood cells on the stained smear:

   a. Anisocytosis
   b. Poikilocytosis
   c. Spherocytosis
   d. Hemolysis

7. This type of cell appears as small,   Outcome 12-10
   purple, circular, or ovoid fragments on the stained blood smear.

   a. White blood cell
   b. Red blood cell
   c. Platelet
   d. Band cell

8. An increased white blood cell count may be evident with which disease?   Outcome 12-4

   a. Thrombocythemia
   b. Anemia
   c. Leukopenia
   d. Leukemia

9. Microcytosis is a word used to describe: Outcome 12-9

   a. Large red blood cells
   b. Large white blood cells
   c. Small red blood cells
   d. Small platelets

10. A hemocytometer is used to: Outcome 12-1

   a. Measure a hematocrit level
   b. Perform manual white blood cell counts
   c. Perform staining of peripheral blood smears
   d. Measure hemoglobin concentrations

Case Study 12-1: Clinical significance

Mr. Smith, a 67-year-old patient, presented to the office with symptoms of a cough, a little tightness in his chest, and complaints of a slight fever. The medical assistant took Mr. Smith's vital signs and wrote his results and chief complaint in his chart. When the physician examined the patient, he believed that Mr. Smith was suffering from a respiratory infection. His plan was to prescribe an antibiotic if the infection turned out to be caused by bacteria, so he asked the medical assistant to draw blood for a CBC.

The medical assistant performed a venipuncture on Mr. Smith and processed the sample for pickup by the reference laboratory for testing later that day. She explained to Mr. Smith that the results should be back in the office in the morning and if the CBC results indicate the presence of a bacterial infection, the physician will call in a prescription for an antibiotic to his pharmacy. She told the patient that she would call him in the morning.

The next morning these results were faxed to the office:

◄ CB LABORATORY ►

ID Number: 09123	Seq#: 43210	Type:	
		Mode:	Blood
Patient ID: 98789		Date:	10-14-2012
		Time:	10:45 AM
Name: James Smith		Sex:	Male
Address: 3456 Waterview Terrace		Age:	67
Seattle, WA 98103			

CBC RESULTS

TEST	PATIENT RESULTS	REFERENCE RANGE		
Hemoglobin	14.2 g/dL	13	18	male
		12	16	female
Hematocrit	43%	45	52	male
		37	48	female
Red blood cell count	$5.7 \times 10^6/mm^3$	4.6	6.2	male
		4.2	5.9	female
White blood cell count	$12,000/mm^3$	4,300	10,800	
Neutrophils	48%	54	65	
Lymphocytes	48%	25	40	
Monocytes	2%	2	8	
Eosinophils	1%	1	4	
Basophils	1%	0	1	
Platelet count	$320 \times 10^3/mm^3$	150	450	

Continued

The medical assistant highlighted the abnormal results, retrieved James Smith's chart, and took the laboratory report and chart to the physician. The doctor reviewed the results and asked the medical assistant to contact Mr. Smith to let him know that he would not be prescribing antibiotics at this time.

The medical assistant called Mr. Smith and explained that the results were not consistent with a bacterial infection. She told Mr. Smith that no antibiotics would be prescribed at this time, but to check back in a week if the symptoms had not gotten better or if things appeared to be worse.

1. What color tube was used for the blood sample?
2. What out-of-range laboratory results should the medical assistant have highlighted for the physician?
3. Are the abnormal laboratory results consistent with a bacterial infection?

RESOURCES AND SUGGESTED READINGS

"QBS Star"
   Provides an overview of the function of the QBC Star hematology analyzer http://www.qbcdiagnostics.com

Chapter 13

Hemoglobin and Hematocrit

Nikki A. Marhefka, EdM, MT(ASCP), CMA (AAMA)

CHAPTER OUTLINE

Learning Outcomes
After reading this chapter, the successful student will be able to:

13-1 Define the key terms.

13-2 Describe the structure and function of a hemoglobin molecule.

13-3 State the type of normal adult hemoglobin and list other types present with various hemoglobinopathies.

13-4 Analyze the general principle of and sources of error associated with CLIA-waived testing of hemoglobin.

13-5 Evaluate the concept of the hematocrit.

13-6 Identify the layers into which the blood sample has separated in a spun hematocrit specimen.

13-7 Examine the general principle of and sources of error associated with CLIA-waived hematocrit procedures.

13-8 Recognize the normal reference ranges for hemoglobin and hematocrit.

13-9 Define *anemia* and examine its clinical significance.

13-10 List the various types of anemia and explain how they are classified.

CAAHEP AND ABHES STANDARDS

 CAAHEP 2008 Standards

I.C.I. Anatomy and Physiology #6: Identify common pathology as it relates to the interaction of body systems.
I.C.I. Anatomy and Physiology #7: Analyze pathology as it relates to the interaction of body systems.
I.P.I. Anatomy and Physiology #12: Perform hematology testing.

 ABHES 2010 Standards

10. Medical Laboratory Procedures, b. CLIA-waived tests, Graduates: 2. Hematology Testing.

KEY TERMS

Anemia	Hemoglobinopathy	Pernicious anemia
Anisocytosis	Hemolysis	Poikilocytosis
Aplastic anemia	Heterozygous	Protoporphyrin
Bilirubin	Homozygous	Sickle cell anemia
Cyanmethemoglobin	Hypochromic	Sickle cell disease
Erythropoiesis	Interstitial fluid	Sickle cell trait
Hematocrit (hct)	Intrinsic factor	Splenomegaly
Hb A	Iron-deficiency anemia	Target cell
Hemoglobin (hgb)	Macrocytic	Thalassemia
Hemoglobin and hematocrit (H&H)	Microcytic	Urobilinogen
Hemoglobin electrophoresis	Packed cell volume	

Two of the most important hematology test procedures are for **hemoglobin (hgb)**, a protein responsible for oxygen transport, and the percentage of the space occupied by red blood cells compared to the entire blood volume known as the **hematocrit (hct)**. Measurement of the **hemoglobin and hematocrit** (abbreviated as **H&H**) is commonly performed in all laboratories and physician offices. The results of these two tests may be used to help diagnose or monitor the progress of treatment for **anemia**, a condition in which the oxygen-carrying capacity of the blood is reduced. This chapter presents additional information about the clinical significance of the hemoglobin and hematocrit measurements, and provides details of testing methods for these parameters.

HEMOGLOBIN

As was established in previous chapters, mature red blood cells are filled with fluid as they are released from the bone marrow. The intracellular fluid is primarily made up of hemoglobin. Oxygen attaches to this protein complex for subsequent transport to the tissues of the body, where it is needed for the production of energy. The primary function of hemoglobin (and thus, the red blood cells) is to transport oxygen to the tissues of the body. Hemoglobin is composed of four molecules of heme within a globin protein chain. Each of these heme molecules has one atom of iron, and one molecule of oxygen can attach to each of these iron atoms. Thus, one red blood cell can transport four molecules of oxygen.

Hemoglobin production begins in the erythroid precursor cells of the bone marrow. The heme is synthesized by the mitochondria of the bone marrow cells, and the globin chains are constructed by the ribosomes of the cells as they mature in the bone marrow. Most of the hemoglobin is formed by the early precursor cells, which are nucleated, but the production continues even after these cells have lost their nucleus until they are released into the general circulation (Fig. 13-1).

Test Your Knowledge 13-1

Hemoglobin is made up of one molecule of _____ and four molecules of _____.   (Outcome 13-2)

Test Your Knowledge 13-2

What is the function of hemoglobin?   (Outcome 13-2)

The hemoglobin molecule becomes oxygenated in the lungs where the oxygen concentration is very high. As the red blood cells leave the pulmonary circulation, the affinity of tissues for the oxygen carried by the hemoglobin molecule will cause the oxygen to diffuse through the red blood cell membrane and across capillary walls to enter the tissues. After the oxygen has left the red blood cells, the cells are capable of transporting carbon dioxide back to the lungs to be expelled. With the delivery of oxygen and transport of

HEMOGLOBIN

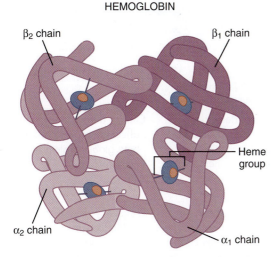

Figure 13-1   A hemoglobin molecule. Note the polypeptide changes with the heme molecules in the center of the complex.

carbon dioxide, the hemoglobin molecules of the red blood cells help the body control the acid-base balance that is necessary for survival.

Mature red blood cells have a life span of approximately 120 days. During their lifetime, they must travel constantly through the cardiovascular system, remaining flexible enough to pass through capillary beds to perform their duties. Eventually, worn-out red blood cells are removed by the tissue macrophage system in the spleen and the hemoglobin is degraded into iron, **protoporphyrin**, and globulin. Protoporphyrin is included in the heme portion of the hemoglobin molecule, and is necessary to make the iron functional and available to attach to the oxygen. The iron released by the breakdown of old red blood cells is removed from the heme, and transported to the bone marrow to be used again. The globulin is degraded into amino acids to be used by the body for creation of protein. Protoporphyrin is converted into **bilirubin**, which combines with albumin for transport to the liver. The liver cells further process the bilirubin and it is excreted as bile, which enters the intestines where bacteria convert it to **urobilinogen** to be excreted in the feces.

HEMOGLOBINOPATHIES

The normal adult hemoglobin is denoted as **Hb A**. Hemoglobin in red blood cells of the fetus and the newborn is Hb F. There are genetic hemoglobin variants present in the population, in which the structure of the globin part of the molecule is altered. The presence of an abnormal hemoglobin is known as a **hemoglobinopathy**. The hemoglobinopathies are a result of genetic changes that may be inherited or caused by mutations. Both the **homozygous** form in which the patient has two identical genes for the same characteristic or the **heterozygous** form that contains two genes for abnormal hemoglobin variants can lead to a mild or severe anemia. If Hb A is present in the cells as well as the abnormal hemoglobin, the abnormality may be masked and no symptoms will be evident. **Sickle cell disease** and **sickle cell trait** are a result of the presence of Hb S. Other hemoglobinopathies may be asymptomatic, whereas others can lead to severe anemia.

▼ **POINT OF INTEREST 13-1**
Hemoglobinopathies

The hemoglobin molecule must have a very specific structure in order to function optimally. Any change in the structure of the globin chains in the hemoglobin molecule may be classified as a hemoglobinopathy. Many of these abnormalities remain undetected because they are not clinically significant. Others, however, will have a significant effect on the body's ability to transport oxygen.

- **Methemoglobinemia:** For the hemoglobin molecule to function appropriately, it is necessary for the iron molecule to be ferrous. This means that the iron molecule is positively charged with two more protons than electrons present in the molecule. If the iron is present in a state other than this, the hemoglobin molecule has a poor affinity for oxygen. This results in a state of cyanosis for the body, because the red blood cells cannot deliver the oxygen appropriately if they do not pick it up as they should in the lung tissues.
- **Hemoglobinopathies with decreased oxygen affinity:** Certain abnormalities of the hemoglobin molecule may create a situation in which there is a pronounced decrease in the affinity for oxygen. This means that the molecules do not pick up the oxygen as they should in the lungs. This type of hemoglobinopathy is characterized by cyanosis. Hb Seattle and Hb Vancouver are examples of this type of hemoglobinopathy.
- **Increased oxygen affinity:** Erythrocytosis is a common symptom of hemoglobinopathies with increased oxygen affinity. In this situation, the molecule holds on so tightly to the oxygen molecules that they cannot be deposited throughout the

Continued

body. The kidneys will increase their secretion of erythropoetin because of the reduced oxygen in the tissues of the body. Hb Chesapeake is an example of this type of hemoglobinopathy.

- **Hemolytic hemoglobinopathies:** Hb S and Hb C are abnormalities of the hemoglobin molecule structure that affect the integrity of the red blood cell molecule as well as the hemoglobin molecule. These abnormalities occur because of the way that the globin chains are interconnected. The red blood cell membranes have increased hemolysis because the hemoglobin molecule formation is unstable. This has a profound effect on the life span of the red blood cell. The high levels of hemolysis lead to a constant state of anemia, jaundice, and cholelithiasis.

Hb S (sickle cell) also may cause the vessels of the body to become occluded due to the distinct shape of the red blood cells. The abnormal crescent shape becomes lodged in the small capillaries of the body, with multiorgan effects.

Thalassemias are a group of inherited disorders in which abnormal hemoglobin is present in the red blood cells. In thalassemia, anemia results either from a defective production rate of the alpha or beta globin chains that make up the globin portion of the normal hemoglobin molecule. Without these chains, it is not possible for the red blood cell precursors to build Hb A, the normal hemoglobin present in the adult red blood cell. Those who are homozygous for the defective gene have severe hypochromic, microcytic anemia, and a variety of other issues related to the severe anemia (Table 13-1).

Test Your Knowledge 13-3
List two abnormal types of hemoglobin.   (Outcome 13-3)

When a hemoglobinopathy is suspected, identification of the hemoglobin variant present in the red blood cells can be accomplished through **hemoglobin electrophoresis.** In this technique, blood for examination is placed on a cellulose acetate gel support medium that is capable of transmitting an electrical current. An alkaline electrolyte solution is added, and an electrical current is applied to the support medium. Each hemoglobin subtype moves across the support medium at a different rate and creates a distinctive pattern. The bands of hemoglobin are detected by staining and identified by their placement on the medium as they have moved.

TABLE 13-1
Thalassemias

Alpha Thalassemias	Beta Thalassemias
Insufficient alpha globin protein produced	Insufficient beta globin protein
Clinical defect: A gene or genes related to the alpha globin protein of hemoglobin is/are missing or changed	**Clinical defect:** Gene defects affect the production of the beta globin protein of hemoglobin
Frequency: Found in persons of Southeast Asian, Middle Eastern, Chinese, and African descent	**Frequency:** Found in persons of Mediterranean descent, and to a lesser extent in Chinese, other Asians, and African Americans
Subtypes • Major Hydrops fetalis—babies die before or shortly after birth • Hemoglobin H disease, moderate to severe anemia • Minor: Called alpha thalassemia trait, mild anemia. • Alpha thalassemia silent carrier has the abnormal gene, but it is not evident because these genes are heterozygous.	**Subtypes** • Major Cooley's anemia—severe anemia • Intermediate, moderate anemia • Minor: Called beta thalassemia trait

*Thalassemia is a genetic defect in the protein portion of the hemoglobin molecule and affects alpha or beta globin protein production. Both globin proteins are necessary to create healthy hemoglobin. Thalassemia causes the body to make fewer healthy red blood cells because they are hemoglobin deficient and are not as well equipped to transport oxygen as normal hemoglobin.

This is a sophisticated test that is performed in reference or hospital laboratories.

HEMOGLOBIN TESTING

Hemoglobin testing is one of the most frequently performed laboratory procedures. The results can be used to detect anemia and provide information to determine its severity. Hemoglobin testing may also be used to monitor the treatment for anemia. Hemoglobin

TABLE 13-2

Hemoglobin Reference Ranges (Normal Values)	
Age/Gender	Hgb (g/dL)
Adult male	14–18
Adult female	12–16
Newborn	17–23
Two-month-olds	9–14
Child, 1–14 years	11.3–14.4

reference ranges vary by age and gender of the patient (Table 13-2). The normal reference ranges for the adult male are 13 to 18 g/dL, and the reference ranges for the adult female are 12 to 16 g/dL. Women of child-bearing age have a lower normal reference range than do men due to the blood loss experienced as a result of the monthly menstrual cycle. Infant hemoglobin values are significantly lower than those of adults, with an average of 11 to 14 g/dL. Children's hemoglobin values gradually increase from infancy levels to adulthood.

Hemoglobin is usually converted to another compound, called **cyanmethemoglobin,** for measurement. Cyanmethemoglobin is a colored pigment, so the change in color once this conversion has been accomplished can be measured as absorbance by a spectrophotometer, using a wavelength of 540 nm. To release the hemoglobin from the cells to be converted and measured, the red blood cell membranes must be broken or dissolved, a process called **hemolysis.** The cyanmethemoglobin reagents used for hemoglobin testing contain a surfactant that promotes rapid hemolysis and formation of the cyanmethemoglobin moledule. Large complex analyzers used in reference and hospital laboratories as well as CLIA-waived point of care testing methods use this basic procedure.

CLIA–Waived Hemoglobin Testing

The CLIA-waived hemoglobin procedures are performed by handheld, point-of-care instruments. These analyzers have been approved by the U.S. Food and Drug Administration (FDA) for performance of hemoglobin testing. Each instrument determines the hemoglobin values with minimal steps involved in the testing process. The HemoCue Hb instrument (manufactured by HemoCue Inc.), and i-STAT (manufactured by Abbott) are examples of common CLIA-waived hemoglobin analyzers used in physician offices (Fig. 13-2).

There are similarities in the testing methods for all the CLIA-waived hemoglobin testing procedures. These include the following:

1. For most of these instruments, blood is collected by capillary puncture and placed on a reaction chamber. The reaction chamber includes the necessary chemicals to lyse the red blood cells and allow the conversion of the hemoglobin to cyanmethemoglobin. For many of these procedures, blood may also be taken from a tube containing anticoagulant.
2. The reaction chamber is placed into the analyzer, and the color intensity is read by a spectrophotometer to determine hemoglobin content.
3. The handheld instruments require very little maintenance or calibration procedures to produce reliable results. However, it is imperative that the operator follow all manufacturer recommendations for calibration and quality control procedures. These results must be logged appropriately, and must all be within an acceptable range before patient testing is performed on the instrument.
4. Test results are available as a digital readout on the instrument. In addition, some of the instruments may be connected to a computer for result storage and printout.
5.
6.

Potential Errors in Hemoglobin Testing

Even though the hemoglobin testing procedure is straightforward, it is still possible to make errors that may have significant impacts on the results. Potential

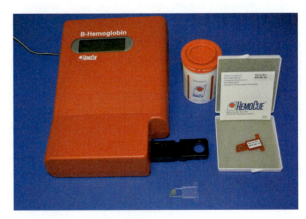

Figure 13-2 A hemoglobinometer.

Procedure 13-1: CLIA-Waived Hemoglobin Testing Using the HemoCue Hemoglobin Analyzer

Hemoglobin analysis is one of the most common CLIA-waived tests performed in physician office laboratories and larger, more complex laboratories. For the HemoCue method, capillary, venous, or arterial blood may be used. Hemoglobin results may be used to screen or monitor the progress of the treatment for anemia.

TASK

Accurately perform hemoglobin testing using a Hemo-Cue hemoglobin analyzer.

CONDITIONS

- Hand-washing supplies and/or alcohol-based hand sanitizer
- Disposable gloves
- Lancet for capillary punctures
- Alcohol prep pad

- Gauze pads
- Biohazardous sharps container
- HemoCue hemoglobin analyzer
- HemoCue microcuvettes
- HemoCue calibration cuvette
- HemoCue control solution
- Disinfectant wipes for cleaning work area

CAAHEP/ABHES STANDARDS

 CAAHEP Standards

I.P.I.12. Perform Hematology Testing

 ABHES Standards

- Perform selected CLIA-waived tests that assist with diagnosis and treatment: 2. Hematology testing

Procedure	Rationale
1. Sanitize hands, allow them to dry completely, and apply gloves.	Gloves must be worn for any procedures in which exposure to blood or other potentially infectious materials is anticipated.
2. Turn on the HemoCue instrument, and wait until the digital printout on the screen indicates that the instrument is ready for testing.	The HemoCue instrument will complete a set of internal verification procedures. Once this has been successfully completed, the digital readout on the screen will indicate that the instrument is ready.
3. Verify the expiration printed on the microcuvette container.	Expired supplies are never to be used for control or patient testing.
4. Open the microcuvette bottle, and remove a microcuvette. Close the bottle securely as soon as the desired microcuvette is removed.	The microcuvette container must stay closed securely. These microcuvettes are very sensitive to moisture exposure.
5. Using the quality control material that is designed for this instrument, verify that the instrument is working correctly. Follow the manufacturer's instructions for use and frequency of testing these materials. Fill the microcuvette with the control material, then insert the cuvette into the holder and push into the instrument for analysis. Note the digital readout when ready, and compare the results to those designated as acceptable for this control material.	The quality control material comes with a set of acceptable result ranges. There are materials available to test at low, medium, and high levels of hemoglobin concentration. Verify that the readout on the digital display indicates a result within the acceptable range for that level of control before performing patient testing. Document the result for this quality control material.

Procedure	Rationale
6. Perform a capillary puncture, using appropriate technique. Wipe away the first drop of blood.	Appropriate capillary puncture procedure includes disinfection of the draw site, allowing the alcohol to dry, using an appropriate site, performing the puncture perpendicular to the fingerprints on the finger, and wiping away the first drop of blood that forms. This drop of blood is contaminated with interstitial fluid and if used for the analysis, can produce erroneous results.
7. Touch the open end of the HemoCue microcuvette to the drop of blood. The microcuvette will fill by capillary action to the appropriate level. 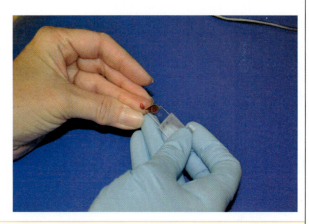	Don't touch the capillary puncture site with the microcuvette; it should be placed into the drop of blood. The microcuvette will not overfill.
8. Wipe off any excess blood from the bottom and sides of the microcuvette with a gauze pad, then place the microcuvette in the cuvette holder and push the holder into the instrument for analysis. 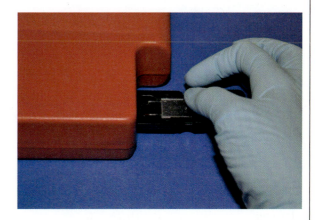	It is important to wipe away excess blood. However, do not allow the gauze to absorb blood from the interior of the cuvette. The interior of the microcuvette is coated with a chemical that lyses the red blood cells, and converts the hemoglobin present to cyanmethemoglobin to be measured in the instrument.

Continued

Procedure 13-1: CLIA-Waived Hemoglobin Testing Using the HemoCue Hemoglobin Analyzer—cont'd

Procedure	Rationale
9. The digital display will present a result within 10 to 20 seconds. Document this hemoglobin result.	The result will continue to be displayed until the cuvette holder is pulled out of the instrument.

Procedure	Rationale
10. After recording the hemoglobin result, pull out the cuvette holder and remove the cuvette. The used cuvette must be discarded as a biohazardous material.	The blood contained in the microcuvette is still considered to be infectious, so it must be disposed of appropriately.
11. Clean and disinfect the work area, then remove gloves and sanitize your hands.	The work area should always be cleaned after use to prepare it for the next user, and hands must always be sanitized afte removing gloves.
12. Document the procedure in the patient's chart if it is available.	In a physician office laboratory, this procedure should be documented in the patient's chart. If the medical assistant is working in a laboratory setting where the chart is not available, this step is not necessary.

Date	
4/2/2012:	Hemoglobin test performed. QC within range. Hgb 13.3 g/dL
09:30 a.m.	Connie Lieseke, CMA (AAMA)

sources of error to take into consideration include the following:

- Adequate blood flow during the capillary collection is necessary to get a homogeneous (well mixed) sample without clots.
- To avoid diluting the blood sample with **interstitial fluid** (the fluid between cells), there should be no squeezing during capillary sample collection and the first drop or two of blood present after the puncture must be wiped away before the blood is applied to the testing chamber or device. If the sample is diluted by interstitial fluid, the hemoglobin value will be erroneously lowered.
- There should be no air bubbles or spaces in the collecting device.

- As is the case with all automated instruments, the reagents and supplies must not be expired when used, and storage requirements for all reagents and samples must be followed as directed.
- The test should be performed within the appropriate time limits after specimen collection as indicated on the instructions for the analyzer.
- All instructions for use of the analyzer must be followed exactly as described.
- Internal and external quality control must be performed at the intervals recommended by the manufacturer, and the results must be within the desired ranges before patient results are reported.

TABLE 13-3	
Hematocrit reference ranges (normal values)	
Age/Gender	hct Value (%)
Adult male	45–52
Adult female	37–48
Newborn	50–62
Two-month-olds	31–39
Child, 1–6 years	30–40

Test Your Knowledge 13-4

Are hemoglobin tests performed on intact red blood cells?   (Outcome 13-4)

Test Your Knowledge 13-5

List two potential errors in performing hemoglobin testing.   (Outcome 13-4)

HEMATOCRIT

The hematocrit is the percentage of space occupied by red blood cells as compared to the entire blood volume in a sample of whole blood. It may also be called the **packed cell volume.** The hematocrit is an indirect test that provides important information about the concentration of red blood cells in the circulating blood. The space occupied by the red blood cells depends on the size of the cells and the total number of cells present. If there is an appropriate amount of red blood cells with a normal hemoglobin concentration in a specimen, the hematocrit will be in the normal reference range. If the red blood cells are small with insufficient hemoglobin or the number of red blood cells is decreased, the hematocrit value will be below the normal reference range.

The normal reference ranges for hematocrit vary with gender and age of the patient (Table 13-3). Newborns have a very high hematocrit value, but it decreases quickly after birth. The reference range for a child is less than that of an adult, but it continues to increase as they approach adulthood. Adult men have a normal range of 45% to 52%, and adult women have a normal range of 37% to 48%. Hematocrit values are decreased with the various forms of anemia, and may be elevated in situations with an overproduction of red blood cells, such as in polycythemia.

CLIA-waived procedures for hematocrit testing are manual methods requiring centrifugation of the specimen. Hematocrit values may also be derived by using moderately or highly complex automated instruments. These analyzers will use the hemoglobin concentration and the mean corpuscular volume (MCV) to calculate a hematocrit result.

Test Your Knowledge 13-6

Define *hematocrit*.   (Outcome 13-5)

CLIA–Waived Hematocrit Testing

In typical hematocrit testing, the red blood cells are forced to the bottom of the tube by centrifugation (Fig. 13-3). This tube may be known as a capillary tube or a microhematocrit tube because the tube is very small and designed to be spun in a small centrifuge. After centrifugation, the tube is compared to a reading device to measure the hematocrit value. The hematocrit is always reported as a percentage, indicating the volume of red blood cells in the sample as compared to the total blood volume.

There are some variables in the testing process, but the following common components are present in all the CLIA-waived manual hematocrit procedures:

- Two hematocrit tubes are always filled from each patient. Both tubes are centrifuged and results are measured from both tubes. The final result reported will be an average of the two tubes, as long as they are within 2% of each other. If the results from the two tubes are more than 2% apart, the sample will need to be recollected and respun.
- The hematocrit tubes must contain anticoagulant (the tube interior is coated with heparin) if they are to be used for capillary samples drawn directly from the

HEMATOCRIT = % OF RBCs

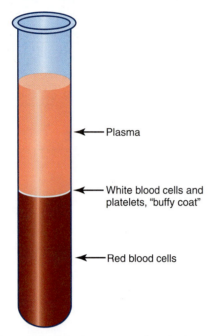

Plasma

White blood cells and platelets, "buffy coat"

Red blood cells

Figure 13-3 Layers of the hematocrit tube. The bottom layer is made up of red blood cells covered with a very thin layer of buffy coat, which represents the white blood cells in the specimen. The uppermost layer is made up of plasma. There is air at the very top of the tube.

patient. If anticoagulant is not used, the blood will clot in the hematocrit tube and the results will be erroneous. It is also possible to use plain tubes (without anticoagulant) if the hematocrit sample is taken from an EDTA lavender top tube.

- Glass tubes should not be used for this process in consideration of employee safety. Safety coated glass tubes are available, which have a glass interior and are covered with a Mylar coating to keep them from breaking. Plastic tubes are also available.
- The sample must be well mixed prior to filling the hematocrit tube (if utilizing an EDTA anticoagulated sample). If a capillary sample is to be used, the site must not be squeezed, as this will add too much interstitial fluid to the sample. The additional fluid may result in a falsely decreased hematocrit result.
- As the tube is filled, air bubbles should be avoided. The addition of bubbles in the specimen can cause the tube to fill insufficiently, in which case it may not be possible to measure the results after centrifugation.
- The end of the hematocrit tube will be plugged with sealing clay to keep the sample from leaving the tube during the centrifugation process.

- Follow the manufacturer's recommendations for the centrifugation times necessary, which may vary with each type of centrifuge.
- Read the results immediately after centrifugation using a built-in reader, or another device designed for hematocrit results. Following centrifugation, the blood in the tube will have been divided into three layers. The hematocrit result is read at the top of the red blood cell column, which is the bottom layer in the tube. There is a thin area called a buffy coat (lighter in color and made of the white blood cells and platelets in the sample) that is visible at the top of the red blood cells, and the plasma makes up the rest of the volume of the sample in the tube (see Fig. 13-3).
- The moderately complex automated procedures available for hematocrit testing are often used in the physician office laboratory. An example of a common instrument is the i-STAT analyzer, made by Abbott Laboratories. The process requires only a few drops of blood. This instrument uses individual cartridges to which the blood sample is added. The hematocrit level is determined by use of an electrical current. As is the case with all CLIA-waived testing procedures, all instructions and quality control procedures recommended by the manufacturer must be followed.

Potential Errors in Hematocrit Testing

The hematocrit testing process may be considered simplistic. However, it is possible to negatively affect the results if not paying close attention to detail. The following are some of the most common errors encountered when using the manual hematocrit procedure:

- If a capillary specimen is used for the procedure, the sample must be collected from free-flowing blood from a skin puncture. If the area is squeezed, interstitial fluid (tissue fluid) may contaminate the sample or the red blood cells can be broken open (hemolysis). The first drop of blood from the skin puncture must be wiped away, as this contains some interstitial fluid as the lancet cut through tissue.
- If the plasma appears pink or reddish, cells may have been hemolyzed during collection. Excessive hemolysis can decrease the value of the hematocrit. Hemolysis may occur during the collection process or as a result of intravascular hemolysis in severe disease states.
- The hematocrit tube must be filled appropriately. If too little blood is added to the tube, it will not be possible to read the result using a reading device after centrifugation. Conversely, the result for a tube that is overfilled cannot be measured using a reading device.

Procedure 13-2: CLIA–Waived Hematocrit Testing Using the StatSpin CritSpin Microhematocrit Centrifuge and Digital Reader

Hematocrit testing is a common CLIA-waived test that is performed in physician office laboratories and larger, more complex laboratories. Spun hematocrit analysis is relatively inexpensive, requires a small amount of blood, and takes only a few minutes. Although capillary spun microhematocrit testing is the most common method, venous blood may also be used for testing. Hematocrit results may be used to screen for or monitor the progress of the treatment for anemia.

TASK

Accurately perform microhematocrit analysis utilizing the StatSpin CritSpin microhematocrit centrifuge and digital reader. The process must be completed within 15 minutes.

CONDITIONS

- Hand-washing supplies and/or alcohol-based hand sanitizer
- Disposable gloves

- Lancet for capillary punctures
- Alcohol prep pad
- Gauze pads
- Biohazardous sharps container
- StatSpin CritSpin microhematocrit centrifuge and digital reader
- Plastic heparinized microhematocrit tubes
- Sealing clay
- HemoCue control solution
- Disinfectant wipes for cleaning work area

CAAHEP/ABHES STANDARDS

 CAAHEP Standards

I.P.I.12. Perform Hematology Testing

 ABHES Standards

- Perform selected CLIA-waived tests that assist with diagnosis and treatment: 2. Hematology testing

Procedure	Rationale
1. Sanitize hands, allow them to dry completely, and apply gloves.	Gloves must be worn for any procedures in which exposure to blood or other potentially infectious materials is anticipated.
2. Use the quality control material that is designed for this procedure and this instrument, and verify that the instrument is working correctly. Follow the manufacturer's instructions for use and frequency of testing these quality control materials.	The quality control material comes with a set of acceptable result ranges. There are materials available to test at low, medium, and high levels of hematocrit results. Verify that the result is within the acceptable range for that level of control before performing patient testing. Document the result for this quality control material.
3. Remove two heparinized microhematocrit tubes from the container, and set them on a piece of gauze in the work area.	The tubes need to be within easy reach for the next step of the process. Heparinized tubes must be used for capillary samples because the blood must be anticoagulated to avoid clotting within the tube.

Continued

Procedure 13-2: CLIA–Waived Hematocrit Testing Using the StatSpin CritSpin Microhematocrit Centrifuge and Digital Reader—cont'd

Procedure	Rationale
4. Perform a capillary puncture, using appropriate technique. Wipe away the first drop of blood.	Appropriate capillary puncture procedure includes disinfection of the draw site, allowing the alcohol to dry, using an appropriate site, performing the puncture perpendicular to the fingerprints on the finger, and wiping away the first drop of blood that forms. This drop of blood is contaminated with interstitial fluid and if used for the analysis, can produce erroneous results.
5. Hold the microhematocrit tube by the end with the color-coded band. Touch the opposite end of the tube to the drop of blood. The blood will enter the tube via capillary action. Fill the tube until the blood reaches the colored band at the opposite end.	For best results, do not allow air bubbles to form in the tube. The tube should be filled to the colored band to allow for accurate reading of the results. 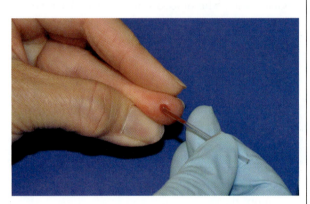
6. Remove the tube from the blood source, and tilt the tube until the blood is halfway between the colored band and the end of the tube.	This step is important to allow for room for the sealing compound at the end of the tube.

Procedure	Rationale
7. Hold the microhematocrit tube horizontally and push the end of the tube with the color-coded band into the sealing clay. Twist the tube and remove from the sealing clay. Wipe away any excess blood that may have leaked from the opposite end of the tube.	If the microhematocrit tubes are not sealed in this way, the blood will leak out of the tubes during the spinning process.
8. Place the tube with the sealed end toward the outer rim of the rotor.	If the sealed end of the tube is not placed to the outer edge of the rotor, all the blood will leak out of the tube when it is spinning.
9. Repeat steps 5 through 8 with another microhematocrit tube. After it is placed in the rotor, screw the rotor cover in place securely.	There should always be two tubes spun for each result to verify the accuracy of the result.
10. Holding the black knob in the center of the rotor, place it in the rotor holder in the centrifuge.	The rotor must be seated securely in place to avoid malfunction of the centrifuge.
11. Close the cover on the centrifuge and start the centrifuge. The StatSpin CritSpin centrifuge requires 2 minutes to fully pack the cells in the microhematocrit tubes.	The time allowed for the centrifugation will vary by method used.
12. When the rotor stops spinning, remove the rotor and place it in the digital reader.	The digital reader is an optional device. A circular or card reader may also be used to read the results.
13. Line up the pointer on the digital reader with the bottom of the cells in the microhematocrit tube and press the "zero" on the reader. Then line up the pointer with the top of the plasma column and set the "100" status on the reader. The final reading is accomplished at the top of the red blood cell column. The result is displayed on the digital reader.	All three steps must be followed to allow for accurate reading of the hematocrit results. Note: If a digital reader is not available, line up the tube with the bottom of the red blood cell column at the "zero" line on a hematocrit reader card, after which the top of the plasma column is to be aligned at the "100" on the card. Read the hematocrit result at the top of the red blood cell column.

Procedure 13-2: CLIA–Waived Hematocrit Testing Using the StatSpin CritSpin Microhematocrit Centrifuge and Digital Reader—cont'd

Procedure	Rationale
14. Record this result.	The result must be recorded before removing the rotor from the system, or going on to read the second tube.
15. Following the same procedure, read the hematocrit result on the second tube.	The results must be within 2% of each other for this to be a valid result. If they are not, the process must be repeated. Report the mean (average) of the two tubes read.
16. Remove the microhematocrit tubes from the rotor and dispose of them as biohazardous sharps.	Although these are plastic tubes, they should still be disposed of in a puncture-resistant container.
17. Clean and disinfect the work area, then remove gloves and sanitize your hands.	The work area should always be cleaned after use to prepare it for the next user, and hands must always be sanitized after removing gloves.
18. Document the procedure in the patient's chart if it is available.	In a physician office laboratory, this procedure should be documented in the patient's chart. If the medical assistant is working in a laboratory setting where the chart is not available, this step is not necessary.

Date	
4/2/2012:	Hematocrit test performed. QC within range. Hct 41%
09:50 a.m.	Connie Lieseke, CMA (AAMA)

The required volume of blood for the hematocrit analysis is determined by following the procedure as written.

- The test may be affected if the timing or the speed of the centrifuge is insufficient. The cells will not pack at the bottom of the tube fully, which may cause the results to be falsely elevated.
- Inaccurate alignment when reading the result will cause errors. The employee must be careful to read only the red blood cell column, and to have the tube placed appropriately against the reading device for accurate results.
- If the sealing clay has not adequately filled the end of the tube, some of the blood will leak out during centrifugation and will affect the result. The end of the tube that is filled with clay is placed to the outside of the centrifuge so that the clay keeps the blood in the tube as the specimen is spun.
- The hematocrit value may be inaccurate immediately after excessive blood loss or following transfusion. Excess plasma may be trapped between the red blood cells in macrocytic, hypochromic, or sickle cell anemias. The cells will not pack as well because of the area occupied by the trapped plasma.

Test Your Knowledge 13-7

What is used to create the layers in the blood sample in manual CLIA-waived hematocrit procedures?

(Outcome 13-6)

THE RELATIONSHIP OF HEMOGLOBIN AND HEMATOCRIT VALUES

Hemoglobin and hematocrit testing is often ordered together as H&H. To verify the validity of the results, it is important to compare the hematocrit and hemoglobin value of the patient's sample. The hematocrit value is approximately three times that of the hemoglobin value in a normal specimen. The hemoglobin value multiplied times three should be within two of the hematocrit results. In addition, the hemoglobin value is about three times that of the red blood cell count. By checking these relationships each time these tests are performed, the medical assistant can verify that the samples are all from the same patient and that the test procedures were performed correctly. Lipemia, hemolysis, and other clinical conditions can make these comparisons inaccurate. If the sample results don't fall within these parameters, the tests should be repeated.

ANEMIA

Anemia is a disorder characterized by the decreased oxygen-carrying capacity of the blood. The following three clinical scenarios may be evident with anemia:

1. A decreased total red blood cell count
2. A decrease in the hemoglobin content of each cell
3. A dysfunctional abnormal hemoglobin content that is not capable of transporting oxygen as it should

To treat anemia, practitioners will attempt to identify the cause. The problem may be chronic inadequate red blood cell production, red blood cell destruction or loss, or the inability of the bone marrow to react to blood loss adequately. Patients with anemia may exhibit signs of fatigue, pallor (pale skin), tachycardia (rapid heartbeats), or dyspnea (difficult breathing). Difficulty with concentration and memory issues may also be common symptoms. These symptoms are all related to the decreased oxygen-carrying capacity of the blood, which starves the cells of the body.

Test Your Knowledge 13-8

Name the disorder where the oxygen-carrying capacity of the blood is reduced. (Outcome 13-9)

Diagnosis and classification of the type of anemia may be accomplished with physical examination results, patient history, and laboratory tests. Patients with anemia may have decreased red blood cell counts, hemoglobin concentrations, or hematocrit values. Some types of anemia exhibit low values in more than one of these parameters, whereas others may demonstrate only one abnormal result. Anemia is often characterized by red blood cell indices that are outside of the normal range as well as specific red blood cell morphology changes.

Red blood cell morphology is observed on the stained blood smear utilized for the white blood cell differential by a trained laboratory technologist. **Anisocytosis** (red blood cells which appear in various sizes) and **poikilocytosis** (red blood cells which appear in various shapes) may be present. The red blood cells of anemic patients will appear abnormal, and may be **microcytic,** (small) **macrocytic** (large), or **hypochromic** (pale in color).

Impaired red blood cell production may be idiopathic (cause unknown) or due to toxins or infection. Anemia may also occur when there is defective synthesis of the heme of the hemoglobin molecule. Acute or chronic hemorrhage may cause anemia when the body is incapable of making enough cells to make up for the loss. Hemolytic anemia occurs with excessive lysis of the red blood cells intravascularly. This can be the result of red blood cell membrane disorders, hemoglobin disorders, metabolic disease, chemical toxins, extensive burns, malaria, or autoimmune destruction of the erythrocytes. A few specific types of anemia are presented below:

- **Iron-deficiency anemia** occurs when there is insufficient iron available for adequate hemoglobin formation. This is a hypochromic, microcytic anemia, as each cell has a reduced amount of hemoglobin. Iron deficiency may be caused by many situations: the body's supply of iron may be low, the absorption of the iron may be impaired, or the demand may be high. As our body breaks down old red blood cells, most of the available iron present in the system is in the tissue macrophage/reticuloendothelial tissue of the spleen. Dietary iron is absorbed in the small intestines.

  Clinical features of iron deficiency anemia may include sores on or a burning sensation of the tongue, ulcers at the corner of the mouth, "pica" (craving for dirt or ice), or chronic gastritis. "Milk anemia" is often a cause in 6- to 24-month-old children, as their diet may not contain sufficient iron. Other causes may include gastrectomy (total or partial) or prolonged treatment of peptic ulcers or acid reflux. Rapid growth during childhood and increased red blood cell production during pregnancy may be causes as well.

- **Aplastic anemias** result from decreased hematopoiesis in the bone marrow that leads to decreased red blood cell production. Only the red blood cells can be affected (**erythropoiesis**) or all blood cell production can be decreased. Radiation, medications, chemicals, or viral infections may be the cause. Chemotherapy agents and radiation treatment for cancer are examples. In most cases, no specific reason for the decreased production of red blood cells is determined. The red blood cell count will be low, and the red blood cell morphology may show anisocytosis and poikilocytosis. If platelet formation is decreased in addition to the low number of red blood cells, bleeding gums and nosebleeds may also be apparent.

- **Pernicious anemia** results from inadequate secretion of **intrinsic factor** by the parietal cells of the stomach lining. Intrinsic factor is necessary for absorption of vitamin B_{12}, which is necessary for red blood cell formation in the bone marrow. The symptoms of pernicious anemia may include pallor, slight jaundice (pale yellow skin), tongue sores, and tingling feelings in the extremities. The red blood cells of the circulating blood are often macrocytic. Autoantibodies to intrinsic factor may be present. The defective absorption of B_{12} may also be associated with celiac disease, malnutrition, or inflammatory disease of the small intestines. Patients with pernicious anemia who lack the intrinsic factor will need to receive B_{12} injections regularly to meet the body's needs.

- **Sickle cell anemia** is caused by a hemoglobinopathy. These patients are homozygous for Hb S; the majority of their hemoglobin is the S variant. The red blood cells of patients with sickle cell anemia are misshapen; they appear crescent or sickle shaped. The red blood cells are destroyed because of their abnormal shape during changes in oxygen tension, The Hb S also causes the cells to be more rigid, which increases their rate of destruction as they try to squeeze through capillaries.

  Sickle cell disease causes **splenomegaly** (an enlarged spleen), as blood pools in the spleen. Patients' hands and feet are sometimes swollen, and patients have increased chance of infection and exhibit joint pain. The abnormally shaped red blood cells become stuck in the blood vessels, causing pain and poor delivery of oxygen to tissues. The red blood cell morphology will include sickle and **target cells** if examined under the microscope.

Test Your Knowledge 13-9

What laboratory tests may be ordered by a physician to verify whether a symptomatic patient may be anemic?   (Outcome 13-8)

Test Your Knowledge 13-10

List four examples of specific anemias. (Outcome 13-10)

SUMMARY

Hemoglobin in the erythrocytes is the molecule to which oxygen attaches and travels in the blood to every cell in the body to be available for energy production. The normal hemoglobin of adults is designated as Hb A. The hemoglobin concentration can be measured by analyzers spectrophotometrically, by measuring color change accomplished as the hemoglobin in the red blood cells is changed to cyanmethemoglobin. The type of hemoglobin present in cells can be identified by hemoglobin electrophoresis performed in reference or hospital laboratories.

The hematocrit is the amount of space occupied by red blood cells as compared to the whole sample, expressed as a percentage. Hematocrit values can be calculated by automated analyzers or directly read from a hematocrit tube after spinning in a centrifuge. The hemoglobin and hematocrit tests are the most frequently ordered procedures used to monitor the oxygen-carrying capacities of the body. If these values are below the normal reference range, anemia is suspected, and health-care professionals will use addition information to plan a course of treatment. Anemia is diagnosed by the history and physical examination of the patient, as well as laboratory test results. The results of laboratory tests that describe the volume and other characteristics of erythrocytes are used to classify the type of anemia present and establish a course of treatment.

TIME TO REVIEW

1. A degradation product of hemoglobin is: Outcome 13-1
   a. Anisocytosis
   b. Intrinsic factor
   c. Bilirubin
   d. Polycythemia

2. _____ from the tissues can   Outcome 13-1
   contaminate hemoglobin or hematocrit specimens
   and decrease the result.
   a. Anemia
   b. Interstitial fluid
   c. Intrinsic factor
   d. Erythropoiesis

3. Hemoglobin is made of chains   Outcome 13-2
   of globin and four molecules of:
   a. Heme
   b. Sodium
   c. Cyanmethemoglobin
   d. Urobilinogen

4. _____ attaches to the   Outcome 13-2
   hemoglobin and travels from higher oxygen concentration levels in the lungs to the cells of the body
   with increased oxygen need.

   a. Iron
   b. Vitamin B_{12}
   c. Glucose
   d. Oxygen

5. The type of hemoglobin normally   Outcome 13-3
   seen in adults is _____.
   a. Hb A
   b. Hb C
   c. Hb F
   d. Hb S

6. Hemoglobin analyzers determine   Outcome 13-4
   hemoglobin concentration by using:
   a. Electrophoresis
   b. Spectrophotometry
   c. Centrifugation
   d. Visual examination of the cells

7. Restate the adult reference ranges   Outcome 13-8
   for hemoglobin and hematocrit testing.

8. Packed cell volume is a   Outcome 13-5
   synonym for _____.
   a. Hemoglobin
   b. Hematocrit
   c. Sickle cell trait
   d. Polycythemia

9. List the layers of the blood sample   Outcome 13-6
   of a spun hematocrit.

10. Anemia may be the result of: Outcome 13-9
    a. Excessive blood loss
    b. Inadequate red blood cell production in the
       bone marrow
    c. Abnormal hemoglobin molecule structures
    d. All of the above

11. Name the anemia caused by   Outcome 13-10
    an insufficient iron supply in the body.
    a. Hemolytic anemia
    b. Iron-deficiency anemia
    c. Pernicious anemia
    d. Sickle cell anemia

12. A substantial decrease in red blood   Outcome 13-10
    cell production may lead to a(n) _____ anemia.
    a. Iron-deficiency
    b. Aplastic
    c. Pernicious
    d. Sickle cell

Case Study 13-1: Why am I so tired?

A 35-year-old male patient came to the medical office with complaints of being weak, lethargic, and unable to focus on tasks. The health-care provider assessed the symptoms and ordered a hemoglobin and hematocrit test to be performed. The results were Hgb 12.3 g/dL and Hct 38%.

Based on the result, the physician ordered another blood draw for iron studies.

1. What disorder was indicated by the results?
2. Why did the physician order the iron studies?

RESOURCES AND SUGGESTED READINGS

Hemoglobal organization; details about thalassemia http://www.hemoglobal.org/whatisthalassemia.html
Mayo Clinic information about anemia http://www.mayoclinic.com/health/anemia/DS00321
Information about the various HemoCue testing instruments http://www.HemoCue.com

Chapter 14

Erythrocyte Sedimentation Rate

Nikki A. Marhefka, EdM, MT(ASCP), CMA (AAMA)

CHAPTER OUTLINE

Learning Outcomes

After reading this chapter, the successful student will be able to:

14-1 Define the key terms.

14-2 Analyze the effect of plasma proteins on erythrocyte sedimentation rates.

14-3 Describe the effects of abnormally shaped red blood cells in normal and abnormal erythrocyte sedimentation rates.

14-4 Recognize normal reference ranges for erythrocyte sedimentation rates for males and females.

14-5 List the pathological and nonpathological states that may exhibit an increased sedimentation rate.

14-6 Describe the CLIA-waived testing methods for the erythrocyte sedimentation rate.

14-7 Correctly perform an erythrocyte sedimentation rate.

14-8 Highlight procedural errors that can cause erroneous erythrocyte sedimentation rate results.

CAAHEP AND ABHES STANDARDS

 CAAHEP 2008 Standards

I.P.I.12: Anatomy and Physiology: Perform Hematology Testing

I.C.I.6: Identify common pathology related to each body system

 ABHES 2010 Standards

Medical Laboratory Procedures; Perform selected CLIA-waived tests that assist with diagnosis and treatment; #2: Hematology Testing

KEY TERMS

Albumin	Fibrinogen	Rouleaux
Aliquot	Globulin	Wintrobe
Erythrocyte sedimentation rate (ESR, sed rate)	Inflammation	Westergren
	Pipette	

The erythrocyte sedimentation rate is one of the oldest laboratory tests still performed today. The test provides a measurement indicating how far the red blood cells settle in a specimen over a given period of time. The proteins present in the plasma and the specific conditions of the red blood cells in the specimen influence this rate. The erythrocyte sedimentation rate test may be performed using automated methods in hospital and reference laboratories or using CLIA-waived manual methods, which may be performed in any laboratory. The presence of **inflammation** (the protective reaction of the body's tissues to injury or irritation), acute or chronic infection, or neoplasms may be characterized by elevated ESR results. However, normal physiology may also cause the erythrocyte sedimentation rate to be elevated.

ERYTHROCYTE SEDIMENTATION RATE

The erythrocyte sedimentation rate (also known as the **ESR** or **sed rate**) is used (in addition to other more specific laboratory tests and patient history) to screen for inflammatory processes in the body. The results of an ESR are nonspecific; an abnormal result does not provide information about the type or cause of the inflammation, but only that it is present. In most situations, an EDTA (lavender top) anticoagulated venous blood sample is used for the test. (Some test methods require a different type of tube, specified later in the chapter.) A long, hollow, plastic tube (**pipette**) is filled with blood (an **aliquot**) which has been diluted with a citrate or saline solution, and the tube is placed upright on a stable, vibration-free, level surface. Gravity causes the red blood cells to settle out of solution and fall to the bottom of the pipette. After 1 hour, the amount that the red blood cells settled is measured in millimeters. The results of the ESR are reported in millimeters per hour (mm/hr).

> **Test Your Knowledge 14-1**
>
> What is measured by the erythrocyte sedimentation rate?
>
> (Outcome 14-1)

PLASMA PROTEINS AFFECTING THE ERYTHROCYTE SEDIMENTATION RATE

Blood plasma normally contains the proteins known as **albumin**, **globulin**, and **fibrinogen**. Inflammatory processes or infection may cause an increase in the levels of globulin and fibrinogen in the body. When these protein levels are elevated, this will increase the value of the erythrocyte sedimentation rate. Elevated amounts of globulin and fibrinogen decrease the negative charge on the surface of the red blood cells, which means that the cells are not as repelled from one another as they would be normally. This causes the cells to become somewhat "sticky," allowing the red blood cells to stack on top of one another like coins (Fig. 14-1). This configuration is known as **rouleaux** formation. Rouleaux are not uncommon occurrences, but the increase in plasma protein concentrations will cause it to become more pronounced. The increased rouleaux will cause the ESR result to be elevated because these stacked cell formations fall faster than single cells. The plasma proteins influence the settling most when the patient's hematocrit is between 30% and 40%.

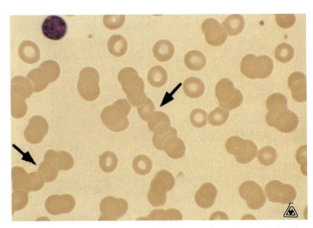

Figure 14-1   Rouleaux formation. Note how the red blood cells "stack" on top of one another, resembling stacks of coins. *From the College of American Pathologists, with permission.*

> **Test Your Knowledge 14-2**
>
> What happens to the red blood cells in the rouleaux formation? (Outcome 14-1)

> **Test Your Knowledge 14-3**
>
> What plasma proteins contribute to the formation of rouleaux when increased in concentration?
> (Outcome 14-2)

> **Test Your Knowledge 14-4**
>
> Why do red blood cells in rouleaux formation settle faster than single red blood cells? (Outcome 14-3)

THE INFLUENCE OF THE RED BLOOD CELLS ON THE ERYTHROCYTE SEDIMENTATION RATE

When the ratio of red blood cells to plasma is lower than normal, the potential for rouleaux formation increases and will increase the speed that the red blood cells settle. For example, someone with anemia may have an elevated erythrocyte sedimentation rate, because his sample has fewer red blood cells as compared to the total sample volume than would be present normally. The presence of macrocytes (large cells) in the specimen will also cause the ESR to be greater than normal.

Erythrocyte sedimentation rates below the normal range may be present when the sample has a lot of microcytes (small red blood cells) or spherocytes (small, dense red blood cells) present. Sickle cells will also cause a decrease in the ESR, as the cells do not stack together as they would normally, so they will not settle out as expected. Patients with polycythemia will demonstrate a decreased erythrocyte sedimentation rate because of the excess number of red blood cells. Excessive leukocytosis (as in the case of chronic myelogenous leukemia) will also cause a decreased ESR result.

When the ESR values are out of the normal range because of the sizes or shapes of the red blood cells, the results may not change rapidly with treatment. Red blood cells live for approximately 120 days in the circulation, and the ESR result will not be significantly changed until the red blood cells present in the body have been replaced by healthy cells. It also takes time for the protein levels in the blood to change significantly with treatment. This means that the erythrocyte sedimentation rate is used more often for initial screening for inflammation or infection than it is to monitor the immediate effects of treatment.

REFERENCE RANGES

The normal reference ranges for the ESR vary by gender and by age. This is partly caused by the difference in the normal number of circulating red blood cells for men and women. The reference ranges are also elevated in adults over the age of 50. The normal reference ranges are listed in Table 14-1.

> **Test Your Knowledge 14-5**
>
> List normal ESR values for men and women younger than the age of 50. (Outcome 14-4)

CLINICAL SIGNIFICANCE OF ERYTHROCYTE SEDIMENTATION RATE TESTING

Inflammatory processes and acute infection with tissue breakdown increase the amount of fibrinogen and globulins present in the bloodstream. These proteins will interact with the red blood cells and cause the erythrocyte sedimentation rate to be elevated. The ESR can be used to diagnose a disease or condition, monitor an ongoing disease process or treatment, or assist with a differential diagnosis in certain disorders. For instance, the ESR will be elevated when a patient has recently experienced a myocardial infarction, but will not be elevated with angina pectoris. The ESR is not as sensitive to

TABLE 14-1		
Reference ranges for the Westergren erythrocyte sedimentation rate		
	Male	**Female**
Younger than 50 years of age	Less than 15 mm/hr	Less than 20 mm/hr
Older than 50 years of age	Less than 20 mm/hr	Less than 30 mm/hr
Older than 85 years of age	Less than 30 mm/hr	Less then 40 mm/hr

changes in treatment as some other laboratory tests may be, but it still may be used to monitor treatment over an extended period of time.

It is important to remember that nonpathological issues may also cause the ESR to appear elevated. Pregnancy is a normal physiological process that will exhibit an elevated ESR. By the 12th week of pregnancy, the ESR result will have increased above the normal range, and will remain so through the first month postpartum. Women who are menstruating may also have an elevated erythrocyte sedimentation rate.

The disorders of polymyalgia rheumatica (an inflammatory condition of the muscles) and temporal arteritis (inflammation and damage to the blood vessels that supply the head) are the only two disease conditions for which an elevated ESR is the primary means of diagnosis. The test may also be used (in addition to other clinical information and laboratory tests) to evaluate septic arthritis, pelvic inflammatory disease, and appendicitis. Rheumatoid arthritis, chronic infection, collagen disease (systemic lupus erythematosus [SLE]), and certain neoplasms (especially prostate or kidney cancer) are characterized by increased ESR results. Erythrocyte sedimentation rates may be used to the monitor the efficacy of therapy in osteomyelitis. The ESR results may be misleading in patients with osteoarthritis, as these patients may have ESR results within normal range even with the presence of inflammation in the joints. The ESR results may also offer valuable information to help determine the risk associated with coronary artery disease.

Test Your Knowledge 14-6

If an ESR is elevated, what process is occurring in the body?

(Outcome 14-5)

POINT OF INTEREST 14-1
Seditainer procedure

Becton, Dickinson has created the Seditainer system, a unique setup for the erythrocyte sedimentation procedure. It is designed to measure the erythrocyte sedimentation rate without transferring the blood to a separate tube. This eliminates the potential for exposure to blood products while transferring the specimen, as well as the possibility of adding bubbles to the specimen during the ESR setup. In the Seditainer system, the evacuated tubes used for drawing blood during the venipuncture have a black top, and they contain 1.25 mL of a sodium citrate solution. The

tube needs to be filled to the point at which the vacuum is exhausted, and the specimen needs to be well mixed. The tube is placed in a special Seditainer stand, and the knob on the stand is used to adjust the top of the blood column to the "0" level. Each spot in the Seditainer stand is marked with a scale used to read the ESR level at the end of 1 hour. The tubes are then discarded without ever being opened.

ERYTHROCYTE SEDIMENTATION RATE DETERMINATION

There are two methods used for performing the ESR. The oldest method is the **Wintrobe** method. To perform the Wintrobe ESR, well-mixed blood from a tube containing EDTA anticoagulant is transferred directly to a Wintrobe tube using a pipette with a long, slim end. The Wintrobe tube is short, with graduated markings up to 100 mm. The ESR result is read after the sample has been allowed to sit undisturbed for 1 hour. It is important that the ESR is not vibrated or disturbed during the time that the test is performed.

The Wintrobe method is not used as widely as is the **Westergren** method. The Westergren method involves the dilution of the EDTA-anticoagulated blood with a sodium citrate solution or saline before the blood is added to the pipette. The Westergren pipette is also smaller in diameter and taller than the Wintrobe tube.

Most offices use a CLIA-waived modified Westergren method that uses a "closed system," allowing the blood to be added to the pipette with a minimal amount of exposure to the specimen for the employee. The test is performed on an EDTA-anticoagulated venous blood sample. A specified amount of room-temperature, well-mixed blood is diluted with a premeasured citrate solution and introduced into a hollow column. The column is marked off into millimeters for ease of reading the results. The top of the sample must be at the "0" mark when the timing is started as a point of reference. The column is placed in a rack so that it is exactly level, and timing begins immediately. The column must not be disturbed during the timing process, and the specimens must be kept out of direct sunlight. At exactly 1 hour, the top of the red blood cell column is noted. The ESR result is documented as the millimeters per hour that the cells have settled. The result is compared to the reference ranges for the patient, based on gender and age.

During the 60 minutes of the testing process, the settling of the red blood cells occurs in three stages. The first stage takes place within the first 10 minutes of the testing period. Rouleaux formation (the stacking of red blood cells) is beginning to occur so there is little sedimentation, even in abnormal samples. The second stage occurs in the next 40 minutes, during which there is a constant rate of settling as the rouleaux are set up (if present). The "stacks" of cells fall rapidly during this time because of the increased volume to surface area. The final stage occurs in the last 10 minutes of the testing process. At this time the settling is slowing as the cells are forming the packed cell volume at the bottom of the column.

CLIA-Waived Erythrocyte Sedimentation Rate Methods

There are various modified Westergren ESR systems available for use in the laboratory. Sediplast (manufactured by Polymedco) is one of the most common kits. An EDTA-anticoagulated venous blood sample of 0.8 mL is pipetted into a vial containing 0.2 mL of 3.8% sodium citrate diluting solution. The vial is then gently inverted to mix and placed into the accompanying rack. A 100-mm marked tube is gently pushed into the vial until it sits on the bottom of the small vial containing the blood. The tube is designed for autozeroing, as the blood mixture will reach the "0" mark and any extra will enter into an overflow area. The timing must begin immediately and continue for exactly 60 minutes. The sedimentation rate in mm/hr is read at the top of the red blood cell column. This closed system minimizes potential exposure to the sample while setting up the procedure and also prevents the potential for splashing when disposing of the setup after testing. This process is expanded and detailed in Procedure 14-1.

POINT OF INTEREST 14-2
The C-reactive protein

The erythrocyte sedimentation rate is elevated when inflammation occurs within the body. However, the ESR does not react quickly when inflammation first starts, and the result does not change immediately when treatment begins. The C-reactive protein (CRP) is also elevated with systemic inflammation processes in the body. The CRP is also known as an acute phase protein. The level of the CRP is elevated with infection, cardiovascular disease, and the formation of atherosclerosis. Because the level of CRP is affected immediately with treatment that reduces inflammation, this test may be a better choice than the ESR with which to monitor a course of treatment.

Although the Wintrobe method is not used as often as is the modified Westergren method, the Wintrobe method is still a CLIA-waived procedure carried out some laboratories. The Wintrobe method requires a special pipette to add the specimen to the tube used for the test, and the method is not considered as safe for the employee because it provides an opportunity for more potential exposure to bloodborne pathogens as the blood is added to the tube.

Test Your Knowledge 14-7
List two CLIA-waived ESR procedures.   (Outcome 14-6)

Automated Erythrocyte Sedimentation Rate Methods

For laboratories that perform high volumes of testing, there are automated ESR analyzers available. These instruments automatically perform the dilutions (if necessary), set up the ESR tubes, and have internal readers that detect the color change present at the top of the red blood cell column when the designated time has passed. Some determine the ESR in less than the 60 minutes required for the manual methods. Polymedco makes the Sedimat and the Sedten analyzers. The Ves-matic, manufactured by Diesse, uses the EDTA lavender top tube directly to perform the ESR measurement. Many of these analyzers are capable of processing multiple ESR tests at one time.

POTENTIAL SOURCES OF ERROR FOR THE ERYTHROCYTE SEDIMENTATION RATE PROCEDURE

The ESR test must be performed very carefully; procedural errors will directly affect the results. The first consideration is the collection of the blood sample to be used. If the blood is allowed to clot, the ESR will be falsely decreased because the fibrinogen in the sample will be used forming the blood clot. Samples will ideally be used for the ESR within a few hours of the blood draw. Most laboratories state that the sample may be used for the test if it is kept at room temperature (20° to 25°C) for up to 24 hours. Refrigeration may cause irreversible changes in the way the cells interact in the sample, so the process must occur within 12 hours if the sample is refrigerated. The blood must be at room temperature at the time the test is performed.

Procedure 14-1: Perform CLIA–Waived Sediplast Westergren Erythrocyte Sedimentation Rate

Erythrocyte sedimentation rates are one of the oldest, easiest, and least expensive testing procedures performed in laboratories. The Westergren method is the most common CLIA-waived manual system employed.

- Biohazardous disposal bag
- Face shield and laboratory coat
- Transfer pipette
- Test tube rack

TASK

Perform an erythrocyte sedimentation rate using the Sediplast system, and read and record the results correctly.

CONDITIONS

- Hand-washing supplies and/or alcohol-based hand sanitizer
- Disposable gloves
- Sediplast Modified Westergren ESR reservoir tube, pipette, and rack
- Lavender top (EDTA) tube filled with blood

CAAHEP/ABHES STANDARDS

 CAAHEP 2008 Standards

I.P.I.12 Anatomy and Physiology; Perform Hematology Testing

 ABHES 2010 Standards

- Medical Laboratory Procedures, b. Perform selected CLIA–waived tests that assist with diagnosis and treatment;
- #2: Perform Hematology Testing

Procedure	Rationale
1. Sanitize hands (allow them to dry), then apply gloves, laboratory coat, and face shield.	Gloves must be worn for any procedures during which exposure to blood or other potentially infectious materials is anticipated. This procedure has an increased risk for exposure to blood products, so a laboratory coat and face shield should also be worn.
2. Gather testing supplies. Check the expiration of the ESR kit components. Verify that the necessary quality control has been performed prior to testing the patient sample.	Expired products must never be used for testing. If the required quality control has not been performed, this needs to be accomplished (and the results verified) before the patient test results are reported.
3. Verify the test ordered and that the sample is appropriately identified.	The test and patient identity should always be verified before any testing procedure is started.
4. Verify that the EDTA tube is at room temperature.	The blood must always be at room temperature for the ESR test result to be valid.
5. Invert the EDTA tube 8 to 10 times to mix the sample.	The specimen must be well mixed or it will provide erroneous test results.
6. Carefully remove the rubber stopper on the top of the EDTA blood tube. Avoid aerosol formation by removing the top slowly. Place the stopper top down on the tabletop, and place the blood tube in a test tube rack.	If the stopper is removed too quickly, a fine "mist" of blood may be released, increasing the potential for exposure.

Procedure	Rationale
7. Remove the pink cap from the prefilled reservoir vial provided with the test kit. Be careful not to spill any of the solution.	The proper amount of diluent in the tube is vital for the dilution factor to be correct and the results to be valid.
8. Using the transfer pipette, add blood to the reservoir vial until it reaches the fill line. Avoid bubbles or air spaces in the reservoir vial. Recap the EDTA blood tube.	It is important to add the necessary volume of blood to the diluent to allow for the correct dilution ratio and to provide enough specimen for an accurate ESR reading.
9. Replace the pink cap on the reservoir vial and invert fully at least 8 times.	The specimen must be mixed thoroughly with the diluent for the results to be accurate.
10. Place the vial in the rack on a level surface. Insert the marked ESR pipette through the pink cap and push down until it comes to the bottom of the vial. The blood will rise to the "0" mark within the ESR pipette, and any excess blood will enter the overflow reservoir.	The blood must reach the "0" mark or the test will not be valid. This process should be accomplished fairly slowly to make certain that the blood reaches the top of the ESR pipette.
11. Make certain that the rack is in a place where it will not be disturbed and where it is not in direct sunlight. Set a timer for 1 hour.	Vibrations, movement or direct sunlight may affect the ESR results. A timer is necessary for appropriate timing of the procedure.

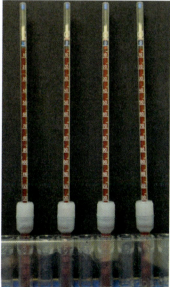

Courtesy of Fisher HealthCare, Inc.

Continued

Procedure 14-1: Perform CLIA–Waived Sediplast Westergren Erythrocyte Sedimentation Rate—cont'd

Procedure	Rationale
12. After 1 hour, note the number at the top of the red blood cell column. This will be in mm marked on the side of the ESR tube. Note this number as the result in mm/hr, and document the result on the log sheet or the patient's chart.	The marks should be relatively easy to read, and are read from the top of the pipette down. 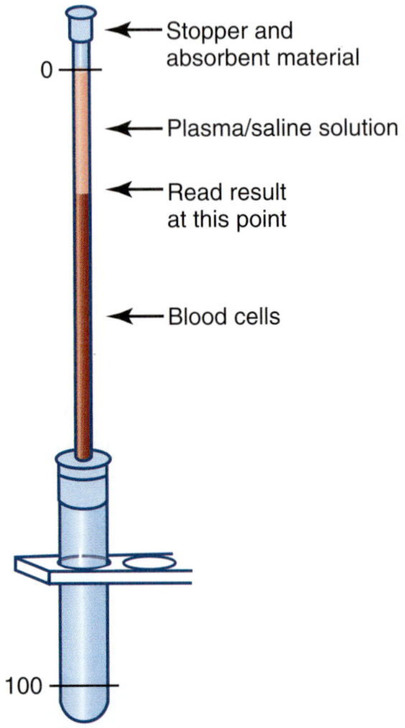 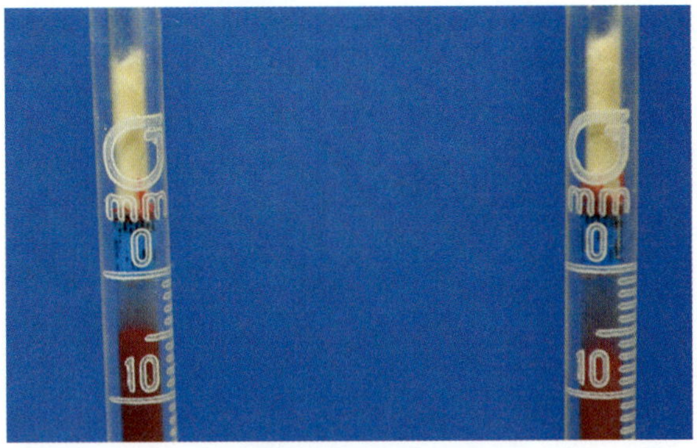

Labels on diagram:
0
Stopper and absorbent material
Plasma/saline solution
Read result at this point
Blood cells
100

Procedure	Rationale
13. Dispose of the ESR setup and the transfer pipette in the biohazardous garbage. Disinfect the work area.	There is blood in the transfer pipette and the ESR setup, so both must be disposed of in the biohazardous garbage.
14. Remove gloves and sanitize hands. Remove face shield.	Hands must always be sanitized after removing gloves. The face shield is not necessary for all procedures, so should be removed until needed again.

Procedure	Rationale
15. Document the ESR results in the patient's chart if not completed previously. If necessary, also log the lot number and expiration of the kit components on the log sheet.	All procedures must be appropriately documented in the patient's chart.

Date	
1/18/2020:	ESR 22 mm/hr. ~~~~~~~~~~~~~~~~
1100 a.m.	~~~~~~~~~~~~~~~~ Connie Lieseke, CMA (AAMA)

The tube of venous blood must be well mixed so that the aliquot removed for the test is representative of the sample. Before removing the blood for the test, the tube is gently inverted at least eight times. After the blood is added to the diluent, adequate mixing is again imperative. When reading the results, if there is not clear definition at the top of the red blood cells in the plasma, the result is to be read at the point when there is a definitive border to the red blood cells in the column.

There can be no bubbles in the column of blood or diluted blood. The tube (column) must be exactly vertical during the testing process, so the holding rack into which it is placed must be level as well. Many of the racks come with leveling devices at the corners so that this can be verified. Movement (such as vibrations) can alter the results, so it is important that this test is not performed on a counter next to a centrifuge or a printer. The timing must be exact for accurate readings, so a timer is usually employed rather than a watch or a clock.

Test Your Knowledge 14-8

List two testing procedure errors that can affect the value of the ESR.   (Outcome 14-7)

SUMMARY

The erythrocyte sedimentation rate is a test that screens for the presence of inflammation. The ESR results can be altered as a result of infection, autoimmune disease, or growth of neoplasms in the body. With inflammation, there is a change in the levels of plasma proteins with an increase in fibrinogen and some globulins. This protein change can cause the red blood cells to form excessive rouleaux, which settle out of solution faster than do single red blood cells. The observance of this sedimentation of red blood

cells in 60 minutes constitutes the test procedure. The CLIA-waived procedures include manual Westergren and Wintrobe methods. There are also automated testing systems available for laboratories that perform a high volume of testing or desire the results in less than 1 hour. The erythrocyte sedimentation rate is used as a tool to aid in diagnosis, monitor disease process, follow treatment, and assess prognosis of certain disorders.

TIME TO REVIEW

1. Rouleaux formation is: Outcome 14-1
   a. An abnormal collection of proteins in the circulating blood
   b. The test for inflammation
   c. A group of red blood cells stacking together like coins
   d. None of the above

2. Examples of proteins that   Outcome 14-2
   are increased in the plasma when the sedimentation rate is elevated include:
   a. Albumin and fibrinogen
   b. Fibrinogen and globulins
   c. Globulins and albumin
   d. Globulin and tyrosine

3. A 30-year-old male patient   Outcome 14-4
   has an ESR of 38 mm/hr. The result of this test for this patient is _____ _____.
   a. Within the reference range for the patient's gender and age
   b. Elevated for the patient's gender and age
   c. Within range for his age, but not his gender
   d. Below the reference range

4. An 87-year-old woman has a   Outcome 14-4
   sedimentation rate of 38 mm/hr. The result for this
   patient is _____ because of this patient's gender
   and age.

   a. Normal
   b. Elevated
   c. Elevated
   d. Decreased

5. An elevated ESR indicates the   Outcome 14-5
   presence of:

   a. Inflammation
   b. Erythropoiesis
   c. Albumin
   d. Renal disease

6. A/an _____ anticoagulated   Outcome 14-6
   venous blood sample is used for the erythrocyte
   sedimentation rate.

   a. Citrate
   b. Heparin
   c. EDTA
   d. Fluoride

7. True or False: Westergren and   Outcome 14-6
   Wintrobe are CLIA-waived erythrocyte sedimentation
   procedures.

8. _____ is measured to determine the   Outcome 14-7
   ESR value.

   a. The ratio of proteins in the blood
   b. The rouleax formation of red blood cells
   c. The settling of the red blood cells
   d. The presence of red blood cells in the bone
      marrow

9. Examples of potential errors when   Outcome 14-8
   performing an ESR include:

   a. Insufficient sample added to diluent
   b. Insufficient mixing of sample and diluents
   c. Reading result at 50 minutes
   d. All of the above

Case Study 14-1: **Cutting corners**

Margaret Lindon is a new employee, and she was nervous on her first day alone in the laboratory. One of the first orders she received was to collect a specimen and perform an ESR test. She had been trained on this procedure the week before, and remembered that it was not very difficult. The requisition indicated that a lavender top tube was to be drawn, and Margaret knew where the ESR supplies were kept. As Margaret was collecting the blood sample, the blood flow stopped, and she could not get it to continue. She discontinued the blood draw with a partial lavender top tube filled.

After the patient left, Margaret began to set up the ESR test. She added the blood to the reservoir tube containing the citrate solution, but realized that she did not have quite enough specimen to fill it to the required line. She inserted the ESR pipette, and the blood-citrate solution came almost to the top of the pipette, but was shy by a few millimeters. After 1 hour, Margaret read the results of the ESR, and reported out that it was 28 mm/hr.

1. Was the correct specimen drawn for the ESR order?
2. What were the potential sources of error for this scenario? Was this result of 28 mm/hr a valid result?

RESOURCES AND SUGGESTED READINGS

"Polymedco Products"
    Information about the various clinical diagnostic test kits and educational materials provided by Polymedco. http://www.polymedco.com/products-pages-7.php
"Diesse USA Product Line"
    Products from Diesse USA including an ESR system. http://www.diesse-usa.com/products.html

Chapter 15

Coagulation Studies

Constance L. Lieseke, CMA (AAMA), MLT, PBT(ASCP)

CHAPTER OUTLINE

Learning Outcomes

After reading this chapter, the successful student will be able to:

15-1 Define the key terms.

15-2 Explain the purpose of coagulation studies.

15-3 Describe the process of coagulation.

15-4 Compare the formation of a thrombus to that of an embolus.

15-5 Compare and contrast the disorders diagnosed or monitored with laboratory coagulation testing.

15-6 Examine how the prothrombin test and INR calculation are used together to monitor coagulation status for a patient.

15-7 Successfully perform a CLIA-waived PT/INR test.

15-8 Explain appropriate use of a PTT test for monitoring coagulation.

15-9 Evaluate the use of platelet counts in coagulation testing.

15-10 Explain why bleeding time tests are not performed as frequently as PT and PTT tests.

15-11 Describe other tests of platelet function.

15-12 List other coagulation tests that may be ordered.

15-13 List the requirements for coagulation specimen collection and potential sources of error for the various tests.

CAAHEP/ABHES STANDARDS

 CAAHEP Standards

None

ABHES Standards

None

KEY TERMS

Afibrogenemia

Aggregate

Antiphospholipid syndrome

Atrial fibrillation

Clotting cascade

Clotting factor

Coagulation

Coumadin

D-dimer

Deep vein thrombosis (DVT)

Disseminated intravascular coagulation (DIC)

Dysfibrinogenemia

Embolus

Endothelial cell lining

Extrinsic pathway

Fibrin degradation products (FDPs)

Fibrinogen

Fibrinolysis

Fibrinolytic drugs

Hemophilia

Hemostasis

Heparin

Hypofibrinogenemia

International normalized ratio (INR)

Intrinsic pathway

Occlude

Partial thromboplastin time (PTT)

Pathological thrombosis

Plasmin

Platelet count

Prophylactic

Prothrombin time (PT)

Stroke

Thrombin

Thrombocytes

Thrombocytopenia

Thrombosis

Viscous

Warfarin

von Willebrand's factor

When most of us receive a paper cut or other minor injury, we take for granted that this minor blood vessel injury will stop bleeding and heal within a short period of time. The process of blood clotting, known as **coagulation,** and the breakdown of these clots within the body are monitored by use of various coagulation testing procedures. Platelets, fibrinogen, thrombin, and 13 other clotting factors are all involved in the process of clot formation, which is necessary for repair of blood vessel damage. The blood vessels also play a role. In addition, chemicals are produced by the body to break down the clots when they are no longer needed. This process is known as **fibrinolysis.** Coagulation studies include quantitative and qualitative analysis of the various components, as well as their function.

PURPOSE OF COAGULATION STUDIES

Coagulation studies are performed in the laboratory when the various elements in the clotting process appear to be imbalanced or malfunctioning. These defects can cause excessive bleeding, bruising, or unwanted blood vessel occlusion (blocking of the vessel) with formation of blood clots in the bloodstream. Anticoagulant medication use is also closely monitored with laboratory coagulation testing. Laboratory tests may include quantitative analysis of certain plasma proteins involved in the clotting process, as well as analysis of platelet count and function. Coagulation studies are often performed prior to surgical procedures to verify that the balance between bleeding and clotting in the body is at a desirable level. **Hemostasis** is the word used to describe the processes needed to balance clot formation and fibrinolysis in the body.

MECHANISMS OF BLOOD CLOTTING

The balance between blood clotting and excessive bleeding involves numerous factors. These include the blood vessels of the body (including the cells that line those vessels); the platelets (**thrombocytes**) circulating in the bloodstream; and numerous coagulation factors present in the circulation as enzymes, substrates, inhibitors, and plasma proteins. The study of coagulation and hemostasis focuses on two major systems. The primary coagulation system includes the action of the platelets and the vascular response to vessel injury. The actions of the plasma proteins and other chemicals in the circulation make up the secondary coagulation system, and complete the coagulation process.

When damage occurs to a blood vessel, the **endothelial cell lining** of that artery, vein, or capillary is disrupted. The first response of the body is to constrict the damaged blood vessel and other vessels in the vicinity, limiting the blood flow to the area so that platelet aggregation can begin. In small arterioles, venules, and capillaries, this may stop the bleeding without moving to the next step. In larger vessels, however, this will not be enough.

When intact, the blood vessel lining does not attract platelets; in fact, the two repel each other. However, when the endothelial cell lining is damaged, the exposed collagen layer underneath the endothelial cells attracts the platelets to **aggregate** and begin the process of coagulation. Fibrinogen and *von Willebrand's factor* assist in the adhesion of the platelets to one another. The following are some of the next steps involved in primary coagulation:

1. The platelets in the area of the damaged vessel change shape and begin to adhere tightly to one another.
2. Platelets are filled with granules in their cytoplasm. As they aggregate and change shape, they release the

content of these granules into the plasma. This chemical causes the platelet plug to become more stable and the connections between the platelets to be very tight.
3. The platelets release a compound known as *proaccelerin,* or *labile factor,* that works with vitamin K to start the rest of the changes necessary for a permanent fibrin clot to form.

Secondary coagulation includes a series of events described as the **clotting cascade.** This cascade involves continuous feedback and interaction in which each **clotting factor** affects other clotting factors to achieve the formation of a solid fibrin clot over the area of the damaged vessel. All of the clotting factors are produced in the liver and introduced into the bloodstream. Some of the clotting factors are also produced by endothelial cells in the vessel lining and megakaryocytes in the bone marrow. There are at least 10 clotting factors, and they are designated by Roman numerals. They work in two different pathways, the **intrinsic pathway** and the **extrinsic pathway,** to accomplish the same goal. The intrinsic pathway involves chemicals that are all present in the bloodstream naturally, whereas the extrinsic pathway is initiated by release of chemicals into the bloodstream by the subendothelial cells exposed during the vessel injury. Table 15-1 lists the clotting factors with their Roman numeral numbers, alternative names, and the laboratory tests used to monitor their activity in the body.

It is important to keep in mind that the balance of bleeding and clotting in the body must be regulated naturally by clotting processes, as well as by fibrinolysis (the breakdown of the formed clots when they are no longer needed) and inhibitors that keep the system from overreacting to damages to the vessel walls. Any natural or acquired interference in this balance will negatively affect hemostasis.

TABLE 15-1

Clotting factors with alternative names and common tests used to monitor levels or detect deficiencies*

Clotting Factor	Alternative Name	Laboratory Test
I	Fibrinogen	Fibrinogen level
II	Prothrombin	Prothrombin time (PT)
III	Thromboplastin	PTT
IV	Ionized calcium	Ionized calcium levels
V	Proaccelerin or labile factor	PT and PTT
VII	Proconvertin or stable factor	PT
VIII	Antihemophilic (also linked to von Willebrand's factor)	PTT
IX	Plasma thromboplastin component	PTT
X	Stuart-Prower	PT and PTT
XI	Plasma thromboplastin antecedent	PTT
XII	Hageman factor	PTT
XIII	Fibrin stabilizing factor	PT and PTT

*There is no factor VI.

DISORDERS DIAGNOSED OR MONITORED WITH LABORATORY COAGULATION TESTS

Coagulation testing is used to diagnose or monitor a variety of diseases or disorders. Some of the results provide information that will help the health-care provider to anticipate problems (such as those performed prior to surgical procedures), whereas other laboratory values are used to achieve a diagnosis or monitor the progress of a disease.

Thrombosis

Thrombosis is the clot formation that occurs naturally in the body. However, there may also be times when **pathological thrombosis** occurs. Clots may form in any vessel of the body related to different risk factors and exhibiting different symptoms dependent on the location of clot formation. Arterial thrombosis can be caused by hypertension, atherosclerosis, blood that is too **viscous,** or thick, and by functional platelet abnormalities. Clots in the arteries usually include a small amount of fibrin and more white cells than thromboses formed in the other vessels.

Pathological thrombosis in the venous system is usually made up of red blood cells and large amounts of fibrin. Deep vein thrombosis (DVT) may be caused by impaired (slow) blood flow, especially in those patients who are recovering from surgery and are therefore

inactive. Other factors that may contribute to formation of venous thrombi include impaired breakdown of clots (fibrinolytic deficiency) and inadequate levels of clotting inhibitors that keep the body from excessive thrombosis formation. A very serious complication of deep vein thrombosis occurs when pieces of the blood clot dislodge from the vessel of formation and enter the bloodstream. This is called an **embolus,** and if it becomes lodged in the pulmonary tissues, it may be fatal.

> **Test Your Knowledge 15-5**
> How is an embolus different from a thrombus?
> (Outcome 15-4)

Atrial Fibrillation

Atrial fibrillation is a condition in which there are erratic electrical signals sent through the atria, which are the upper chambers of the heart. Because of these erratic signals, the heart does not beat with the correct rhythm or at the correct speed. This causes turbulence, or a disrupted blood flow through the heart, and an increased risk of blood clot (thrombus) formation within the atria. This is especially common in the left atria. If a thrombus is present, the patient is at a very high risk of embolus formation as well, as the blood travels through the heart and may pick up pieces of the clot. The emboli often travel to the brain, where they **occlude** (block) the small vessels and cause a **stroke.** A stroke (also known as a cerebrovascular accident) is the result of a blockage of blood flow to an area of the brain. Patients who have chronic atrial fibrillation are often prescribed **warfarin** as a lifelong treatment option, as warfarin is a drug that interferes with the extrinsic clotting factor system of the body, and decreases the risk of blood clots forming in the atria.

Postsurgical Prophylaxis

Because the opportunity for thrombosis formation is heightened when the blood flow to a specific area of the body is slowed, those who are immobile or recovering from surgery are at high risk of blood clot development in their legs, especially. This is called a **deep vein thrombosis, or DVT.** Increased passive exercise (when possible) helps to reduce this risk, and is often started the same day or one day postsurgery with the assistance of a member of the physical therapy team. However, this may not always be enough to keep clots from forming in the deep veins of the legs. Many patients who anticipate extended hospitalization after surgery will be placed on heparin during or immediately after the procedure as a **prophylactic** measure, treatment in anticipation of a potential problem, as opposed to treatment after the blood clot has occurred. Heparin is fast acting, is given via IV or injection, and affects the intrinsic clotting system of the body. Heparin is a very good choice for inpatient treatment, but as patients near discharge, they are usually started on oral warfarin treatment, as this is easier to maintain in the home environment.

Disseminated Intravascular Coagulation

Disseminated intravascular coagulation (DIC) occurs when the blood clotting system is activated throughout the body, rather than just at a site with injury to a blood vessel. Small thrombi form everywhere, including within organs and capillary beds. That patient's coagulation factors are used up after a time, as well as the substances that break down blood clots. This often results in uncontrolled bleeding. DIC can be a process that is slow to develop, and in this situation the individual usually has systemic thrombi develop, but no uncontrolled bleeding. In acute (or rapid-acting) DIC, the patient develops the multiple thrombi, but they also may hemorrhage because of the rapid use of the coagulation factors within their body.

There is *always* an underlying cause for patients who exhibit disseminated intravascular coagulation. Many times (especially in acute cases) if the underlying situation is addressed and resolved, the DIC will also resolve.

Potential causes of disseminated intravascular coagulation include the following:

- Systemic infection with bacteria or fungi
- Severe trauma
- Solid tumors or hematological cancers
- Obstetrical complications such as placental abruption or amniotic fluid emboli
- Aortic aneurysms or other vascular disorders
- Systemic inflammatory responses, such as those that occur with transfusion reactions

The first course of treatment for DIC is to resolve the underlying problem, if possible. However, in situations in which the initial disease process cannot easily be resolved, or cannot be resolved quickly enough, the symptoms of disseminated intravascular coagulation may be treated with transfusions of platelets, coagulation factors contained in fresh frozen plasma, and fibrinogen as provided in cryofibrinogen precipitate.

> **Test Your Knowledge 15-6**
> How are DIC and DVT similar?   (Outcome 15-5)

Thrombocytopenia

In **thrombocytopenia,** the patient does not have enough platelets circulating to coagulate effectively when necessary. Certain medications or other underlying hematology disease states may cause this condition. Because of the low numbers of platelets, the clots that form in response to vascular damage will not be adequate. In addition to thrombocytopenia, patients may exhibit disorders of platelet adhesion, where the platelet count is normal for the patient, but their platelets lack the ability to stick to other platelets and form the aggregate plug that is necessary to stop the bleeding with vascular injuries.

> **Test Your Knowledge 15-7**
> How is thrombocytopenia different from the other disorders presented thus far in this chapter?
>   (Outcome 15-5)

Antiphospholipid Syndrome

Antiphospholipid syndrome is a condition in which small systemic blood clots form, presenting potential risk for embolism or organ failure. Because the blood clots can form anywhere, the patient is at a high risk for stroke, or total occlusion of blood vessels providing circulation to internal organs.

Hemophilia

Hemophilia is a sex-linked inherited disorder that affects approximately 1 in 5,000 males. There are two types of hemophilia: type A and type B. Those affected with type A hemophilia lack the clotting factor VIII. Those with type B lack the clotting factor IX. Both groups of patients may bleed excessively and experience vascular damage, in addition to internal bleeding in the elbows, knees, and other joints. Not all patients with hemophilia are affected to the same extent; the disorder may express itself with mild to moderate symptoms. It is also possible to develop hemophilia in response to chemotherapy treatment or other disease states. In those situations, the patients actually develop antibodies to the clotting factors, which render them useless when needed within the body. Patients with all types of hemophilia will need to be treated with the missing clotting factors to avoid excessive bleeding. The clotting factors may be derived from human donated plasma, or they may be created in a laboratory without human elements.

LABORATORY TESTS USED TO DIAGNOSE COAGULATION DISORDERS OR MONITOR ANTICOAGULANT THERAPY

As we have learned, certain disease states may cause a patient to be more prone to thrombosis formation, whereas other pathologies may cause excessive bleeding. For those who have disorders causing excessive bleeding, the coagulation tests associated with diagnosis and monitoring of the conditions are usually performed at a hospital or reference laboratory. These tests may include the prothrombin time (PT), the activated partial prothrombin time (PTT), fibrinogen levels, fibrin degradation products (FDPs), and D-dimer. Health-care providers may also request levels of specific clotting factors. Table 15-2 contains information about the tests covered in this chapter, why they are commonly ordered, and the specimen types required. Medical assistants may perform PT/INR tests, and will be involved in the specimen collection process for the tests performed outside the physician office, so they will benefit from the basic knowledge about the specimen requirements and clinical significance of the various test results.

TABLE 15-2

Common coagulation tests, clinical indication or significance, and specimen requirements

Test Name	Abbreviation	Test Use	Specimen Type
Activated partial prothrombin time	PTT or PTT	Screening for coagulation dysfunction; intrinsic system of blood coagulation. Also used to monitor heparin anticoagulant use.	Light blue top tube with citrate anticoagulant; must be filled completely.
Fibrin degradation products	FDP	Monitoring of breakdown products from blood clot dissolution	Special FDP tube for plasma levels; may also use red top tubes for serum levels.
D-dimers	D-dimers	Fibrin breakdown products from blood clot dissolution	Citrated plasma from full light blue top tube. Plasma should be frozen if the test cannot be performed immediately.
Fibrinogen level	Fib	Measures amount of circulating fibrinogen in bloodstream	Plasma from full light blue top citrate tube.
Bleeding time	BT	Platelet function	Test performed on patient
Platelet count	Plt Ct	Assessment of number of platelets available for blood coagulation	Lavender top tube with EDTA anticoagulant. Test performed on whole blood.
Platelet function assay 100	PFA 100	Assessment of platelet function; clotting ability of platelets	Full light blue top citrated tube; whole blood is used for the assay.

TABLE 15-2

Common coagulation tests, clinical indication or significance, and specimen requirements—cont'd

Test Name	Abbreviation	Test Use	Specimen Type
Prothrombin time	Prothrombin time or PT	Screening for coagulation dysfunction; specifically extrinsic blood clotting cascade. Also used for monitoring oral anticoagulant use.	Full light blue top citrate tube or capillary sample if performed with point-of-care testing.
International normalized ratio	INR	Factor used for monitoring oral anticoagulant use; standardizes results using various reagents and testing methods	Full light blue top citrate tube or capillary sample if test is performed with point-of-care testing instrument

Prothrombin and International Normalized Ratio

The **prothrombin time (PT)** is a test that measures the efficacy of the extrinsic coagulation process. Prothrombin is a clotting factor that is manufactured by the liver, and the change of prothrombin to **thrombin** is one of the last steps to forming a clot when a vessel is damaged. The action of clotting factors I, II, V, VII, and IX may be monitored with the prothrombin time test result. The prothrombin time may be elevated in patients who have insufficient amounts of these clotting factors, as well as those who are deficient in vitamin K. Patients suffering from liver disease may also have an increased prothrombin time result because of the inability of the liver to create the clotting factors as needed.

The PT is reported in seconds, as it is a measurement of the amount of time needed for a clot to form in the specimen after the addition of thromboplastin and calcium to a sample of platelet-poor plasma. PT tests are often performed as part of a coagulation screen before surgical procedures or when a patient shows signs of excessive bleeding or bruising. Prothrombin times may be used to screen for initial coagulation disorders. The PT is also used to help monitor oral anticoagulant use, as the result is elevated when a patient is being treated with these oral anticoagulants.

POINT OF INTEREST 15-1
History of warfarin

As the population in the United States grew dramatically in the early 1900s, so did the demands for farming. The Midwest was farmed extensively, growing crops to feed the U.S. population as well as the food to feed dairy and beef cattle. Once the "natural" feed products of the area were exhausted (such as wheat and grasses native to the region), it was necessary to research other crops that might suffice to feed the animals. Sweet clover was introduced, as the protein content and digestibility was similar to that of alfalfa. However, sweet clover was more prone to spoilage than the other food sources had been because of issues related to its high moisture content.

Soon, there were reports of unexplained hemorrhage and sickness in cattle that had been fed from the sweet clover after harvest. Through analysis, it was found that the spoilage of the clover created dicoumarol. Dicoumarol attached itself to the vitamin K present in the intestines of the cattle. Vitamin K is essential for several blood clotting mechanisms, so these cattle would bleed excessively, as the necessary vitamin was no longer usable.

In 1948, warfarin was created as a derivative of dicoumarol, and in 1952 it was introduced to the world as a type of rat poison. A young navy recruit decided that he wanted to end his life, and ingested a large dose of this warfarin rat poison. Remarkably, he did not die, although his blood clotting processes were definitely affected. This situation prompted more research into how warfarin could be used to treat humans, and in 1954, it was first authorized for human use as an oral anticoagulant. In 1955, President Eisenhower was treated with warfarin after a heart attack.

Warfarin (brand name Coumadin) is the most common drug prescribed worldwide. It is taken by those who have a prior history of blood clots or heart disorders such as atrial fibrillation and heart valve deformities, as well as given to surgical patients. The efficacy of warfarin can be affected by ingestion of foods that are high in vitamin K, such as cabbage, cauliflower, spinach, soybeans, and broccoli.

A CLIA-waived PT test procedure is used to monitor the anticoagulant effects of medications such as **warfarin** (Coumadin) in the physician office laboratory. These drugs are used by patients who are at a high risk for blood clot formation. Close monitoring of the effects of oral anticoagulants is necessary, as patients who have too much in their bloodstream run the risk of excessive bleeding, whereas those with too little could develop thrombosis.

A calculation called the **international normalized ratio (INR)** is reported with the PT result. The INR is a factor that allows for standardization of prothrombin tests performed with different methodologies and/or reagents. Prothrombin tests performed with different lot numbers of reagents or different methodologies may differ by 10% to 20% from one laboratory to another. This can be problematic when adjusting oral anticoagulant dosages based on PT test results. In 1983 the World Health Organization proposed a calculation (the INR) to standardize the variables that are present when performing prothrombin testing with various instruments and lot numbers for reagents. For an individual who is not on oral anticoagulants, the INR would be approximately 1, and for those who are being treated with warfarin or Coumadin, the INR should be 2 to 3. Decisions to change medication levels are based on the INR result, not the PT result that may be reported with the INR. Reference ranges for the prothrombin time may vary between laboratories, but they are approximately 11 to 13 seconds.

> **Test Your Knowledge 15-8**
>
> True or False: Is the INR used when screening for potential coagulation defects?   (Outcome 15-6)

The Coaguchek S, manufactured by Roche Diagnostics, is a CLIA-waived PT/INR testing method often used in the physician office laboratory. This type of analyzer is a point-of-care test (POCT) that allows for immediate results. Performance of this test in the office can benefit the patient by allowing the results to be available to the health-care provider within minutes. This allows the patient to receive any necessary instruction about medication changes warranted by the results while still in the office. The test requires only 10 microliters of blood (approximately one drop), and the sample may be obtained through a capillary puncture or a venipuncture.

In situations in which the PT and INR are ordered as part of a coagulation screen or when the testing is performed at a reference laboratory, a full, well-mixed, light blue top sodium citrate tube is required for the test.

Procedure 15-1: CLIA–Waived Prothrombin Time/INR Testing Using the CoaguChek S Instrument

TASK

Perform PT/INR testing utilizing the CoaguChek S instrument and document the results appropriately. Complete all steps within 10 minutes.

CONDITIONS

- Hand sanitization supplies
- Gloves
- Completed patient requisition form and patient chart
- CoaguChek S instrument
- Test strips
- Quality control material
- Test strip code chip
- Bulb and capillary provided with instrument for application of sample
- Gauze or cotton balls
- Alcohol pad for sanitization

- Lancet device or venipuncture supplies
- Biohazardous disposal container
- Biohazardous sharps container

Note: This test may be performed on a capillary blood sample or a sample obtained through venipuncture. Be certain to have the necessary supplies available for the method used for sample collection, as well as a biohazardous sharps disposal container and gloves.

CAAHEP/ABHES STANDARDS

 CAAHEP 2008 Standards

None

 ABHES 2010 Standards

None

Procedure	Rationale
1. Verify test ordered on requisition form. Greet and identify patient.	The requisition should always be examined to be certain which test is ordered, and the patient identity must always be verified before proceeding.
2. Sanitize hands, allow them to dry, and apply gloves.	Gloves protect the hands from exposure to potential bloodborne pathogens. Gloves should always be applied in the presence of the patient.
3. Gather necessary supplies. Test strips must be at room temperature for at least 5 minutes prior to use. Compare the number on the code chip (located in a small compartment at the top of the box of test strips) to the last three numbers after the lot symbol on the test strip pouch. If these numbers do not match, this code chip may not be used with these strips.	Supplies must be within reach before starting the process so that the timing of the testing is accurate. The code chip must be the correct number for the reagent strip for the test result to be accurate.
4. Verify whether quality control (QC) testing needs to be performed on the instrument. If so, perform QC testing and verify validity of results before proceeding with patient testing.	The frequency of the QC testing is based on the manufacturer's and individual laboratory recommendations.

5. Determine the method to be used for specimen collection.
  a. If a capillary sample is to be used, prepare the lancet. Roche manufactures a capillary tube and bulb to aid with specimen collection, as well as a lancet specifically designed to be used with the CoaguChek system. Assemble the capillary tube and bulb if desired. The blood may also be applied directly to the test strip without the aid of the capillary tube.
 	
  b. Blood obtained through venipuncture is acceptable, as long as it is collected into a preservative-free plastic syringe using a 21- to 23-gauge needle. The specimen would need to be applied to the strip immediately after the collection has been completed.
	The capillary sample is the most common method of testing used in the physician office laboratory.
	
	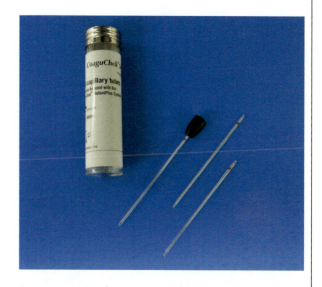
	
	Preservatives and/or anticoagulants are not acceptable for this testing method. The blood cannot be allowed to clot before application on the test strip, or the results will be inaccurate.

Continued

Procedure 15-1: CLIA–Waived Prothrombin Time/INR Testing Using the CoaguChek S Instrument—cont'd

Procedure	Rationale
6. Insert the code chip into the machine, and place the instrument on a flat, vibration-free surface. Turn on the power, and make certain that the code displayed on the screen matches the numbers printed on the foil wrapper enclosing the test strip.	If the codes do not match, the instrument will not provide a test result.
7. The test strip icon will flash on the CoaguChek S display screen. Open the foil pouch and insert a test strip into the instrument by sliding it (printed side up) into the tray on the front of the instrument in the direction of the arrows. Continue to push the test strip into the instrument until it stops. Test strips must be used within 4 minutes of removal from the foil package.	For most of the testing process, the CoaguChek S display screen will guide your next steps. 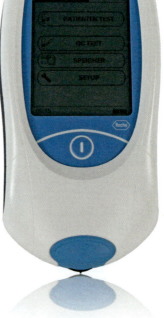 *Courtesy of Roche Diagnostics.*
8. Prepare the appropriate site for the capillary puncture, or obtain the blood sample via venipuncture.	Once the test strip is placed into the instrument, the time will be limited for the specimen to be collected and applied for the testing process.
9. Monitor the display screen; at this point, a test strip icon should be visible as well as a flashing clock icon. Do not apply the sample until the icon for a blood drop appears on the screen.	If the sample is applied too soon, the instrument will not process the sample and the screen will display an error.

Procedure	Rationale
10. Once the flashing blood icon appears on the screen, a countdown for 180 seconds begins. The instrument will beep every 30 seconds until an adequate sample has been applied to the test strip. The sample must be applied before the countdown reaches 0.	A countdown of 180 seconds should be adequate time to obtain the capillary sample, or to prepare to apply the venipuncture specimen.
11. Utilizing appropriate capillary or venipuncture procedure, obtain the blood sample. Apply a drop of blood to the test strip directly over the flashing yellow light. This flashing light indicates where the sample is to be applied.	For this procedure, the first drop of blood obtained from a capillary sample is to be used; do not wipe away the first drop of blood as you would customarily do for other types of collections. For samples obtained through venipuncture, the first four drops of blood are to be discarded from the end of the needle, after which the next drop is to be applied to the sample area. Do not allow bubbles to form when applying the sample.
12. After specimen application, the screen will display a clock icon. Do not touch the instrument or the test strip during this time. The result will be available on the screen (and stored in the memory of the instrument) within 1 minute.	The clock icon is displayed during the entire testing procedure.
13. Document the result on the instrument log sheet.	Once the test strip is removed from the machine, the result is no longer displayed on the screen, so it is best to record it immediately.
14. Discard the test strip by pulling it out of the instrument and discarding it into a biohazardous waste container.	The test strip is contaminated with blood and must be disposed of accordingly.
15. Sanitize the work area and put away supplies.	Be sure to refrigerate the test strips right after use.
16. Remove gloves and sanitize hands.	Hands must always be sanitized after removing gloves.
17. Document the test results in patient chart.	All results must be documented in the patient's chart.

Date	
04/18/2013:	PT/INR test performed from capillary puncture. PT result 23.2 seconds, INR 2.1
	Connie Lieseke, CMA (AAMA)

Activated Partial Thromboplastin Time/ Partial Thromboplastin Time

Activated partial thromboplastin time is abbreviated PTT. The PTT is a measurement of the efficacy of the intrinsic coagulation pathway. This pathway includes the actions of clotting factors VIII, IX, XI, and XII. The PTT is measured in seconds, just as the PT is. Technically it is the amount of time that the blood sample takes to clot when phospholipid and calcium are added to the specimen. The PTT test may be ordered (with the PT) as part of a presurgical screen, when a patient has excessive bleeding or bruising, or to monitor the use of **heparin** therapy. Heparin is a fast-acting anticoagulant that affects the factors in the intrinsic blood-clotting pathway. Heparin is used to treat patients who are at high risk for thrombosis and to treat those who have already developed blood clots, especially in postsurgical settings. Heparin is not a medication commonly used in the home setting, because it must be administered IV or by subcutaneous injection multiple times per day. Reference ranges for the PTT are 25 to 31 seconds, and the specimen must be a full light blue top sodium citrate tube.

Test Your Knowledge 15-9

Which medication is monitored by using the PTT?
    a. Coumadin
    b. warfarin
    c. heparin
    d. aspirin   (Outcome 15-8)

Platelet Count

One of the first steps in the coagulation process is the aggregation of platelets at the site of the vessel injury. For this reason, it is imperative that platelets are present in sufficient numbers and also that they function appropriately in order for the body to repair vessel damage as it should. Platelets are produced by the bone marrow, and when the blood vessels are injured, they adhere to the site of the injury and to other platelets. This primary "plug" helps to protect the body from excess blood loss, and also starts the clotting cascade, which ends with a more permanent fibrin mesh at the site to allow for the damage to heal.

Insufficient platelet amounts (thrombocytopenia) will put the patient at risk for excessive bleeding with vessel injury. A **platelet count** is performed to monitor the number of platelets present in the general circulation. Platelet counts are routinely performed as part of a complete blood count, and may also be ordered as part of a coagulation screen. The specimen required is a lavender top EDTA tube, and the reference range is 150,000 to 450,000 mm³.

Fibrinogen

Fibrinogen is a "sticky" substance manufactured by the liver that is an essential part of the blood-clotting process. It is naturally dissolved in plasma, and is the precursor to fibrin. Fibrin is necessary for effective blood clot formation. Fibrinogen is also known as clotting factor I. The presence of adequate levels of fibrinogen is essential to platelet aggregation. Levels of fibrinogen may be decreased in the presence of genetic disorders, resulting in a diagnosis of **afibrinogenemia** or **hypofibrinogenemia. Dysfibrinogenemia** is a rare

genetic disease that causes abnormal fibrinogen activity; the fibrinogen created in the liver is not able to convert to fibrin correctly to complete blood clot formation. Low levels of fibrinogen may contribute to excessive bleeding, and conversely, levels that are above the normal range may contribute to formation of small intravascular blood clots. Fibrinogen levels may be elevated in any condition that causes inflammation including pregnancy, acute infection, cancer, coronary heart disease, myocardial infarction (MI), and stroke. These increased levels of circulating fibrinogen will make the patient more prone to pathological blood clot formation, so the fibrinogen level test is often performed with the PT, PTT, and platelet count assays to screen for coagulation dysfunction. Reference ranges for fibrinogen are approximately 20 to 400 mg/dL, but may vary with the method used for testing by any individual laboratory. Fibrinogen requires a full light blue top sodium citrate tube.

Test Your Knowledge 15-10

If fibrinogen levels are decreased, what might a potential outcome be for the patient?   (Outcome 15-11)

Fibrin Degradation Products

Clot creation and subsequent breakdown must remain in balance for the body to maintain a healthy coagulation response. Once a damaged vessel has healed, **plasmin** (an enzyme designed to dissolve blood clots) and other chemicals in the plasma immediately begin to dissolve the fibrin mesh forming the clot so that it does not become too large. The by-products of fibrinolysis may be measured in the laboratory with an assay that measures **fibrin degradation products (FDPs).** FDPs are essentially fragments that are released as blood clots are dissolved. These fragments are released when fibrinogen (the precursor of fibrin) or fibrin is broken down by plasmin. The amount of fibrin degradation products increase in disseminated intravascular coagulation, pulmonary embolism, and with some obstetrical complications. In most laboratories, the FDP test is performed on plasma collected in a light blue top tube with sodium citrate anticoagulant. If the test is to be performed within 4 hours, the tube is to remain at room temperature. If the sample must be transported elsewhere for testing and the processing takes more than 4 hours, the tube should be spun down and the plasma must be frozen. Serum FDP assays may also be performed, which may require specific tubes that contain thrombin to clot the blood and chemicals to prevent fibrinolysis within the tube. Normal reference ranges for FDP are based on the testing procedure, and may vary.

D-Dimer

The FDP test measures all the breakdown products created as blood clots dissolve. One of these by-products is very specific for certain cross-linked components of the fibrin clot, and that can be measured by performing a **D-dimer** test. D-dimers are a specific type of breakdown product that indicates the dissolution of fibrin, rather than just fibrinogen. The D-dimer test is currently replacing the FDP analysis in many laboratories. D-dimers are always present in small amounts in the blood, but elevated levels may be indicative of disseminated intravascular coagulation, pulmonary embolism, or deep vein thrombosis. The body increases the amount of D-dimers produced as soon as a clot begins to form because the clot dissolution process starts almost simultaneously to keep the blood clot from growing larger than necessary. Surgical procedures may elevate D-dimer levels, as well as pregnancy, inflammation, some types of cancer, and liver disease. Use of **fibrinolytic drugs** (also called clot busters) will also increase the amount of FDP and D-dimers in the bloodstream, so these tests may be used to monitor fibrinolytic medication therapy as well. The reference ranges for D-dimers are based on the testing method used for the assay. The D-dimer analysis requires platelet-poor citrated plasma, drawn in a light blue top tube. The specimen must be spun in a typical benchtop centrifuge for at least 10 minutes before separation of the plasma from the cells. In addition, there are specialized centrifuges that are specially equipped to create platelet-poor plasma in less than 10 minutes for tests that require this type of specimen.

Bleeding Time Test

A bleeding time test is performed to evaluate how well platelets function to form a plug in the capillary beds with induced damage. It is not a test performed from a blood sample, but is a measurement performed directly on the patient. Because there are other tests used to monitor the different parts of the coagulation cascade, the bleeding time is generally used to identify platelet function abnormalities, and it may also detect deficiencies of **von Willebrand's factor,** which is part of the factor VIII used for blood clotting. The platelet count and all other clotting factors may be within the

normal reference ranges, but if the platelets do not perform as they should, the patient may still have issues with prolonged bleeding. In the past, the bleeding time test was a common presurgical laboratory order, but the true ability of the bleeding time to detect potential surgical hemorrhage has been called into question in recent years.

Bleeding times have been performed using various methods since they were first developed approximately 85 years ago. Many of these procedures were not standardized, so it was difficult to reproduce the results or to establish reliable normal reference ranges. Historically, the procedures all included a "stab" into soft tissues of the body (usually the earlobe) and monitoring the wound until bleeding had stopped. A lancet or surgical blade was used, but there was a lack of uniformity concerning the depth or length of the incisions created.

> **Test Your Knowledge 15-11**
>
> List two reasons that the bleeding time test is not considered to be the test of choice for platelet function analysis as it once was.   (Outcome 15-10)

Most modern facilities that perform bleeding times today use a modified Ivy method. This method includes the use of the Surgicutt, a spring-loaded lancet device manufactured by the International Technidyne Corporation. The blade in the lancet device has a depth of 1 mm and a width of 0.5 mm. The device is easy to use, and the blade retracts after use so that there is minimal opportunity for accidental employee exposure to patient fluid. The standardized depth and width of the incision has assisted in the determination of reliable reference ranges and safety for the patients. There are also special lancet devices available for use on infants.

Bleeding times are used to determine how long it will take for a patient to stop bleeding after a superficial puncture or incision is made into the skin. The bleeding time procedure requires an incision device (such as the Surgicutt), a sphygmomanometer (blood pressure cuff), an antiseptic wipe, sterile filter paper provided in circles, and an adhesive bandage. Figure 15-1 shows the supplies necessary to perform a bleeding time test. The performance of a bleeding time is a unique procedure and includes the following concepts:

1. It is essential to ask the patient about aspirin use within the past week. Even one aspirin, or other products that include aspirin, can profoundly affect the results obtained with the bleeding time.

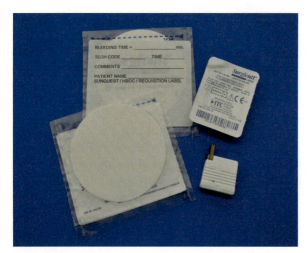

Figure 15-1 Bleeding time supplies including Surgicutt lancet and filter paper.

The patient should be asked whether he or she is under therapy with heparin or oral blood thinners such as warfarin. If the patient has taken any of these medications, you must check with the physician before performing the test, as the validity of the results may be affected. Long-term use of other NSAIDs (such as ibuprofen) may also increase the bleeding time.

2. The bleeding time is to be performed 2 to 3 inches below the bend of the elbow on the skin of the forearm. Visible veins, moles, tattoos, scars, bruises, shunts, or fistulas and edematous areas should be avoided, as well as areas with excessive hair growth. Clean the site thoroughly with an alcohol antiseptic wipe and allow the alcohol to dry completely before continuing with the procedure.

3. Apply a blood pressure cuff above the elbow to the arm to be used, and inflate the cuff to 40 mm Hg.

4. The bleeding time device (a Surgicutt lancet) is to be applied to the arm in a horizontal manner, and pressure must not be used when making the incision. Start the stopwatch as soon as the incision is made. At 30-second intervals, wick away excess blood with filter paper, taking care not to disturb the actual incision site. Rotate the filter paper as the blood is blotted away each time so that each wicking session is definitive.

5. When no more blood can be blotted away, stop timing the process and release the blood pressure cuff. The time that has elapsed since the incision was made is the bleeding time. Normal results are usually 1 to 9 minutes. If the results are less than 1 minute or

more than 9 minutes, some laboratories will require that the test be repeated, as there may be procedural errors that contributed to the result.

Bleeding times are not used as frequently as they once were, and many laboratories no longer offer this test as an option. It has been shown that the correlation of an elevated bleeding time to the risk of excessive surgical bleeding is not always conclusive, and the results for bleeding times are not reproducible. The procedure often causes a scar at the site of the incision, which can be a significant consequence to some patients. In addition, the use of NSAIDs (such as ibuprofen or Advil) may affect the bleeding time, in addition to aspirin or aspirin-containing products. The effect of the drugs on the bleeding time result is not predictable; the bleeding time may be extended, but it is difficult to predict the amount that it will be affected. Other variables may be the result of incorrect technique; if the incision is too deep or too shallow, the results will not be accurate. Also, when blotting away excess blood, if the incision is touched, the bleeding time may be falsely elevated.

It is important to realize that the PTT and PT tests are ordered much more commonly than the bleeding time test. These tests have fewer variables that could cause erroneous results than the bleeding time does, and abnormal results are mapped more specifically to the various coagulation factors. The bleeding time technique also requires specific training, whereas the PT and PTT tests require a more common capillary or venipuncture procedure. In addition, the bleeding time requires 10 to 20 minutes to complete, which may be too time intensive for busy practice or laboratory settings.

Other Tests Used to Assess Platelet Function

Platelet function cannot be measured just by counting the number of cells, and screening for platelet dysfunction is not as precise or easily performed as is a platelet count. The bleeding time test may help to identify gross platelet function abnormalities, but it is not sensitive or specific enough to identify all issues. Many reference and hospital laboratories are now using the Platelet Function Analyzer 100 (PFA-100), manufactured by Siemens Corporation. This machine tries to simulate the bleeding process that occurs in the body by using a tube of blood obtained through a venipuncture. The testing process involves the addition of whole blood into a tube that is coated with additives that promote platelet adherence and aggregation in order to mimic these actions within the human body. The machine measures the amount of time that is necessary for a blood clot to form within this treated tube, and this is reported as a closure time (CT).

There are other types of automated platelet function tests available, but they are not used as widely as is the PFA-100. Controversy still exists about whether these new automated tests are as useful for predicting overall platelet function assessment as the bleeding time once was, even though the bleeding time test is no longer performed in many institutions.

SPECIMEN REQUIREMENTS FOR COAGULATION TESTING

With the exception of CLIA-waived point-of-care PT testing, when collecting samples for coagulation testing, a light blue top tube with sodium citrate is used for most coagulation tests ordered. This includes the fibrinogen test, PTT, PT, and sometimes the FDP test. Some laboratories use a special FDP tube that only requires 2 mL of blood in a 5-mL tube.

- Evacuated light blue top vacuum tubes may include different concentrations of citrate (with the same volume of fluid anticoagulant in the tube), so it is important to clarify which type should be drawn for the testing method used in the laboratory where the testing will occur. The light blue top tubes may be available with 3.2% citrate or 3.5% citrate. In all situations, a ratio of one part anticoagulant to nine parts blood must be maintained, or the result will be erroneous because of specimen dilution.
- The citrate tube must be filled until the vacuum has been exhausted; no short samples can be tested. If the evacuated tube is not filled until the vacuum is exhausted, the clotting time (and subsequently the testing results) will be falsely elevated because of the dilution factor with the anticoagulant in the tube.
- Tubes are spun in the centrifuge before the test is performed, and the plasma is tested immediately or separated from the cells. Ideally, the sample will be tested within 1 hour of collection, or within 4 hours if the specimen has been refrigerated.
- For patients who have a hematocrit measuring above 55%, it is necessary to reduce the amount of anticoagulant used in the tube to avoid prolonged clotting times because of the change in the ratio of plasma to anticoagulant. Laboratories will have an established procedure for the performance of this process.

- It is critical that samples used for coagulation testing remain free of IV fluid or other contaminating substances. Many times the samples are drawn as part of the dialysis process, so it is especially critical to clear the line of all other fluids before the specimen is obtained.
- Clotted or hemolyzed samples will also not be acceptable for coagulation testing, as the results will be inaccurate. To avoid microclot formation in the tube, it is very important that the tubes used for coagulation studies are inverted at least eight times as soon as possible after collection.

> **Test Your Knowledge 15-12**
>
> True or False: Light blue top tubes collected for coagulation studies may be partially filled with no negative effects. (Outcome 15-13)

A lavender top tube with EDTA anticoagulant is used for platelet counts. Platelet counts may be performed as part of a complete blood count, or they may be ordered separately when needed. As in the case with the light blue top citrate tube, it is very important that the lavender top tube be mixed thoroughly right after the blood draw to avoid microclot formation. Platelet counts are performed on whole blood, so the specimen is not centrifuged after collection.

SUMMARY

Coagulation and clot dissolution are vital processes to maintain homeostasis in the human body. The repair of damaged blood vessels within the body is a complex process that includes platelets and a variety of chemical reactions to work efficiently. Coagulation studies determine whether there are enough platelets and other chemicals present for the process to be successful, as well as evaluating the efficiency of the clotting process to predict excessive bleeding or unnecessary blood clot formation. Other disease processes may be complicated by formation of small blood clots, so patients may be medicated with anticoagulant drugs to avoid potential problems. This medication use must be monitored closely with the use of coagulation tests on a regular basis. The anticoagulant medications target the various aspects of the clotting cascade and require different testing mechanisms to monitor their levels. Common tests used to monitor coagulation processes in the body and medications that affect the clotting mechanisms include the PT/INR test, platelet counts and platelet function tests, and the activated partial thromboplastin time. Other tests may be performed to evaluate the amount of clot dissolution or fibrinolysis occurring in the body. Coagulation testing may be performed in the physician office laboratory as well as in hospital and reference laboratories.

TIME TO REVIEW

1. *Aggregate* is a word used to describe: Outcome 15-1

   a. Platelet adhesion and clumping
   b. Consolidation of clotting factors
   c. Deep vein emboli
   d. Fibrinolysis

2. Which of these terms might be used   Outcome 15-1
   to define FDP?

   a. The factors necessary to form a clot
   b. Products produced as a clot dissolves
   c. Platelet count
   d. Clotting time

3. A substance that is viscous may also   Outcome 15-1
   be described as:

   a. Runny
   b. Thin
   c. Syrupy
   d. Dry

4. Fibrinolysis is an important part of   Outcome 15-3
   hemostasis because:

   a. Fibrinolysis helps to control the number of unwanted blood clots in the body
   b. Fibrinolysis is the first step in coagulation
   c. Fibrinolysis helps to keep the blood viscous
   d. None of the above

5. True or False: A diagnosis of atrial   Outcome 15-5
   fibrillation increases the risk of unwanted blood clot formation.

6. True or False: Postsurgical prophylactic   Outcome 15-5
   treatment is provided only to patients with hemophilia.

7. Platelet counts may be ordered as part   Outcome 15-8
   of a coagulation workup because:

   a. Adequate numbers of platelets are necessary for hemostasis
   b. Platelets play a very important role in the repair process for damaged vessels

   c. Extremely high numbers of platelets can contribute to excessive clot formation
   d. All of the above

8. What are two potential sources of   Outcome 15-7
   error for the CLIA-waived PT/INR test procedure?

9. How are D-dimers and fibrin   Outcome 15-12
   degradation products similar?

Case Study 15-1: Presurgical puzzle

Mr. Hammond will be having a total hip replacement next week. His physician orders a coagulation screen, including a PT, PTT, platelet count, fibrinogen level, and a bleeding time. All results are within the normal range except for the bleeding time, which at 12 minutes is elevated slightly.

1. What may be an explanation for this situation?

Case Study 15-2: Relative values?

Cindy Lou is a new medical assistant who has just started to work in the laboratory. She has experience a high volume of patients this morning, and she feels a bit overwhelmed. Later in the day, the physician office receives a call from the laboratory with abnormal PT and PTT results for one of the patients that Cindy drew that morning. The results for both tests are elevated, but the patient has no signs of excessive bruising or bleeding. These tests were ordered as a screen prior to an elective surgery that the patient was to have done next week.

The physician asks Cindy to contact the laboratory and see if the results for the platelet count are available. Cindy talks to the technician performing the hematology testing, and she is told that the specimen for the platelet count needs to be redrawn because it was clotted.

1. How do you think the specimen condition for the platelet count and the other tube used for the PT/PTT testing might be related?
2. How does this situation with the clotted tube relate to the elevated results for the PT and PTT?

RESOURCES AND SUGGESTED READINGS

"Atrial Fibrillation and Warfarin"
Excellent explanation of the risks involved with atrial fibrillation as related to blood clots, and the use of warfarin for treatment http://www.patient.co.uk/showdoc/23068883

"D-dimers and Fibrin Degradation Products"
Information about coagulation studies performed at Massachusetts General Hospital; great information about the differences between FDP and D-dimers http://www2.massgeneral.org/pathology/coagbook/CO002700.htm

"Disseminated Intravascular Coagulation (DIC); Consumption Coagulopathy; Defibrination Syndrome"
Details about disseminated intravascular coagulation disease. http://www.merck.com/mmpe/sec11/ch136/ch136c.html

"Hemophilia, Factor VIII Deficiency"
Facts about bleeding and clotting disorders http://www.hemophilia.org/NHFWeb/MainPgs/MainNHF.aspx?menuid=179&contentid=45&rptname=bleeding,

"Warfarin and Chinese Medicine"
Details about the development of warfarin, plus lots of information related to herbs and Chinese medications that affect bleeding tendencies. http://www.itmonline.org/arts/warfarin.htm

"ITC, The Point of Care, Surgicutt Bleeding Time Device"
Detailed information about the Surgicutt device and procedure for bleeding time testing. http://www.itcmed.com/Products/Surgicutt

Hematology and Coagulation
What Does It All Mean?

As you can see, hematology and coagulation testing provides invaluable information to physicians and other primary health-care providers. Now, let us revisit our Case in Point for this section and see what it all means.

Case in Point

At the beginning of this section we met M.J., a 38-year-old male patient who was worked into the doctor's schedule because he felt tired and weak and experienced bleeding gums after brushing his teeth. Patient history revealed that M.J. received a blood transfusion following a tractor accident several weeks prior to this appointment. Upon your encounter with M.J., you noted that he seemed very pale. The doctor ordered a CBC, PT, and PTT to help assess the situation. Upon examination of the results obtained (located on page 258), no wonder M.J. felt so poorly.

M.J. is suffering from a condition known as disseminated intravascular coagulation (DIC). *Disseminated*, in this case, means "widespread over the body." *Intravascular* refers to taking place within blood vessels, and *coagulation* means "the clotting of blood." Under normal conditions, the human body has built-in mechanisms to clot blood when injury occurs and to dissolve clots when appropriate. This balance between clotting and bleeding is known as *hemostasis*. However, when the clotting and bleeding balance is disrupted, individuals experience abnormal bleeding, as noted when M.J. bled while brushing his teeth, and clotting. This imbalance can cause serious injury to the organs of the body. Individuals become anemic, as evidenced by M.J.'s complaints of being tired and weak, as well as the observation of the patient being pale. This anemia results because of the incredible loss of blood, which in turn results in an inability of red blood cells to transport oxygen to the tissues. If the condition is left untreated, death may result. Fortunately, in M.J.'s case, he recognized the abnormal situation taking place in his body and sought help.

Although laboratory results are important in confirming the diagnosis and monitoring of DIC, physicians often make the initial diagnosis based primarily on clinical symptoms. Unfortunately there is no single laboratory test that is diagnostic for DIC; a battery of tests must be performed and the results examined in concert with each other rather than independently. In addition to the tests presented in this case study there are additional laboratory tests that may be performed to provide more information about the clinical situation when DIC is suspected. A further discussion of these additional tests is beyond the scope of this text.

On the Horizon

A wide variety of substances, often referred to as analytes, make up the test menu available in the chemistry section of the clinical laboratory. Likewise, the test methodologies that may be used to determine these analytes are many. Some tests are performed on complex instruments, whereas others are conducted using relatively simple-to-operate equipment. The results obtained from such tests provide healthcare team members with a wealth of knowledge in the diagnosis and monitoring of numerous diseases and conditions.

Relevance for the Medical Assistant

Medical assistants (MAs) typically assume one or both of these roles associated with chemistry laboratory tests: (1) specimen collection and processing and (2) performance of select chemistry tests. In addition to performing CLIA-waived tests, MAs may also perform moderate-complexity tests with appropriate training. Further, MAs may also review patient charts while performing their other duties and in the process may examine laboratory results (from this area as well as all areas of the laboratory). Familiarity of common laboratory tests and their significance allows MAs to take the information obtained from such reviews into account as they work with their patients.

Case in Point

You are working at a health fair being conducted at Acme Innovations, Inc. Part of the health fair consists of collecting blood for a fasting blood glucose level. The following result was obtained on Carrie W., a 34-year-old female Acme employee:

Test	Patient Result	Reference Range
Fasting blood glucose	215 mg/dL	70–100 mg/dL

Questions for Consideration:

- What does the word fasting refer to in this case?
- What is the purpose of the fasting blood glucose test?
- What laboratory test could be ordered to help assess this patient and to monitor Carrie's condition?
- Suppose that Carrie is pregnant and her doctor wishes to assess her for gestational diabetes. What laboratory test could be ordered in this situation?

Clinical Chemistry On the Horizon

The content in this section is limited to three chapters and serves as an overview of the chemistry section of the clinical laboratory:

Chapter 16: Overview of Clinical Chemistry introduces the reader to the scope of the chemistry section of the clinical laboratory, including the identification and brief description of specimens upon which this testing is performed. A brief overview of some of the more common individual chemical analytes, including glucose and cholesterol as well as groups of tests known as profiles, are covered.

Chapter 17: Glucose Testing covers the physiology and pathophysiology associated with blood glucose. The various glucose tests available, including venous blood samples, hemoglobin A1c, glucose tolerance tests, and capillary puncture glucose testing, are described. Suggested procedures and quality control considerations are also covered.

Chapter 18: Other Select Chemistry Tests covers the physiology and pathophysiology associated with the following representative chemistry tests: cholesterol, lipids, and electrolytes. Proper collection and testing technique, reference ranges, quality control issues, sources of error, and test interpretation are included.

Chapter 16

Overview of Clinical Chemistry

Constance L. Lieseke, CMA (AAMA), MLT, PBT(ASCP)

CHAPTER OUTLINE

Learning Outcomes

After reading this chapter, the successful student will be able to:

16-1 Define the key terms.

16-2 Relate how serum differs from plasma.

16-3 Describe common substances dissolved in plasma.

16-4 Examine the reasons that glucose testing is performed in the physician office laboratory.

16-5 Cite the tests included in a lipid panel.

16-6 List common analytes included in an electrolyte panel.

16-7 Differentiate which organ system is evaluated using a blood urea nitrogen test and creatinine test.

16-8 Evaluate the purpose of ordering tests in a panel format rather than individually.

16-9 Describe the tests commonly ordered as cardiac enzymes.

16-10 Explain the rationale for serial cardiac enzyme blood specimen collections.

16-11 Restate the liver profile tests most commonly ordered by physicians.

16-12 Outline the parameters that must be taken into account when considering reference ranges for clinical chemistry tests.

16-13 Examine potential sources of error for chemistry testing procedures.

CAAHEP/ABHES STANDARDS

  CAAHEP Standards

None

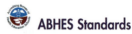 ABHES Standards

None

KEY TERMS

Analytes

Atherosclerosis

Basic metabolic panel (BMP)

Blood urea nitrogen (BUN)

Brain natriuretic peptide (BNP)

Cholesterol

Clinical chemistry

Comprehensive metabolic panel (CMP)

Creatine kinase (CK)

Creatinine

Diabetes mellitus

Electrolytes

Endogenous cholesterol

Exogenous cholesterol

Gestational diabetes

Glycosylated hemoglobin (Hb A1c)

High-density lipoprotein (HDL)

Hemolysis

Hepatic function panel

Homeostasis

Hyperlipidemia

Hyperthyroidism

Hypothyroidism

Icteric

Ischemia

Jaundice

Lipemia

Lipid

Lipoproteins

Low-density lipoprotein (LDL)

Lytes

Myocardial infarction

Myoglobin

Occlude

Physiology

Plaque

Plasma

Quality not sufficient (QNS) specimen

Qualitative

Quantitative

Serially

Serum

Thyroid-stimulating hormone (TSH)

Thyroxine (T4)

Triiodothyronine (T3)

Troponin

Very low-density lipoprotein (VLDL)

CLINICAL CHEMISTRY

When scientists first began to study the human body, their focus was on anatomy. Science was not able to analyze what could not be seen with the naked eye, so much of the **physiology** (or function) of the body was unknown. Many hypotheses were formed, but it took a very long time before they could be proved or disproved. It was obvious that the human body functioned best when in a state of **homeostasis** (internal balance), and the scientists could recognize some of the more visible means by which this balance was achieved. It was easy to see how the iris in the eye constricted when exposed to

bright light or when perspiration was formed on the forehead in hot weather. However, many of the small changes within the human body were not so obvious; they are based on adjustments to the levels of chemicals needed to keep our body functioning appropriately. It was not until the 19th century that scientists began to realize how closely the appropriate balance of these chemicals in the body was linked to overall health.

Clinical chemistry includes the **quantitative** analysis of the various **analytes** (substances being analyzed; in this case, chemicals) dissolved in the fluids of our bodies. Quantitative tests provide an actual number that represents the amount of a substance present in the body.

Qualitative testing, which indicates the presence or absence of specific chemicals, may also be performed in the clinical chemistry department in the laboratory. Chemical elements are present in our bodies at all times, but increases or decreases in the levels of certain analytes may be indicative of a disease process. Clinical chemistry testing allows the health-care provider to evaluate these changes and use them to diagnose and prescribe treatment. Procedures used to monitor drug levels for some prescription drugs or to identify substances that may be present in the body in the case of environmental or drug poisoning are also performed in the clinical chemistry area of the laboratory.

Test Your Knowledge 16-1

How are qualitative tests different from quantitative tests? (Outcome 16-1)

Reference laboratories may offer hundreds of clinical chemistry tests on various types of specimens. Although all these tests are clinically significant, many of them are only used in the presence of specific disease states. In this chapter, we concentrate on the most commonly performed clinical chemistry tests using blood, urine, and stool specimens.

SPECIMEN TYPES USED FOR CLINICAL CHEMISTRY ANALYSIS

Common specimens in clinical chemistry testing include urine, **serum,** and **plasma.** Many other fluid specimens, including cerebrospinal fluid, synovial fluid taken from the joints of the body, semen, amniotic fluid, and peritoneal fluid from the abdominal cavity, are analyzed for quantitative chemistry. Occasionally chemistry testing may be performed using whole blood. This is usually done in physician office laboratories using CLIA-waived testing methods. In larger laboratories, most clinical chemistry testing is performed on plasma or serum specimens separated from the sample after centrifugation. Serum is obtained from clotted blood and plasma comes from whole blood.

Plasma

As presented in Chapter 8, plasma is the liquid portion of the blood in our body in which the blood cells are suspended. This liquid makes up more than 50% of the total blood volume. We also use the word *plasma* to describe the liquid portion of the blood when collected in a tube containing anticoagulant. Plasma is made up of at least 90% water, in which there are many dissolved substances and gases. There are too many chemical compounds present in plasma to list them all separately, but general categories include the following:

- **Plasma proteins:** Plasma proteins are large molecules that are not excreted as waste products and which are designed to remain in the blood. These include antibodies (immunoglobulins), as well as blood-clotting proteins (fibrinogen and prothrombin) and albumin.
- **Medications:** If an individual must take medication, it is transported throughout the body in the plasma.
- **Electrolytes:** Electrolytes are compounds that have a positive or negative charge when dissolved in water, and are capable of transmitting an electrical impulse within the body.
- **Hormones:** Endocrine glands throughout the body secrete hormones directly into the bloodstream. Hormone tests are commonly ordered to verify the function of the various endocrine glands, such as the pituitary gland and thyroid gland.
- **Lipids:** Fat molecules such as cholesterol are transported through the bloodstream.
- **Enzymes:** Protein-based molecules that catalyze (speed up) chemical reactions are known as enzymes.
- **Food:** When digestion is complete, the food we eat has been broken into components that can be easily used by our body for energy or building blocks for other molecules. These breakdown products are absorbed into our bloodstream and dissolve in the plasma for transportation. Fatty acids, proteins, and simple sugars are carried as food in the plasma. In addition, essential trace elements such as minerals and vitamins are also present.
- **Dissolved gases:** CO_2 is present in plasma as a by-product of metabolism. Other dissolved gases include oxygen (even though it is attached to the red blood cells) and nitrogen.
- **Waste:** Cell metabolism creates waste products that are processed in the liver and removed from the body through the urinary system.

Serum

Serum is the liquid portion of blood that has been collected into a tube that does not contain anticoagulant. Plasma and serum are very similar; however, when a specimen is drawn in a tube without an anticoagulant, the proteins and other blood clotting factors are utilized as the blood clot forms. The lack of coagulation factors dissolved in the liquid limits some of the tests that may be performed on a serum specimen.

Test Your Knowledge 16-2

Which of these are present from a centrifuged tube containing no anticoagulant?
   a. Serum
   b. Plasma
   c. Whole blood
   d. None of the above   (Outcome 16-2)

Other Specimen Types Used for Clinical Chemistry Testing

As mentioned previously in this chapter, clinical chemistry testing may be performed on numerous specimen types. In the physician office laboratory, whole blood may be used for CLIA-waived procedures such as glucose or cholesterol testing, providing a quantitative result.

Urine chemical testing is performed as part of a routine random urinalysis with semiquantitative results reported that indicate a range for the analyte values. In some disease states, it is necessary to obtain results that are more specific, with a specific number reported for the chemical concentration rather than a range. This type of quantitative urine chemistry testing is performed at reference or large hospital laboratories, but not in physician office laboratories. These quantitative urine tests may be used to screen for kidney damage caused by diabetes, hypertension, or other disease processes. Urine may also be analyzed to research the cause of renal calculi (kidney stone) formation. Common quantitative tests performed on urine specimens include microalbumin, total protein, and creatinine. A timed urine specimen (such as a 24-hour urine specimen) is generally used for these tests.

For all clinical chemistry testing, it is important to keep in mind that reference ranges are based on certain specimen types. For instance, serum and plasma look identical once the liquid has been removed from the blood specimen, but the reference ranges for some chemicals are very different in the two specimen types. It is essential to collect the correct type of tube for the analysis when performing a blood collection, and also to label the specimen type if the liquid is removed from the original collection container to avoid any potential problems. Other types of specimens may have a similar appearance if they are transported in an unlabeled specimen container.

CLIA–WAIVED CLINICAL CHEMISTRY TESTS

Glucose Testing

The most common type of CLIA-waived clinical chemistry test performed in the clinic setting is glucose testing. This test may be used to screen for **diabetes mellitus** (type 2 diabetes) or to monitor the glucose levels of patients who have already been diagnosed and are under treatment. **Gestational diabetes** in pregnant women may also be diagnosed with tests performed in the physician office laboratory. It is beneficial to the patient to have these tests performed on site, as the results are available within minutes. Abnormal glucose levels may be reported to the health-care provider immediately, allowing for additional tests to be ordered or for further patient interaction to be initiated if necessary. CLIA-waived glucose testing methods use whole blood specimens, usually obtained from a capillary puncture. The glucose levels may be ordered as fasting, random, or timed specimens.

Test Your Knowledge 16-3

List two reasons that glucose testing might be performed in a physician office laboratory.   (Outcome 16-4)

Diabetic patients may also be monitored with a **glycosylated hemoglobin,** or **Hb A1c,** test. Hemoglobin is present in all the red blood cells of the body, and one subunit of this hemoglobin molecule is hemoglobin A. When hemoglobin A is exposed to excessive levels of glucose, it becomes glycosylated, which means that the glucose molecules bind to the hemoglobin A irreversibly. The Hb A1c test can measure the amount of glycosylated hemoglobin present, and because red blood cells live for approximately 3 months in the body, Hb A1c results may be used indirectly as an indication of the overall blood sugar levels for the past few months. Hb A1c may be performed as a CLIA-waived test in the physician office laboratory or automated testing may be performed in a reference laboratory. Whole blood is used for this analysis; capillary samples are used for the CLIA-waived methods, and an EDTA lavender top tube is used for the reference laboratory methods.

Cholesterol and Lipid Testing

Lipids are substances including oils and fats that are insoluble in water and soluble in organic solvents. **Cholesterol** is an example of a lipid, but there are other types of fats in our bodies as well. Our digestive system breaks down ingested fats into fatty acids, which are transported through the bloodstream to the liver, where they are used to manufacture lipids. Because lipids do not dissolve in water, the body attaches lipids to a protein molecule for transport to the cells of the body to be used. These complexes are called **lipoproteins.** Lipids are used as an alternative source of energy when glucose is not readily available, and they are also necessary for hormone production, cell wall integrity, utilization of fat-soluble vitamins, hunger satiation, maintenance of appropriate body temperature, and skin health.

In the laboratory, the two types of lipids most commonly analyzed are cholesterol and triglycerides. Total blood cholesterol and total triglyceride counts provide valuable information to health-care providers about cardiovascular health and potential risk factors for the future. However, more information can be gained by breaking down the relative amounts of lipids according to subtype. These categories are **HDL (high-density lipoproteins), LDL (low-density lipoproteins),** and **VLDL (very low-density lipoproteins).** Elevated total cholesterol, triglyceride, and LDL levels may are considered to be risk factors for coronary heart disease. Chapter 18 provides more in-depth information about lipid testing.

Test Your Knowledge 16-4

Which of these tests is included in a lipid panel?
  a. LDH
  b. LDL
  c. VLDL
  d. ALT   (Outcome 16-5)

Cholesterol

Cholesterol is essential for the human body to function properly. Cholesterol is used for hormone production, absorption of vitamin D, bile production, and cellular membrane structure, and is also used as part of the covering (the myelin sheath) on some of the nerves in the body. The liver creates all the cholesterol that we need to function normally. This is called **endogenous cholesterol** because it is manufactured within the body. **Exogenous cholesterol** comes from our diets. When cholesterol builds up in the body it can lead to **plaque** formation within the blood vessels, a condition known as **atherosclerosis.** Plaque buildup may eventually **occlude** (block) blood vessels, or pieces of plaque may break away from the vessel lining and travel as an embolus, lodging elsewhere in the body and causing a blood clot.

Cholesterol levels ordered individually do not require fasting samples. However, cholesterol levels are often ordered as part of a lipid panel with the triglyceride,

HDL, LDL, and VLDL levels. These additional tests do require a fasting sample, so patients should be advised to abstain from eating for 12 hours prior to the blood draw.

Triglycerides

Patients who have a diet that is high in carbohydrates may have elevated triglyceride levels. Most of the fat in our bodies is made up of triglycerides. When a person takes in more calories than are needed for energy, the excess calories are converted into triglycerides and stored as fat for use later as an energy source. Those who have diabetes, hypertension, or excess alcohol intake are especially prone to high triglyceride levels. **Hyperlipidemia** is the word used to describe high levels of lipids (cholesterol and triglycerides) in the plasma. Patients who have elevated triglyceride levels may have plasma or serum that appears "milky" because of all the fat molecules present. The presence of the fat molecules suspended in the blood is called **lipemia.** Because triglyceride levels do rise after ingestion of food, triglyceride testing usually requires a fasting blood draw.

Lipid Panels

A lipid panel commonly includes a total cholesterol level, a triglyceride level, HDL, LDL, VLDL, and a total cholesterol : HDL ratio. These values will provide the health-care provider with valuable information concerning the risk factors for coronary artery disease.

POINT OF INTEREST 16-1
Cholesterol testing

Cholesterol testing is performed to assist the health-care provider in evaluating the patient for potential heart disease. The total cholesterol level consists of high-density lipoproteins (HDL) and low-density lipoproteins (LDL). The HDL is considered to be "good cholesterol" because it actually cleans excess cholesterol from the blood vessels in the body and carries it away in the bloodstream. Ideally, the patient will have a higher concentration of HDL in the bloodstream than LDL. Elevated levels of LDL may lead to heart disease, as the low-density lipoproteins will deposit cholesterol on the walls of the blood vessels.

There is a direct correlation of elevated cholesterol results and/or an imbalance of HDL and LDL results and atherosclerosis. The following individuals are at higher risk than others:

• Smokers
• Those diagnosed with diabetes mellitus

Continued

- Patients with hypertension
- Men over 45 and women over 55
- Family history of heart disease
- Obesity

Laboratory tests usually place the patient in one of three categories:

High risk: Having a total cholesterol level of 240 mg/dL or above

Borderline high: Having a cholesterol result of 200 to 239 mg/dL. Often the health-care provider will order additional testing to see if the elevated level is the result of the presence of the LDL (bad cholesterol) or HDL (good cholesterol).

Desirable or normal: Having a total cholesterol level less than 200 mg/dL is considered normal, and places the patient at a low risk of heart disease.

Triglyceride testing is often performed with the cholesterol assay in the laboratory as part of a lipid panel. Triglycerides are a form of fat, and are often carried by another lipoprotein, very low-density lipoprotein (VLDL). Elevated levels of triglycerides in the bloodstream may also lead to heart disease. Poor diet and low levels of exercise may lead to elevated triglyceride levels.

Electrolytes

Routine blood screening often includes an order for **electrolytes.** Electrolytes (often abbreviated as **lytes**) include several minerals that are essential for normal body function. They carry an electrical charge (positive or negative charge) when dissolved in water. Sodium, potassium, chloride, and CO_2 are usually included in an electrolyte assay. Additional tests may also be included by some laboratories, such those for as magnesium and calcium. Electrolyte assays may provide information to the health-care provider about the acid-base balance of the body, causes for edema, or additional information about the status of kidney dysfunction. Electrolyte levels may also be altered by certain drugs, dehydration, and overhydration. The tests within the electrolyte panel may be ordered individually, or as a group. CLIA-waived automated procedures are available for electrolyte testing, but these tests may also be performed at hospital laboratories and reference laboratories. More information is available about the specific testing methods for electrolytes and the clinical significance of the analytes in Chapter 18.

Test Your Knowledge 16-5

Which of these analytes is not included in an electrolyte panel?
   a. Sodium
   b. Potassium
   c. Chloride
   d. Cadmium   (Outcome 16-6)

OTHER COMMON CLINICAL CHEMISTRY TESTS

So far, we have focused on clinical chemistry tests that may be performed in the physician office laboratory as well as reference laboratories. In this section of the chapter, we focus on some of the most commonly ordered clinical chemistry tests that are not usually performed in the physician office laboratory. These tests would all be performed on serum or plasma in a hospital or reference laboratory. Many of these commonly performed tests are ordered as profiles or panels rather than individual tests. The panels are beneficial to the health-care provider because the tests included in a panel may evaluate various aspects of a specific organ system; in the case of the **basic metabolic panel (BMP)** and **comprehensive metabolic panel (CMP),** they evaluate parameters of several organ systems. Obtaining all the results at once can allow for a differential diagnosis, and also may save the patient time and money by not having to return to the laboratory for separate blood draws. Charges for the tests included in a Medicare-approved panel may not legally surpass the costs of ordering the tests individually, so it is cost effective to perform multiple tests at one time.

Test Your Knowledge 16-6

List two advantages of ordering tests as a panel rather than individually.   (Outcome 16-8)

Blood Urea Nitrogen

As protein is broken down by the body, it produces urea as a by-product. Nitrogen is part of this urea molecule. Urea should be cleared from the blood by the kidneys, so if the level blood urea nitrogen is elevated, it may be an indication that the patient has impaired renal function. **Blood urea nitrogen (BUN)** is a measurement of the amount of urea in the bloodstream. This test is often ordered in conjunction with a creatinine test.

Creatinine

Creatinine is a by-product of muscle metabolism. As in the case with the blood urea nitrogen, creatinine should be cleared from the blood by the kidneys. Elevated creatinine levels may indicate impaired kidney function. Creatinine levels may be performed on urine samples to correlate the levels with those obtained from testing the serum or plasma. This provides more in-depth information about potential kidney dysfunction.

Test Your Knowledge 16-7

True or False: BUN and creatinine tests are routinely ordered to evaluate kidney function. (Outcome 16-7)

Thyroid Panels

The thyroid gland secretes several very important hormones directly into the bloodstream. These hormones, **thyroxine (T4)** and **triiodothyronine (T3)** are essential for regulation of cellular metabolism. The thyroid gland also secretes thyrocalcitonin, which helps to stimulate calcium storage in the bones of the body. Many laboratories offer thyroid panels that include the T3 and T4. Another hormone that affects thyroid function is the **TSH (thyroid-stimulating hormone),** which is secreted by the pituitary gland. Thyroid-stimulating hormone is necessary for the thyroid to be "stimulated" to produce the T3 and T4. For the thyroid gland to function normally, there must be a source of iodine in the diet. Iodine can be ingested with iodized salt, seafood, or vegetables that were grown in soil with supplementary iodine. **Hypothyroidism** is a condition in which the thyroid gland does not produce enough of the hormones necessary to stimulate cell metabolism at a normal level. Patients may also suffer from **hyperthyroidism,** in which case the thyroid gland is producing hormones at a level that is above normal, resulting in overstimulation of cell metabolism. TSH levels outside of the normal range may cause under- or overstimulation of the thyroid gland, resulting in an imbalance; for this reason, the TSH may also be included in some thyroid panels.

Comprehensive Metabolic Panel and Basic Metabolic Panel

The CMP is a set of 14 tests that screen for problems with the kidneys, glucose metabolism, liver, and acid-base balance of the body. The CMP may be used as a general screening test during a routine office visit, or the panel may be ordered to monitor medication use or

changes in a disease process. The tests included in this panel are BUN, creatinine, sodium, potassium, chloride, carbon dioxide, calcium, albumin, total protein, bilirubin, alkaline phosphatase (often abbreviated as ALP), alanine aminotransferase (also called SGPT or ALT), aspartate aminotransferase (which may also be known as SGOT or AST), and glucose. The CMP is a panel that has been approved for payment by the Center for Medicare & Medicaid Services (CMS), so it is acceptable for it to be ordered as a diagnostic test for patients with Medicare coverage.

The BMP includes eight tests that will help to identify problems with electrolytes, kidney function, glucose metabolism, and acid-base balance. The basic metabolic panel may be used as a diagnostic tool, or used to monitor medication use or patient progress with ongoing treatment. The BMP includes glucose, calcium, sodium, potassium, carbon dioxide, BUN, and creatinine levels. The BMP has also been approved for payment as a panel by the CMS, so patients who have Medicare as their primary insurance may have this test ordered knowing that its cost is reimbursable.

Cardiac Enzymes

Cardiac enzymes are ordered in situations in which the health-care provider suspects damage to the heart, as in the case of **ischemia** (a temporary decrease of blood flow to the heart muscle) or in the case of trauma to the heart muscle from a **myocardial infarction** (heart attack). The profile usually includes a total **creatine kinase (CK)** and a CK-MB, in addition to other tests such as **troponin** or **myoglobin.** Creatine kinase is found in muscles other than the heart muscle; therefore, if the total CK level is elevated, additional testing must be performed to identify the source of the abnormal result. CK isoenzymes are subtypes of the creatine kinase analyte. The CK-MB (creatine kinase myocardial band) isoenzyme is a specific marker for heart muscle damage. The CK-MB levels will start to rise in the bloodstream approximately 4 hours after a myocardial infarction, and will peak approximately 18 hours after the event. Troponin levels will be elevated with heart muscle damage, but not with other types of muscle trauma. Troponin I levels are especially sensitive to myocardial damage. Troponin testing may be performed on a STAT basis when a myocardial infarction is suspected because these levels become elevated sooner and remain elevated longer than the CK-MB after a heart attack. This allows for earlier diagnosis and appropriate treatment. It is recommended that the troponin levels are tested every 2 to 4 hours for the first 24 hours after a cardiac event. Myoglobin may also be used as an indicator for a myocardial infarction, because it will be elevated in the bloodstream sooner after a cardiac event than troponin will be. Myoglobin is found in cardiac and skeletal muscles, so the levels may be elevated in the bloodstream in situations other than myocardial infarction because it is not specific to the heart muscle.

When a patient has chest pain and a myocardial infarction is suspected, the cardiac enzymes are ordered **serially,** because the levels of the various components will change with time if there was damage to the heart muscle. Specimens are usually collected every few hours, and the health-care provider looks for a pattern in the elevation of the different components to rule out or differentially diagnose damage to the heart muscle as a result of a heart attack. If the specimens are not drawn several times within the first 24 hours, it is not possible to establish whether a heart attack really occurred. The myoglobin is usually the first test to be elevated, but most health-care providers like to have more information before proceeding with a differential diagnosis. It is important to remember that other diagnostic procedures (such as an electrocardiogram) will also assist with the diagnosis as well.

Another common cardiac analysis is the **brain natriuretic peptide (BNP)** test. BNP is synthesized in the ventricles of the heart. The BNP secretion rate is increased under conditions of additional myocardial stretch and abnormal wall tension. The test is used to differentiate whether dyspnea (difficulty breathing) is the result of pulmonary conditions or cardiac dysfunction. An excessively elevated BNP level is indicative of heart failure.

Test Your Knowledge 16-8

Why are cardiac enzymes ordered as a series of blood draws rather than just once?　(Outcome 16-10)

Hepatic or Liver Profile

Disorders of hepatic (liver) function may be diagnosed using a **hepatic function panel.** Many of the hepatic enzymes are also found in other tissues of the body. The use of a panel may be helpful to the provider for a differential diagnosis. Patients with elevated liver enzymes often exhibit **jaundice** (yellowing of the skin and eyes), nausea and vomiting, or urine that is dark in color. Specimens obtained from patients with liver disease or damage may have plasma or serum that appears **icteric.** Icteric samples have a dark yellow or greenish tint to the fluid portion of the blood, which often correlates to an elevated total bilirubin level. Hepatic function panels may also be used to monitor liver function when patients are taking medication

that is known to cause hepatic damage. This panel usually includes at least seven tests that may be elevated with liver dysfunction: ALT (alanine aminotransferase), alkaline phosphatase, AST (aspartate aminotransferase), bilirubin, total protein, and albumin.

Hepatic function panels may include additional tests in some laboratory settings. However, if there are additional tests added to those listed above, Medicare may not pay for the tests performed.

Test Your Knowledge 16-9

Which of these tests are included in a hepatic function panel?
- a. AST
- b. Total protein
- c. ALT
- d. None of the above
- e. All of the above　　　　(Outcome 16-11)

REFERENCE RANGES

It is important to realize that the reference ranges for clinical chemistry tests are based on the technique used by the laboratory performing the test, the age and gender of the patient, the test preparation, and sometimes even by the time of the day that the specimen was drawn. Occasionally there may be a difference in reference ranges for the plasma versus serum samples as well. It is important always to document the details of the blood draw and patient preparation carefully when collecting the blood sample so that the reference ranges will be accurate. It is also essential that the medical assistant learn how to read the laboratory report so that abnormal results are recognized immediately. The reference ranges for the laboratory tests listed in this chapter are included in Table 16-1 and Table 16-2.

POTENTIAL SOURCES OF ERROR

The most common sources of error for clinical chemistry tests occur in the preanalytical area. These include improper patient preparation, inappropriate specimen collection techniques, and errors in specimen processing. Specific sources of specimen processing errors include the following:

- **Hemolysis:** A sample can be hemolyzed (the red blood cells broken open) during specimen collection or afterward during processing. Examples of procedures that may cause **hemolysis** include a traumatic blood draw, using a needle that is too small for the collection process,

TABLE 16-1

Reference ranges for glucose testing

	Fasting Plasma Glucose	2-Hour Postprandial Glucose
Normal	70–100 mg/dL	Less than 140 mg/dL
Prediabetes	101–125 mg/dL	141–199 mg/dL
Diabetes	126 mg/dL or above	200 mg/dL or above

Data from American Diabetes Association.

TABLE 16-2

Reference ranges for common chemical analytes (listed alphabetically)

Analyte	Normal Range (Adults)
Albumin (Alb)	3.5–5 g/dL
Alkaline phosphatase (ALP)	42–136 U/L
Alanine aminotransferase (ALT)	10–35 U/L
Aspartate aminotransferase (AST)	0–35 U/L
Bilirubin, total (TBili)	0.3–1 mg/dL
Blood urea nitrogen (BUN)	10–20 mg/dL
Brain natriuretic peptide (BNP)	0–100 ng/L
Calcium (Ca)	8.2–10.5 mg/dL
Carbon dioxide (CO_2)	22–30 mEq/L
Chloride (Cl)	96–106 mEq/L
Cholesterol, total (Chol)	Less than 200 mg/dL
Creatinine (Creat)	0.6–1.2 mg/dL
Creatine kinase (CK) aka Creatine Phosphokinase (CPK)	55–170 U/L
High-density lipoprotein (HDL)	Greater than 50 mg/dL
Lactate dehydrogenase (LD, LDH)	100–190 U/L
Low-density lipoprotein (LDL)	Less than 100 mg/dL
Myoglobin	Less than 90 µg/L
Potassium (K)	3.5–5.0 mEq/L
Sodium (Na)	136–145 mEq/L
Thyroid-stimulating hormone (TSH)	0.4–4.2 µU/mL
Thyroxine (T4)	4.5–11.2 µg/dL
Triglyceride (Trig)	Less than 150 mg/dL
Triiodothyronine (T3)	75–220 ng/dL

shaking a tube after collection rather than using gentle inversion, or subjecting the whole blood sample to extreme heat or cold temperatures. Hemolysis may also result if a tube without anticoagulant is centrifuged before the specimen is allowed to clot adequately. Any activity that causes the red blood cells in the specimen to be agitated unnecessarily may potentially cause the red blood cells to be broken. Hemolysis causes the serum or plasma to take on a red color, which interferes with many testing methods. Figure 16-1 shows a specimen

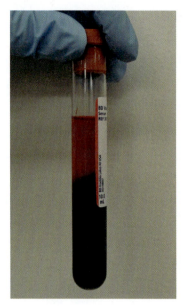

Figure 16-1   A centrifuged blood specimen with hemolysis evident in the serum.

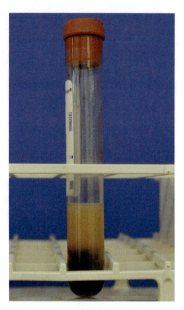

Figure 16-2   A centrifuged blood specimen with lipemia evident in the serum.

with visible hemolysis. Hemolysis may also increase levels of certain analytes in the plasma (potassium or iron, for instance) that are not normally present in high concentrations. The reference ranges for these chemicals are based on nonhemolyzed specimens, so it may appear that the patient needs treatment for an imbalance when the result is erroneous due to hemolysis.

- **Lipemic specimens:** Lipemia is present in a specimen when there are too many lipoproteins in the blood circulation. The excessively high levels of lipoproteins may be caused by hereditary hyperlipidemia or chronic liver disease. Malabsorption disorders may also cause lipemia to be evident. More often, lipemia results when a patient has not followed the instructions for specimen preparation by not fasting as directed before the blood draw. Lipemic specimens have a "milky" appearance that may be visible immediately after collection or after centrifugation. These fatty particles suspended in the specimen will interfere with many clinical chemistry assays. Some testing may be possible if the specimen is "cleared" using a special centrifugation process, but often the laboratory will ask that the specimen be redrawn if the lipemia is severe. Lipemia is evident in the specimen included in Figure 16-2.
- **Specimen collection errors:** The medical assistant who is performing specimen collection needs to keep the difference between plasma and serum samples in mind. If a test calls for a serum sample, a tube without anticoagulant must be used for the collection. In

addition, certain test results may also be affected if a tube with serum/plasma separator gel is used for the collection. Specifics about the type of specimens that are acceptable and unacceptable for a particular test would be listed in the laboratory directory, which provides collection specifics for the tests offered by that laboratory. This SST restriction is most common when collecting specimens for medication levels.

Another potential source of error when collecting clinical chemistry specimens is the incorrect timing of the collection. Tests may be ordered as a series of blood draws, as in the case of the cardiac enzymes. Medication levels may also be ordered at specific times as peak and trough draws. It is important to understand the process involved in these timed collections so that the specimens are properly labeled and the reference ranges are matched to the specimen type. In the case of medication levels, it is important to find out if there are restrictions concerning the length of time between the last dose and the specimen collection so that the health-care provider will receive results that allow for proper treatment of the patient.

In addition to the incorrect type of specimen collection and the incorrect timing, another potential source of error is the order in which the tubes are collected. Carryover of anticoagulant from one tube to another may cause changes in the levels of certain analytes when the testing procedures are performed. Potassium levels, for example, may be elevated if the lavender top tube is collected before the green top tube and a carryover of anticoagulant results.

- **Quantity not sufficient:** Laboratory directories provide information about the volume needed for testing procedures, and they may also provide a minimum volume accepted for the test. A **QNS specimen** (one that does not have the quantity necessary for testing) will require a re-collection, which delays potential treatment for the patient. These volume requirements must be taken into consideration before the sample is collected; they can affect the choices made concerning which type of collection setup to use and how many tubes to draw. The stated minimum volumes usually allow the test to be performed *only once;* this means that if there are any errors during the analysis or an extremely high or low result, retesting the sample will not be possible. Sometimes it is necessary to retest the sample using dilutions to obtain a true value, but this would also not be possible if only the minimum volume is submitted to the laboratory.
- **Exposure to light:** Some analytes (bilirubin and ferritin, for example) will deteriorate when exposed to light after collection. These samples need to be covered immediately (usually wrapping foil around the tube will suffice) and centrifuged as soon as possible. The plasma or serum to be analyzed should be separated into a tube designed to protect the specimen from light exposure. Figure 16-3 shows an amber plastic transfer tube that is designed to minimize the light exposure for a specimen.
- **Exposure to air:** Once a specimen has been centrifuged, it may be necessary to remove the rubber top of the tube and separate out the plasma or serum. The exposure to air should be minimized, as the concentration for some analytes will change with the exposure. Alcohol analysis is an excellent example of this; the longer the tube is open, the lower the alcohol concentration may become in the specimen. Carbon dioxide is another common analyte that may decrease with continued exposure to air.
- **Specimen processing:** Careful adherence to specimen processing is essential for clinical chemistry tests. Many of the chemical concentrations will change when left at room temperature for extended periods of time, so researching the specimen requirements prior to processing is important. If there is a question about how to handle a specimen, the laboratory directory should be consulted, and if necessary, the testing laboratory should be contacted for clarification *before* the specimen is collected. Plasma or serum may require freezing or refrigeration within a certain amount of time after collection to maintain the integrity of the sample. It is also necessary to prechill specimen collection tubes for some analytes.

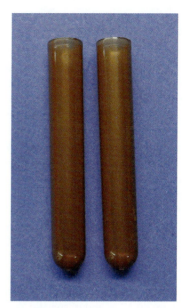

Figure 16-3   Amber transfer tubes designed to minimize specimen exposure to light.

- **Delayed processing:** Blood specimens to be used for clinical chemistry should be centrifuged as soon as possible so that the plasma or serum can be removed from the cells in a timely manner. Serum tubes must be allowed to clot completely before centrifuging. Delayed separation of cells from plasma or serum will allow analytes that are in a higher concentration within the cells than outside the cells to "leak" out of the cells and cause erroneous test results. This can result in an inaccurate diagnosis and/or unnecessary treatment for the patient. Conversely, glucose that is present in the plasma or serum will continue to be used by the cells in the specimen as an energy source if the serum or plasma is not removed from the cells in a timely manner. Therefore, the longer that the cells remain in contact with the fluid portion of the blood, the lower the glucose levels will become in the plasma or serum. This can make it appear that the patient has a very low plasma glucose level when the specimen is tested in the laboratory.

Test Your Knowledge 16-10

Which of these potential sources of error are related to high levels of lipids in the bloodstream?
   a. Lipemia
   b. Hemolysis
   c. Erroneous low glucose levels
   d. QNS specimens   (Outcome 16-13)

SUMMARY

Clinical chemistry is a complex component of laboratory testing. There are hundreds of tests that may fall into this category, and the specimen collection and processing requirements will vary depending on the testing method and laboratory policies. Some clinical chemistry tests may be performed in physician office laboratories; most of these will use whole blood specimens for analysis. Common clinical chemistry tests performed in the physician office laboratory include glucose and cholesterol testing. Clinical chemistry tests performed at reference laboratories are usually performed on plasma or serum specimens rather than whole blood specimens. Many of these tests may be ordered as panels or profiles. There are numerous sources of error in specimen collection and processing for clinical chemistry tests, so the medical assistant has to remain diligent about specific specimen requirements to provide appropriate specimens for meaningful laboratory results.

TIME TO REVIEW

1. Atherosclerosis is: Outcome 16-1
   a. Hardening of the arteries due to age
   b. A buildup of waxy plaque on the lining of blood vessels
   c. A condition related to high glucose levels
   d. The presence of occult blood in the stool

2. Creatinine is present in the blood   Outcome 16-1
   as a by-product of:
   a. Protein metabolism
   b. Heart damage
   c. Muscle metabolism
   d. Glucose metabolism

3. Myoglobin and troponin are   Outcome 16-1
   examples of:
   a. Tests included in a typical hepatic function panel
   b. Tests included in a typical renal function panel
   c. Tests included in the BMP
   d. Tests included in an order for cardiac enzymes

4. True or False: Plasma is the liquid   Outcome 16-2
   portion of the blood separated after centrifugation from a tube that does not contain anticoagulant.

5. True or False: Hemoglobin is a   Outcome 16-3
   substance that is dissolved in blood plasma.

6. Which of these tests are not   Outcome 16-5
   included in a typical lipid panel?
   a. Total cholesterol
   b. Total triglyceride
   c. VLDL
   d. Creatinine

7. An electrolyte panel typically   Outcome 16-6
   includes which of these tests?
   a. BUN
   b. CPK
   c. ALT
   d. Potassium

8. True or False: A panel of laboratory   Outcome 16-8
   tests costs more for the patient than ordering all the tests in the panel individually.

9. Which of these tests are not   Outcome 16-9
   usually included in a cardiac panel?
   a. ALT
   b. CK-MB
   c. CK
   d. Myoglobin

10. Which of these factors may be   Outcome 16-12
    taken into consideration when evaluating reference ranges for a test?
    a. Age and gender of the patient
    b. Testing methodology
    c. Time of day for specimen collection
    d. All of the above

11. True or False: Hemolysis is avoidable   Outcome 16-13
    when collecting a blood sample.

Case Study 16-1: What order?

Mr. Oliver arrived early for his blood draw one Monday morning. The medical assistant was running late that day, and seemed to be a bit distracted as she prepared for the blood draw. Mr. Oliver's physician had ordered a CBC (to be collected in a potassium EDTA tube) and a potassium level (to be collected in a green top heparinized tube). The MA completed the blood draw, and thanked Mr. Oliver for his time.

The next day, the physician's office called Mr. Oliver and asked him to come in to have his potassium level rechecked, as it was elevated on the test from the day before. This was not an expected result, as usually Mr. Oliver's potassium level was decreased below the reference range. The specimen was drawn and checked on a STAT basis, and the result was in the low end of the reference range. The physician told Mr. Oliver that the previous result was elevated because of a laboratory error.

1. What are two sources of error that could cause the potassium result to be erroneously elevated in this scenario?

RESOURCES AND SUGGESTED READINGS

"Modern Technology Helps Shed Light on Illness in Artists of the Past"
A summary of an article by Paul L. Wolf, MD, which appeared in the November 2005 edition of the *Archives of Pathology and Laboratory Medicine,* a publication of the College of American Pathologists. Very interesting information concerning the way that illnesses and drugs have influenced the work of many famous artists and composers. http://www.newswise.com/articles/view/516145/

"Cholesterol"
Excellent presentation on cholesterol and the effects that it may have on the cardiovascular system; also includes information about lifestyle changes and symptoms of myocardial infarction and stroke http://www.americanheart.org
"Diseases and Conditions Index, Coronary Artery Disease"
National Heart, Lung and Blood Institute; National Institutes of Health
Excellent information about coronary artery disease including illustrations. http://www.nhlbi.nih.gov/health/dci/Diseases/Cad/CAD_WhatIs.html
"Third Report of the Expert Panel on Detection, Evaluation, and Treatment of High Blood Cholesterol in Adults (Adult Treatment Panel III)"
National Heart, Lung and Blood Institute: National Institutes of Health
Includes recommendations for lipid testing and desirable ranges and treatment options. http://www.nhlbi.nih.gov/guidelines/cholesterol/index.htm

Chapter 17

Glucose Testing

Constance L. Lieseke, CMA (AAMA), MLT, PBT(ASCP)

CHAPTER OUTLINE

Learning Outcomes

After reading this chapter, the successful student will be able to:

17-1 Define the key terms.

17-2 Explain how insulin and glucagon work together to maintain healthy blood sugar levels.

17-3 List three ways that insulin secretion affects the body.

17-4 Compare and contrast type 1 and type 2 diabetes.

17-5 Describe how gestational diabetes is different from type 1 and type 2 diabetes.

17-6 List potential problems that may develop with uncontrolled diabetes.

17-7 Explain why it is important to diagnose and treat gestational diabetes.

17-8 Examine the differences between the random and fasting glucose testing.

17-9 Explain the procedure for postprandial glucose testing.

17-10 Describe the steps involved in a glucose tolerance test.

17-11 Identify the clinical significance of the Hb A1c test.

17-12 Explain how the results for capillary whole blood glucose testing may compare to those tested on a plasma sample.

17-13 Describe common maintenance and quality control issues that may need to be addressed in home and laboratory glucose testing methods.

17-14 Perform CLIA-waived glucose testing.

17-15 Perform a CLIA-waived Hb A1c test.

CAAHEP/ABHES STANDARDS

 CAAHEP Standards

I.P.13. Perform chemistry testing

 ABHES Standards

- 10. Medical Laboratory Procedures, b. CLIA-waived tests
- Graduates: b. Perform selected CLIA-waived tests that assist with diagnosis and treatment, #3 Chemistry Testing

KEY TERMS

Albumin	Glucose challenge test	Islets of Langerhans
Autoantibodies	Glucosuria	Ketones
Autoimmune response	Glycated hemoglobin	Ketonuria
Body mass index (BMI)	Glycemic control	Macrosomia
Carbohydrates	Glycogen	Metabolic syndrome
Diabetes	Glycogenolysis	Microalbumin
Diabetes insipidus	Glycolysis	Microalbuminuria
Diabetes mellitus	Glycosylated hemoglobin	Oral glucose tolerance test (OGTT)
Diabetic ketoacidosis	Hb A1c	
Diabetic neuropathy	Hyperglycemia	Polydipsia
Etiology	Hypoglycemia	Polyphagia
Fasting blood sugar (FBS)	Impaired fasting glucose (IFG)	Polyuria
Fasting plasma glucose (FPG)	Impaired glucose tolerance (IGT)	Postprandial
Gestational diabetes	Insulin	Prediabetes
Glucagon	Insulin dependent	Type 1 diabetes
Glucose	Insulin resistance	Type 2 diabetes

History has provided us with many detailed observations of patients with **diabetes.** The ancient physicians documented the symptoms related to diabetes, such as frequent excessive urination and weight loss; however, they were not able to effectively treat the condition. In the first century AD, a physician in ancient Greece named this malady *diabetes,* based on the Greek word for "siphon," as it seemed to him that the liquid taken in by the body was just "siphoned" through and came directly out as urine. Other ancient civilizations provide examples of urine from ill patients that attracted ants because of the sweetness of the fluid. In the 1700s, physicians discovered that the urine and blood from patients exhibiting diabetic symptoms tasted sweet, like sugar, and this became an accepted means of diagnosing diabetes in symptomatic patients.

The treatment of diabetes remained ineffective because physicians could not determine the cause or source of the dysfunction responsible for the symptoms. Some thought there was a problem with digestion in these patients, whereas others thought it must be a disease of the kidneys because there was so much urine produced. It was not until the late 19th century that scientists discovered evidence that the pancreas was involved in the process. In 1889, two physicians who were studying fat digestion and utilization discovered that the removal of the pancreas caused the animals in the experiment to exhibit the symptoms of diabetes. In 1922, Frederick Banting and Charles Best experimented with extracts from the pancreas to isolate **insulin,** an enzyme that is necessary for the proper utilization of glucose by the cells of the body. Insulin became available in the 1920s as injected medication to treat diabetes, with immediate lifesaving results for those afflicted.

In 1935, scientist Roger Himsworth presented evidence that diabetes was actually two separate diseases: "insulin sensitive" (today's type 1 diabetes) and "insulin insensitive" (now known as type 2 diabetes). This discovery provided the opportunity for a deeper understanding of the disease and its treatment, as well as the development of an oral medication for "insulin-insensitive" type of diabetes, which became available in the 1950s.

Even though the cause and types of diabetes are now understood and more treatment options are available, diabetes is still a very serious, widespread, and expensive health problem. According to statistics from the Centers for Disease Control and Prevention (CDC), approximately 8% of the population of the United States has diabetes, and in 2007 it was the sixth leading cause of death. Common complications of diabetes include cardiovascular disease, increased stroke risk, poor healing, hypertension, blindness, kidney disease, nervous system dysfunction, amputations, and dental disease. Diabetes can also contribute to complications of pregnancy and causes increased susceptibility to other illnesses. Because of the severity of this disease and the number of those afflicted, **glucose** testing has become a very common procedure performed in physician office laboratories and reference laboratories. Health-care providers and patients must work closely together to manage the disease and provide appropriate treatment to avoid the onset of life-threatening complications.

GLUCOSE UTILIZATION AND CONTROL MECHANISMS

Glucose is a type of simple sugar that is needed as an energy source by all living things. When **carbohydrates** are digested, glucose enters into the bloodstream as a by-product. As the blood glucose levels rise, the body reacts in several ways:

- Some of the glucose goes directly to the brain tissues, where it is needed for normal function. Cells of the brain do not require insulin to take in glucose for energy.
- The increased levels of glucose in the blood trigger the pancreas to release insulin, which is produced by clusters of specialized beta cells in the pancreatic **islets of Langerhans.** Insulin is required for glucose to enter most of the cells of the body so that it can be used as an energy source. The cells of the body have a receptor that interacts with the insulin molecule. This interaction allows glucose to pass through the cell membrane. Insulin may be considered as a "key" to open the doors on the cells to allow the glucose to enter. The cells accept as much glucose as needed for normal function.
- Because a meal may provide more glucose than is needed immediately, insulin triggers the body to store the excess glucose in the muscles and liver as **glycogen,** which is essentially a long string of glucose molecules. When the demand for glucose increases past what is in the bloodstream, this glycogen is broken down and released for use as glucose. The increased glucose demand may also result in the transmission of a message to the brain encouraging the body to take in food. Additional unneeded glucose may be stored as fat.

Test Your Knowledge 17-1
What is glycogen? (Outcome 17-1)

Once the glucose has entered the cells of the body, the blood glucose levels begin to return to normal. The goal of the body is to keep a consistent level of glucose in the bloodstream at all times while providing the necessary energy to the cells. Glucose continues to be used by the cells constantly, and with increased activity the glucose demands are heightened. The increased demand causes the glucose levels in the bloodstream to decrease below the normal range as the glucose molecules move into the cells. When this occurs, another cell type (alpha cells) in the pancreatic islets of Langerhans secrete a hormone called **glucagon,** which counteracts the effects of insulin. (See Fig. 17-1 for more details about the pancreas and the islets of Langerhans.) Glucagon causes the pancreas to reduce insulin production, and signals the liver, muscles, and adipose tissues of the body to release some of the glucose that is stored there into the bloodstream to increase blood glucose levels. This process of glycogen breakdown is called **glycogenolysis**. Figure 17-2 demonstrates the balance between glucose, insulin, and glucagon.

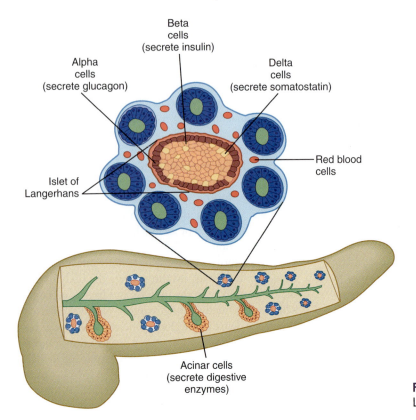

Figure 17-1   Pancreas and islets of Langerhans; note the alpha and beta cells.

The intricate balance of the blood sugar levels, insulin secretion, and glucagon secretion is essential for the body to function normally. Insulin is required for most of the cells in the body to take in glucose to be used for energy, and insulin also triggers the formation of glycogen and triglycerides from the excess blood glucose so that the body has a backup source of energy between meals or during times of increased need. In addition, the secretion of insulin stimulates the liver and muscle cells to absorb amino acids introduced into the bloodstream during digestion and use these to create proteins. Insulin also stimulates the cells to take in fatty acids from the bloodstream so that there is not an excessive buildup.

Test Your Knowledge 17-2

Which of these processes is triggered by the secretion of insulin?
   a. Formation of glycogen
   b. Increase of blood glucose
   c. Formation of glucose
   d. Secretion of glucose   (Outcome 17-3)

PATHOPHYSIOLOGY OF GLUCOSE METABOLISM

Prediabetes

According to the American Diabetes Association, there are approximately 57 million Americans that have **prediabetes,** which is defined as a condition in which the blood glucose level is elevated, but not high enough to be indicative of a diagnosis for type 1 or type 2 diabetes. Those who have prediabetes may already be experiencing some of the adverse effects of **hyperglycemia** (elevated blood glucose) and are at a greatly increased risk of developing diabetes within the next few years.

Those with prediabetes have some degree of insulin resistance, usually associated with obesity, a sedentary lifestyle, and poor eating habits. Patients with increased abdominal fat and an elevated **body mass index (BMI)** (a measurement of weight in relationship to height) are at an increased risk, as well as those with a history of type 2 diabetes in their immediate family. In addition, diabetes is more common in certain ethnic groups. Latinos,

REGULATION OF BLOOD GLUCOSE LEVELS
Control center–Pancreas

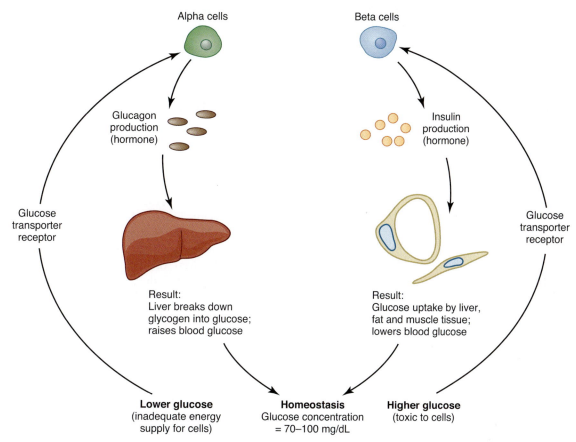

Figure 17-2   Representation of the balance between blood glucose, insulin, and glucagon. When blood glucose is increased, the body produces insulin to allow the glucose to enter the cells. This decreases the blood glucose levels, which triggers glucagon to be released if the level drops too low. The glucagon then decreases the absorption of glucose into the cells, and increases the breakdown of glycogen, if necessary.

African Americans, Native Americans, Asian Americans, and Pacific Islanders have an increased presence of diabetes in their populations. The elderly also have a disproportionate amount of diabetes present. Because these groups have more diabetes in their midst, prediabetes is also more likely.

Prediabetes is detected by testing the blood glucose level. The desirable **fasting plasma glucose (FPG)** result tested after approximately 12 hours of fasting is below 100 mg/dL. Prediabetes is indicated by an FPG of 100 to 125 mg/dL, and patients with diabetes usually demonstrate an FPG of 126 mg/dL or above. Prediabetics with an FPG of 100 to 125 mg/dL are

said to have **impaired fasting glucose (IFG).** The prediabetes diagnosis may also be based on an abnormal **oral glucose tolerance test (OGTT)** result. The result at 2 hours during this procedure for prediabetics will be between 140 and 200 mg/dL, and for diabetics it will be over 200 mg/dL. (The OGTT procedure is detailed later in this chapter.) Prediabetics with glucose levels at 2 hours between 140 and 200 mg/dL are said to have **impaired glucose tolerance (IGT).**

Those diagnosed with prediabetes do not always proceed to develop diabetes. Studies have shown that if patients with prediabetes make a concentrated effort to increase physical activity and reduce their weight by 5%

to 10%, they may not develop diabetes, or at the very least, they may delay the onset of diabetes for a few years. These lifestyle changes will also stop any undesirable effects of the hyperglycemia on the cells of the body. The American Diabetes Association strongly recommends counseling and follow-up for this group to assist with lifestyle changes.

Diabetes

The word *diabetes* is used to refer to a group of disorders that all exhibit **hyperglycemia,** or elevated blood glucose. These may also be known as different types of **diabetes mellitus,** or "sweet" diabetes, because of the glucose content in the urine of those diagnosed. There are actually three different types of diabetes associated with hyperglycemia, which differ by their **etiology** (cause) and by their treatment. These include **type 1 diabetes,** which previously was known as insulin-dependent diabetes or juvenile-onset diabetes. **Type 2 diabetes** was previously known as non-insulin-dependent diabetes. **Gestational diabetes** is a disorder of glucose metabolism that only affects those who are pregnant. A diagnosis of type 1 or type 2 diabetes is usually only assigned to a patient after confirmation of the abnormal blood levels.

Type 1 Diabetes

Patients with type 1 diabetes have a lack of insulin. The beta cells of the islets of Langerhans in the pancreas have been destroyed and are not capable of creating enough insulin to keep the body healthy. Type 1 diabetes is present in approximately 5% to 10% of all diabetic patients, and presents most often in children or adolescents. Adults may also be afflicted, although this is not as common as it is in those under the age of 20. The destruction of the beta cells responsible for insulin production is most commonly associated with an **autoimmune response,** in which the patient's body develops **autoantibodies** that attack the cells in the islets of Langerhans. There seems to be a genetic predisposition to this condition, although it appears that there is usually some sort of "trigger" that brings on the autoantibody production. Viral infections and environmental factors have been linked to the progression of the disease.

Type 1 diabetes may develop over a few weeks; the onset of the disease is often quite rapid as compared to type 2 diabetes, which has a gradual progression. Type 1 diabetes patients commonly exhibit fatigue, increased urination and increased thirst, nausea and vomiting,

and weight loss in spite of an increased appetite. During the initial onset of symptoms, the patient may have periods of hyperglycemia as well as **hypoglycemia** (low blood sugar). If the diagnosis and treatment are not established early in the disease process, the body will react to the shortage of insulin by using fatty acids as an energy source instead of depending on glucose. The use of fatty acids may cause a buildup of **ketones** in the bloodstream. Ketones are a by-product of fat metabolism, and because they are acidic in nature, they will change the pH of the body over a period of time. Initial symptoms of **diabetic ketoacidosis** include abdominal pain, nausea, and vomiting. As the condition progresses, the patient may have increased shallow respirations, which is the body's way of attempting to change the acidic blood pH. The patient may have difficulty thinking and communicating clearly, and may eventually become comatose. It is at this point that the diagnosis of type 1 diabetes is often assigned, as the patient is admitted to the emergency room or hospital once he or she becomes critically ill.

Treatment of type 1 diabetes requires frequent insulin injections. Insulin cannot be administered orally, as it is not effective once it has been digested. There are many different types of insulin; some act quickly and stay in the circulation for a short period of time, and others are designed to be longer lasting. Patients who are **insulin dependent** monitor their blood glucose level several times daily and adjust their insulin intake accordingly.

Type 2 Diabetes

Type 2 diabetes is characterized by a lack of insulin activity on the cells of the body. This may be due to **insulin resistance,** in which the cells have a diminished ability to interact with insulin as they should. Because the insulin no longer acts on the cells of the body to allow the glucose to pass through into the cells, the blood glucose levels remain elevated. Type 2 diabetes may also be the result of a decreased production of insulin by the beta cells of the pancreas. In situations in which the patient exhibits insulin resistance, the body will try to produce more insulin to overcome the resistance, but after a period of time the demand is excessive and the production cannot keep up with the needs of the body. Those who have type 2 diabetes often have high levels of insulin in the bloodstream as well as high levels of glucose. In addition to the high levels of blood glucose that result because of ineffective cellular transport, the body also tries to accommodate the imbalance by breaking down additional glycogen in the liver, which adds additional glucose to the bloodstream and complicates the situation further.

Type 2 diabetes is the most common form of the disease, affecting approximately 95% of all diabetics. The CDC has declared type 2 diabetes to be at an epidemic level, as the numbers of those diagnosed increase every year. The etiology (cause) of type 2 diabetes is complicated. There is a direct correlation with obesity and individuals who have been diagnosed with **metabolic syndrome** (a group of risk factors that occur together and increase the risk of coronary heart disease, stroke, and type 2 diabetes), as well as a family history of type 2 diabetes and a sedentary lifestyle. Women with a history of polycystic ovary syndrome or gestational diabetes also have an increased chance of developing type 2 diabetes. Those older than age 40 are at a higher risk than those who are younger, although there has been a sharp increase in the number of obese children diagnosed with type 2 diabetes in the past few years. Certain ethnic groups are at a higher risk, such as Native Americans and those of Asian or African descent.

Diagnosis of type 2 diabetes may be delayed for years after the first onset of symptoms as this type of diabetes develops slowly. As with type 1 diabetes, many patients diagnosed with type 2 diabetes demonstrate increased urination and increased thirst. Some other common symptoms include unexplained weight loss or weight gain, flu-like symptoms with fatigue and nausea accompanied by a loss of appetite, changes in vision, and poor healing. Patients may also find that they are more susceptible to other illnesses, such as the common cold. Having frequent urinary or yeast infections may also be an indicator of type 2 diabetes. Another clinical indicator may be a change in oral health, because diabetes may cause inflammation that leads to infection in the gums. In addition, some patients experience tingling or loss of sensation in the fingertips or toes, which is caused by damaged nerve endings from the high levels of glucose in the body.

Type 2 diabetes is first treated with lifestyle changes. Most patients diagnosed with this type of diabetes are overweight, so the first goal is to lose approximately 8% to 10% of the total weight. Diabetics are also encouraged to exercise for at least 150 minutes per week to improve their health. Oral medications that enhance the ability of the body to react to insulin or stimulate the beta cells of the pancreas to produce more insulin may also be used. If these measures are ineffective in accomplishing **glycemic control** (appropriate blood glucose levels), the patient with type 2 diabetes may be treated with insulin injections.

Untreated or uncontrolled type 1 or type 2 diabetes may lead to hypertension and other serious cardiovascular diseases, as well as **diabetic neuropathy**; nervous system damage; eye and kidney tissue damage; poor healing; foot and skin complications; and gastroparesis, a disorder in which the stomach takes too long to empty after eating. Those with diabetes are at an increased risk of developing depression. Patients with type 1 diabetes may also have an increased risk of developing celiac disease (a chronic digestive disorder caused by the inability to metabolize gluten) or a painful musculoskeletal condition known as "frozen shoulder," in which the individual loses movement of the shoulder for a period of time.

Test Your Knowledge 17-3

List one way that type 1 and type 2 diabetes are similar.
(Outcome 17-4)

Test Your Knowledge 17-4

List two potential consequences of uncontrolled or untreated diabetes.
(Outcome 17-6)

Gestational Diabetes

Gestational diabetes (sometimes abbreviated as GDM) is similar to type 2 diabetes because it is a form of glucose intolerance rather than a reduction in insulin production. Approximately 4% of all pregnant women develop gestational diabetes. It is more frequent among Hispanic Americans, African Americans, Native Americans, Asian Americans, indigenous Australians, and Pacific Islanders. Obesity, previous delivery of an infant weighing more than 9 pounds, and a positive family history of diabetes also increase the risk of developing gestational diabetes. Women who have gestational diabetes will usually demonstrate it in subsequent pregnancies, and are at an increased risk of developing type 2 diabetes later in life.

Although the exact cause of gestational diabetes is not clear, it is thought that the insulin resistance present in gestational diabetes is demonstrated as a result of the additional hormones present in the body during pregnancy. The placenta produces high levels of hormones (such as cortisol and estrogen) to support and sustain the pregnancy. These hormones block or reduce the action of insulin on the cells of the mother's body, which causes her blood glucose levels to become elevated.

The high levels of hormones are not usually a problem until late in the pregnancy, as the mother's pancreas normally responds to the additional insulin demands early in the pregnancy. As the pregnancy continues, the additional maternal insulin production cannot overcome the effects of the hormones produced by the placenta, and the mother will exhibit sustained elevated blood glucose levels.

Gestational diabetes is a serious health risk because of the additional glucose in the mother's bloodstream. Glucose passes through the placenta to the fetus, causing a condition known as **macrosomia.** *Macrosomia* means "fat baby." In this condition, the additional glucose passed on to the baby from the mother causes the baby's body to produce excessive fat cells in response to the additional unneeded glucose. The baby may become excessively large, which can cause complications during delivery. Many babies born to mothers with gestational diabetes must be delivered using a cesarean delivery, as their excessive size does not allow a vaginal birth. If a vaginal birth is attempted, these babies are at a high risk of shoulder damage during the delivery. Studies have shown that babies born to mothers with gestational diabetes have increased risk of becoming obese as children, as well as an increased risk of developing type 2 diabetes later in life.

In addition to the risks from excessive size, infants born to mothers with gestational diabetes have an increased risk of breathing problems, as well as extreme hypoglycemia (low blood glucose levels) after birth. During the pregnancy, the infant has been producing enough insulin to process the glucose created by his or her own body, as well as the additional glucose supplied by the circulation of the mother. When the additional maternal glucose supply is discontinued at birth, there is too much insulin in the infant's bloodstream, resulting in low levels of blood glucose. Without careful monitoring, this situation can become life threatening. These babies may also be at an increased risk for other chemical imbalances in the first few days of life.

Test Your Knowledge 17-5

Is gestational diabetes more like type 1 or type 2 diabetes? Why?
(Outcome 17-5)

Test Your Knowledge 17-6

How is macrosomia related to gestational diabetes?
(Outcome 17-7)

POINT OF INTEREST 17-1
Another type of diabetes

There is another disease that shares the name diabetes, but it is not associated with hyperglycemia. **Diabetes insipidus** is an endocrine disease characterized by a lack of the hormone vasopressin, which acts on the kidneys to reduce urinary output and allow for concentration of the urine. Vasopressin is produced by the pituitary gland, and those with this disease either do not produce enough vasopressin, or they have developed a resistance to the actions of vasopressin to concentrate urine. A patient with diabetes insipidus produces excessive amounts of urine each day, and often sees the physician because of symptoms associated with bed-wetting, dehydration, and/or electrolyte imbalances. Diabetes insipidus has very little in common with the other forms of diabetes discussed in this text, except for the initial common symptoms of increased urination and increased thirst.

TYPES OF GLUCOSE TESTS PERFORMED

The role of the laboratory in diabetes care is to assist the health-care provider in the initial diagnosis, differentiation about the type of diabetes present, and monitoring the progress of the treatment once it has started for the patient. There are several types of glucose test procedures performed that provide necessary information to the health-care provider.

Fasting Blood Glucose Test

The glucose level performed in a laboratory on a fasting blood specimen is known as a fasting plasma glucose (FPG). The term **fasting blood sugar (FBS)** may also be used. Most laboratories perform blood glucose levels on plasma or serum, rather than on whole blood. To prepare for this test, the patient needs to fast for 12 hours and should not smoke, drink anything but water, or take medication before the test. (Sometimes the medication is a *must;* this should be cleared with the physician before the specimen is drawn.) The World Health Organization recommends the use of plasma obtained from a venipuncture for this test. If the test cannot be performed within an hour of the blood draw, a gray top tube should be used for the specimen. The additives in the gray top tube reduce **glycolysis** (utilization of the glucose in the specimen by the living cells present) for up to 24 hours at room temperature. The desirable fasting plasma or serum glucose level is 70 to 100 mg/dL

Patients with FPG of 100 to 125 mg/dL have impaired fasting glucose, and are prediabetic. A result equal to or above 125 mg/dL is indicative of diabetes.

Random Glucose Test

A random blood glucose test is one that is taken at any time of the day without regard for the time of the last meal. A patient who is symptomatic for diabetes, perhaps exhibiting **polyuria,** (excessive urination) **polyphagia,** (excessive hunger), or **polydipsia** (excessive thirst) and unexplained weight loss may have a random glucose test ordered. According to the criteria established by the American Diabetes Association, if the random glucose result for a symptomatic patient is equal to or greater than 200 mg/dL, then the patient is classified as a diabetic.

Test Your Knowledge 17-7

Which of these best describes a random glucose?
  a. A glucose level drawn 1 hour after eating
  b. A glucose level drawn after 12 hours of fasting
  c. A glucose level drawn at any time of the day without any previous preparation
  d. A glucose level drawn just before eating

(Outcome 17-8)

Postprandial Glucose Test

Postprandial refers to something done after eating or after mealtime. Glucose testing that is performed postprandial may mean that the blood specimen was collected a specific amount of time after a meal, or it may mean that the specimen was drawn at a certain interval after ingestion of a glucose-rich beverage. Diabetics who are striving to achieve close glycemic control will test their blood glucose levels at home 1 or 2 hours postprandial to see how their body has handled the meal. Most diabetic educational materials provide target ranges for 2-hour postprandial blood glucose levels. Ideally, the blood glucose should not go above 140 mg/dL for non-diabetic patients; for diabetics the level should remain below 180 mg/dL 2 hours after eating.

Initial screening procedures for gestational diabetes may also use postprandial glucose testing. This may be called a **glucose challenge test.** Patients do not need to fast before this procedure. When they arrive at the laboratory or physician office, they are given a drink that contains 50 g of glucose. This drink must be ingested within 5 minutes for the test to be valid. A blood specimen is drawn exactly 1 hour after ingestion of the glucose solution. Patients with gestational diabetes will demonstrate a postprandial blood glucose level at 1 hour that is greater than or equal to 140 mg/dL. If this glucose challenge result is elevated, then the health-care provider will usually order a 3-hour oral glucose tolerance test.

Test Your Knowledge 17-8

True or False: A laboratory postprandial glucose test is drawn at a specific time interval after ingestion of a drink high in glucose or ingestion of a meal.

(Outcome 17-9)

Oral Glucose Tolerance Testing Procedures

According to the National Institutes of Health, the oral glucose tolerance test is more sensitive to the detection of prediabetes than the fasting glucose test level. The OGTT is used primarily for the diagnosis of diabetes mellitus. This test may be performed on a patient with an abnormal FPG, assuming that the result of the FPG was less than 200 mg/dL. If the fasting result was equal to or more than 200 mg/dL, an oral glucose tolerance test is not indicated because the high FPG level is indicative of diabetes. This test may also be ordered for patients who are being evaluated for gestational diabetes, or those who had an abnormal 1-hour postprandial glucose result.

- A patient preparing for an oral glucose tolerance test should have a carbohydrate-rich diet for at least 3 days prior to the scheduled test. Diets that restrict carbohydrate intake may produce erroneous results. The patient must fast for 12 hours prior to the test. During this time, no food or liquid other than water is to be consumed. The patient should also avoid smoking and strenuous exercise.

- Upon arrival at the laboratory or the clinic, the patient will have a fasting plasma glucose specimen drawn. This specimen should be analyzed for glucose content before continuing with the process; if the fasting plasma glucose results are elevated above 126 mg/dL, the test will not continue. Also, some laboratories will collect a urine specimen with each blood draw; this helps to provide more information about the glucose that may be "spilled" into the urine specimen. Usually a blood glucose of 170 mg/dL or greater will cause glucose to be present in the urine specimen, as the body cannot handle these high levels.

- After the fasting specimen has been drawn, the patient will be given a solution with 75 or 100 g of glucose dissolved in water. (For a patient who is not pregnant,

75 g are used; when testing for gestational diabetes, 100 g are used.)

- Blood specimens (and urine if that is the policy of the laboratory) will be collected at least three more times during the procedure: 1 hour, 2 hours, and 3 hours after the initial dose of glucose drink has been ingested. Some laboratories will also collect a blood specimen half an hour after ingestion to provide more information about how the body is utilizing the glucose in the specimen.

- Occasionally, patients will feel nauseous, tired, cold, and perspire while undergoing this test. It is important that patients are kept calm, and that they stay in an area where they can be monitored while waiting. Sometimes a patient will vomit shortly after ingestion of the glucose solution; if this occurs early in the process (prior to 1 hour after drinking the sweetened drink), then the procedure should be discontinued and rescheduled, as the results may be inaccurate. Also, if a patient loses consciousness or exhibits symptoms of slurred speech and impaired thought processes, the test should be discontinued and the physician or emergency personnel should be notified immediately. These could be signs of hypoglycemia that require immediate treatment.

The interpretation of the test results is different when screening for diabetes mellitus than it is for gestational diabetes. For gestational diabetes screening with a 100-g glucose solution, if there are two abnormal results in the various timed blood draws, the patient is diagnosed with gestational diabetes, whether or not she is symptomatic. According to the American Diabetes Association, these results are considered abnormal for a pregnant woman:

- Fasting plasma glucose: greater than or equal to 95 mg/dL
- 1-hour plasma glucose: greater than or equal to 180 mg/dL
- 2-hour plasma glucose: greater than or equal to 155 mg/dL
- 3-hour plasma glucose: greater than or equal to 140 mg/dL

For suspected diabetes mellitus in patients who are not pregnant, a 75-g glucose solution is used. The American Diabetes Association has established these parameters for a diagnosis of diabetes in nonpregnant individuals:

- Fasting plasma glucose: greater than or equal to 126 mg/dL
- 1-hour plasma glucose: greater than or equal to 200 mg/dL
- 2-hour plasma glucose: greater than or equal to 200 mg/dL

- 3-hour plasma glucose: greater than or equal to 200 mg/dL (the 3-hour sample is not always included in the procedure for non-gestational-diabetes patients)

> **Test Your Knowledge 17-9**
>
> How many times (at a minimum) is the blood drawn for a patient completing a 3-hour glucose tolerance test?
> (Outcome 17-10)

Glycosylated Hemoglobin

As presented in Chapter 16, elevated blood glucose levels will eventually change the hemoglobin molecule present in the red cells of the body by irreversibly binding glucose to the hemoglobin A subunit. This compound is known as **glycosylated** or **glycated hemoglobin,** and is abbreviated as **Hb A1c.** The typical red blood cell survives in the body for 90 to 120 days. Because the changes to the hemoglobin molecule are constantly occurring whenever the blood glucose level becomes elevated (whether the patient is aware of the elevation or not) the Hb A1c level is an excellent way to measure glycemic control over a 2- to 3-month period. The Hb A1c test is not recommended as a diagnostic tool for diabetes, but is an excellent tool for monitoring the management of the disease.

The American Diabetes Association has provided guidance regarding the frequency of this test and the interpretation of the results. A nondiabetic patient will have Hb A1c levels below 6%. For diabetic patients, the goal is to remain below 7%, as it is understood that there may be spikes in the blood glucose that are unavoidable. As part of the management of diabetes, those who have unstable blood sugars should have their Hb A1c tested quarterly; those who appear to have good glycemic control should be checked at least two times per year. In addition, the recommendation includes performance of an annual lipid profile and urine **microalbumin** testing to screen for renal damage. Microalbumin testing is discussed in more detail later in this chapter.

> **Test Your Knowledge 17-10**
>
> The Hb A1c test may be used to monitor the overall glycemic control for a patient for which of these time intervals?
>   a. 1 month
>   b. 6 weeks
>   c. 3 months
>   d. 6 months
> (Outcome 17-11)

TABLE 17-1

Types of diabetes, diagnostic test procedures, and treatment methods

Type of Diabetes	Symptoms	Clinical Presentation	Diagnostic Test Procedures	Treatment
Diabetes insipidus	Excessive amount of urine production; dehydration and electrolyte imbalance as a result of fluid loss	Lack of vasopressin production by pituitary gland or kidney resistance to vasopressin	Medical history, physical examination, urinalysis, magnetic resonance imaging and/or CAT scan of the brain, fluid deprivation testing	Vasopressin (usually a nasal spray) and fluid replacement if necessary
Type 1 diabetes	Hyperglycemia, fatigue, dehydration, nausea, vomiting, weight loss	Autoantibodies destroy pancreatic cells that produce insulin, resulting in reduced or absence of insulin	Medical history, physical examination, abnormal blood glucose levels with verification of fasting plasma glucose above 126 mg/dL or random plasma glucose above 200 mg/dL	Insulin injections
Type 2 diabetes	May be asymptomatic for years; usually develops slowly. Hyperglycemia, fatigue, dehydration, nausea, vomiting, weight loss	Cells of the body develop resistance to insulin; keeps glucose from entering cells so the plasma glucose levels become elevated	Medical history, physical examination, abnormal blood glucose levels with fasting plasma glucose or glucose tolerance test	Lifestyle changes, oral medication; insulin injections may become necessary if oral medications don't accomplish desired glycemic control
Gestational diabetes	Often asymptomatic; may develop symptoms like those of diabetes mellitus	Increased levels of hormones from pregnancy increase cellular resistance to insulin	Abnormal glucose challenge test and/or abnormal glucose tolerance test	Lifestyle changes, oral medications, or insulin injections (if needed for glycemic control) until birth of infant

POINT OF INTEREST 17-2
New Testing procedures for monitoring diabetes

There is a new procedure available for monitoring the glycemic control of diabetes patients. The GlycoMark blood test measures the level of a substance naturally present at a consistent level in the bloodstream. This molecule is known as 1,5-anhydro-D-glucitol (1,5 AG), which is a monosaccharide that is very close in chemical structure to glucose. When the glucose level of a diabetic patient rises above 180 mg/dL, the kidneys are not able to reabsorb the 1,5 AG molecule because the glucose blocks the sites for this molecule to be reabsorbed. Thus, when the glucose level rises (with poor glycemic control) the 1,5 AG concentration decreases below the reference range.

This procedure provides an opportunity to monitor the glycemic control for diabetic patients for the past 1 to 2 weeks. As a comparison, the Hb A1c test provides a measurement of the glycemic control over the past 3 months. Many physicians feel that this new testing method may allow them to treat their newly diagnosed diabetics more efficiently, because the results will be affected by poor glycemic control very quickly.

Blood Ketone Testing

Many home glucose meters are now capable of testing ketones as well as glucose levels in the bloodstream. Elevated levels of ketones in the blood are indicative of fluctuations in the blood glucose levels. Although close attention to diet, exercise, and medication will help to ensure that a diabetic patient maintains appropriate glycemic control, there may be situations that stress the body and allow the diabetes to become out of control, such as the following:

- Patients with preexisting diabetes who become pregnant
- Patients who are ill for several days, especially if they are vomiting or have diarrhea
- Situations of unusually high stress
- Blood glucose levels equal to or greater than 300 mg/dL
- Symptoms of hyperglycemia such as nausea, fatigue, and vomiting that are not associated with another disease process

Some ketone testing procedures will provide qualitative results indicating the presence or absence of ketones in the blood. Other testing methods provide quantitative results, indicating the level of ketones present. Patients should discuss their situation with a health-care provider before testing for the presence of blood ketones.

Capillary Sample Testing and Correlation to Plasma Glucose Levels

The World Health Organization recommends that the plasma glucose level (rather than whole blood testing) is used for diagnosis and monitoring of diabetic patients. However, this is not always possible, even in a laboratory or clinic setting. Some rural areas in the United States do not have laboratory facilities that meet these standards. Outside of the United States it can become even more problematic. These rural or underserved areas often have a glucose meter available, which is designed to perform whole blood glucose testing rather than plasma glucose testing.

Plasma glucose levels are 10% to 15% higher than those of whole blood obtained via a capillary procedure. Because the glucose levels for diagnosis of prediabetes and diabetes are very specific, it may be necessary to calculate the plasma glucose level using a whole blood capillary result. Many of the new glucose meters include this calculation in their results when reported; for instance, instead of the number on the screen indicating the glucose level in the whole blood specimen that was just tested, a calculation will have already been included and the number is actually indicative of the plasma glucose level. If the meter in use does not use this calculation, many of the glucose meter manufacturers' websites will provide more information to correlate whole blood glucose to plasma glucose levels.

This discrepancy between plasma and whole blood glucose is not often explained to patients who are self-monitoring their levels at home. It is important to mention that their results may not compare to the laboratory results because the reference ranges and testing methods are different. The health-care provider and any diabetes educators who are working with the patients need to help them develop parameters to use for self-monitoring from the testing instrument that they are using at home.

Glucose may also be tested using serum samples. This is not recommended for diabetes screening because the glucose level in the specimen can change slightly during the time period required for the blood to clot. If the specimen is centrifuged immediately after clotting, with immediate separation of the serum from the cells, then the glucose result will be very similar to that of a plasma specimen. However, if there is a delay in the processing of the specimen, the serum glucose result will be much lower than a plasma result would have been for that patient.

> ### Test Your Knowledge 17-11
> If a whole blood glucose and a plasma glucose were collected on the same patient at the same time, which of the results would be expected to be higher?
>
> (Outcome 17-12)

Urine Testing for Diabetics

Urine testing is not used as a diagnosis tool for diabetes or prediabetes. The threshold for each individual for the amount of glucose tolerated in the bloodstream may be different. Usually anyone who has a blood glucose level above 170 mg/dL will have glucose present in the urine as well, a condition known as **glucosuria.**

The urine of diabetic patients may also be monitored for other chemical substances. The presence of ketones in the urine (**ketonuria**) may be an indicator of poor glycemic control. When the glucose in the bloodstream cannot enter the cells of the body to be used for energy, the body will break down fatty acids as an alternative energy source. This process is natural, and occurs in our body during fasting periods and times when our energy needs are accelerated. Ketones are a by-product of fatty acid metabolism, and if they are present in the urine, it may indicate excessive use of fatty acids for energy. This means that there is not enough insulin (or the cells are resisting the insulin that is present) to allow the glucose to be metabolized as it should by the cells of the body.

Glucose molecules are large, and are not designed to be passed into the urine in measurable amounts. When a patient has high levels of blood glucose over an extended period of time, these large molecules are forced through the filtration system of the nephron, causing damage because of their large size. The damaged glomerulus will now allow other large molecules present in the blood to enter the urine. The presence of these substances in the urine is considered to be abnormal and indicative of damage to the kidney. One of these large molecules is a plasma protein called **albumin.** Approximately 20% to 40% of all diabetics develop renal disease, and the first sign that the kidneys have been damaged may be the presence of **microalbuminuria.** This means that there are small amounts of albumin present in the urine; the levels are just above normal ranges. When the albumin levels in the urine are still low, it may be possible to eliminate further kidney damage by increasing efforts for glycemic control. If the levels increase to macroalbuminuria (large amounts of albumin in the urine), it is a sign that the renal disease has progressed with more severe damage to the filtration system of the kidneys. It is recommended that all diabetics be tested for urine microalbumin levels at least annually.

GLUCOSE TESTING METHODS

There are many different types of instruments used to perform glucose testing. The equipment varies from machines that analyze hundreds of specimens per hour to those that test one specimen at a time as a CLIA-waived test.

Home Glucose Testing Instruments

Blood glucose monitors are the most common self-testing products sold in the world. They are an essential part of diabetes education and monitoring, and allow diabetic patients a degree of freedom and control of their disease that previously was not possible. Blood glucose meters are all similar in function; a small testing strip is inserted into the instrument, a drop of blood is applied, and a result appears on the screen on the front of the instrument within seconds. However, these instruments may vary in size, complexity, cost of operation, and necessary quality control measures. These are some considerations to take into account when choosing an instrument for home glucose monitoring, including the following:

1. What type of diabetes is being monitored? For those who have type 1 diabetes and use an insulin pump, a continuous glucose monitor may be the most appropriate choice of device. These monitors have a sensor that is placed just under the surface of the skin that samples the blood glucose level 24 hours per day. These results are transmitted to a recording device with a memory, or to an insulin pump. If the continuous glucose monitor is paired with an insulin pump, the amount of insulin injected will be automatically matched to the glucose readings. A health-care provider and/or diabetes educator would be able to help the patient decide if this is the best method for a particular patient.

2. A patient should not take the first testing instrument that is offered and assume that they are all alike. Some instruments require a larger specimen volume than do others, and other machines have a code that must be verified whenever a new bottle of test strips are opened. Some patients prefer instruments that don't need a code to be entered, and some are most interested in a small instrument that can take samples from different areas of the body in addition to the fingertips. If possible, patients should sample several types of instruments when they meet with their health-care provider to discuss the need for blood glucose testing. Diabetes educators are another good resource.

3. Instruments may vary by cost of operation. The blood glucose meters themselves are often quite inexpensive; sometimes they are even free. However, the testing strips can be quite expensive. A typical diabetic patient who is self-monitoring will use at least two or three strips per day. Some insurance plans will help to pay only for specific brands of instruments and strips, so it is best to investigate this early in the process.

4. Patients should be certain that they can read the results displayed on the instrument used. For those with impaired vision, meters are available that display the result in larger numbers. Also, the lighting on the screen may vary, which might make certain models less appealing for some patients with specific vision needs.

Quality Control and Common Errors

Many diabetic patients have been self-monitoring for more than a decade. Unfortunately, they may not have been offered the resources that are now available when they started the process, and their home testing methods may not be providing accurate results. It is important to remember that the glucose meters used by patients at home are an essential tool for their health maintenance. Education about quality control methods for the instrument, storage and use of strips, and record-keeping options should be offered.

- Periodically, patients should bring in their home glucose meter and compare plasma glucose levels from the laboratory to those that they obtain at the same time using their own instrument. Although these results may vary as much as 10% to 15% from one another, this process can identify meters that are not testing accurately, or help the clinic staff to identify problems with the way the patient is performing the test on his or her meter while observing the patient.
- Quality control solution may be purchased and tested periodically to assure that the results obtained by the meter are accurate. Desirable ranges for the quality control solution are usually printed on the box or bottle containing the solution, and the patient can immediately verify the accuracy of the result. Explain to patients that if the machine is not testing within these ranges, they need to correct the situation before continuing use of the meter.
- Cleaning and proper storage of the instrument is essential, but often overlooked.
- Reagent strips must be stored as directed by the manufacturer, and need to be discarded if they are discolored or expired. Many patients leave the bottle open between tests, which causes the strips to absorb moisture and provide erroneous results.
- Reviewing the troubleshooting section of the meter instructions with patients can help them to understand error codes and possible courses of action when the instrument is not performing as expected. Much of this information is available online as well.
- Patients who are self-monitoring blood glucose levels must keep careful records in order for their efforts to be meaningful to their care. Educating the patients about different ways to accomplish this goal can be beneficial. Some of the meters available on the market have the capacity to store a great deal of information that may be downloaded to a computer to be printed or transmitted to a health-care provider. Patients may prefer to keep a handwritten log; if so, they should be provided with blank copies for their use.
- Ask patients about the type of lancet they are using, and how they are disposing of the used devices. Many of the newer automatic lancets may be adjusted according to the depth of the puncture, which is beneficial to those who test often. Lancets should never be used more than once, and should not be disposed of in the regular home trash. Some offices allow the patients to bring in their lancets in an appropriate biohazardous sharps container for disposal; others do

not. To assist patients with proper disposal methods, find out what the recommendations are in your area for disposal of this type of waste, and provide that information to your diabetic patients.

> **Test Your Knowledge 17-12**
>
> What is one area in which a medical assistant may need to offer education and assistance for diabetics who are performing home monitoring of their glucose levels?
>
> (Outcome 17-13)

Laboratory Glucose Testing and Potential Sources of Error

When glucose testing is performed in a large laboratory on an automated instrument, plasma or serum is tested. There are several different enzymatic methods available for glucose testing with similar reference ranges based on the type of specimen. Fasting samples will have different results from random specimens or those that were drawn as part of a glucose tolerance test.

Glucose testing may also be ordered on cerebrospinal fluid (CSF). The reference range for this test is approximately two-thirds of the blood glucose level for the same patient collected at the same time as the cerebral spinal fluid sample. When the CSF glucose levels are low as compared to the plasma glucose, it may be indicative of meningitis.

Because a specimen drawn for plasma or serum glucose testing in a laboratory must be processed before it is analyzed, there exists opportunities for error in the pre-analytical phase. The following are some considerations that must be addressed to avoid potential problems:

- The timing of the blood draw is critical. For instance, if the specimen is to be drawn fasting, it is imperative that the patient is informed and the preparation is verified before the collection occurs.
- Glucose continues to be metabolized by the cells present in the blood specimen after it is added to the collection tube. If the specimen is not processed by centrifugation and tested within 1 hour of collection, the plasma or serum glucose level may not indicate the actual amount of glucose present in the bloodstream of the patient; instead, it will be indicative of the amount left in the tube after the glucose has been utilized by the cells. If there will be more than a 1-hour delay in testing after collection, a tube with sodium fluoride or potassium oxalate additives should be used for the specimen collection. This slows down the utilization of glucose by the cells, and allows the

plasma glucose to remain stable for approximately 24 hours at room temperature.

- Reference ranges for glucose levels are generally stated as plasma levels. However, serum may also be drawn for glucose testing, as long as the serum is separated from the cells within 1 hour. The reference

ranges are usually the same for plasma and serum glucose.

- CLIA-waived testing for blood glucose is not designed to be performed with plasma samples. It is important to read the directions for the CLIA-waived methods to ensure that the results will be accurate.

Procedure 17-1: Performance of Hb A1c Test Using Bayer's A1c Now+ System

TASK

Correctly perform an Hb A1c test using Bayer's A1c Now+ testing system.

CONDITIONS

- Gloves
- Laboratory coat
- Hand sanitization supplies
- A1c Now *plus* monitor
- Sample dilution kit pouch
- Test cartridge pouch
- Whole blood from capillary puncture or well-mixed heparinized blood sample
- Gauze pad
- Biohazardous waste container
- Quality control materials

CAAHEP/ABHES STANDARDS

 CAAHEP Standards

I.P. Anatomy and Physiology, #13 Perform chemistry testing

 ABHES Standards

- 10. Medical Laboratory Procedures, b. CLIA-waived tests
- Graduates: b. Perform selected CLIA-waived tests that assist with diagnosis and treatment, #3 Chemistry Testing

Procedure	Rationale
1. Greet and then identify patient using at least two unique identifiers.	All patients must be identified properly before collecting samples or performing laboratory testing.
2. Verify test ordered, and explain procedure to patient.	All laboratory test orders should be verified by checking the chart and/or requisition form more than once. A quick explanation of the procedure for the patient will ensure more cooperation.
3. Verify that all samples, reagents, and monitor are at room temperature.	Test results may not be valid if the sample and/or reagents are not at room temperature.
4. Wash hands and apply gloves.	Hands should always be washed between patients and before starting any procedures. Gloves are appropriate personal protective equipment (PPE) for this procedure.
5. Assemble necessary equipment.	Various steps in this procedure require careful adherence to limits in time. Materials that are organized will assist in the process of following the directions properly.

Continued

Procedure 17-1: Performance of Hb A1c Test Using Bayer's A1c Now+ System—cont'd

Procedure	Rationale
6. Prior to performance of test, verify whether a quality control (QC) specimen needs to be tested, and if so, complete that test *before* the patient's test is performed.	Liquid QC should be used to verify the test results at these times: a. With a new shipment b. Whenever a new lot number of reagents or QC is put into use c. New operator; someone who is being trained on the procedure d. Problems with storage, instrument, reagents, etc. e. To ensure that storage conditions are fine, QC should be performed at least once monthly.
7. Verify that all lot numbers match on the monitor, the sample dilution kit pouch, and the test cartridge pouch.	If the lot numbers do not match, the monitor will not provide a valid test result upon completion of the test.
8. Verify that the kit has not expired.	The Bayer's A1c Now+ kit may be kept at room temperature for 4 months, but then any unused materials must be discarded. If kept refrigerated, the supplies may all be used until the printed date of expiration.
9. Open the sample dilution pouch and remove the dilution device.	The dilution device should not be removed until just before the test is performed.
10. Perform the capillary puncture following appropriate procedure, or mix the whole blood sample to prepare for next step.	Whole blood specimen may be obtained from fingerstick capillary puncture, or a green top heparinized sample may be used as long as it has not been at room temperature for more than 8 hours, or refrigerated for more than 14 days. Lithium heparin or sodium heparin are acceptable sample types.
11. Add a 5-μL blood sample to blood collection device.	It is not necessary to measure the blood added to the collection device; however, take care that the sample area on the collection device is filled, but not overfilled. If it appears to be underfilled, add more sample; if overfilled, wipe away excess. Do not allow excess blood to remain on the outside of the collection device.
12. Plug blood collection device into the sampler body. Push firmly so that there is no gap on insertion.	If a gap is present, the sample will not combine with the dilution solution inside the sampler body, and the results will be invalid.

Procedure	Rationale
13. Shake the device six to eight times to mix the dilution solution with the sample thoroughly.	Solution must be well mixed to break down the blood sample for appropriate testing.
14. Set sample assembly on the tabletop as the test cartridge is prepared.	
15. Tear open the test cartridge pouch and ensure that the code number on the cartridge matches the code number printed on the instrument.	This system is set up so that the monitor has a definitive number of uses available; all the supplies need to be from the same serial number and cartridge code numbers for the results to be valid.
16. Insert the test cartridge into the monitor until it is seated firmly and an audible click is heard.	If the test cartridge is not seated firmly, no test procedure will occur.
17. Verify that the instrument screen display reads WAIT.	The instrument undergoes a series of internal self-checks before the testing process proceeds.
18. When the instrument screen displays SMPL, pick up the sampler device and remove the base piece, exposing the plunger.	The base piece must be removed so that the sample can be added to the testing device. The sample must be added within 2 minutes.
19. Deliver the sample by pressing the plunger gently and firmly into the corresponding sample application area on the cartridge. Remove after 1 second.	The sample application must occur all at once, but excessive force is not necessary. The application device must be removed for the testing process to proceed.
20. The instrument screen will display a countdown from 5 minutes to 0. Do not move the monitor during this time.	The testing process takes 5 minutes to complete. Moving the monitor may cause inaccurate or invalid test results.
21. The results will display as a percentage on the screen. Record results appropriately in computer, on log sheet, and/or in chart if available.	Results must be recorded immediately so that they are reported correctly.
22. Following office protocol, allow the patient to leave the testing area, or consult with the health-care provider.	If results are far outside of the normal range, it may be office policy that the health-care provider speaks with the patient before he or she leaves the office.
23. Dispose of sample dilution cartridge and test cartridge as biohazardous trash, and disinfect work area.	The work area must always be clean and disinfected after each procedure.
24. Remove gloves and sanitize hands.	Hands must always be sanitized after removing gloves.
25. Document the test results in patient chart.	All results must be documented in the patient's chart.

Date	
8/30/2014:	*Hb A1c 6.9%* ~~~~~~~~~~~~~~~~~~~~~~~~ *Connie Lieseke, CMA (AAMA)*
12:45 p.m.	~~~~~~~~~~~~~~~~~~~~~~~~~~~~~~~~~~~~~~

Procedure 17-2: Performance of Whole Blood Glucose Testing

TASK

Correctly perform a blood glucose test using the HemoCue Glucose 201 Analyzer.

CONDITIONS

- Gloves
- Laboratory coat
- Hand sanitization supplies
- HemoCue Glucose 201 Analyzer
- HemoCue Glucose microcuvettes
- HemoCue Glucose Control Cuvette
- Capillary puncture supplies
- Biohazard sharps container
- Gauze or laboratory wipes
- Biohazardous waste container
- Quality control materials

CAAHEP/ABHES STANDARDS

 CAAHEP Standards

I.P. Anatomy and Physiology, #13 Perform chemistry testing

 ABHES Standards

- 10. Medical Laboratory Procedures, b. CLIA-waived tests
- Graduates: b. Perform selected CLIA-waived tests that assist with diagnosis and treatment, #3 Chemistry Testing

Procedure	Rationale
1. Greet and then identify patient using at least two unique identifiers.	All patients must be identified properly before collecting samples or performing laboratory testing.
2. Verify test ordered, and explain procedure to patient.	All laboratory test orders should be verified by checking the chart and/or requisition form more than once. A quick explanation of the procedure for the patient will ensure more cooperation.
3. Wash hands and apply gloves.	Hands should always be washed between patients and before starting any procedures. Gloves are appropriate personal protective equipment (PPE) for this procedure.
4. Assemble necessary equipment, and verify that all reagents are within the posted expiration dates.	Glucose microcuvettes must be stored refrigerated, as well as the glucose control solution, but they must be removed from the refrigerator and placed within reach before the process begins. Materials that are organized will assist in the process of following the directions properly.
5. Turn on the HemoCue instrument. When the LCD display reads READY, the instrument is ready to be used.	The HemoCue instrument undergoes a series of self-checks when it is turned on.
6. Place the HemoCue Control Cuvette on the cuvette holder and push the holder into the instrument.	The control cuvette is designed to check the function of the instrument and detect any interference with the testing method. It should be used at least once per day.

Procedure	Rationale
7. Verify that the values displayed on the instrument screen are within the acceptable ranges provided with the Control Cuvette.	The ranges are specific per cuvette and are designed specifically for each instrument. If the results are out of range, try cleaning the cuvette and testing again. If they continue to be out of range, the instrument cannot be used for patient testing and the manufacturer must be notified.
8. Prior to performance of test, verify whether a quality control (QC) specimen needs to be tested, and if so, complete that test *before* the patient's test is performed.	Liquid QC should be tested following laboratory protocol and manufacturer's recommendations. Examples of when QC should be used to verify the test results include the following: a. With a new shipment b. Whenever a new lot number of reagents or QC is put into use c. New operator; someone who is being trained on the procedure d. Problems with storage, instrument, reagents, etc. e. To ensure that storage conditions are fine, QC should be performed at least once monthly
9. Perform a capillary puncture, using appropriate technique. Wipe away the first drop of blood.	The first drop of blood should be discarded, as it may be contaminated with interstitial fluids resulting in an erroneous result.
10. Remove a microcuvette from the container. Hold the open end of the microcuvette to the drop of blood obtained from the capillary puncture. Approximately 5 µL of blood will enter the microcuvette.	The blood will enter the microcuvette by capillary action. It is not possible to overfill the microcuvette. Avoid air bubbles as the microvuvette is filled.
11. Wipe away any excess blood on the outside of the microcuvette.	If excess blood is present on the outside of the microcuvette, it may interfere with the testing process and cause erroneous results or an instrument error while processing the specimen.
12. Place the filled microcuvette on the holder and push it into the instrument for processing.	The microcuvette will fit only when placed on the holder in a certain direction.
13. Within a few seconds, the glucose result will appear on the display screen in mg/dL. Record this result appropriately, in the computer, the patient log sheet, and/or the patient's chart.	The result will stay on the screen until the microcuvette holder is pulled from the instrument for the next sample to be added. It is important to record it as soon as it is evident on the screen.
14. Following office protocol, allow the patient to leave the testing area, or consult with the health-care provider.	If results are far outside of the normal range, it may be office policy that the health-care provider speak with the patient before he or she leaves the office.
15. Pull the microcuvette holder back out, remove the microcuvette, and discard in the biohazardous trash.	The microcuvette contains blood, so it must be discarded as a biohazardous substance.

Continued

Procedure 17-2: Performance of Whole Blood Glucose Testing—cont'd

Procedure	Rationale
16. Turn off the instrument, and disinfect the microcuvette holder.	The microcuvette holder can be completely removed from the instrument for cleaning with alcohol or soap and water.
17. Be sure to dispose of the capillary puncture device in a sharps container and any other equipment that may be contaminated with blood in a biohazardous container.	It is vital to always properly dispose of biohazards.
18. Disinfect the work area.	It is important to keep the work area clean and organized.
19. Remove gloves and sanitize hands.	Hands must always be sanitized after removing gloves.
20. Document the test results in the patient's chart.	All results must be documented in the patient's chart.

Date	
8/17/2014: 10:50 a.m.	Fasting blood glucose 85 mg/dL ~~~~~~~~~~~~~~~~~~~ Connie Lieseke, CMA (AAMA)

SUMMARY

Diabetes is disease that has reached epidemic proportions. It requires early diagnosis and consistent monitoring for successful treatment. Consequences of untreated diabetes include cardiovascular disease, loss of vision, poor healing, diabetic neuropathy, and permanent renal damage. Prediabetes can now be identified, and early intervention has helped to stop the progression of the disease for those who make appropriate changes to their diet and exercise habits. There are various testing procedures that may be used to diagnose prediabetes and diabetes, and to monitor treatment once it is under way. Type 1 diabetes must be treated with insulin injections, and the dosage is directly related to the amount of glucose present in the body at the time. Type 2 diabetes is managed with lifestyle changes and oral medication. Frequent blood glucose monitoring assists with treatment for this type of diabetes as well. Gestational diabetes is developed by pregnant women and may be identified toward the end of the pregnancy. Gestational diabetes that is untreated may lead to pregnancy complications as well as serious health issues for the unborn child. Several different timed glucose tests allow an opportunity to identify and classify the diabetic patient, including fasting plasma glucose, and postprandial glucose testing. Hb A1c testing is also useful to monitor the progress of the disease. Self-management testing performed at home by diabetic patients helps to achieve glycemic control between visits to the health-care provider.

TIME TO REVIEW

1. Glycogenolysis is: Outcome 17-1
   a. The breakdown of glycogen to be used for energy
   b. The formation of glycogen as a means of storing energy for later use
   c. The breakdown of glucose
   d. The breakdown of glucagon

2. What does a BMI tell us about a   Outcome 17-1
   patient?
   a. A calculation comparing the height and weight of a patient
   b. A calculation used to compare glucose and body weight

c. A calculation of Hb A1c
d. None of the above

3. When is the term *impaired*   Outcome 17-1
   fasting glucose used?

   a. When the fasting glucose level is over 200 mg/dL
   b. When the fasting glucose level is between 100 to 125 mg/dL
   c. When the fasting glucose level is below 100 mg/dL
   d. When the fasting glucose level is between 100 to 124 mg/dL

4. Does the release of glucagon   Outcome 17-2
   raise or lower blood glucose levels?

   a. Glucagon raises blood glucose levels
   b. Glucagon decreases blood glucose levels

5. True or False: Type 1 diabetes   Outcome 17-4
   is treated with insulin injections whereas type 2 diabetes is treated with oral medications and lifestyle changes.

6. True or False: A patient who is   Outcome 17-5
   diagnosed with gestational diabetes had diabetes before she became pregnant.

7. Which of these body systems may   Outcome 17-6
   be affected by diabetes?

   a. Cardiovascular
   b. Integumentary
   c. Nervous
   d. Eye
   e. All of the above

8. How long should a patient go   Outcome 17-8
   without food and drink before a fasting plasma glucose is drawn?

   a. 8 hours
   b. 16 hours
   c. 12 hours
   d. 10 hours

9. True or False: A postprandial   Outcome 17-9
   glucose sample is always drawn after drinking a glucose-rich beverage.

10. What is the correct number of   Outcome 17-10
    times that a patient drinks the glucose solution while completing a 3-hour glucose tolerance test procedure?

    a. One
    b. Two
    c. Three
    d. Four

11. True or False: The Hb A1c   Outcome 17-11
    test is used to establish a diagnosis of diabetes.

12. How may the serum glucose   Outcome 17-13
    level be affected if the sample is drawn into a tube with no additive and the tube is allowed to sit for 3 hours before centrifugation and processing?

    a. The glucose level may increase
    b. The glucose level may decrease
    c. There will be no effect on the glucose level
    d. It will be impossible to test the glucose level

Case Study 17-1: Use of the Hb A1c

Rose Grace is a patient who has been treated successfully for type 2 diabetes for many years with oral medication and lifestyle changes. The past few months have been especially stressful for her, and she has not been monitoring her diet, exercise, or blood glucose levels consistently during this time. A week before her quarterly appointment with her physician she starts to watch her diet carefully and catch up with some of her glucose monitoring to prepare for the visit. When she sees the physician, she is pleased to have her random glucose at 145 mg/dL, and she does not share all the activities of the past few months with her health-care provider, as it appears that her blood glucose is fine. However, when the Hb A1c result is available, Rose's physician calls her and tells her that she needs to come in for another visit to discuss additional treatment options.

1. What did the Hb A1c result tell the health-care provider that was not apparent with the blood test performed at the initial visit?

RESOURCES AND SUGGESTED READINGS

"National Diabetes Information Clearinghouse"
   Provides in-depth information about the various types of diabetes, diagnosis, and management http://www.diabetes.niddk.nih.gov/
"American Diabetes Association website"
   Information about risk factors, managing diabetes, and support for those who have diabetes; website provides information for providers, patients, and family members http://www. diabetes.org
"Executive Summary: Standards of Medical Care in Diabetes—2009"
   Diabetes Care 32, no. S1 (January 2009): S6–S12, doi: 10.2337/dc09-S006.

Standards of diabetic medical care developed by worldwide consensus and adopted by the World Health Organization, National Institutes of Health, and the American Diabetes Association. Includes parameters for diagnosis and treatment.

"2007 Diabetes Fact Sheet"
National Center for Chronic Disease Prevention and Health Promotion;
Provides statistics for diabetes morbidity and mortality in 2007
http://www.cdc.gov/diabetes

Chapter 18

Other Select Chemistry Tests

Constance L. Lieseke, CMA (AAMA), MLT, PBT(ASCP)

CHAPTER OUTLINE

Lipid Testing
    Cholesterol
        Cholesterol Metabolism Within
        the Body
        Types of Cholesterol
        Risk Factors, Desired Ranges, and Clinical
        Interpretation of Abnormal Lipid Results
        Triglycerides
        Metabolic Syndrome
        Reference Ranges and Clinical Interpretation of
        Abnormal Results
    Lipid Panels

Electrolytes
    Function of Electrolytes and Consequences of
    Electrolyte Imbalances
        Testing Preparation and Common Testing Methods
    Reference Ranges
Summary
Time to Review
Case Study
Resources and Suggested Readings

Learning Outcomes

After reading this chapter, the successful student will be able to:

18-1 Define the key terms.

18-2 Identify dietary sources of cholesterol.

18-3 Compare and contrast the different types of lipoproteins tested in a lipid panel.

18-4 Provide the desired range for cholesterol levels.

18-5 Describe the effects of elevated cholesterol levels on the body.

18-6 Explain how the body uses triglycerides.

18-7 Describe the appearance of lipemia in a blood specimen.

18-8 Evaluate the potential health issues that are caused by high levels of triglycerides.

18-9 List the components of common lipid panels.

18-10 Explain the patient preparation necessary before a specimen is collected for a lipid analysis.

18-11 Perform a CLIA-waived cholesterol test.

18-12 Describe how electrolytes are used by the body.

18-13 Summarize the consequences of untreated electrolyte imbalances.

18-14 List the common analytes included in an electrolyte panel.

18-15 Perform a CLIA-waived electrolyte test.

CAAHEP/ABHES STANDARDS

 CAAHEP 2008 Standards

I.P.I.13. Perform Chemistry Testing
I.A.I.2. Use language/verbal skills that enable patients' understanding

 ABHES Standards

• 10. Medical Laboratory Procedures, b. CLIA-waived tests
• 10. Medical Laboratory Procedures, b. 3) Chemistry Testing

KEY TERMS

Acidosis	Fibrates	Lipemia
Alkalosis	Hyperkalemia	Lipoproteins
Anions	Hypernatremia	Malabsorption
Apolipoproteins	Hypokalemia	Metabolic syndrome
Buffer	Hyponatremia	Niacin
Cations	Intracellular	Statins
Extracellular	Ions	

Clinical chemistry includes the quantitative chemical analysis of various body fluids, as introduced in Chapters 16 and 17 in this text. Because this area of the laboratory performs so many different testing procedures, it is not possible to cover them all in detail in this book. This chapter provides more details about lipid testing and provides additional information about the role of electrolytes in the body. Cholesterol analysis and some electrolyte testing are commonly performed in physician office laboratories, as well as hospital and reference laboratories.

LIPID TESTING

Lipid testing includes the quantitative analysis of cholesterol levels, differentiation of the different types of lipoproteins that transport cholesterol in the body, and analysis of total triglyceride levels. Heart disease is the most common cause of death in the United States, and because the presence of elevated cholesterol (hypercholesterolemia) or hyperlipidemia is a risk factor for many serious cardiovascular complications, frequent monitoring of lipid levels is very important.

Cholesterol

Cholesterol is a white, soft, waxy substance that is present in all the cells of humans. Although humans use cholesterol to form cell membranes, create hormones, and perform other vital body functions, too much cholesterol is very damaging to the blood vessels within our body. It is recommended by the National Cholesterol Education Program that all adults have their cholesterol levels checked at least once every 5 years. The cholesterol level for any individual is dependent on

many factors, including genetics, sex, diet, level of physical activity, social habits, and age.

Cholesterol Metabolism Within the Body

The cholesterol that is needed by our body is manufactured in the liver, but cholesterol is also ingested with animal products, dairy products, and hidden in processed foods. This excess cholesterol is deposited within the blood vessels, causing plaque buildup. The plaque on the interior of the arteries causes them to harden and lose elasticity, a condition known as *atherosclerosis*. The vessels may eventually fill with sticky, hard cholesterol and become occluded (blocked) so that the blood flow is disrupted. The blood that is trapped by the plaque buildup may become clotted. Pieces of the plaque may also break away from the vessel walls and travel to other areas of the body as emboli.

> **Test Your Knowledge 18-1**
>
> The human body produces adequate cholesterol to meet its needs. Additional cholesterol is added as part of our diets. What is one primary source of ingested cholesterol?   (Outcome 18-2)

Types of Cholesterol

Cholesterol is a type of lipid that does not dissolve in blood plasma. It must be attached to another molecule for transport throughout the body. The molecules used for cholesterol transport are also created in the liver, and are called **apolipoproteins.** These are special types of protein that are designed to attach to a lipid molecule, becoming a **lipoprotein.** As introduced in Chapter 16, there are three types of lipoproteins present to transport cholesterol in the bloodstream:

- **High-density lipoprotein (HDL):** A carrier molecule that is known as the "good cholesterol" because it transports cholesterol through the vascular system without contributing to the buildup on the vessel walls. In fact, HDL has been shown to help remove some of the cholesterol that has accumulated in the vascular system. A high level of HDL appears to protect the body from heart disease, and a low level (below 40 mg/dL for men and 50 mg/dL for women) increases the risk for heart disease and stroke.
- **Low-density lipoprotein (LDL):** The major lipoprotein cholesterol transport molecule present in the bloodstream. This is often referred to as the "bad cholesterol" because the lipoprotein has a higher fat content than does the HDL and actually sticks to the blood vessel walls and adheres to the waxy buildup, leading to vessel occlusion. This waxy buildup (plaque) creates a unique environment in which blood cells may bind to one another and form a blood clot. When a blood clot or an occlusion occurs in one of the coronary vessels that supplies blood to the heart, a heart attack may result. Blocked blood flow to the brain results in a stroke (also known as a cerebrovascular accident [CVA]). According to the American Heart Association, LDL cholesterol levels above 160 mg/dL greatly increase the chance of heart disease.
- **Very Low-Density Lipoprotein (VLDL):** Present in smaller amounts than the other transport molecules. Elevated VLDL levels are directly related to the formation of plaque from sticky cholesterol deposits, which increases the risk of heart disease and stroke.

Test Your Knowledge 18-2

Which classifications of lipoproteins are considered as contributors to plaque buildup?   (Outcome 18-3)

Risk Factors, Desired Ranges, and Clinical Interpretation of Abnormal Lipid Results

Total cholesterol screening assists with identification of those who are at high risk for cardiovascular disease. According to the Centers for Disease Control and Prevention (CDC), approximately 17% of the adults in the United States have total cholesterol levels above the desired range. Cholesterol levels may be elevated in certain diseases, such as diabetes, hypothyroidism, and kidney or renal disease. However, more commonly the elevation of total cholesterol is the result of risk factors such as a

sedentary lifestyle, poor diet, cigarette smoking, heredity, and obesity. The presence of two or more risk factors for a specific patient may double the risk of a heart attack. Native Americans and African Americans are at an exceptionally high risk because of genetic factors.

HDL levels may be increased in women because of the natural presence of estrogen in their bodies. Testosterone has been shown to lower HDL levels. Cigarette smoking, sedentary lifestyles, and obesity all contribute to lower HDL levels. It is possible to change the relative levels of LDL and HDL in the body through diet and exercise. The goal of treatment is to decrease total cholesterol, increase HDL levels and decrease LDL levels. Increased exercise, smoking cessation, and weight loss can elevate HDL levels and decrease LDL levels. Early detection, immediate lifestyle changes, and oral medications may have a profound effect on these analytes. LDL levels may be decreased with the use of a class of medications called **statins.**

Test Your Knowledge 18-3

True or False: Elevated HDL levels are desirable in a healthy adult.   (Outcome 18-4)

Cholesterol reference ranges are based on fasting specimens. According to the CDC, the recommended cholesterol levels are the following:

- Total cholesterol levels below 200 mg/dL
- LDL cholesterol level below 100 mg/dL
- HDL cholesterol at 40 mg/dL or above
- Triglycerides below 150 mg/dL

Test Your Knowledge 18-4

Sally Seashore has her fasting cholesterol test performed as a part of her yearly physical. Her total cholesterol level was 205 mg/dL. Is this within the desirable range?   (Outcome 18-4)

It is not only adults who have elevated cholesterol levels. Children who have parents or grandparents who developed heart disease before they were age 55, or those who have other risk factors such as race and obesity should have their cholesterol levels monitored closely, as it is now clear that the development of plaque buildup in the blood vessels may begin very early in life.

Test Your Knowledge 18-5

Why are elevated LDL levels considered to be a health risk?   (Outcome 18-5)

Procedure 18-1: Cholesterol Testing Using the Cholestech LDX System

TASK

Perform CLIA-waived cholesterol testing using the Cholestech LDX System

CONDITIONS

- Gloves
- Laboratory coat
- Hand sanitization supplies
- Cholestech LDX analyzer
- Cholestech thermal label printer
- Liquid controls (level 1 and level 2)
- Test cassettes in foil wrap
- Optics test cassette and holder
- Capillary puncture supplies
- Cholestech capillary tubes and black plungers for collection and application of blood samples
- Biohazardous sharps container
- Gauze or laboratory wipes
- Biohazardous waste container

- Liquid quality control materials (two levels)
- Acrylic safety shield (if using lithium heparin vacuum tubes rather than capillary samples for the testing process)

CAAHEP/ABHES STANDARDS

 CAAHEP Standards

I.P.I. Anatomy and Physiology, #13. Perform Chemistry Testing   **I.A.I.** Anatomy and Physiology, #2. Use language/verbal skills that enable patients' understanding

 ABHES Standards

- 10. Medical Laboratory Procedures, b. CLIA-waived tests
- 10. Medical Laboratory Procedures, b. 3) Chemistry Testing

Procedure	Rationale
1. Greet and then identify patient using at least two unique identifiers.	All patients must be identified properly before collecting samples or performing laboratory testing.
2. Verify test ordered, and explain procedure to patient. Verify whether patient has prepared properly.	All laboratory test orders should be verified by checking the chart and/or requisition form more than once. A quick explanation of the procedure for the patient will ensure more cooperation. Cholesterol testing requires the patient to fast for at least 12 hours prior to the blood draw. It is important that the patient understands the meaning of a 12-hour fast to verify whether he or she has followed the necessary preparation instructions.
3. Wash hands and apply gloves.	Hands should always be washed between patients and before starting any procedures. Gloves are appropriate personal protection equipment (PPE) for this procedure, as well as a laboratory coat.
4. Assemble necessary equipment, and verify that all reagents are within the posted expiration dates. Allow all reagents to come to room temperature.	The Cholestech LDX cassettes are stored in the refrigerator, but must come to room temperature before use. It is recommended that they be removed from the refrigerator for at least 10 minutes prior to use. Organization of materials will make it easier to follow the procedure specified by the manufacturer properly.

Procedure	Rationale
5. Plug in the analyzer and allow it to initialize. Verify that the printer has paper attached to the testing instrument correctly.	The analyzer must be allowed to initialize before use.
6. Perform an optics check using an optics check cassette. When testing the optics test cassette, the following procedures are followed: a. Press RUN. The analyzer will then perform a self-test, and display a Self-Test OK message on the screen. The drawer will then automatically open, and a message of Load Cassette and Press Run will appear on the screen. b. Use the optics check cassette by inserting the cassette into the open drawer of the instrument. Be careful not to touch the dark areas of the cassette; it should be handled only by the edges and by touching the clear parts of the cassette. c. Press RUN again. The drawer will shut and the testing process for the optics check will begin. d. A series of numbers will be displayed on the screen. These are the results of the optics check. The results must all fall between 80 and 105, and they must also be within the ranges provided with purchase of the optics check to be a valid test. e. Verify that the results are as desired before continuing with the testing process. If the results are not within range, the instrument will display an error code (Optics Test Fail), and it will not be possible to process patient samples until a valid optics check is performed.	The optics check cassette is to be used as directed by the manufacturer and laboratory policy to verify that the four optic channels of the instrument are working correctly. This should be used at least once daily before patient samples or quality control samples are tested. An optics test should also be completed after the machine is moved or cleaned. Acceptable ranges will be provided with the cuvette upon purchase. If the results do not fall within the acceptable range, the instrument may not be used for specimen testing until the cause has been identified and the problem has been identified and solved. Troubleshooting tips will be available in the user manual and/or manufacturer insert.
7. Remove the optics check cuvette from the instrument and place it back in the designated container.	The cuvette must be stored in the designated container to keep it from being damaged. Exposure to moisture or damaging the cuvette may affect the performance.
8. Prior to patient testing, verify whether a quality control (QC) specimen needs to be tested, and if so, complete that process before the patient's test is performed. Patient testing cannot be performed unless the quality control values are within the established ranges.	Liquid QC should be tested following laboratory protocol and manufacturer's recommendations. Examples of when QC may be utilized to verify the test results include the following: a. With a new shipment b. Whenever a new lot number of reagents or QC is put into use c. New operator; someone who is being trained on the procedure d. Problems with storage, instrument, reagents, etc.
9. Tear open the foil package and set the testing cassette on a level nonabsorbent surface.	The cassette needs to be ready for the application of the sample as soon as the blood collection is complete.

Continued

Procedure 18-1: Cholesterol Testing Using the Cholestech LDX System—cont'd

Procedure	Rationale
10. Perform a capillary puncture, using appropriate technique. Wipe away the first drop of blood.	The first drop of blood should be discarded, as it may be contaminated with interstitial fluids resulting in an erroneous result.
11. Remove a capillary tube and a black plunger from the container. Insert the black plunger into the capillary tube, and then hold the open end of the capillary tube to the drop of blood obtained from the capillary puncture. The capillary tube will fill with sample, and this should be completed within approximately 10 seconds.	The blood will enter the capillary tube without further action if the capillary tube is kept level while the end is immersed in a drop of blood. Avoid air bubbles as the capillary tube is filled.
12. Introduce the blood into the sample well on the cassette. Be careful not to touch the dark areas of the cassette. Use the black plunger to empty the capillary tube into the testing well.	Blood on other areas of the cassette apart from the sample well may interfere with the testing process.
13. Place the filled cassette into the drawer as soon as the sample has been added. If the drawer has closed, press the RUN button again and the drawer will open.	The cassette needs to be processed immediately for accurate results. Do not allow the filled cassette to be moved excessively. It should be kept horizontal as it is placed in the drawer.
14. Within a few seconds, the cholesterol result will appear on the display screen in mg/dL. Record this result on the patient log sheet.	The result will stay on the screen until the RUN button is pushed to open the drawer for the next test sample to be added. It is important to record the result as soon as it is evident on the screen. The result will print if the instrument is attached to a printer.
15. Following office protocol, allow the patient to leave the testing area, or consult with the health-care provider about the test results.	If results are far outside of the normal range, the office policy may be that the health-care provider speaks with the patient before he or she leaves the office.
16. Discard the capillary tube and plunger and contaminated cassette in the biohazardous garbage.	The capillary tube, plunger, and cassette contain blood, so they must be discarded as a biohazardous substance.
17. Turn off the instrument if there are no further tests needed and disinfect the work area. Discard any other waste appropriately.	The work area should always be disinfected after use.
18. Remove gloves and sanitize hands.	Hands must always be sanitized after removing gloves.
19. Document the test results in patient chart.	All results must be documented in the patient's chart.

Date	
8/17/2014:	*Fasting cholesterol 195 mg/dL* ~~~~~~~~~~~~~~
2:15 p.m.	~~~~~~~~~~~~~~~~~~~~~~~~~~ *Connie Lieseke, CMA (AAMA)*

Triglycerides

Triglyceride levels are usually included in lipid panels as an additional indicator for evaluating the risk of cardiovascular disease. Triglycerides are the end product of the fats that we ingest. When a person takes in more calories than are needed for energy, some of the excess calories are also turned into triglycerides and stored as fat for use later as an energy source. These are then stored in the liver and the adipose cells of our body, and may also sometimes be stored in the muscle tissue. A patient who often eats more calories than those used by the body may develop elevated blood triglyceride levels.

Test Your Knowledge 18-6

What leads to a buildup of triglycerides in the adipose tissue of the body?
   a. Consumption of excess calories
   b. Pancreatitis
   c. Elevated LDL levels
   d. Plaque buildup   (Outcome 18-6)

Metabolic Syndrome

Elevated triglyceride levels unaccompanied by other risk factors are not linked as closely to cardiovascular disease as are high cholesterol levels. However, the high triglyceride levels may be part of a group of conditions that are known as **metabolic syndrome.** Metabolic syndrome includes hypertension, hyperglycemia, excessive fat deposits around the waistline, low HDL levels, and high triglyceride levels. Patients who simultaneously exhibit most of these conditions in the metabolic syndrome have an increased risk for cardiovascular disease, as well as a greater potential for developing diabetes. Oral medications may be prescribed to lower triglyceride levels. **Niacin** is commonly used, as is a classification of drugs called **fibrates.** If the triglyceride levels are elevated as well as total cholesterol and LDL levels, a combination of drugs may be used to lower the various lipid levels.

Reference Ranges and Clinical Interpretation of Abnormal Results

Hyperlipidemia is the word used to describe elevated levels of cholesterol and triglycerides in the bloodstream, and as introduced in Chapter 16, patients with hyperlipidemia may have cloudy or "milky" plasma and/or serum apparent after a sample of their blood is spun in a centrifuge.

This appearance is known as **lipemia,** and it is caused by suspended fat particles, which can cause interference for many testing procedures. Large reference laboratories may have specialized centrifuges designed to clear the excess fats from the plasma or serum so that testing can continue on these specimens.

Test Your Knowledge 18-7

Lipemia is a suspension of _____ , visualized in the liquid portion of the blood after centrifugation:
   a. Hemolyzed red blood cells
   b. Excess fat particles
   c. Plaque
   d. Milk   (Outcome 18-7)

According to the CDC, triglyceride levels should be drawn as fasting samples, because the blood levels become elevated with the ingestion of food. Triglyceride levels may be categorized as the following:

- Normal: below 150 mg/dL
- Borderline high: 150 to 199 mg/dL
- High: 200 to 499 mg/dL
- Very high: equal to or greater than 500 mg/dL

Lipid Panels

A lipid panel commonly includes a total cholesterol level; a triglyceride level; the HDL, LDL, VLDL; and a total cholesterol/HDL ratio. These values provide the health-care provider with valuable information to determine whether the cholesterol levels for a patient indicate a risk factor for coronary artery disease. The lipid panel also provides information that is useful for monitoring patients who are taking medication to treat high cholesterol or triglycerides. Current recommendations from the National Institutes of Health's National Cholesterol Education Program include the performance of a screening fasting (at least 12 hours) lipid panel at least once every 5 years. For patients with elevated LDL levels and/or triglyceride or total cholesterol levels that are too high, lifestyle changes and possible drug treatment should be started immediately. The fasting lipid panel should be rechecked once every 6 weeks until the established goals have been met for a patient, and a fasting lipid panel should continue to be performed every 4 to 6 months while completing treatment.

Fats are essential to homeostasis, but ingestion of too much can be quite harmful. Most Americans take in an excess of fat on a daily basis. According to the Centers for Disease Control and Prevention (CDC), fats should not make up more than 35% of our caloric intake each day. In addition to controlling the amount of fat ingested, we can benefit from monitoring the types of fats we eat, because certain types of fats cause much more harm to our cardiovascular systems than others. Polyunsaturated and monounsaturated fats are healthier for the body than *trans* fats, saturated fats, and cholesterol. The unhealthy fats are "hidden" in many of the processed foods that we eat. To avoid an unhealthy diet, it is important to be educated about the types of fats in our diets:

- *Trans* **fats:** It is required that all products containing *trans* fats have them listed on their nutrition labels. This type of fat actually starts as a liquid; a process called hydrogenation changes the oils into a solid fat. *Trans* fat helps processed foods last longer without spoilage, but the presence of *trans* fats increases LDL cholesterol levels and decreases HDL cholesterol levels. Many processed baked goods (such as pies, cookies, crackers, and cakes) include *trans* fats to extend their shelf life. *Trans* fats may also be present in solid margarine products. Nutritionists recommend soft margarine over solid margarine whenever possible.
- **Saturated fats:** The current recommendation is to restrict our daily caloric intake from saturated fats to less than 10%. This type of fat comes from meat and high-fat dairy products. It is also present in palm and coconut oils, which can be included in a many processed foods. Choosing low-fat products, fat-free milk, and lean meats can help to control the amount of saturated fats ingested. Check labels to reduce the amount of saturated fats (and *trans* fats) whenever possible. Removing the skin from meats before cooking, and skimming off visible fat from soups and stews can also help to reduce dietary intake. Diets that are high in saturated fat are believed to contribute to cardiovascular disease.
- **Cholesterol:** Cholesterol is usually found in the same type of products as those having high levels of saturated fat. Meat, eggs, and dairy products contain high levels of cholesterol. Steps that lower the intake of saturated fat will also help to control cholesterol in the diet because they appear in similar foods. Remember, genetics also plays a role in total blood cholesterol content; many patients will have high levels of cholesterol even with excellent diets and active lifestyles. In this case, patients will usually need to be treated with oral medications to keep their cholesterol level at a reasonable level.
- **Monounsaturated and polyunsaturated fats:** These fats are considered the most "healthy" fats. They come from ingestion of fish, vegetable oils, and nuts. All sources of fat are high in calories, but polyunsaturated and monounsaturated fats do not pose as high a cardiovascular threat as do the other types.

ELECTROLYTES

In Chapter 16, electrolytes are defined as substances that are capable of conducting an electrical charge when dissolved in water. Particles that are positively or negatively charged because of the loss or gain of electrons are called **ions,** and all electrolytes fall within this description. Positively charged ions are called **cations,** and those ions with a negative charge are called **anions.** The most common cations in the body are sodium and potassium. Sodium has a high **extracellular** concentration, which means that it has a higher concentration outside the body's cells, in the plasma. Potassium is higher in concentration inside the cells, in the **intracellular** environment. The most common anions present in the body are chloride and bicarbonate. Bicarbonate (HCO_3^-) is an ion created when carbon dioxide reacts with water. Most electrolyte panels measure Na^+, K^+, Cl^- and bicarbonate. Figure 18-1 illustrates the distribution of the most common electrolytes inside and outside red blood cells. Bicarbonate may be measured directly or by analysis of total CO_2, as most of the carbon dioxide present in the blood is found as bicarbonate molecules. Additional electrolytes present in the body include magnesium, calcium, phosphate, and sulfate; however, these are not included in most electrolyte panels.

> **Test Your Knowledge 18-8**
> True or False: Electrolytes are neutral; they neither exhibit a positive nor negative charge when dissolved in water.
> (Outcome 18-1)

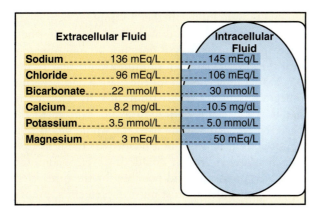

Extracellular Fluid	Intracellular Fluid
Sodium .... 136 mEq/L	145 mEq/L
Chloride .... 96 mEq/L	106 mEq/L
Bicarbonate ...... 22 mmol/L	30 mmol/L
Calcium .... 8.2 mg/dL	10.5 mg/dL
Potassium .... 3.5 mmol/L	5.0 mmol/L
Magnesium .... 3 mEq/L	50 mEq/L

Figure 18-1   Major intracellular and extracellular electrolytes.

Function of Electrolytes and Consequences of Electrolyte Imbalances

Appropriate amounts of the various electrolytes in the body are essential to maintain homeostasis and acid-base balance. The electrolytes are also responsible for transmission of nervous impulses, and they play a major role in contraction and relaxation of the muscle fibers present throughout the body. The presence of the various intracellular and extracellular electrolytes in appropriate concentrations also allows for cells to keep their shape so that they can function properly. More specific electrolyte functions include the following:

- **Sodium (Na⁺):** Sodium is the electrolyte found in highest concentration outside the cells of the body. We take in sodium through our diets, and the amount retained by the body is controlled by the kidneys. Sodium loss also occurs through perspiration. Sodium is essential for controlling the amount of fluid retained in the cells of the body. When the sodium levels are too low (a condition known as **hyponatremia**) in relation to the amount of fluid present in the body, the patient may exhibit drowsiness and confusion. If the condition worsens, it can lead to muscle twitches, seizures, coma, and even death. Hyponatremia can occur with various renal disorders, endocrine imbalances that the amount of antidiuretic hormone (ADH) produced, excessive water intake, or retention of fluids from various disease processes. Certain prescription drugs may also contribute to low sodium levels. **Hypernatremia** (elevated sodium levels) results when the concentration

of sodium is elevated as compared to the amount of fluid in the body. Essentially, a patient with hypernatremia has too little water in the body for the amount of sodium that is present. This can be the result of severe vomiting and/or diarrhea with fluid loss, or excessive sweating without fluid replacement. Hypernatremia may also occur with severe burns, and is a risk for those with disease states that cause excessive urine to be produced. Sodium levels that are outside the reference range may lead to lethargy, confusion, muscle twitches, seizures, coma, and death if not treated promptly.

- **Potassium (K⁺):** Potassium is present in high concentrations within the cells of the body, but normally is quite low in the blood plasma. The kidneys control the amount of potassium excreted from the body, and dietary intake helps to keep the necessary balance for healthy function. The presence of potassium is essential for cardiac function, as well as the transmission of nervous impulses to other muscles of the body. **Hyperkalemia** is the word used to describe elevated levels of potassium in the blood, and **hypokalemia** is the word used to describe diminished levels of potassium. Both conditions may be caused by renal dysfunction or certain hormonal imbalances. Reduced dietary intake may also contribute to hypokalemia, as well as use of prescription medications that contribute to increased urination. Diseases that cause gastrointestinal **malabsorption** (problems with the absorption of nutrients from food ingested) will also cause hypokalemia. Potassium imbalances are not tolerated well by the body, and may result in cardiac arrhythmias or other symptoms of muscle weakness.

- **Chloride (Cl⁻):** Chloride is an anion, which means that it has a negative charge when dissolved in water. It is a very important extracellular presence, as chloride contributes to homeostasis by participation in acid-base balance. Chloride moves into and out of the cells of the body in response to the transfer of hydrogen and carbon dioxide through the cellular membrane. When chloride levels become imbalanced, the acid-base neutrality of the body's tissues may be affected, and **acidosis** (increase in acidity of the blood) or **alkalosis** (increase in alkalinity of the blood) may result.

- **Bicarbonate (HCO₃⁻):** Bicarbonate is formed when carbon dioxide combines with water present in blood plasma. As is the case with chloride, bicarbonate plays an essential role in acid-base balance of the body. It acts as a **buffer,** which means that the presence of bicarbonate helps to keep the body's pH at a neutral level by interacting with substances capable of changing the pH. Most of the bicarbonate in the body is found outside the cells, but there is a small amount present intracellularly. Bicarbonate may be indirectly measured in the laboratory by analyzing the amount of total CO_2 present in the blood. Abnormal amounts of bicarbonate (directly tested or analyzed by measuring total carbon dioxide levels) may contribute to acidosis or alkalosis.

Test Your Knowledge 18-9

A patient who has been treated with diuretics for the past few months develops an arrhythmia and is seen in the ER. When the patient has his blood tested, which electrolyte level may be outside of the reference range?

(Outcome 18-13)

Testing Preparation and Common Testing Methods

Specimen collection for electrolyte testing does not require any specific preparation, but it is important to collect the sample using appropriate phlebotomy technique to avoid erroneous results. Electrolyte testing performed in hospital and reference laboratories usually requires plasma or serum samples, which need to be separated from the blood cells in the specimen within an hour of collection. Electrolyte results can easily be affected by poor preanalytical procedures. Because potassium is at such a high concentration within blood cells and exhibits such a low extracellular concentration, any specimen collection or processing errors that contribute to hemolysis will cause the plasma potassium values to be falsely elevated. Excessive hemolysis may also cause the plasma sodium and chloride results to be decreased because of a dilution effect from all the intracellular contents released when the cells are broken. Contamination of the specimen with IV fluids will also alter the plasma electrolyte results; the effects will vary depending on the type of fluids being administered. CLIA-waived electrolyte procedures use whole blood for testing. The samples may be obtained by capillary puncture or by venipuncture, using a lithium heparin (light green top tube) or sodium heparin (dark green top tube). It is not possible to determine whether a sample is hemolyzed at the time of the blood draw by looking at the whole blood specimen; hemolysis does not become apparent until the sample has been spun in a centrifuge or until it has sat long enough for the plasma and/or serum to begin to separate visibly from the cells. This means that it is especially critical to avoid damage to the specimen when it will be used for whole blood testing, because it will not be evident that the cells have been hemolyzed, which could cause erroneous test results for potassium and possibly for the other electrolytes. The phlebotomist must implement appropriate venipuncture technique, including the use of the correct needle size, with complete insertion of the bevel into the interior of the vein. The tourniquet should not be applied for longer than 1 minute, and pumping of the fist should not be encouraged. Also, the blood sample should be gently inverted (not shaken).

There are many instruments that have been approved for CLIA-waived electrolyte testing. These instruments are capable of performing all the tests included in most electrolyte panels, including sodium, potassium, chloride, and bicarbonate. The testing instruments are present in physician office laboratories, but may also be used as a STAT testing method in other environments. These include the Abaxis Piccolo Blood Chemistry Analyzer and the Abbott i-STAT System. (See Fig. 18-2.)

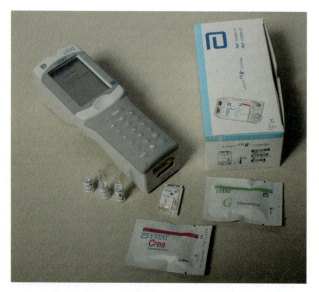

Figure 18-2 Abbott i-STAT analyzer. *Courtesy of Abbott Point of Care, Princeton, NJ.*

Test Your Knowledge 18-10

Which of these tests is not part of a typical electrolyte panel?

a. Sodium
b. Potassium
c. Nitrogen
d. Chloride

(Outcome 18-14)

Reference Ranges

It is important to realize that the reference ranges for any analyte may vary according to the method used for testing. The following are approximate ranges established for adults for plasma samples:

- Sodium: 135 to 145 mmol/L
- Potassium: 3.5 to 5.0 mmol/L
- Chloride: 98 to 108 mmol/L
- Bicarbonate: 22 to 30 mmol/L

Procedure 18-2: Electrolyte Testing Using an Abbott i-STAT Chemistry Analyzer

TASK

Perform CLIA-waived whole blood electrolyte testing using an i-STAT analyzer.

CONDITIONS

- Gloves
- Laboratory coat
- Hand sanitization supplies
- I-STAT chemistry analyzer
- I-STAT analyzer electrolyte (panel or individual test) cartridges
- Capillary puncture supplies or venipuncture supplies and green top tubes
- Biohazardous sharps container
- Gauze or laboratory wipes
- Biohazardous waste container
- Quality control materials

CAAHEP/ABHES STANDARDS

 CAAHEP Standards

I.P.I. Anatomy and Physiology, #13. Perform Chemistry Testing **I.A.I.** Anatomy and Physiology, #2. Use language/verbal skills that enable patients' understanding

 ABHES Standards

- 10. Medical Laboratory Procedures, b. CLIA-waived tests
- 10. Medical Laboratory Procedures, b. 3) Chemistry Testing

Procedure	Rationale
1. Greet and then identify patient using at least two unique identifiers.	All patients must be identified properly before collecting samples or performing laboratory testing.
2. Verify test ordered, and explain the testing procedure to the patient.	All laboratory test orders should be verified by checking the chart and/or requisition form more than once. A quick explanation of the procedure for the patient will ensure more cooperation.

Continued

Procedure 18-2: Electrolyte Testing Using an Abbott i-STAT Chemistry Analyzer—cont'd

Procedure	Rationale
3. Assemble necessary equipment, and verify that all reagents are within their expiration dates. For an electrolyte panel to be performed, it may be necessary to use a cartridge that tests for other analytes in addition to those in the electrolyte panel, due to the cartridge packaging.	i-STAT cartridges are to be stored at 2° to 8°C until their printed expiration. Cartridges must be removed from the refrigerator and allowed to be at room temperature for at least 5 minutes before use. A cartridge expires 2 weeks after it is removed from the refrigerator, and it is not to be put back in the refrigerator once it has reached room temperature. Materials that are organized will assist in the process of following the directions properly.
4. Wash hands and apply gloves.	Hands should always be washed between patients and before starting any procedures. Gloves are appropriate personal protective equipment (PPE) for this procedure.
5. Turn on the analyzer. If necessary, use the electronic simulator cartridge to verify that the instrument is operating correctly.	An internal electronic simulation occurs after every 8 hours that the instrument is in use. It may also be necessary to use an external electronic simulator cartridge if the internal test is not successful or if the laboratory policy dictates the use of this additional step. This cartridge is stored at room temperature. To use, insert the cartridge into the instrument with the I facing upward. If the test is successful, the LED screen will display a PASS message.
6. Prior to performance of test, verify whether a quality control (QC) specimen needs to be tested, and if so, complete that test before the patient's test is performed. It is recommended that two levels of quality control be tested every time QC is run.	Liquid QC should be tested following laboratory protocol and manufacturer's recommendations. Examples of when QC should be used to verify the test results include the following: a. With a new shipment b. Whenever a new lot number of reagents or QC is put into use c. New operator; someone who is being trained on the procedure d. Problems with storage, instrument, reagents, etc. e. To ensure that storage conditions are fine, QC should be performed at least once monthly
7. Remove the cartridge from the foil pouch. Be careful to handle the cartridge only by the edges, and place it on a level, clean surface until use.	If the contact points of the cartridge are scratched or damaged before the test is performed, it may have an adverse effect on the test results. The cartridge should be removed from the pouch before the sample is collected just to save time.
8. Perform a capillary puncture, using appropriate technique. Wipe away the first drop of blood. Use a heparinized capillary tube to collect a blood sample, avoiding the formation of air bubbles in the tube.	The first drop of blood should be discarded, as it may be contaminated with interstitial fluids, resulting in an erroneous result.

Procedure	Rationale
9. Hold the end of the filled capillary tube to the sample well. The well will fill with blood through capillary action. Fill the well to the indicated fill mark.	The blood will enter the cartridge well by capillary action. It is acceptable to slightly overfill the well, but if the well is grossly overfilled or if blood is smeared on the cartridge outside of the well, the instrument will give an ERROR code when the assay is performed. Avoid air bubbles as the sample well is filled.
The sample may also be taken from a sodium heparin– or lithium heparin–evacuated blood tube, or from a sterile syringe without additives.	If an evacuated blood tube is used, a plain plastic capillary tube can be used to transfer the specimen to the cartridge. If a sterile syringe is used for the venipuncture, it is important to apply the sample immediately to the cartridge to avoid clots in the specimen.
10. The analyzer will request an operator ID and a specimen/patient identification number. Enter these according to laboratory policy.	These identification methods allow for better documentation and tracking.
11. After the analysis has completed, the result will be displayed on the LED screen for 45 seconds. It may be recorded directly on the patient log sheet and transferred to the patient chart when ready.	The result may be recalled before running the next specimen by pushing DIS (display) on the instrument. Sample results are also kept in the analyzer memory, and some laboratories will have the instrument interfaced with their patient data system for direct documentation in the patient record.
12. Following office protocol, allow the patient to leave testing area, or consult with the health-care provider.	If results are far outside of the normal range, office policy may be that the health-care provider speaks with the patient before he or she leaves the office.
13. Remove the used cartridge from the instrument, and discard it as biohazardous trash.	The cartridge contains blood, so it must be discarded as a biohazardous substance.
14. Turn off the instrument or prepare to run the next specimen.	If numerous specimens are waiting to be assayed, leave the instrument turned on between samples.
15. Dispose of the capillary puncture device or used venipuncture supplies in a sharps container immediately after use. Any other equipment that may be contaminated with blood must be disposed of as a biohazard.	It is vital to always properly dispose of biohazards.
16. Disinfect the work area.	It is important to keep the work area clean and organized. Prompt disinfection helps to stop the cycle of infection.
17. Remove gloves and sanitize hands.	Hands must always be sanitized after removing gloves.
18. Document the test results in patient chart.	All results must be documented in the patient's chart.

Date	
8/17/2014:	Electrolyte test performed: Sodium 140 mmol/L, Potassium 3.7 mmol/L, Chloride 100 mmol/L, TCO2 25 mmol/L
11:29 a.m.	~~~~~~~~~~~~~~~~~~~~~~~~~~~ Connie Lieseke, CMA (AAMA)

SUMMARY

Clinical chemistry is a complex laboratory department where a wide variety of tests may be performed. This chapter focused on some of the clinical chemistry tests that might be performed in a physician office laboratory as well as in larger reference laboratories. These include lipid panels, electrolyte analysis, and fecal occult blood testing. Lipid testing is very important, as elevated levels of total cholesterol, LDL, and triglycerides may be indicative of potential damage to the cardiovascular system and subsequent myocardial infarction or stroke. Electrolytes are responsible for conduction of nerve impulses and maintenance of homeostasis with acid-base balance. Imbalances of sodium, potassium, chloride, and bicarbonate can be life threatening, and may indicate an ongoing disease process elsewhere in the body.

TIME TO REVIEW

1. Hypernatremia is: Outcome 18-1
   a. Elevated sodium concentration in the blood
   b. Elevated potassium concentration in the blood
   c. Decreased sodium concentration in the blood
   d. Decreased potassium concentration in the blood

2. Statins are used to treat: Outcome 18-1
   a. Electrolyte imbalances
   b. Anemia
   c. Elevated triglyceride levels
   d. Elevated cholesterol levels

3. True or False: Cholesterol levels are   Outcome 18-2
   increased by excessive ingestion of carbohydrates.

4. True or False: When evaluating   Outcome 18-9
   cholesterol levels, the total cholesterol is not the only level considered by the practitioner.

5. Which type of lipoprotein is   Outcome 18-3
   considered to be the "good cholesterol"?
   a. HDL
   b. VLDL
   c. Triglyceride
   d. LDL

6. Elevated lipid levels in the   Outcome 18-8
   bloodstream increase the chance of:
   a. Plaque formation on the blood vessel walls
   b. Myocardial infarction
   c. Liver damage
   d. Electrolyte imbalances

7. Which of these are included in the   Outcome 18-1
   metabolic syndrome?
   a. Elevated triglyceride levels
   b. Hypertension
   c. Hyperglycemia
   d. Excessive fat deposits around the waistline
   d. All of the above

8. Which tests are included in a lipid   Outcome 18-9
   panel?
   a. Total cholesterol, HDL, LDL, VLDL, triglyceride
   b. HDL, GLDL, LDL, BUN
   c. Total cholesterol, triglyceride, HDL, anion gap
   d. None of the above

9. How should a patient prepare for a   Outcome 18-10
   lipid panel specimen collection?
   a. No preparation is necessary
   b. The patient must fast for 12 hours
   c. The patient should follow a carbohydrate-restrictive diet for a week prior
   d. The patient should follow a protein-rich diet for a week prior

10. What is a consequence of elevated   Outcome 18-13
    or decreased bicarbonate levels?
    a. Loss of cellular membrane shape
    b. Cardiac arrhythmia
    c. Acidosis or alkalosis
    d. Muscle tremors

Case Study 18-1: Difficult draw

Kim Babado, CMA (AAMA), is working in the laboratory area of an internal medicine clinic. She has the responsibility of drawing blood on most of the patients in the practice, performing some point-of-care testing, and processing blood and other samples to prepare them for transport to a large reference laboratory across town. The second patient of the morning has an order for an electrolyte panel. When Kim examines the patient's arm, she has a difficult time finding a suitable site for the blood draw. The patient has very small veins that seem to roll away every time Kim touches them. Kim's first attempt is unsuccessful. On her second try, Kim does successfully puncture the vein, but obtains a slow blood flow that fills the tube approximately half full. After the blood specimen is spun in the centrifuge, Kim notes a light pink shade to the plasma.

1. Do you think that the specimen is appropriate for electrolyte testing?

Case Study 18-2: Dietary effects

A patient has a lipid panel drawn on Monday afternoon, and his results include an elevated triglyceride level. The ordering physician asks for the specimen to be redrawn to verify the results before meeting again with the patient.

1. What is a possible explanation for the elevated triglyceride level for this patient?
2. What might be important information to give the patient before the next blood draw?

RESOURCES AND SUGGESTED READINGS

"Colorectal Cancer Screening"
   Colorectal cancer screening information and recommendations from the Centers for Disease Control and Prevention http://www.cdc.gov/cancer/colorectal/basic_info/screening/
"Hemoccult's Newest Gold Standard in FOBTs-Hemoccult ICT"
Beckman Coulter Hemoccult ICT test information http://www.hemocultfobt.com/sales/sales_Hemo_ICT.htm
"Hemoccult Fecal Occult Blood Tests"
   Provides links to overview for all of Beckman Coulter Hemoccult products http://www.hemoccultfobt.com/
"Tests Granted Waived Status Under CLIA"
   List of all CLIA-waived tests, including CPT code for reimbursement http://www.cms.hhs.gov/CLIA/downloads/waivetbl.pdf
"Cholestech"
   Detailed information about the Cholestech analyzers available for lipid testing. http://cholestech.com
"Abbott Point of Care"
   Detailed information about the Abbott i-STAT analyzer and other point-of-care testing instruments manufactured by Abbott http://abbottpointofcare.com

Clinical Chemistry
What Does It All Mean?

As the chapters in this section clearly point out, there is a plethora of tests that are typically performed in the clinical chemistry area of the laboratory. These tests may be ordered and performed on an individual basis or may be ordered and tested in groups known as profiles. Physicians and other primary care providers such as nurse practitioners and physician assistants make these important ordering decisions.

Case in Point

At the beginning of this section we met 34-year-old Carrie W. A fasting blood glucose test was performed on her as part of a health fair sponsored by Carrie's employer, Acme Innovations, Inc. Her value was significantly higher than the highest number in the normal range for this test. The fact that this test was done after a period of fasting indicates that her ability to process glucose is likely impaired.

Glucose serves as the body's main source of energy. Under normal circumstances, glucose is metabolized and the resulting products are used by the body for the many functions it performs on a daily basis. An unusually high glucose level suggests that the body is unable to metabolize glucose properly. The most likely condition associated with this scenario is diabetes mellitus. Individuals with diabetes mellitus typically either do not produce the substance insulin that is necessary for glucose metabolism or they produce insulin but its function is impaired. In either event, glucose is not being properly used and eventually builds up in the body, thus causing increased blood glucose levels. Because the body can count on glucose for energy, it resorts to fat. Incomplete fat metabolism ensues. A by-product of incomplete fat metabolism is a substance known as ketone.

Once the body has reached its saturation point of glucose and ketones, excess amounts of both substances are deposited into the urine for disposal from the body. Thus, along with high blood glucose levels, individuals with diabetes mellitus typically also have high levels of glucose and ketones in the urine (urine testing is covered in detail in Chapter 21).

In some instances a change in diet stabilizes the blood glucose levels to the point that the diabetes mellitus can be manageable without taking other steps. However, there are instances when treatment with insulin is indicated.

On the Horizon

Perhaps the easiest, most noninvasive specimen type for analysis from humans is urine. In fact, the concept of analyzing urine has been noted in drawings on ancient history walls. Early analyzers determined that if urine from a diabetic individual is spread on the ground, then because of its sweet smell, ants would gravitate to it. At one point, a group of so-called self-taught urine analyzers, known as the "pisse prophets," marketed their services to individuals. Patients who submitted their urine and paid a fee received an analysis of their urine without ever being examined by a physician.

There have been many advances in urine analysis over the years, one of the more notable being the advent of plastic strips impregnated with chemical pads, known as a dipstick. Today, a test that incorporates the dipstick technology, known as a urinalysis, screens for a number of abnormalities. In many instances, such abnormalities may be detected through urinalysis testing, often before the patient experiences any symptoms. This section focuses on the urinalysis test, as it is crucial in the diagnosis and monitoring of disease as well as in the monitoring of select treatment regimens. The occult blood test is also covered in this section.

Relevance for the Medical Assistant (Health-Care Provider)

As with so many other aspects of laboratory testing, medical assistants and other health-care support personnel are often involved in the collection of samples for urinalysis testing by assisting the patient in the process or providing the patient with collection instructions. Furthermore, medical assistants often perform urinalysis and occult blood testing along with appropriate quality control. Medical assistants are also responsible for completing the documentation associated with this testing.

Continued on page 390.

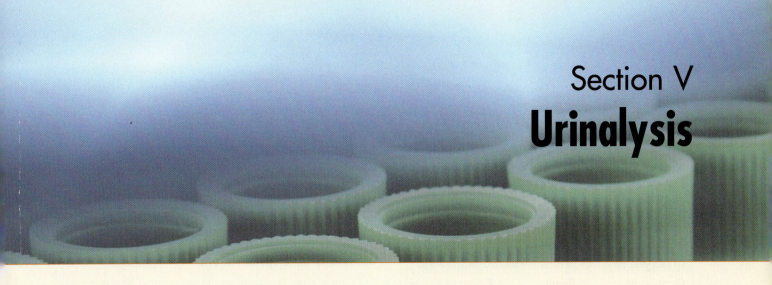

Section V
Urinalysis

On the Horizon

Chapter 19: Urinalysis introduces the reader to key anatomical parts associated with the urinary system. A brief overview of the formation of urine detailing the functions of the anatomical parts of the urinary system is presented. An overview of the routine urinalysis test including quality control is described.

Chapter 20: Physical Characteristics of Urine covers the color, clarity, volume, and odor of urine samples. The measurement of specific gravity and testing for it using a urinometer and refractometer are introduced. Proper technique, normal test reference range, sources of error and interference, and test interpretation are described.

Chapter 21: Chemical Examination of Urine and Feces identifies and describes 10 chemical tests that comprise a typical urine dipstick. The occult blood test is introduced and described. Proper technique, normal test reference range, sources of error and interference, and test interpretation are covered.

Chapter 22: Microscopic Examination of Urine introduces the reader to the most commonly seen microscopic "formed elements" found in urine. Proper technique, normal test reference range, sources of error and interference, and test interpretation are covered.

Continued from page 388.

Case in Point

Three-year-old Johnny is rushed to the doctor's office after he drank antifreeze in the family garage. As the medical assistant on duty at the time, you are asked to give instructions to Johnny's mother so she can help the young boy collect a urine sample. Once the sample is collected, you are asked to conduct the physical and chemical examination portions of a urinalysis test on it. You obtain the following results:

Urinalysis Physical Examination

Component	Result	Reference Range
Color	Amber	Yellow
Clarity	Cloudy	Clear

Urinalysis Chemical Examination (Dipstick)

Component	Result	Reference Range
Glucose	Negative	Negative
Bilirubin	Negative	Negative
Ketone	Negative	Negative
Specific gravity	1.005	1.005–1.030
Blood	Trace	Negative
pH	6.0	4.5–8.0
Protein	100 mg/dL	Negative–trace
Urobilinogen	0.2 mg/dL	0.2–1 mg/dL
Nitrite	Negative	Negative
Leukocyte esterase	Negative	Negative

Questions for Consideration:

- What key points would you make when giving directions to Johnny's mother when she helps Johnny collect a urine sample?
- What is the purpose of the physical examination of urine?
- What is the purpose of the chemical examination of urine?
- What is the third portion of the urinalysis test that has not yet been done?
- What is the purpose of the chemical examination portion of the urinalysis test?

Chapter 19

Urinalysis

Constance L. Lieseke, CMA (AAMA), MLT, PBT(ASCP)

CHAPTER OUTLINE

Learning Outcomes
After reading this chapter, the successful student will be able to:

19-1 Define the key terms.

19-2 Describe the function of the urinary system.

19-3 Differentiate the parts of the urinary system.

19-4 Explain how urine is formed in the kidneys.

19-5 Describe the route followed as urine is excreted from the body.

19-6 Discuss the clinical significance of urinalysis results.

19-7 Compare and contrast the different types of testing involved in routine urinalysis.

19-8 Describe common quality assurance procedures used for the analysis of urine.

19-9 Describe the personal protective equipment necessary to process urine samples.

CAAHEP/ABHES STANDARDS

 CAAHEP Standards

I.C.I.5: Describe the normal function of each body system.

 ABHES Standards

None

KEY TERMS

Afferent arteriole	Loop of Henle	Renal tubule
Aliquot	Macroscopic	Retroperitoneal
Anterior	Microscopic	Rugae
Bladder	Micturition	Secretion
Bowman's capsule	Nephrons	Specific gravity
Calyx	Peritoneum	Ureters
Distal convoluted tubule	Pisse prophets	Urethra
Efferent arteriole	Proximal convoluted tubule	Urinalysis
Filtration	Reabsorption	Urinary meatus
Glomerular filtration	Reagent dipstick	Urine microscopic
Glomerulus	Renal cortex	Uroscopy
Hilum	Renal medulla	
Kidneys	Renal pelvis	

HISTORICAL PERSPECTIVE OF URINALYSIS

Urine has been used as a primary diagnostic tool by those who practice medicine for thousands of years. The first recorded observation of the characteristics of urine was written over 6,000 years ago. Ancient physicians could only make assumptions utilizing the color, appearance, smell, and sometimes taste of urine because their knowledge of human anatomy and physiology was very limited. Urine observation and analysis was known as **uroscopy.** Some of these early diagnostic theories resulting from uroscopy proved to be quite accurate, whereas others were later shown to be complete fallacies.

Unfortunately, the type and amount of information that could be derived from urine became exaggerated, and examination of urine without the presence of the patient or any other clinical information became popular. The analysis of urine lost medical credibility for a time, as the examination of urine became a tool used by uneducated individuals who pretended to diagnose disease and predict the future using urine specimens. This type of uroscopy was a profitable venture until 1637, when Thomas Brian published a book that labeled these practitioners as **pisse prophets.** The book discredited their practices and led to the demise of this profession.

Today, the analysis of urine is a valuable tool used by health-care practitioners to screen for potential abnormalities or monitor disease processes and the efficacy of treatment. A urinalysis may provide important information to assist with the diagnosis of diabetes or kidney damage, or detect a potential urinary tract infection. Urinalysis is a relatively inexpensive, noninvasive CLIA-waived procedure that is commonly performed in physician offices by medical assistants. The analysis of urine includes observation of the physical characteristics of the urine specimen that may be seen or measured with the naked eye. The physical characteristics of the urine include documentation of the color and appearance of the urine specimen. Urinalysis procedures also include procedures such as the measurement of urine **specific gravity** (a measurement of the density or concentration of the urine specimen), or measurement of the specimen volume when needed for reference. Additional analysis for the presence of various chemical components is another part of the testing process. Analysis of urine may also include a **microscopic** component, which uses a microscope to look for formed elements in the urine specimen. Urine microscopic analysis is not a CLIA-waived test, but medical assistants often prepare and set up the specimen on the microscope for examination by a practitioner or other qualified professional. Additional training may allow for medical assistants to perform microscopic examination of urine specimens as well.

Test Your Knowledge 19-1
How are procedures used to document the physical characteristics of the urine different from the microscopic procedures?   (Outcome 19-7)

It is important to adhere to the proper collection procedure for urinalysis specimens. Ideally, urinalysis is performed on clean-catch midstream urine specimen samples, and if the procedures for this collection are not followed carefully, erroneous results may be reported to the physician. Inadequate cleansing before collection will introduce contaminants into the specimen that can alter the results. In addition, if a culture is added to the specimen after initial testing, it is important that the specimen be collected using the clean-catch midstream method. Ideally, approximately 50 mL of urine will be submitted for urinalysis testing, but according to the Clinical Laboratory and Standards Institute, the minimum volume for accurate results is 12 mL.

ANATOMY AND PHYSIOLOGY OF THE URINARY SYSTEM

The urinary system includes two **kidneys**, two **ureters**, the **bladder**, and the **urethra**. (These structures can be seen in Fig. 19-1.) The functions of the urinary system include filtration of the blood, excretion of excess waste, and the regulation of fluid and acid-base balance within the body. The kidneys also help to regulate blood pressure, and they produce erythropoietin, a hormone that stimulates production of red blood cells.

Test Your Knowledge 19-2
What is the function of the urinary system?
                                           (Outcome 19-2)

The Kidneys

The kidneys are considered the most important organs of the urinary system because they are responsible for the formation of urine. They are bean-shaped structures located to the back of the abdominal cavity on either side of the vertebral column. The **peritoneum**, or membrane that lines the abdominal cavity, covers only the **anterior** (front) side of the kidneys, which means that they are **retroperitoneal**, or behind the peritoneum. The left kidney is located a bit higher than the right kidney. A thick renal capsule consisting of connective tissue

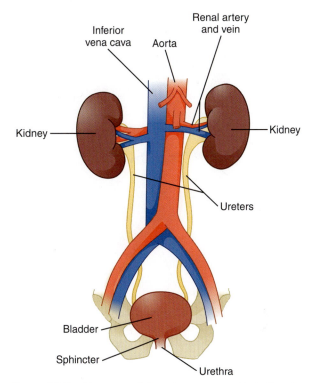

Figure 19-1   The parts of the urinary system, including the kidneys, ureters, urinary bladder, and the urethra.

and fat surrounds and protects each kidney. The indented (concave) portion of the kidney is known as the **hilum**, the region where the renal artery enters the kidney and the renal vein and ureter leave the kidney.

Test Your Knowledge 19-3
Which of these best describes the kidneys?
   a. Located in front of the peritoneum
   b. Pear-shaped organs
   c. Located on either side of the vertebral column with one slightly lower than the other
   d. Covered with hilum   (Outcome 19-3)

The kidneys are made up of an outer **renal cortex** and an inner **renal medulla**. The renal medulla may be visualized as a series of structures known as *pyramids,* as is evident in Figure 19-2. Each pyramid drains into a **calyx,** which serves as a collection tubule for the urine as it is created. The area of the kidney where the calyces join is called the **renal pelvis,** which is connected to the ureter leaving the kidney.

Each kidney contains approximately 1 million **nephrons.** Nephrons are known as the functional unit of the

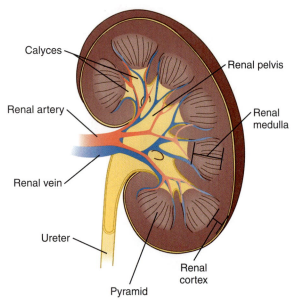

Calyces

Renal pelvis

Renal artery

Renal medulla

Renal vein

Ureter

Renal cortex

Pyramid

Figure 19-2 A cross section of a kidney, showing the renal vein and artery, ureter, renal pelvis, renal medulla, renal pyramids, and renal cortex.

kidneys, because these microscopic structures filter the blood and create urine utilizing filtration, reabsorption, and secretion, as described later in this chapter. The vast majority of the nephrons in the kidneys are *cortical nephrons,* located in the outer cortex layer of the kidney. All nephrons function to filter blood and create urine, but the cortical nephrons are responsible primarily for removal of waste products and reabsorption of nutrients. *Juxtamedullary nephrons* are longer, and extend deep into the medulla. These nephrons specialize in concentration of the urine.

Test Your Knowledge 19-4

Why are the nephrons called the functional units of the kidneys?   (Outcome 19-3)

Almost one-quarter of the body's blood supply is in the kidneys at any given time. The kidneys are incredibly vascular to allow for adequate processing of the blood supply and production of at least 1 liter of urine each day. To understand how this process occurs, it is important to look closely at the anatomy and physiology of the nephrons, as they perform **filtration, reabsorption,** and **secretion** to create urine. A nephron is shown in Figure 19-3.

Blood enters the nephrons through a small vessel called the **afferent arteriole.** The blood continues to

flow through a complex tangled tuft of capillaries that makes up the **glomerulus.** The capillaries rejoin, and the blood passes through the **efferent arteriole** as it leaves the glomerulus. The efferent arteriole is much smaller than the afferent arteriole, which causes a great deal of pressure to build up within the glomerulus. This hydrostatic pressure pushes out fluid from the blood as it travels through the tuft of capillaries. The cell lining of these capillaries is different from those in other places in the body, as it contains pores that allow small molecules to pass through and facilitates the passage of fluid at a high rate. This process is called **glomerular filtration.**

The fluid that is forced from the capillaries during glomerular filtration is collected by a tubule that surrounds the tuft of capillaries. This is called the **Bowman's capsule.** The Bowman's capsule is the beginning of the **renal tubule,** a hollow structure that contains the blood filtrate. Not all the fluid forced from the capillaries is excreted from the body as urine; if it were, the body would be depleted of vital electrolytes and fluid very quickly. Approximately 99% of the fluid and electrolytes are reabsorbed by capillaries that surround the renal tubules. Additional substances are also secreted into the filtrate before it leaves the kidneys as urine.

The renal tubules form a V-shaped complex, including the **proximal convoluted tubule,** the **loop of Henle,** and finally the **distal convoluted tubule** on the other side of the V. (See Fig. 19-3.) This complex of tubules is surrounded by capillaries, which allows for essential exchanges to occur between the blood and the filtrate within the tubules. The primary reabsorption of fluid and electrolytes occurs in the proximal convoluted tubule. More water, sodium, and chloride are reabsorbed into the blood from the filtrate in the loop of Henle at the bottom of the V-shaped complex. Most of the final adjustments are accomplished in the distal convoluted tubule to create urine from the glomerular filtrate. Urine that has passed through the renal tubules flows into the collecting duct, which then drains into the calyx area of the kidney. The calyces open up to form the renal pelvis, and the urine leaves the kidneys through the ureter.

Test Your Knowledge 19-5

What processes occur in the renal tubules?

(Outcome 19-4)

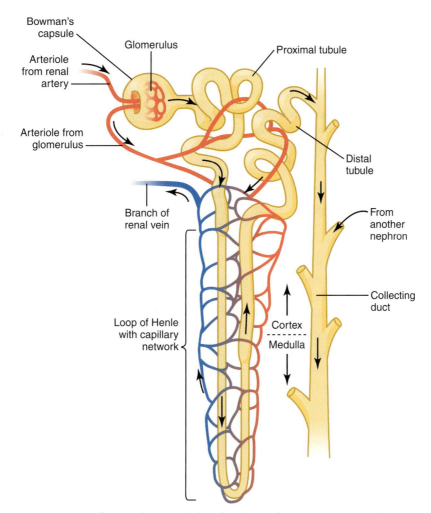

Figure 19-3   The components of the nephron, including the glomerulus, Bowman's capsule, proximal convoluted tubule, loop of Henle, and distal convoluted tubule.

Ureters

The ureters are flexible hollow tubes that connect the kidneys to the bladder. Urine flows from each renal pelvis through the ureter by peristaltic waves created by the muscular ureter walls. Each ureter is approximately 12 in. long, which allows enough length for them to pass behind the abdominal cavity before entering the bladder.

Test Your Knowledge 19-6

Are the ureters involved in the production of urine?

(Outcome 19-4)

Bladder

The bladder is a hollow muscular sac that is designed to store urine. The size and shape of the bladder differ according to the amount of urine being stored at any time. The interior lining of the empty bladder forms **rugae,** which are folds that allow for the bladder to expand when filled with urine. Typically, the adult bladder can hold about 500 mL of urine, but the urge to urinate can be felt when the bladder contains approximately 150 mL of urine. The release of urine from the bladder (**micturition**) involves the interaction of the micturition reflex center in the sacral region of the spinal cord and the voluntary muscles that surround the urethra.

Urethra

When the urine leaves the bladder, it travels through a hollow tube called the urethra as it leaves the body. The urethra varies in length according to the patient's gender. The male urethra is approximately 21 cm in length, whereas the female urethra averages only 4 cm. In males the urethra also is used by the reproductive system to transport semen. The opening at the distal (far) end of the urethra where it leaves the body is called the **urinary meatus.**

SEQUENCE OF URINE PRODUCTION AND EXCRETION

Each part of the urinary system plays an important role in the formation and excretion of urine. The process begins as the blood is filtered in the glomerular capillaries and ends as the urine passes through the urinary meatus.

- Blood is forced through the glomerular capillaries with sufficient pressure to force most of the liquid portion of the blood out through the pores in the capillaries to form the glomerular filtrate.
- The glomerular filtrate is collected in the Bowman's capsule that surrounds the glomerulus.
- The glomerular filtrate continues to pass through the renal tubules, including the proximal convoluted tubule, the loop of Henle, and the distal convoluted tubule.
- The refined filtrate (now known as urine) enters the collecting ducts.
- The collecting ducts join to drain into the calyces, which are part of the renal pelvis.
- The urine leaves the renal pelvis through the hilum into the ureter.
- The ureter transports the urine into the urinary bladder.
- Urine leaves the body through the urethra.
- The distal end of the urethra where the urine leaves the body is known as the urinary meatus.

CLINICAL SIGNIFICANCE OF URINE TESTING RESULTS

Urinalysis is one of the most common tests performed in physician offices and laboratories. The test is fast, simple, and relatively inexpensive to perform. Urine testing is considered reliable to detect or monitor the progress of numerous disease states. Disorders of carbohydrate metabolism, urinary tract infections, and abnormal pH changes in the body may all be detected through analysis of urine. The malfunction of the kidneys or liver may also be evident in a urine specimen. Urinalysis is also commonly performed as a screening procedure for asymptomatic disease. The analysis of urine has several parts: physical examination, chemical testing, and a microscopic examination of the urine sediment for detection of formed elements present in the specimen.

Test Your Knowledge 19-7

True or False: Urinalysis is performed only to confirm a clinical diagnosis.   (Outcome 19-6)

POINT OF INTEREST 19-1
Bladder cancer testing

Bladder cancer is one of the most prevalent cancers in the United States. It is most common in men over the age of 60. The risk of developing bladder cancer is greatly elevated in those who smoke, and patients who have experienced chemical exposure (such as dry cleaning chemicals) are also at a high risk for bladder cancer. One of the first symptoms of bladder cancer may be the presence of blood in the urine (hematuria), as well as increased urinary frequency, irritability, and pelvic pain. If detected early, bladder cancer is highly treatable.

As of June 2004 the Department of Health and Human Services U.S. Preventive Services Task Force recommends against routine screening for bladder cancer for asymptomatic patients without the presence of risk factors. However, there are various tests for patients who show symptoms of bladder cancer, or for those who have multiple risk factors. One of these is cystoscopy, which is a visual examination of the bladder using a scope. Biopsies that are obtained during a cystoscopy may also provide valuable information.

In addition to these screening procedures, the health-care provider may choose to test the patient's urine specimen for the presence of the *nuclear matrix protein*, which is often elevated in the presence of bladder cancer. The NMP22 Bladder Chek test (manufactured by Matritech Corporation) is the only U.S. Food and Drug Administration–approved, CLIA-waived test for the screening of urine for potential bladder cancer. For patients who have been previously diagnosed with bladder cancer, the BTA Stat test (manufactured by Polymedco) may be used to detect bladder cancer cells. The BTA Stat test has not been approved for use as a screening mechanism. A positive result with either of these tests will lead to further investigative procedures to establish the presence of cancer cells and define the severity of the condition.

Physical Examination

The first step taken when analyzing a urine specimen is to perform a direct observation of the urine specimen. The color and appearance of the urine specimen may be noted, depending on the policies and procedures of the laboratory. Some laboratories will also allow for documentation of any unusual specimen odor, because an ammonia-like odor may indicate an old urine specimen that has not been properly preserved. In addition, the physical examination may include the documentation of the urine specific gravity, using a refractometer. The specific gravity measurement provides information about the amount of dissolved substances present in the urine specimen. The physical examination, as well as the rest of the procedures included in a urinalysis, should be performed on fresh urine specimens within 1 hour of collection. If there will be a delay in the testing, the specimen needs to be refrigerated at 4° to 6°C or added to a preservative tube as directed by laboratory policy. If refrigerated, the specimen needs to be brought back to room temperature before testing.

> **Test Your Knowledge 19-8**
>
> What is observed and recorded during the physical examination of a urine specimen?   (Outcome 19-7)

Chemical Examination

After the initial physical examination has been performed and recorded, the urine specimen will be tested with a **reagent dipstick,** a thin piece of plastic covered with reagent pads that will change color depending on the concentration of specific chemicals in the urine specimen. Reagent dipsticks are commonly used to test for glucose, ketones, pH, bilirubin, urobilinogen, red blood cells, white blood cells, nitrites, albumin, and protein. Specific gravity may also be measured using this method. Chemical testing may be performed manually with visualization of the color changes on the reagent pads, or an instrument may be used to evaluate the changes in color

and assign values. More details about the chemical testing of urine are presented in Chapter 21.

Microscopic Examination

The final test performed as part of a urinalysis is the **urine microscopic** examination. An **aliquot** (small sample) of the urine specimen is centrifuged. At least 12 mL of urine are required to obtain an appropriate specimen for microscopic examination. The sediment formed at the bottom of the tube during centrifugation is placed on a slide and viewed under the microscope. The laboratory professional will document the formed elements present when the specimen is examined. Cells commonly present in the urine specimen include squamous epithelial cells as well as red and white blood cells. Bacteria and fungi may be observed along with many other microscopic structures. Chapter 22 focuses more specifically on the microscopic urine examination and the significance of the results.

> **Test Your Knowledge 19-9**
>
> Which part of the urinalysis procedure uses reagent test strips?
> a. Observation of color and clarity
> b. Microscopic examination
> c. Chemical analysis
> d. Culture   (Outcome 19-7)

POINT OF INTEREST 19-2
HIV urine testing

According to the Centers for Disease Control and Prevention, every year there are more than 16 million people in the United States who are tested for potential HIV infection. Many of these patients will have a rapid test performed in the physician office, using an oral sample (from the mucosal surface of the mouth) or a capillary blood sample. Most patients are not aware that urine may also be tested for HIV antibodies. Urine HIV testing has not been approved as a rapid test method, but Calypte Biomedical Corporation manufactures a urine screening test that has been approved by the U.S. Food and Drug Administration for HIV testing. It is important to remember that urine is not considered to be an infectious material for HIV; however, antibodies may be present in urine. Urine testing for HIV has been shown to be a little less sensitive and specific for HIV antibodies

Continued

than the testing performed on blood or oral samples. Any positive results should be rechecked two times, and if the result is positive, the specimen must be sent out for confirmation with a western blot confirmatory test before the patient is to be considered HIV positive.

QUALITY ASSURANCE FOR URINE TESTING PROCEDURES

Urine analysis involves several different processes, some of which may be performed manually or by means of instrumentation. Quality assurance methods for handling and testing urine specimens include the following:

- Appropriate explanation of collection techniques should be provided to patients. A clean-catch midstream urine collection technique is best for urinalysis testing to provide a sample that is contaminant free.
- A sterile collection container with appropriate labeling should be provided to the patient. This allows the specimen to remain contaminant free in case there is a culture added to the specimen after the urinalysis is performed.
- Testing should occur within 1 hour of collection whenever possible. If this is not feasible, refrigeration or preservation of the sample at 4° to 6°C must occur within 1 hour.
- Calibration of and use of quality control specimens on the refractometer if used for specific gravity testing must be implemented.
- Staff training must be ongoing for standardization of terms used to report the physical examination and other results.
- Use of external quality control specimens must occur; a positive and negative quality control specimen should be processed for all parameters reported on patient specimens. The frequency of testing is dependent on the number of urinalysis tests performed, the manufacturer's recommendations, and the adopted laboratory policies.
- Reagent strips must be stored properly; they are to remain in the original container with the dessicant as packaged, and they should remain out of direct light and be protected from humid environments. The cap must stay on the container to keep moisture from affecting the strips, which would result in erroneous results.

- Centrifuges used to spin urine specimens should be calibrated regularly.
- Commercial quality control specimens should be processed by all who perform urine microscopic examination. Slides and pictures used for proficiency testing may also be useful.

STANDARD PRECAUTIONS USED WHEN ANALYZING URINE SPECIMENS

As introduced in Chapte 3, Standard Precautions combine the principles of Universal Precautions with those of Body Substance Isolation. Universal Precautions state that all blood and other potential infectious body fluid specimens should be treated as if they are infectious for HIV, hepatitis B, and other bloodborne pathogens. Body Substance Isolation procedures specify how employees are to be protected from other pathogens that may be present in a specimen. Essentially, when testing urine using the Standard Precautions, it is important for the employee to be shielded from potential exposure to the pathogens that may be present in the urine specimen. This protection may be accomplished by use of gloves when handling the urine specimens and by wearing a laboratory coat to protect against potential splashes or spills. Eye protection should be worn when removing the cover from the tube to protect against aerosols or splashing.

Test Your Knowledge 19-10

Which of these is a type of personal protective equipment (PPE) that should be worn while a medical assistant performs a urinalysis test?
   a. Laboratory coat
   b. Gloves
   c. Respiratory protection
   d. a and b
   e. a, b, and c   (Outcome 19-9)

TYPES OF URINE SPECIMENS

This chapter and the others in this section focus on the collection, processing, and testing of urinalysis samples. A urinalysis should be performed using a clean-catch midstream urine specimen, preferably collected with the first morning void. However, as presented in Chapter 9, urine specimens may be used for other types of testing as well. These samples differ in their collection requirements, analysis procedures, and the clinical significance of the results. Examples of alternative urine specimens include the following:

- Timed specimens, such as postprandial specimens or those collected during a glucose tolerance testing procedure
- 24-hour urine specimens used for specific chemical analysis
- Postprostatic massage specimens
- Urine collected for *Chlamydia* testing
- Urine collected for drug testing

SUMMARY

For many years analysis of urine specimens has been an invaluable tool for providing important clinical information. The urinary system is complex, and is responsible for the filtration of toxins from the body, as well as the acid-base and overall fluid balance that is necessary for homeostasis. The technological advances in testing methods are dramatic, and urine may now be used to identify and/or monitor the progress of many disease states. Urinalysis is commonly performed in physician offices as well as large reference laboratories. A typical urinalysis test includes macroscopic, physical, chemical, and microscopic components. Quality control plays a very important role in every part of urine testing procedures.

TIME TO REVIEW

1. The renal calyx is: Outcome 19-1
   a. A cup-like extension of the renal pelvis
   b. Part of the nephron
   c. The membrane that covers the kidney
   d. A vessel in the Bowman's capsule

2. Specific gravity is a ratio that Outcome 19-1
   compares:
   a. The weight of the urine specimen to a "normal" urine specimen
   b. The weight of the urine specimen to the patient's blood
   c. The weight of the urine specimen to distilled water
   d. None of the above

3. The afferent and efferent arterioles: Outcome 19-2
   a. Enter and exit the bladder
   b. Enter and exit the kidney
   c. Enter and exit the ureters
   d. Enter and exit the glomerulus

4. True or False: The urinary system Outcome 19-2
   is very important for maintenance of the body's normal pH.

5. The urinary bladder: Outcome 19-3
   a. Helps to concentrate the urine
   b. Serves as a storage receptacle
   c. Can stretch to hold more than 1 L of fluid
   d. Is superior to the kidneys in the body

6. The initial filtration of the blood: Outcome 19-4
   a. Occurs in the distal convoluted tubule
   b. Occurs as the blood enters the kidney
   c. Occurs as the blood passes through the glomerulus
   d. Occurs in the ureters

7. True or False: Microscopic Outcome 19-7
   examination of urine specimens is an automated procedure.

8. What is the recommendation for Outcome 19-8
   the use of quality control materials for the reagent strip testing portion of the urinalysis?
   a. Test positive controls only
   b. Test negative controls only
   c. Test positive and negative controls
   d. No quality control materials need to be used for this part of the analysis

9. Why should a laboratory coat be Outcome 19-9
   worn when performing urinalysis testing?

10. True or False: Because blood is Outcome 19-9
    not usually present in urine specimens, it is not necessary to wear gloves when processing urine samples.

Case Study 19-1: Reagent storage requirements

When John arrives at work in the office laboratory on Monday morning, he finds that the lid for the urine reagent strips is not on the container. There was no one in the office over the weekend, and John was not the last person in the laboratory at the end of the day on Friday.

1. Should John use these strips for urine testing? Why or why not?

RESOURCES AND SUGGESTED READINGS

Clinical and Laboratory Standards Institute, Urinalysis: Approved Guideline, ed. 3. CLSI document G16-A3. Wayne, PA, 2009
    Approved laboratory standards for collecting, processing, and testing urinalysis samples
Becton, Dickinson, "Best Practice: Tips for Urinalysis." Lab-Notes, 13, no. 2, 2003
    Online newsletter from Becton, Dickinson and Company. Includes details about urine processing for urinalysis and urine cultures, including information about preservative tubes http://www.bd.com/vacutainer/labnotes/2003 spring/best_practice.asp

Chapter 20

Physical Characteristics of Urine

Constance L. Lieseke, CMA (AAMA), MLT, PBT(ASCP)

CHAPTER OUTLINE

Learning Outcomes

After reading this chapter, the successful student will be able to:

20-1 Define the key terms.

20-2 Describe the clinical significance of abnormal urine color.

20-3 Explain how urine clarity is interpreted and reported.

20-4 Discuss the clinical significance of urine volume and odor.

20-5 Describe the clinical significance of specific gravity results.

20-6 Compare and contrast the different methods used to perform urine specific gravity testing.

20-7 Provide the units used to report specific gravity results.

20-8 List potential sources of error for urine physical examination procedures.

20-9 Analyze and document the physical characteristics of a urine specimen.

CAAHEP/ABHES STANDARDS

CAAHEP Standards

I.P.I.13. Perform Urinalysis

ABHES Standards

- 10. Medical Laboratory Procedures, b. Perform selected CLIA-waived tests that assist with diagnosis and treatment, #1: Urinalysis

KEY TERMS

Anuria	Meniscus	Refractometer
Amorphous phosphates	Myoglobin	Specific gravity
Amorphous urates	Nocturia	Urinary frequency
Clarity	Oliguria	Urinary incontinence
Enuresis	Polyuria	Urinometer
Glycosuria	Pyuria	Urochrome
Hematuria	Refractive index	

PHYSICAL CHARACTERISTICS OF URINE

There are several steps involved in analyzing a urine specimen. Analysis and documentation of the physical properties of urine make up the first procedural step. This analysis includes observation and documentation of the color, appearance, and specific gravity of the urine specimen. Urine odor may also be noted in some cases, but is not part of the standardized reporting procedure. The physical characteristics of urine may provide information for the health-care provider about kidney function and the status of other body systems. Many times the abnormal color or appearance of a urine specimen is the first sign of a serious disorder.

Urine Color

Normally, urine specimens may appear pale yellow (also known as straw) to amber in color. **Urochrome** is the substance that provides the traditional yellow color observed in urine. Urochrome is a pigment that is released continuously as a product of hemoglobin breakdown and normal metabolism. Because the amount of urochrome is consistent, the intensity of the yellow color in the specimen will vary with the patient's hydration status. Urine specimens that are more concentrated (such as the first morning void specimen) will have a darker yellow color than those that are obtained later in the day, as the patient becomes more hydrated.

> ### Test Your Knowledge 20-1
> How is urochrome related to urine color?
>
> (Outcome 20-1)

The terms used to describe the color of urine may vary slightly among laboratories, but it is important that they are standardized within each facility. Simple descriptive terms are best, such as straw, yellow, dark yellow, and amber. Employees should be trained to recognize these colors so that the reporting methods are consistent. It is also important to evaluate urine color on a well-mixed specimen in a clear container, so that the true color can be evaluated. Figure 20-1 shows various colors of urine specimens.

A noticeable change in urine color may be caused by a pathological condition. However, certain foods, vitamins, or medications may also cause an abnormal color. Table 20-1 lists potential causes for various urine colors. The most commonly encountered abnormal colors and their significance are listed here:

- *Dark yellow to amber:* Although these colors are technically within the normal range, sometimes urine will

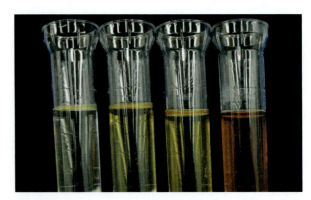

Figure 20-1   Urine color: *left to right,* straw; yellow; dark yellow; amber.

TABLE 20-1

Urine Colors and Possible Causes

Urine Color	Possible Causes	More Information
Colorless to pale yellow	Recent fluid intake, diabetes mellitus, polyuria	Pale yellow and/or colorless urine are not necessarily abnormal, but may be present in some disease states
Dark yellow	First morning specimen, recent strenuous exercise	Usually normal; fluorescent, dark yellow urine may be due to ingestion of multivitamins
Yellow/brown/amber	Hepatitis, dehydration	
Green	Presence of *Pseudomonas* bacterial species in urine specimen	The culture reports will confirm the presence of this bacterium type.
Blue or green	Certain types of drugs or dyes used for contrast studies; ingestion of Clorets breath mints	
Pink or red	Red blood cells, myoglobin, ingestion of fresh beets or fresh blackberries	
Brown or black	Hemoglobin in urine that has been standing or melanin	Melanin may be present in patients with melanoma

appear dark yellow or amber when bilirubin is present in the specimen. This may indicate liver dysfunction, such as in hepatitis, or other conditions that lead to increased red blood cell destruction. Recent strenuous exercise may also cause urine to appear dark yellow.

- *Orange:* Urine may also appear orange when bilirubin levels are elevated in the specimen. However, a more common cause of bright orange urine is the presence of Pyridium (phenazopyridine), a medication used to treat recurrent urinary tract infections. This medication produces a potent orange pigment that will interfere with many of the testing procedures included in a urinalysis.
- *Red to brown:* The presence of red blood cells (**hematuria**) in the urine specimen may cause it to appear pink, red, or even brown. Urinary tract infections or renal dysfunction may allow red blood cells to enter the urinary tract. The presence of hemoglobin from increased red blood cell lysis elsewhere in the body also leads to red urine specimens, although the urine is clearer than it is when intact red blood cells are present. **Myoglobin** is a by-product of muscle destruction, and elevated levels may also cause the urine to appear reddish in color. Many medications, fresh beets, and fresh blackberries may also contribute to a red urine specimen.

- *Blue or green:* Urinary tract infections caused by *Pseudomonas* bacterial genus may cause the patient's urine to appear green in color. Various medications may also cause a green or blue hue.
- *Fluorescence:* Multivitamins may cause the urine to "fluoresce," although the urine color may be normal.
- *Brown or black:* Hemoglobin may turn brown in acidic urine that has been left standing for an extended period of time. Brown or black urine may be evident for patients that have melanoma. This is caused by the presence of melanin and melanogen in the specimen.

Test Your Knowledge 20-2

Ms. Jones has had recurrent urinary tract infections for most of the past year. Her physician has prescribed a medication to treat these infections. On Monday morning, Ms. Jones takes her first dose of the medication. Later that afternoon, Ms. Jones goes to the restroom and is alarmed to see that her urine is bright orange.

Is the bright orange color indicative of a serious problem?

What is the probable cause of the abnormal color in her urine? (Outcome 20-2)

Urine Clarity

The word **clarity** is used to describe the transparency of the urine specimen. A normal urine specimen will be clear when examined in a clear container. The color and the clarity of the specimen are usually evaluated at the same time. As was explained in the section Urine Color, the terms used to describe urine clarity need to be standardized within a laboratory. Common descriptive terms used include clear, hazy, cloudy, or turbid. Figure 20-2 shows the difference in specimen urine clarity. When evaluating urine clarity, it can be helpful to use an object or print behind the specimen; the visibility of the object or print when viewed through the urine specimen will help to determine the clarity that should be reported. Common terms used to describe urine clarity and their clinical significance are listed here:

- *Clear:* A clear specimen has no visible particles and is transparent. Most normal urine specimens appear clear.
- *Hazy:* Hazy specimens may have a few particles floating in the specimen and are not completely transparent. However, it is still relatively easy to see through a hazy specimen. Mucus and other cellular elements may cause the urine to appear hazy.
- *Cloudy:* A cloudy specimen will be difficult to see through because of the particles that are suspended in the specimen. Recently voided specimens may appear cloudy because of **pyuria** (the presence of white blood cells or pus), bacteria, mucus, red blood cells, sperm, yeast, or casts in the specimen. Fat particles suspended in the urine specimen will cause it to be excessively cloudy. Contamination caused by vaginal creams may also cause the urine specimen to appear cloudy. In addition, specimens that have been allowed to stand at room temperature for extended periods of time may develop a cloudy appearance because of the increase in the number of bacteria present in the specimen.

Refrigerated specimens may also become cloudy; this is due to the presence of urates and phosphates in the urine specimen. When the specimen is allowed to cool, these waste products become visible as diffuse (amorphous) particles throughout the specimen, known as **amorphous urates** or **amorphous phosphates.** Amorphous urates are present in acidic urine, and may cause the cloudy urine to appear slightly pink. If there are so many amorphous urates present that the specimen cannot be viewed under the microscope, the urine can be warmed to 60°C to clear the urine. Alkaline urine will result in the formation of amorphous phosphates, with a white, cloudy appearance. The amorphous phosphates can be cleared from the specimen if needed for microscopic examination by adding a drop of acetic acid to the specimen.

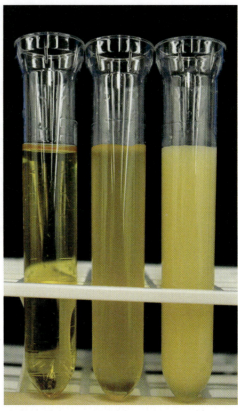

Figure 20-2 Urine clarity: *left to right,* clear; hazy; cloudy.

Urine clarity provides clues concerning the type and number of formed elements present in the specimen. A cloudy specimen has a high concentration of formed elements, whereas a clear specimen usually has a low concentration. The chemical analysis and microscopic examination provide additional information about any chemicals or structures present in the specimen. A clear urine specimen is not always normal, as there may be abnormal chemical constituents present that don't cause the urine to appear abnormally cloudy.

> **Test Your Knowledge 20-3**
>
> Why is it important to place print or something similar behind the urine specimen when evaluating the urine clarity?   (Outcome 20-3)

Specimen Volume

The volume of urine produced in a 24-hour period will vary depending on factors such as the hydration status, general renal health, and dietary habits of a patient. The normal adult urine volume for a 24-hour period is between 750 and 2,000 mL per day. Terms used to describe abnormalities in urine volume or urinary frequency are listed below:

- **Anuria:** The absence of urine production
- **Urinary frequency:** An increase in the urge to urinate
- **Oliguria:** Diminished urinary output of less than 400 mL per day
- **Polyuria:** Excessive urination
- **Enuresis:** The inability to control the flow of urine. This term is used for patients who have involuntary urination after the age at which bladder control should have been established.
- **Nocturia**: Excessive or frequent urination at night
- **Urinary incontinence**: Involuntary urination

To perform a complete urinalysis, most laboratories prefer a specimen of approximately 50 mL; the minimum acceptable volume is usually 12 mL. Those performing the testing procedures on urine specimens with a volume less than 12 mL will need to be mindful of the limited availability for rechecking the results of the analysis if needed.

Test Your Knowledge 20-4

A patient has been ill with vomiting and diarrhea for several days. His urine volume over 24 hours is likely to be:
  a. Increased
  b. Decreased

(Outcome 20-4)

Urine Odor

Routine urinalysis procedures do not include the documentation of urine odor. A normal, recently voided urine specimen has an aromatic odor that is not unpleasant. Abnormal urine odors are generally not considered to be clinically significant, but they may still be associated with certain conditions or characteristics of the urine specimen. Urine specimens that are left at room temperature for an extended period of time will develop an ammonia odor as the urea present in the specimen degrades. Bacterial infections of the urinary tract will result in a urine specimen with a strong foul-smelling odor. A urine specimen with a fruity, sweet odor may indicate the presence of ketones in the urine in a diabetic patient. Other metabolic disorders may give the urine a characteristic odor. For example, patients with phenylketonuria will excrete urine with a characteristic mousy or musty odor. Ingestion of certain foods (such as asparagus, garlic, or onions) can also cause the urine specimen to have an unusual smell.

Test Your Knowledge 20-5

True or False: A urine specimen with a strong odor is always indicative of a urinary tract infection.

(Outcome 20-4)

POINT OF INTEREST 20-1
The odoriferous asparagus

The odor associated with a urine specimen may be attributed to its volume and the concentration of the chemicals present in the urine specimen. For example, within a short period of time after ingesting asparagus, many people have reported that their urine has a "sulfur" smell. It is thought that this distinctive odor is caused by the breakdown of amino acid compounds in the asparagus as it is digested.

However, there is a continuing debate over the production of odoriferous urine because it does not appear to be universal. Some studies have shown that less than half of the population actually excretes sulfurous-smelling urine after asparagus ingestion. It was thought that genetically the two groups differed, and they were labeled as "excretors" and "nonexcretors," based on whether they smelled the sulfur in their urine after asparagus ingestion. This belief is still held by many. However, other scientists believe that all individuals actually excrete the sulfurous odor, but only some individuals are able to detect the odor. Those who cannot detect the smell are not aware of its presence, and may have been misclassified as "nonexcretors" in the original studies. There is not enough scientific evidence available to prove or disprove either hypothesis.

Specific Gravity

Specific gravity measurements are one of the physical examinations performed during a routine urinalysis. Urine specific gravity is defined as the density (or weight) of the urine specimen as compared to the density (weight) of distilled water at the same temperature. The density of the urine specimen is dependent on the amount and size of the dissolved substances present in the urine specimen. These include such substances as glucose, proteins, and electrolytes. The kidneys are responsible for selective reabsorption of essential chemicals and fluid after the blood is filtered. Abnormal specific gravity values may be an early indication of renal dysfunction. Low specific gravity urine is considered to be dilute with very few dissolved substances, whereas urine with a high specific gravity indicates that the urine is concentrated with increased amounts of dissolved substances.

> ### Test Your Knowledge 20-6
> True or False: Urine specimens with high specific gravity results are always cloudy.   (Outcome 20-5)

Because urine specific gravity is measured against distilled water, the results are reported using units that reflect this comparison. Urine specific gravity is reported in units beginning with 1.000 (for distilled water) to amounts above 1.030 (for highly concentrated urine specimens). Urine concentration (as measured by the specific gravity of the urine specimen) may be elevated with congestive heart failure, dehydration, adrenal gland dysfunction, **glycosuria** (the presence of glucose in the urine), high levels of urine protein, or recent use of high molecular weight IV fluids. The urine specific gravity may also be elevated in situations in which the patient has become dehydrated as a result of excessive vomiting or diarrhea. Decreased urine specific gravity may be present in diabetes insipidus, excessive fluid intake, or renal failure. The normal urine specific gravity is 1.005 to 1.030.

> ### Test Your Knowledge 20-7
> A urine specific gravity is documented on the patient's chart as 1.25. Is this correct?   (Outcome 20-7)

Specific gravity may be measured in several ways, but there are three methods used most often in physician office laboratories. These include the use of a **refractometer**, a **urinometer**, or a reagent dipstick.

Refractometer Measurement Technique

An instrument called a refractometer measures the **refractive index** of a solution. This is a measurement of the velocity of light in air as compared to the velocity of light in a solution. The number of dissolved particles present in the solution affect the velocity and the angle at which the light passes through a urine specimen. Clinical refractometers (see Fig. 20-3) used for urine analysis use a prism to direct one distinct wavelength of light for comparison to a special scale. The concentration of the urine specimen has a direct effect on the angle of the light as it passes through to the prism. The refractive index is not identical to the specific gravity of urine, but refractometers are calibrated to provide specific gravity readings.

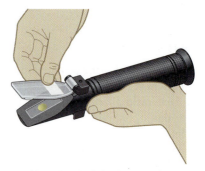

Close the daylight plate gently.

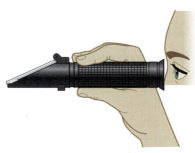

Look at the scale through the eyepiece.

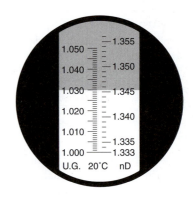

Read the scale where the boundary line intercepts it.

Figure 20-3   Steps to be taken when determining urine specific gravity with a refractometer. *Courtesy of NSG Precision Cells. www.precisioncells.com*

Refractometers are portable, relatively inexpensive, and easily calibrated. This method of measurement uses only a drop of urine, which can be beneficial as compared to other methods. Refractometers must be calibrated regularly with distilled water to achieve a result of 1.000. Five percent NaCl may also be used to check the calibration, and it should read 1.022. Urine quality control samples should also be used to verify that the refractometer is working correctly and that the operator knows how to read the results appropriately. Procedure 20-1 provides detailed instructions for the use of a refractometer to measure urine specific gravity.

Urinometer Measurement Technique

A urinometer is a device that uses a weighted float attached to a scale. This weighted float will displace a volume of liquid relative to its weight. When used with distilled water, the weight will sink until the calibrated scale reads exactly 1.000. Because urine has more dissolved substances present than does distilled water, the urinometer float will displace less fluid. This will result in a higher reading on the urinometer scale. Figure 20-4 includes an example of a urinometer.

Urinometers are rarely used for specific gravity testing. The Clinical and Laboratory Standards Institute does not recommend their use for urine specific gravity, but they may still be used in small physician office laboratories. There are several disadvantages to the urinometer method, including the large volume of urine required for the procedure (10 to 15 mL), the fragility

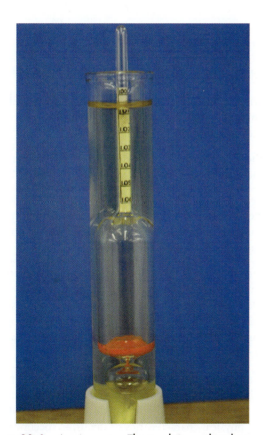

Figure 20-4 A urinometer. The result is read at the top of the urine column (at the meniscus) on the measurement scale printed on the urinometer.

of the weighted float/scale, and the need for a specific container that allows for the displacement of the fluid during the process. In addition, the specific gravity is measured at the **meniscus** (the bottom of the curve at the top of the urine column) of the fluid after the float is added to the urine specimen; the reported results may sometimes be inaccurate because of problems with reading the meniscus properly.

Reagent Strip Methodology

Specific gravity measurements performed by using reagent strips are another indirect measurement of the amount of dissolved substances in the urine specimen. Reagent strip reactions are based on the release of ionic solutes in the specimen. These ions are released for measurement when exposed to the reagent pad on the strip as it is dipped into the urine specimen. A color change occurs on the reagent pads, which can be measured in 0.005 intervals from 1.000 to 1.030. Many facilities have adopted this method of measuring specific gravity because it does not involve an additional instrument for the procedure, as the results are read for specific gravity while reading those for other chemical analytes on the reagent strip.

Test Your Knowledge 20-8

What are three advantages of using the refractometer method for specific gravity testing?   (Outcome 20-6)

POTENTIAL SOURCES OF ERROR

Numerous preanalytical variables may affect the physical characteristics of urine specimens. The assessment procedures for color, clarity, and specific gravity may also be performed incorrectly. The following are some of the most common sources of error:

- *Incorrect or missing identification on the specimen:* Urine specimens must be labeled with the patient's name, birth date, and specimen number or other unique identifier. The date and time of collection must also be noted on the requisition form and on the specimen.
- *Inappropriate specimen storage:* Urine specimens are to be analyzed within 2 hours of collection. If this is not possible, the specimen must be refrigerated or appropriately preserved within 2 hours of collection. Ideally, the color and clarity of the specimen should be determined, but if they were not, the specimen must be allowed to reach room temperature again before assessment.

Procedure 20-1: Observation and Documentation of Urine Physical Properties

TASK

The student will perform an assessment of the physical properties of a urine specimen, including the color, appearance, and specific gravity. A handheld refractometer will be used for the specific gravity measurement.

CONDITIONS

- Gloves, laboratory coat, and protective eyewear
- Freshly voided urine specimen
- Transfer tube
- Refractometer
- Graph paper to be used as "print" for urine clarity comparison
- Distilled water
- Transfer pipettes
- Kimwipes
- Permanent fine-tip pen for marking identification on the transfer tube
- Black pen for documentation on the patient's chart
- Patient's chart
- Biohazardous waste container

CAAHEP/ABHES STANDARDS

 CAAHEP Standards

I.P.I. Anatomy and Physiology, #13. Perform Urinalysis

 ABHES Standards

- 10. Medical Laboratory Procedures, b. Perform selected CLIA-waived tests that assist with diagnosis and treatment, #1: Urinalysis

Procedure	Rationale
1. Wash hands	Hand washing breaks the cycle of infection.
2. Put on gloves.	Wearing proper personal protective equipment (PPE) protects employees from potential exposure to pathogens present in the specimen.
3. Verify test order and assemble necessary equipment and specimen.	Verification of test order eliminates potential errors, and organization of supplies saves time.
4. Verify specimen labeling and identification.	Urine specimens need to be labeled with the name of the patient, the birth date, and the account or specimen number. The date and time of the collection must also be documented.
5. Verify that specimen collection was less than 1 hour before testing or that it was refrigerated and/or preserved appropriately after collection.	Specimens that are allowed to stay at room temperature for more than 1 hour after collection without the addition of preservative may yield inaccurate results because of changes in pH, bilirubin or urobilinogen concentration, glucose levels, and bacterial contamination.
6. Allow any refrigerated specimens to come to room temperature before proceeding.	Specimens that are colder than room temperature may exhibit crystallization of amorphous urates or phosphates, which can interfere with measurement of all the physical characteristics of the urine specimen.

Procedure	Rationale
7. Mix specimen well.	Urine specimens must be mixed well to judge their color and appearance accurately, as well as the specific gravity reading. Without mixing, the formed elements in the specimen will settle to the bottom of the container and may not be considered when determining whether a specimen has an abnormal color or clarity. These substances will also not be reflected in the specific gravity reading.
8. Observe the color of the specimen by visual observation. Report as straw, light yellow, yellow, dark yellow, or amber.	The terms used to describe specimen color need to be standardized throughout the laboratory.
9. Place a printed piece of paper behind the specimen to measure the clarity. Report as clear, hazy, cloudy, or turbid.	Abnormal urine appearance may be linked to a pathological condition. Use of standardized terms is important throughout the laboratory.
10. Pour a small amount of the urine specimen (less than 50 mL) into a transfer tube that has been labeled with the patient's name and/or ID number.	The urine specimen may need to have a culture performed on it; this decision is often not made until the routine urinalysis has been completed. By pouring off specimen into a transfer tube rather than inserting the pipette directly into the urine container, contamination is avoided.
11. Using distilled water, verify the function of the refractometer: a. Open the refractometer cover and place one drop of distilled water on the prism under the cover using a clean transfer pipette. b. Close the cover, and verify that the sample has spread over the entire prism surface. c. Look at the scale through the eyepiece; bright light in the vicinity helps with visualization. d. Read the scale where the line intercepts it. This is where the colors change with a sharp line of division. e. Wipe the sample away from the face of the prism with a Kimwipe laboratory tissue and water.	The refractometer should read 1.000 when the specific gravity of distilled water is tested. If this is not the reading achieved, follow the manufacturer's directions for calibration of the refractometer before testing the urine specimen. Read the scale where the boundary line intercepts it.

Continued

Procedure 20-1: Observation and Documentation of Urine Physical Properties—cont'd

Procedure	Rationale
12. Following laboratory protocol, test a quality control specimen using the refractometer. Use the same procedure outlined in step 10. Chart the results on the quality control log.	The frequency of the quality control measurement will be dependent on the number of tests performed in most laboratories. Be certain that the quality control material reading falls within the acceptable range; if the results are outside the acceptable range, do not use the refractometer for testing the specific gravity of the urine specimen until the accuracy of the instrument has been verified.
13. Using a clean transfer pipette, place one to two drops of the urine specimen (from the transfer tube) on the face of the prism. Following the procedure outlined in step 10 above, read the specific gravity of the specimen.	Reference ranges for urine specific gravity are approximately 1.005 to 1.030.
14. Dispose of the urine left in the transfer tube by pouring it down the sink and flushing it with plenty of water. Dispose of the tube and transfer pipette used for the urine in a biohazard disposal bag. If the urine is not to undergo additional testing immediately, refrigerate it or preserve it accordingly.	
15. Clean the instrument using distilled water and a Kimwipe.	Do not allow the urine specimen to dry on the prism. Do not use harsh cleaners or abrasives to clean the prism or it will become scratched and unusable. Refer to the manufacturer's instructions for more cleaning procedures.
16. Remove gloves and sanitize hands.	Gloves should always be removed immediately after a procedure is performed. Hand sanitization is appropriate before and after gloves are worn.
17. Document results for patient specimen on the chart (if available) and testing log sheet. Be certain to use the correct digits for the documentation.	Documentation needs to occur immediately after the specimen testing is complete.

Date	
10/24/2013	*Urine color: yellow, Clarity: clear, Specific gravity: 1.015*
11:58 a.m.	*Connie Lieseke, CMA (AAMA)*

- *Insufficient specimen volume:* There must be a minimum of 12 to 15 mL of urine submitted for a routine urinalysis to be performed.
- *Use of nonstandardized terms for reporting:* Although there may be various terms used to describe the color and/or clarity of the urine specimen, all laboratory personnel must use the same standard terms within their institution. This allows for normal ranges to be established, and is important when reporting results.
- *Lack of personnel training:* Although the assessment of the urine physical properties is a relatively simple process, there must be documented training for those who perform this task.
- *Use of noncalibrated equipment:* Refractometers must be calibrated regularly using distilled water, and quality control materials should be tested to verify that they are working appropriately.

Test Your Knowledge 20-9

A medical assistant performing urinalysis reported the urine clarity for a specimen as partly hazy. If the laboratory where she works uses the same criteria as that noted in this textbook for specimen clarity, is this the correct way to report this test result?   (Outcome 20-8)

SUMMARY

The physical examination of urine will provide information about the color, clarity, and specific gravity of the specimen. Occasionally, an unusual odor may also be noted during this part of the urine analysis. Results that are outside the reference range for these physical characteristics may be the result of pathological conditions, or they may be caused by medication use or ingestion of certain foods. Accurate results must begin with a specimen that has been collected properly, identified appropriately, and preserved or refrigerated within 2 hours of collection. When reporting the color and clarity of a specimen, it is important to use terms that have been approved by the facility so that the reporting methods are standardized. Instruments used for specific gravity readings must be calibrated and quality control material must be tested at regular intervals to verify the accuracy of the measurement. Medical assistants must also be aware of potential sources of error when performing an assessment of the physical properties of a urine specimen to avoid inaccurate results.

TIME TO REVIEW

1. Which of the following words is used to describe blood in the urine?   Outcome 20-1
   a. Glycosuria
   b. Hematuria
   c. Pyuria
   d. Oliguria

2. Which of the following words is used to describe a slightly cloudy urine specimen?   Outcome 20-1
   a. Hazy
   b. Clear
   c. Turbid
   d. Amber

3. Which of the following is an instrument used to measure the specific gravity of a urine specimen?   Outcome 20-1
   a. Hemoglobinometer
   b. Urochrome meter
   c. Refractometer
   d. None of the above

4. Which of the following may cause urine specimens to exhibit an abnormal color?   Outcome 20-2
   a. Ingestion of rare meat
   b. Ingestion of broccoli
   c. Aspirin use
   d. Ingestion of fresh beets

5. Which of the following is used to describe urine clarity when the specimen has particulate matter suspended in it?   Outcome 20-3
   a. Hazy
   b. Cloudy
   c. Turbid
   d. All of the above

6. A urine specimen with an ammonia-like odor may be caused by: Outcome 20-4
   a. Bacteria in the specimen
   b. Asparagus ingestion
   c. Multivitamin use
   d. Dye studies

7. A urine specimen with a specific gravity reading of 1.035 will demonstrate: Outcome 20-5
   a. High levels of dissolved substances
   b. Low levels of dissolved substances
   c. An amber color
   d. A foul odor

8. Which of the following is not a   Outcome 20-8
   potential source of error for urine testing?
   a. A urine specimen received without a patient name
   b. Observation and documentation of urine color
      and clarity upon specimen receipt
   c. Observation and documentation of urine color
      and clarity immediately after taking the specimen
      from the refrigerator
   d. Use of a container that was not provided by the
      laboratory for the urine collection

RESOURCES AND SUGGESTED READINGS

Clinical and Laboratory Standards Institute, Urinalysis:
   Approved Guideline, ed. 3. CLSI document G16-A3.
   Wayne, PA, 2009
   Approved laboratory standards for collecting, processing,
   and testing urinalysis samples

Case Study 20-1: **Too much to do**

Cindy Collier, CMA (AAMA), is working in the office laboratory for a busy internal medicine clinic. She is about to perform a urinalysis on a specimen that was collected from a patient who is in to see the physician because of blood in her urine. Cindy verifies the identification on the specimen and places it on the counter in the laboratory area. Before she has a chance to do anything else, she is called away to perform a venipuncture and PT/INR on another patient. Approximately 1 hour later, Cindy hurries into the laboratory so that she can start to analyze the urine specimen. She picks up the cup, and documents that the specimen is clear and appears yellow in color. She also notes that there is a red "ring" around the bottom interior of the cup.

1. What did Cindy forget to do before assessing the color and clarity of the specimen?
2. Is her assessment of the specimen's being yellow and clear a correct result for this specimen?

Chapter 21

Chemical Examination of Urine and Feces

Constance L. Lieseke, CMA (AAMA), MLT, PBT(ASCP)

CHAPTER OUTLINE

Learning Outcomes

After reading this chapter, the successful student will be able to:

21-1 Define the key terms.

21-2 Differentiate various disease states related to abnormal urine chemistry results.

21-3 Identify abnormal values for the analytes tested with urine chemistry analysis.

21-4 List potential sources of error for urine chemistry testing, and describe how these errors may be avoided.

21-5 Describe appropriate safety precautions implemented when testing urine.

21-6 Compare the testing methods available for urine chemistry analysis.

21-7 Perform CLIA-waived urine chemistry analysis using a manual and an automated testing method.

21-8 Provide examples of confirmatory tests performed on urine specimens.

21-9 Explain the importance of fecal occult blood testing.

21-10 Detail the necessary patient preparation for fecal occult blood specimen collection.

21-11 Perform a CLIA-waived fecal occult blood test.

CAAHEP/ABHES STANDARDS

 CAAHEP Standards

III.P.III.2. Practice Standard Precautions
I.P.I.14. Perform Urinalysis

 ABHES Standards

- Apply principles of aseptic techniques and infection control.
- Use standard precautions.
- Perform CLIA-waived tests that assist with diagnosis and treatment, Urinalysis.
- Instruct patients in the collection of a fecal specimen.

KEY TERMS

Acidosis	Hematuria	Microalbuminuria
Alkalosis	Hemoglobinuria	Multiple myeloma
Bence Jones protein	iFOB	Myoglobin
Bilirubin	Intravascular lysis	Myoglobinuria
Conjugated bilirubin	Jaundice	Nitrite
Fecal occult blood testing (FOBT)	Ketones	Proteinuria
Glucosuria	Ketonuria	Semiquantitative
Glycosuria	Leukocyte esterase	Sulfosalicylic acid precipitation test
Guaiac method	Leukocytes	Urobilinogen

The chemical testing of urine specimens is the second component included in a complete urinalysis. There have been numerous changes to chemical urine testing procedures through the years, and the most significant changes occurred with the development of reagent test strips. Since the 1950s it has been possible to test numerous chemical analytes at once with disposable reagent test strips. These strips are made of a plastic with absorbent pads attached. (An example is shown in Fig. 21-1.) The pads are impregnated with various chemicals, and each pad is designed to change color as it reacts with a specific analyte present in the urine specimen. The resulting colors on the pads are interpreted by comparing the individual pad to a chart supplied with the reagent strips. An example of a chart used for comparison is shown in Figure 21-1. By comparing the color changes with the reference chart it is possible to perform a **semiquantitative** measurement, providing an approximate value for each of the chemicals being tested. The results may be reported as the milligrams per deciliter present, or by using a semiquantitative reporting method of trace, 1+, 2+, 3+, or 4+. Some of the results may also be reported as positive or negative, which is an example of a *qualitative* test result.

URINE ANALYTES AND THEIR CLINICAL SIGNIFICANCE

A routine urinalysis usually includes testing for bilirubin, blood, glucose, ketones, leukocytes, nitrites, pH, protein, and urobilinogen. The reagent strips most commonly used include testing for specific gravity as well. Many of these chemical substances are normally present in the urine specimen, but the amount of the individual analyte present may change with certain disease states. Other chemicals are not present in the urine specimen normally, and their detection may

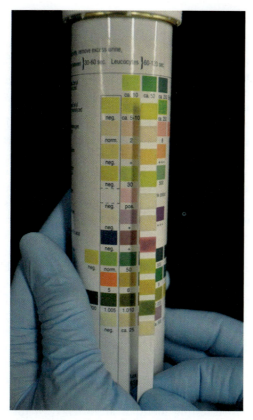

Figure 21-1 Urine chemical reagent testing strip and chart used for comparison when reading urine chemical reagent strip results.

be clinically significant. Chemical analysis of urine specimens may detect dysfunction of carbohydrate metabolism, pH imbalances, red blood cell hemolysis, and liver or kidney problems. The performance of urine chemical testing in the physician office laboratory is beneficial for the patient because abnormalities are quickly detected and appropriate treatment or follow-up testing can be taken care of immediately while the patient is still in the presence of the health-care provider.

There are two primary manufacturers for urine reagent strips. Multistix is manufactured by Siemens Medical Solutions Diagnostics, and Chemstrip is manufactured by Roche Diagnostics. The strips are available with various types of reagent pads, depending on the needs of the health-care provider ordering the urine tests. If testing is performed with an automated system, there may be a recommendation for one brand rather than the other. The manufacturer's insert will include instructions for use and will also include interfering substances for each analyte.

Test Your Knowledge 21-1

True or False: All analytes tested by the urine reagent strips are present in measurable quantities in a normal urine specimen.   (Outcome 21-3)

Bilirubin

Normally, **bilirubin** is not present in the urine. The presence of bilirubin in the urine specimen may be an early indication of liver disease or bile obstruction. Bilirubin is a by-product of red blood cell destruction. As red blood cells are broken down at the end of their 120-day life cycle, hemoglobin is released. This decomposition of red blood cells occurs in the spleen and liver. As the hemoglobin molecules released from the red blood cells degrade further, they are split into smaller components. Bilirubin is created from hemoglobin as part of this degradation process. To travel through the bloodstream, bilirubin must be carried by molecules of albumin (a type of protein) because the bilirubin is not water soluble. The bilirubin-albumin molecule is too large to enter the urine within the kidneys. Instead, the bilirubin-albumin complex is returned for processing in the liver, where the bilirubin becomes water soluble and is separated from the albumin. This water-soluble bilirubin is called **conjugated bilirubin.** Conjugated bilirubin is not usually detected in the urine because it is passed from the liver directly into the bile duct to be secreted into the intestines. The intestinal bacteria further alter the bilirubin, changing it into a compound known as **urobilinogen.** Bile obstruction may lead to the presence of conjugated bilirubin in the urine, and liver dysfunction may also cause bilirubin to be detected in the urine specimen.

Bilirubin is has a strong yellow-orange color. When it becomes elevated in the bloodstream, the patient's skin, sclera of the eye, and plasma reflect this intense yellow color, known as **jaundice.** Excessive hemolysis, liver dysfunction, or bile obstruction may cause jaundice. Just as the bilirubin is elevated in the bloodstream with bile obstruction or liver dysfunction, the levels may also be elevated in the urine specimen, allowing for detection with a chemical analysis.

Test Your Knowledge 21-2

What clinical dysfunction will cause a urine specimen to test positive for bilirubin?   (Outcome 21-2)

Blood

There are three reasons that a urine sample may show a positive result for blood. The presence of intact red blood cells, known as **hematuria,** will cause a positive reaction. Hematuria will often present with a cloudy, red urine specimen with large amounts of red blood cells present. Microscopic examination of the urine specimen will detect red blood cells in the urine sediment.

The presence of hemoglobin without the presence of intact red blood cells (**hemoglobinuria**) will also cause a positive result for blood in a urine sample. Hemoglobinuria may be the result of red blood cell lysis that occurs in the urinary tract, or it can be caused by **intravascular lysis,** which is the breakdown of red blood cells within the vessels. Intravascular lysis occurs in hemolytic transfusion reactions. Hemoglobinuria may also be present with severe burns, malaria, hemolytic anemias, or with some spider or snake bites that cause hemolysis within the blood vessels. The presence of blood in the urine specimen is not normal, except in the case of specimen contamination with menstrual blood or trauma caused by catheter insertion.

Finally, the presence of **myoglobin** in the urine, known as **myoglobinuria,** will result in a positive result for blood. Myoglobin is present in muscle tissues, where it serves as an oxygen-storing molecule. When present in urine, it may cause the urine to appear red-brown in color, but the specimen clarity will remain clear. Myoglobin may be present in the urine when there is trauma to the muscles, convulsions, alcoholism, electrocution, or excessive exercise. Myoglobin is actually toxic to the kidneys; therefore, high amounts present in the urine may be an indicator of concurrent kidney damage. There are many testing methods and comparisons between urine and plasma that may differentiate a positive urine blood result due to hemoglobin from one that is due to myoglobin, because there are very few intact red blood cells present in the urine in both cases.

Test Your Knowledge 21-3

Which of the following will result in a positive test for blood in the urine specimen?
   a. Intact red blood cells
   b. Elevated levels of iron in the blood
   c. Pus in the urine
   d. None of the above   (Outcome 21-3)

Glucose

The presence of glucose in the urine is not a normal result. Blood glucose is normally regulated through hormonal changes and kidney function, including the reabsorption of almost all the glucose filtered out by the glomeruli. However, when the blood glucose concentration becomes excessively elevated (at levels between 160 and 180 mg/dL) the glucose concentration is too high for most of it to be reabsorbed by the tubules, and the glucose "spills" into the urine. **Glycosuria** is a word used to describe the presence of sugar in the urine; **glucosuria** is used when the sugar in the urine is identified as glucose. Glucose is the most common cause of glycosuria, and most reagent strip methods test positive only in the presence of glucose; they do not react with other sugars. However, galactose, lactose, fructose, and pentose are other sugars that may be present in the urine. Point of Interest 21-1 provides more information about additional test procedures that may be performed on the urine specimen to allow for detection of sugars other than glucose. Elevated levels of galactose in the urine of infants may be indicative of a serious condition that needs immediate intervention; therefore, alternative testing methods are often used for urine testing on infants to provide an opportunity to detect galactosuria.

Urine glucose testing can be an invaluable part of diabetes screening. Because the symptoms of diabetes are not clearly defined and do not present themselves in the same way for each individual, there are many patients who are unaware that they are diabetic. For this reason, glucose testing is one of the most common tests performed on urine specimens. Because the blood glucose concentration can fluctuate throughout the day, urine glucose testing done for the purpose of diabetes screening should be performed on fasting specimens. Diabetic patients may also use urine glucose testing to monitor their disease progress; this testing is usually performed on postprandial specimens. Glucosuria may also be present when the reabsorption of the kidney tubules has been compromised, as in the case of renal failure.

Test Your Knowledge 21-4

True or False: All diabetic patients will have a positive urine glucose result at all times.   (Outcome 21-2)

POINT OF INTEREST 21-1
Galactosemia

The glucose test pad on the urine chemical reagent strip is specific for glucose only; other types of sugars that may be present in the urine are not detected by the enzymatic chemical reaction that occurs when this pad is exposed to the urine specimen. However, for infants, this reagent pad test does not provide enough information. Urine specimens that test negative for an infant should have an additional test performed that will detect other types of sugars that may be present in the urine. When an infant ingests lactose (a type of sugar commonly found both in breast milk and formula), the lactose interacts with a naturally occurring enzyme, lactase. Lactase splits the lactose molecule into two smaller sugar molecules, glucose and galactose. Glucose is easily used by the body for energy, but galactose must be metabolized further before the body can make use of it. Hereditary galactosemia is a condition in which the infant is not capable of metabolizing the galactose. The galactose levels in the bloodstream begin to climb, causing initial symptoms of convulsions, irritability, lethargy, poor weight gain, jaundice, and vomiting. If the elevated levels of galactose continue to increase, the liver, brain, kidneys, and eyes may be affected irreversibly. Detection of galactosemia within the first few days of life is critical, as the treatment involves the complete removal of this sugar type from the diet, and these changes must begin immediately.

To ensure that elevated levels of other sugars such as galactose (also known as reducing substances) are detected in urine specimens for infants, an alternate form of testing is used. The Clinitest test manufactured by Bayer Corporation uses a copper reduction testing method, in contrast to the enzymatic method used on test strip reagent pads. The copper reduction test method will detect the presence of all types of sugar, not just glucose. In this test, a few drops of the urine specimen are mixed with a few drops of water, and a reagent tablet is dropped into the tube. A violent reaction ensues, and the resulting color of the mixture in the tube is compared to a chart (provided with the tablets) to interpret the amount of reducing substances present in the specimen. If the test result for the Clinitest is positive, it is assumed that the sugar present is not glucose, as this would have also caused a positive result on the reagent pad reaction.

Care should be taken when performing the Clinitest procedure. Gloves, eye protection, and skin protection need to be worn, as the reaction that occurs within the tube involves boiling the mixture and it is possible to cause damage to the skin, eyes, or mucous membranes. It is important to dispose of the mixture properly as well, as it contains sodium hydroxide and citric acid. The procedure and precautions outlined in the package insert should be followed carefully.

Ketones

Ketones are a product of fat metabolism, and their presence in urine is not considered a normal result. When fat is metabolized, the process usually continues to the point at which the ketones are fully broken down and undetectable. However, if the glucose in the body cannot be readily used for energy, then fat metabolism is increased, and ketones may be present in the blood and in the urine. Uncontrolled diabetes mellitus, malabsorption syndromes, excessive reduction in carbohydrate intake, and vomiting may all lead to the presence of ketones in the urine (**ketonuria**) because these conditions don't allow glucose to be used efficiently as a source of energy.

The word *ketones* is used to describe three different products released into the bloodstream as fat is metabolized: acetone, acetoacetic acid, and beta-hydroxybutyric acid. Reagent strips test specifically for acetoacetic acid. The other two ketone types are actually created by acetoacetic acid, so detection of this compound will provide a clinically significant result, indicating the presence of any type of ketone product.

Urine ketones are often monitored in patients with type 1 diabetes mellitus. When the body does not have enough insulin, the glucose present in the bloodstream cannot be used, and the body will begin to metabolize increasing amounts of fat for energy. If the ketones can be detected early (in the blood and in the urine), the patient may be aware of an impending crisis and the dosage of insulin can be regulated to allow for more efficient glucose metabolism.

Leukocytes

Leukocytes are white blood cells. Their presence in the urine in small amounts is not an abnormal result, but when the number of leukocytes becomes elevated, it is indicative of inflammation or infection of the urinary tract. Reagent strips test for the presence of **leukocyte esterase,** a substance present in granulocytic white blood cells (those that have granules in their cytoplasm), such as neutrophils, basophils, and eosinophils. Leukocyte esterase is also present in monocytes. Neutrophils are the white blood cell type that is most commonly elevated in urinary tract infections. Leukocytes may be visualized with microscopic examination of the urine, but because leukocyte esterase is present even with lysed white blood cells, the presence of leukocytes in the urine specimen may be overlooked if only the microscopic results are considered in the patient assessment.

Test Your Knowledge 21-5

True or False: The leukocyte esterase result will always be positive when white blood cells are present in the urine specimen.   (Outcome 21-3)

Nitrite

Some types of bacteria are capable of converting nitrate, which is normally present in urine, to **nitrite,** which is not usually detectable. *Escherichia coli*, which is the most common cause of bacterial urinary tract infection, is capable of producing nitrites. Many other gram-negative organisms are also capable of this conversion, such as those of the *Klebsiella, Proteus,* and *Serratia* genera. A positive nitrite result is indicative of the presence of bacteria in the urine. However, there are two factors that must be considered when interpreting this result. First of all, not all bacteria are capable of converting nitrate to nitrite, so a negative result does not necessarily mean that the specimen is bacteria free. Second, the bacteria must be present in the urine specimen long enough to accomplish the conversion, and this usually takes 4 to 6 hours. If a nitrite test is to be used as a screening tool for a potential urinary tract infection, a first morning void specimen should be used for the test, because the urine collected with this type of specimen has been in the bladder all night with the bacteria, allowing for an opportunity for the conversion to occur. Specimens collected at other times of the day may or may not have been in the bladder for a long enough period of time for this result to be a positive one, even if the bacteria present are capable of converting nitrate to nitrite.

pH

The pH of normal freshly voided urine may vary from 4.6 to 8.0. The abbreviation pH stands for "parts hydrogen," and the pH of a substance is the measurement of how acidic or alkaline that substance is, based on the concentration of hydrogen ions present. The lungs and the exchange of ions in the urinary tubules of the kidneys primarily control the pH of the human body. The pH of the blood must be maintained between 7.35 and 7.45.

Urinary pH may be abnormal when the body is in a state of **acidosis** (a blood pH of 7.35 or below) or when the blood pH is elevated above 7.45 (known as **alkalosis**). Metabolic issues not related to kidney function may cause an abnormal urine pH. Kidney dysfunction may also lead to alkaline or acidic urine because the exchange of ions occurs in the renal tubules. Medications or nutritive supplements may be used for patients with chronic urinary tract infections to keep the urine slightly acidic, as this environment is not supportive of bacterial growth. This may cause urine pH results that are outside of the normal range, but will not necessarily be interpreted as abnormal for the patient who is undergoing treatment.

Protein

The presence of protein in the urine (**proteinuria**) is most commonly associated with renal disease. A positive result for protein does not always indicate kidney damage, but there should always be additional testing performed to determine whether the proteinuria is indicative of a pathological condition. Normal urine has very little protein present, as most protein molecules are not allowed to enter the urine through the glomerulus because the molecules are too large to leave the plasma. Any that are filtered out are usually reabsorbed by the renal tubules and are not present in the urine specimen.

Protein may be present in the urine when there is no renal disease or damage. This occurs when the total protein level of the plasma is elevated. This elevation is the result of the increased presence of small protein molecules in the plasma that are capable of passing through the pores in the glomerulus. The kidneys will filter out the excess protein, but when they have reached their capacity for protein reabsorption in the renal tubules, protein will be present in the urine specimen. Muscle trauma, fever, or excessive intravascular hemolysis will elevate the blood protein levels. This is usually a transient result that will not continue once the underlying condition has been resolved.

Patients with **multiple myeloma** (a cancer of the bone marrow) may present elevated amounts of **Bence Jones protein** in their plasma. This specific type of protein will be filtered out of the blood, and when the tubular reabsorption capacity has been surpassed, Bence Jones protein will be present in the urine specimen. It is possible to differentiate Bence Jones protein from other types of protein by taking advantage of the different reaction of this specific type of protein when exposed to heat. The Bence Jones protein will coagulate (clump up) when exposed to temperatures between 40°C and 60°C, but it will dissolve back into the solution when exposed to temperatures of 100°C. Other proteins will coagulate at a similar temperature, but will not dissolve at the higher temperatures. The absence of Bence Jones protein in the urine is not a valid means of ruling out multiple myeloma, as many patients with this disease do not excrete levels high enough to be detected in the urine specimen. Protein electrophoresis is a more specific test used for diagnosis.

The most common type of protein present in the urine as a result of damage to the kidneys is albumin. It may be indicative of damage to the glomeruli or to the renal tubules. The presence of albumin may be a transient condition, as in the case of strenuous exercise or dehydration. Patients with hypertension may also present with proteinuria. Positive protein tests in pregnant women (especially in the last trimester of pregnancy) may be indicative of preeclampsia, a serious condition that must be treated immediately. **Microalbuminuria,** or the chronic presence of small amounts of albumin in the urine, is a common occurrence in diabetic patients. It is an indication that the glucose levels in the blood are not stabilized, and the increased workload required of the kidneys to filter out these large molecules has caused the glomeruli to become damaged. The damaged glomerulus allows protein molecules to leak into the urine specimen, presenting as microalbuminuria.

Most reagent strips detect only the presence of albumin. If other types of protein are suspected, it may be necessary to use other testing methods to detect their presence. The **sulfosalicylic acid precipitation test** (SSA test) is a test that will detect all forms of protein in the urine specimen. In this procedure, 3 mL of 3% sulfosalicylic acid is added to an equal volume of centrifuged urine. The specimen is mixed well with the acid, and the degree of turbidity (cloudiness) is measured. The grade or degree of turbidity is correlated to the probable amount of protein present in the specimen. This test may be useful when there is color interference in the urine specimen and a protein test is desired, or when the urine specimen has a very alkaline pH, as this can interfere with the reagent strip results for protein.

> **Test Your Knowledge 21-6**
> Which of these are nonpathogenic causes of proteinuria?
> a. Fatigue
> b. Fever
> c. Vomiting
> d. Ingestion of red meat   (Outcome 21-3)

Urobilinogen

The presence of a small amount of urobilinogen in the urine is normal. However, increased levels may be indicative of liver disease (such as hepatitis or cirrhosis) or hemolytic disorders. Urobilinogen is produced in the intestines by the intestinal bacteria as bilirubin is broken down. Once formed, either it will be reabsorbed into the bloodstream (where it will eventually pass through the kidneys) or it may be excreted in the feces. Some of the urobilinogen in the intestines is further broken down by intestinal bacteria to form urobilin, a pigmented substance that adds color to feces. Urine urobilinogen levels may be elevated because the liver is incapable of processing the urobilinogen in the blood or because there are elevated levels of bilirubin present. In the case of bile duct obstruction, the urine will be positive for bilirubin, but the urobilinogen levels will be normal. Hemolytic diseases may produce a negative bilirubin result with a positive urobilinogen reaction.

Specific Gravity

The clinical significance of the specific gravity test is presented in Chapter 20, as well as several testing methods that are used for specific gravity measurements. Specific gravity tests may be useful in monitoring the hydration status of patients or to measure the ability of the renal tubules to concentrate the urine specimen as needed. The specific gravity pad on the reagent strip takes advantage of the increased amount of ions present in urine specimens having higher concentrations. The greater the number of ions that are present in the urine, the more the color changes when exposed to the specimen. The specific gravity reagent pads are usually sensitive from 1.000 to 1.030 and are semiquantitative. The results may be inaccurate with alkaline urine specimens (falsely decreased results) or when high concentrations of protein are present in the urine specimen (falsely elevated results).

POINT OF INTEREST 21-2
CLIA-waived drug screening tests

Many employers now require their potential employees to have a urine drug screening test performed prior to an offer of employment. These drug screening collections are becoming a common part of the duties for medical assistants and phlebotomists in many offices. In some cases, the drug screenings may be federally mandated. Other employers have developed a drug screening policy to keep the workplace safer. If a drug screening collection is ordered by an employer, the medical assistant will be involved in the collection process, and a chain of custody will be started to document the transportation of the specimen until it is tested in a reference laboratory that specializes in this type of testing. This process requires specific training and a great deal of attention to detail. The employment status of the client depends on these results.

Urine drug screenings may also be ordered to check for illegal drug use in patients for whom this is suspected as part of their clinical diagnosis. These tests may be performed in the office, using CLIA-waived urine drug screening kits. They are available to test for many different drugs of abuse, such as marijuana, cocaine, amphetamines, opiates, oxycodone, and PCP. These tests are generally performed by applying the urine specimen to a reagent stick that will change color if the metabolite of that specific drug is present. In addition, employers who would like to have immediate results may ask for a quick screening test to be performed in the office using these CLIA-waived kits. This is not always conclusive; sometimes the patient may be taking prescription drugs that will cause the screening tests to be positive, because the urine tests are designed to identify the metabolites (breakdown products) of the drug that was ingested, not the drug itself. If a patient has a positive result, it is imperative to follow the office protocol for sending out the specimen for confirmatory testing.

A urine drug screening test may not always detect the presence of the drugs in the system even if the patient has been exposed recently. Each drug has a different time interval for which it can be detected. This can vary depending on the amount of exposure, the size of the individual, his or her unique metabolic rate, the pH of the urine specimen, and the type of drug. Drugs that are lipid soluble (such as marijuana) are detectable for longer periods of time than are many other drugs that are considered to be more dangerous. The product literature for the CLIA-waived testing kit used in the office should be consulted for more information about the sensitivity of the test. Some facilities now request testing of hair samples, as the retention time for the drug in the hair follicles is much longer than its presence in the urine. There are currently no CLIA-waived procedures for hair testing.

In addition, if the urine specimen is very dilute, it is possible that the test may be falsely negative. Most offices that perform drug screening collections and/or testing will have established policies in which specimens that are too dilute will need to be recollected. This decision is based on the specific gravity value of the specimen.

Another CLIA-waived test that may be requested by employers and/or health-care providers tests for the presence of alcohol by testing a saliva sample. Orasure Technologies manufactures a CLIA-waived quantitative saliva alcohol test. If an employer suspects that an employee has been ingesting alcohol while at work, that employer may request this test be performed as a screening tool. A blood alcohol test would be more sensitive, and may also be requested. This would require testing at a reference or hospital laboratory, as there are no CLIA-waived tests available to screen blood for alcohol.

POTENTIAL SOURCES OF ERROR

Some of the most common errors encountered while performing urine chemical testing are the following:

- *Incorrect specimen labeling:* Urine specimens must have the labels affixed to the specimen container, not to the lid of the container. Lids may be removed from multiple specimen containers at once, allowing for confusion when attempting to identify the correct patient name for each specimen. Labeling errors also include specimens that are mislabeled or not labeled at the time of collection.
- *Improper storage:* The reagent strips must be protected from direct light, moisture, and excessive heat. They should also not be stored in an area near volatile liquids, as the pads on the strip may absorb some of the chemicals present in the environment. Strips should not be removed from the bottle until just before use, and the desiccant provided needs to remain in the bottle of strips until they are all used. If the reagent strips

are exposed to moisture, they will become discolored and must be discarded. The lid for the bottle must be replaced immediately after removing reagent strips. The bottles are to be stored at room temperature, and care should be taken not to use the strips after the expiration date printed on the bottle. Reagent strips should never be cut in half or altered in any way.

- *Improper technique:* The manufacturer's instructions state that the urine reagent strip is to be dipped completely into a well-mixed specimen and removed immediately. Excess urine is to be removed from the strip by sliding the edge of the strip along the side of the container as it is withdrawn from the specimen. Inaccurate results are produced when the reagent strip is allowed to remain in the urine for an extended period of time, as the chemicals in the reagent pads will erode, contaminating the urine specimen to produce inaccurate color changes. Once the strip is removed from the urine, it is recommended that any excess urine still present be blotted away with an absorbent pad. Also, many formed elements in the urine specimen will settle to the bottom of the container if the specimen is not well mixed, allowing for potential false-negative results when the strip is inserted into the specimen.

- *Incorrect timing of reactions:* Incorrect timing of reactions is probably the most common error in reagent strip analysis. Each brand of test strips will specify how long the urine should remain in contact with the testing strip before the result is to be read by observing the color change on the pad. This time varies among tests, but all test pads should usually be read within 120 seconds. Unfortunately, the person performing the test commonly dips the reagent strip into the urine specimen, but doesn't follow the timing recommendations when reading the results. This results in an inconsistency within the laboratory and may lead to false-positive test results because of increased reaction times, or false-negative test results because of inadequate reaction times.

- *Incorrect result interpretation:* The reagent strips and color charts used to read the reactions are not interchangeable among manufacturers. For manual procedures, it is important to line up the reagent strip appropriately to the color chart used for comparison, and to report the analyte using the units and reporting methods suggested by each manufacturer. Some tests are reported as qualitative results in which the result is either positive or negative, whereas other tests are reported using a scale of 1+, 2+, and so on. Other analytes are reported using units of measurement, such as 20 mg/dL.

- *Test interference:* Because every reagent pad on the test strip is impregnated with a different chemical, each pad may be affected by different types of interfering substances. Urines that are very alkaline may interfere with several of the pads, as will strong colors (such as those with Pyridium [phenazopyridine] use), the presence of detergents or antiseptics, or high specific gravity. High levels of ascorbic acid (vitamin C) may cause false-negative results for blood, glucose, bilirubin, nitrite and leukocyte esterase. The presence of menstrual blood may cause false-positive results for blood that are not clinically significant. Many diagnostic dyes and medications also can cause interference for some of the testing methods. The manufacturer's insert will provide more detailed information about interfering substances for the various tests.

- *Incorrect urine storage or preparation:* Although this is not technically a potential source of error only for reagent strip testing, it is a common problem that can affect all the urinalysis results. Urine samples should be refrigerated, tested, or properly preserved within 1 hour of collection. Urine that is allowed to remain at room temperature for extended periods of time can undergo chemical changes that were not present at the time of collection.

- *Failure to perform maintenance, calibration, or quality control:* Whether the method used in the laboratory is manual or automated, quality control testing should at least be performed at the frequency specified by the manufacturer. In addition, automated instruments have requirements for calibration and maintenance, and these recommendations must be followed and documented appropriately.

Test Your Knowledge 21-7

What are three ways that reagent strips can be handled incorrectly?   (Outcome 21-4)

Test Your Knowledge 21-8

Which of these is an example of an improper urine chemistry testing technique that may affect results?
  a. Performing the test without wearing gloves
  b. Allowing the reagent strip to remain in the urine for 60 seconds before removal
  c. Mixing the specimen just prior to testing
  d. Allowing the urine specimen to reach room temperature before testing   (Outcome 21-4)

SAFETY PRECAUTIONS

Urine is not considered to be an infectious agent for HIV and other bloodborne pathogens unless it is visibly contaminated with blood. However, it may still be infectious because it is contaminated with other microorganisms, such as bacteria. Mucous membrane exposure is the route of infection most reasonably anticipated for urine specimens being tested for chemical analytes, because of the potential for splashing the urine into the eyes or mouth as the specimen is handled. Standard precautions should be used when handling urine specimens, and appropriate actions should be taken to avoid splashing, spilling, or formation of aerosols when handling the urine specimen. Application of standard precautions for urine specimens include the following:

- Appropriate hand hygiene procedures before and after application of gloves. Also, if accidental exposure to bare skin does occur, this site should be disinfected as soon as possible.
- Glove use when performing testing procedures. Gloves should be removed when leaving the testing area and approaching a clean area of the laboratory or physician office.
- Wearing of long-sleeved, fluid-resistant laboratory coats that are completely buttoned or snapped.
- Occlusive dressings or bandages used over broken skin.
- Use of eye protection and/or face shield when exposure is anticipated.
- Nail biting, smoking, eating, drinking, or manipulating contact lenses is prohibited when handling urine specimens.
- Covering urine specimens before centrifuging.

Test Your Knowledge 21-9

What is the most common route of accidental exposure to urine specimens?   (Outcome 21-5)

QUALITY CONTROL PROCEDURES

The chemical analysis of urine is a CLIA-waived testing procedure. This does not mean, however, that quality control is not an important part of the process. For instance, the package insert for the Bayer Multistix urinalysis test strips suggests that a positive and negative quality control should be tested whenever a new bottle of strips is put into use. This is a minimum frequency suggestion; individual laboratories may require that quality control

samples be checked each day or each shift, depending on workload and/or laboratory policy. Most laboratories will require quality control testing daily. The frequency recommendation for automated urine chemistry testing may be different from the advice given for manual urine testing. There may also be unexpected situations (such as the exposure of the strips to extreme heat and/or cold) that will warrant quality control testing before patient specimens can be analyzed.

Commercial quality control materials are available for purchase. Examples of these include Lyphochek Quantitative Urine Control by Bio Rad, and KOVA-Trol (manufactured by Hycor Biomedical, Inc.). It is suggested that the positive control used for urinalysis procedures be a weakly positive specimen, so that the sensitivity of the testing process can be challenged. (Alternatively, three levels of control can be implemented to verify the sensitivity of the testing process.) It is important to note that water should never be used as a negative control because it does not really resemble urine enough to test the procedure. Some laboratories will freeze aliquots of positive and negative urine specimens to be used as quality control specimens; this is appropriate as long as the desired results are verified with multiple testing procedures and acceptable ranges are established for each test. Ideally, each laboratory will also participate in an external quality assessment survey to evaluate its performance as compared to other laboratories utilizing the same testing procedures. This is not a required component for CLIA-waived tests, but the comparison with other laboratories will allow for more confidence in the test results.

It is important to remember that patient testing should be performed only if the urine quality control results are within the acceptable range. If the results are not as expected, then patient results cannot be analyzed until the reason for the discrepancy has been identified. Troubleshooting steps may include using a new bottle of control material or using a new testing strip from a different bottle or lot number.

URINE TESTING METHODS

Urine reagent strip testing is considered one of the easiest laboratory tests performed. However, it is important to follow the instructions provided by the manufacturer precisely the way that they are written to ensure that the patient results are valid. The strips must be stored properly, and must not be exposed to moisture. Reagent strips must be discarded after their expiration date, and must be used only once. In addition, it is important to adhere to the instructions for timing the reactions and interpreting the results. The color changes for each test pad must be read individually at different time intervals, ranging from 30 to 120 seconds.

The manufacturer's insert for the reagent strips also provides information about potential causes of interference. An example is ascorbic acid (vitamin C), which can cause false-negative results for glucose, blood, and other substances on some reagent strips. Staff who perform chemical urine analysis need to be familiar with the package insert provided for the reagent strips used by their facility, and a copy should be available for reference at all times.

Reagent strips are also available to test for one or two chemical analytes, rather than the entire spectrum that is usually included in a routine urinalysis. Ketones and glucose are some of the most common analytes included on these limited test strips. These can be beneficial for those with type 1 diabetes or for monitoring pregnant women for potential gestational diabetes. Other test strips may be used to monitor protein and creatinine levels in the urine, which can help to detect kidney dysfunction in high-risk patients, or can be used to monitor the progress of kidney disease for patients who have already been diagnosed. Microalbuminuria may be detected by strips designed to pick up very low levels of protein in the urine. The presence of microalbuminuria is a significant factor in the progression of diabetes.

> **Test Your Knowledge 21-10**
>
> True or False: Urine reagent strips manufactured by different companies may be available with different test capabilities.

The reference values for urine chemical strips are the same whether the test is performed manually or by automation. These results are summarized on Table 21-1. It is important to remember that these reference values are obtained by following the manufacturer's instructions precisely; special attention should be given to the timing intervals for reading the results.

Automated urinalysis instruments are designed to read reagent strip reactions at the appropriate intervals. The results are usually printed out and can also be sent automatically through a computer interface for many instruments. The use of automated urinalysis instruments may help reduce errors by eliminating potential sources of error with the timing of reactions and the interpretation of

TABLE 21-1	
Reference ranges for urine chemistry results	
Chemical Analyte	**Normal Finding**
pH	4.6–8.0
Protein	2–8 mg/dL (negative to trace)
Specific gravity	1.005–1.030
Leukocyte esterase	Negative
Nitrite	Negative
Glucose	Negative
Ketones	Negative
Leukocytes	Negative
Blood	Negative
Urobilinogen	0.1–1.0 mg/dL

color changes on the reagent pads. Some of the automated instruments are designed to read one strip at a time, whereas others are capable of processing numerous reagent strips at once. Bayer and Roche Diagnostics both manufacture automated urinalysis instruments, including the Bayer Clinitek models and the Roche Urisys instruments (Fig. 21-2). Various models are available from both of these manufacturers. Calibration and

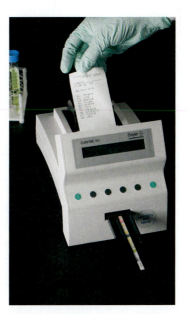

Figure 21-2 Bayer Clinitek urine analyzer with printed results. *From Eagle, S, Brassington, C, Dailey, C, and Goretti, C: The Professional Medical Assistant: An Integrative, Teamwork-Based Approach. FA Davis, Philadelphia, 2009, with permission*

maintenance are necessary for both of these machines, in addition to the testing of quality control specimens at specified intervals. Results are then recorded on a urinalysis report form (Fig. 21-3).

Test Your Knowledge 21-11

What is an advantage of automated urine chemistry testing procedures over manual testing procedures?

(Outcome 21-6)

CONFIRMATORY URINE TESTING

Sometimes the color of a urine specimen may cause color interference with the reagent strip test pads, producing invalid results. It may then be necessary to perform other types of confirmatory tests to provide some reliable information to the practitioner. The following are the most common confirmatory tests performed:

- *Acetest* (Bayer Corporation): The Acetest is used to test for the presence of ketones in the urine specimen. These reagents may be used to test other body fluids if necessary. The Acetest tablet reaction is less affected by the inherent color of the urine specimen, and the color changes are less subtle than they are on the reagent pads on the urine dipsticks. The testing process requires a tablet and an absorbent pad.
- *Ictotest* (Ames Corporation): The Ictotest is used to detect the presence of bilirubin in the urine specimen. This procedure is more sensitive to the presence of bilirubin than the reagent pad test, and is affected less by the strong colors present in some urine specimens. The test involves a tablet and an absorbent pad.

CB LABORATORY
Urinalysis Report Form

Patient Name:_____   Date:_____

Patient ID:_____   Time:_____

Analyte	Result Observed	Reference Value
Glucose		Negative
Bilirubin		Negative
Ketones		Negative
Blood		Negative
pH		4.6 to 8.0
Protein		Negative to trace
Urobilinogen		0.1 to 1.0 mg/dL
Nitrite		Negative
Leukocyte esterase		Negative
Specific gravity		1.005 to 1.030

Comments: _____

Signature/Initial of Operator: _____

Figure 21-3   Urinalysis report form.

Procedure 21-1: CLIA-Waived Chemical Examination of Urine Using Manual Reagent Strip Method

TASK

Performance of a CLIA-waived chemical examination of a urine specimen utilizing the manual reagent strip method.

CONDITIONS

- Gloves, laboratory coat, and protective eyewear
- Urine specimen freshly voided or appropriately preserved
- Clear conical plastic transfer tube
- Reagent strips with color comparison chart for reading results
- Normal and abnormal quality control specimens
- Test tube rack
- Kimwipes or paper towels
- Permanent fine-tip pen for marking identification on the transfer tube
- Urinalysis report form
- Black pen for documentation on the patient's chart
- Patient's chart
- Biohazardous waste container

CAAHEP/ABHES STANDARDS

 CAAHEP Standards

III.P. Psychomotor Skills, III. Applied Microbiology/Infection Control, #2. Practice Standard Precautions
I.P. Psychomotor Skills, I. Anatomy and Physiology, #14. Perform Urinalysis

 ABHES Standards

- Apply principles of aseptic techniques and infection control.
- Use standard precautions.
- Perform CLIA-waived tests that assist with diagnosis and treatment, Urinalysis.

Procedure	Rationale
1. Assemble necessary equipment. Put on eye protection, or position plastic shield in a way that the procedure may be performed behind the shield.	Organization of supplies saves time and helps to avoid errors. Eye protection shields employees from potential biohazard exposure.
2. Wash hands.	Hand washing breaks the cycle of infection.
3. Verify test order and specimen labeling and identification.	Verification of test order and specimen identification eliminates potential errors.
4. Verify that specimen collection was less than 1 hour before testing or that it was refrigerated and/or preserved appropriately after collection.	Specimens that are allowed to stay at room temperature for more than 1 hour after collection without the addition of preservative may yield inaccurate results because of changes in pH, bilirubin or urobilinogen concentration, glucose levels, and bacterial contamination.
5. Allow any refrigerated specimens to come to room temperature before proceeding.	Specimens that are colder than room temperature may exhibit crystallization of amorphous urates or phosphates, which can interfere with measurement of all the physical characteristics of the urine specimen, as well as cause potential interference with the chemical analysis.

Continued

Procedure 21-1: CLIA-Waived Chemical Examination of Urine Using Manual Reagent Strip Method—cont'd

Procedure	Rationale
6. Mix specimen well with a gentle swirling motion.	Urine specimens must be mixed well to provide accurate chemistry results.
7. Pour some of the urine specimen into a labeled clear conical transfer tube. The transfer tube should be at least half full. Place the transfer tube in the tube rack.	Using a transfer tube for the urine to be chemically analyzed eliminates potential contamination of the original specimen by dipping in the reagent strip. If a urine culture is necessary, the original urine specimen will not be contaminated.
8. Prior to performance of patient testing, verify whether a quality control (QC) specimen needs to be tested, and if so, complete that process before the patient's test is performed. Patient testing cannot be performed unless the quality control values are within the established ranges.	Liquid QC should be tested following laboratory protocol and manufacturer's recommendations. Examples of when QC may be used to verify the test results include the following: a. With a new shipment of reagent strips b. Whenever a new lot number of reagents or QC is put into use c. New operator; someone who is being trained on the procedure d. Problems with storage, instrument, reagents, etc.
9. Perform the reagent strip test following these procedures: a. Dip the reagent strip into the well-mixed urine in the transfer tube. Make certain that all the reagent pads are moistened. b. Remove the reagent strip from the urine immediately, running the straight edge of the reagent strip along the top of the tube to remove excess urine. c. Immediately blot the edge of the reagent strip on a paper towel or laboratory wipes. d. Begin the timing for the pad development as the reagent strip is removed from the tube. e. Observe the color changes on the reagent pad at the appropriate time intervals as directed by the manufacturer. Compare the colors to the provided chart for observation, or to the chart provided on the reagent strip bottle. f. Record the results on the urinalysis report form. g. Discard the used reagent strip into a biohazard waste container.	Careful adherence to the procedure will allow for accuracy of results.

Procedure	Rationale
10. Dispose of the urine left in the transfer tube by pouring it down the sink and flushing it with plenty of water. Dispose of the tube and transfer pipette used for the urine in a biohazardous disposal bag. If the urine is not to undergo additional testing immediately, refrigerate it or preserve it accordingly.	
11. Sanitize the work area, remove gloves, and sanitize hands.	Gloves should always be removed immediately after a procedure is performed. Hand sanitization is appropriate before and after gloves are worn.
12. Document results for patient specimen on the chart (if available) and testing log sheet. Be certain to use the correct digits for the documentation.	Results must be recorded immediately after the testing process is complete.

Date	
10/24/2014:	*Chemical Urinalysis: Glucose: negative, Bilirubin: negative, Ketones: negative, Blood: negative, pH: 6.0, Protein:*
	negative, Urobilinogen: 0.1 mg/dL, Nitrite: negative, Leukocyte esterase: negative, Specific gravity: 1.020
11:58 a.m.	*Connie Lieseke, CMA (AAMA)*

Procedure 21-2: Chemical Examination of Urine Using Automated Reagent Strip Method

TASK

Perform a chemical examination of a urine specimen utilizing an automated urinalysis instrument.

CONDITIONS

- Gloves, laboratory coat, and protective eyewear
- Urine specimen freshly voided or appropriately preserved
- Clear conical plastic transfer tube
- Reagent strips and automated testing instrument with paper for result recording
- Normal and abnormal quality control specimens
- Test tube rack
- Kimwipes or paper towels
- Permanent fine-tip pen for marking identification on the transfer tube
- Urinalysis report form
- Black pen for documentation on the patient's chart

- Patient's chart
- Biohazardous waste container

CAAHEP/ABHES STANDARDS

 CAAHEP Standards

III.P. Psychomotor Skills, III. Applied Microbiology/Infection Control, #2. Practice Standard Precautions
I.P. Psychomotor Skills, I. Anatomy and Physiology, #14. Perform Urinalysis

 ABHES Standards

- Apply principles of aseptic techniques and infection control.
- Use standard precautions
- Perform CLIA-waived tests that assist with diagnosis and treatment, Urinalysis.

Continued

Procedure 21-2: Chemical Examination of Urine Using Automated Reagent Strip Method—cont'd

Procedure	Rationale
1. Assemble necessary equipment. Put on eye protection or position plastic shield in a way that the procedure may be performed behind the shield.	Organization of supplies saves time and helps to avoid errors. Eye protection protects employees from potential biohazard exposure.
2. Wash hands.	Hand washing breaks the cycle of infection.
3. Verify test order and specimen labeling and identification.	Verification of test order and specimen identification eliminates potential errors.
4. Verify that specimen collection was less than 1 hour before testing or that it was refrigerated and/or preserved appropriately after collection.	Specimens that are allowed to stay at room temperature for more than 1 hour after collection without the addition of preservative may yield inaccurate results because of changes in pH, bilirubin or urobilinogen concentration, glucose levels, and bacterial contamination.
5. Allow any refrigerated specimens to come to room temperature before proceeding.	Specimens that are colder than room temperature may exhibit crystallization of amorphous urates or phosphates, which can interfere with measurement of all the physical characteristics of the urine specimen, as well as cause potential interference with the chemical analysis.
6. Mix specimen well with a gentle swirling motion.	Urine specimens must be mixed well to provide accurate chemistry results.
7. Pour some of the urine specimen into a labeled clear conical transfer tube. The transfer tube should be at least $1/2$ full. Place the transfer tube in the tube rack.	Use of a transfer tube for the urine to be chemically analyzed eliminates potential contamination of the original specimen by dipping in the reagent strip. If a urine culture is necessary, the original urine specimen will not be contaminated.
8. Prior to performance of patient testing, verify whether a quality control (QC) specimen needs to be tested, and if so, complete that process before the patient's test is performed. Patient testing cannot be performed unless the quality control values are within the established ranges.	Liquid QC should be tested following laboratory protocol and manufacturer recommendations. Examples of when QC may be used to verify the test results include the following: a. With a new shipment of reagent strips b. Whenever a new lot number of reagents or QC is put into use c. New operator; someone who is being trained on the procedure d. Problems with storage, instrument, reagents, etc.

Procedure	Rationale

9. Perform the reagent strip test following these procedures:
  a. Dip the reagent strip into the well-mixed urine in the transfer tube. Make certain that all the reagent pads are moistened.
  b. Remove the reagent strip from the urine immediately, running the straight edge of the reagent strip along the top of the tube to remove excess urine.
  c. Immediately blot the edge of the reagent strip on paper towel or laboratory wipes.
  d. Place the reagent test strip onto the appropriate area to be fed into the urinalysis instrument. Input any specimen ID necessary into the instrument, if possible.
  e. Monitor the instrument as the test is completed, watching for possible errors.
  f. Record the results on the urinalysis report form after they are printed. Some models display the results on a screen; if so, it will be necessary for them to be transposed onto the report form.
  g. Discard the used reagent strip into a biohazardous waste container.
	Careful adherence to the procedure will allow for accuracy of results.

10. Dispose of the urine left in the transfer tube by pouring it down the sink and flushing it with plenty of water. Dispose of the tube and transfer pipette used for the urine in a biohazardous disposal bag. If the urine is not to undergo additional testing immediately, refrigerate it or preserve it accordingly.	Urine does not need to be disposed of in the biohazardous garbage, but it is important to flush the sink well after disposal.
11. Sanitize the work area, remove gloves, and sanitize hands.	Gloves should always be removed immediately after a procedure is performed. Hand sanitization is appropriate before and after gloves are worn.
12. Document results for patient specimen on the chart (if available) and testing log sheet. Be certain to use the correct digits for the documentation.	Results must be recorded immediately after the testing process is complete.

Date	
10/24/2009:	*Chemical urinalysis using Bayer Clinitek 500; Quality control results within range: Glucose: negative, Bilirubin: negative, Ketones: negative, Blood: negative, pH: 6.0, Protein: negative, Urobilinogen: 0.1 mg/dL, Nitrite: negative, Leukocyte esterase: negative, Specific gravity: 1.020*
11:58 a.m.	*Connie Lieseke, CMA (AAMA)*

- *Sulfosalicylic acid precipitation test:* This test involves the addition of an acid to the urine specimen and an observation for the amount of turbidity caused when the acid is added. A semiquantitative assessment of the amount of protein present in the urine specimen may result by measuring the turbidity present. The SSA precipitation test is not affected by the color of the specimen, as the measurement involves the turbidity present, not a color change reaction.
- *Clinitest* (Bayer Corporation): This test is used as a confirmatory test for the presence of glucose and other sugars in the urine specimen. It is not affected as much by the original color of the specimen, although some substances (such as ampicillin and vitamin C) can cause inaccurate results.
- *Microscopic examination:* Chapter 22 details the process used for urine microscopic examinations. In situations in which the color of the specimen prohibits valid results for blood, leukocyte esterase, or nitrites, the examination of the urine sediment for these formed elements may provide additional information for the practitioner.

FECAL OCCULT BLOOD TESTING

Fecal occult blood testing (FOBT) detects blood that is "hidden" in or on feces. Blood in the stool may be clinically significant even though there are only small amounts present. It is not unusual for adults to shed a few milliliters each day in their feces as a result of the natural processes occurring in the stomach and intestines. However, increased blood loss may be due to a pathological condition that needs medical attention. Blood may be present in the stool in the following situations:

- Bleeding hemorrhoids
- Ulcers and/or inflammation of the stomach or duodenum
- Presence of polyps, lesions, or tumors in the intestines
- Nosebleeds
- Bleeding gums
- Diverticulitis, colitis, and/or Crohn's disease
- Parasitic infection
- Colorectal cancer

Stool testing for the presence of occult blood is a simple, noninvasive, and relatively inexpensive screening test. The fecal occult blood test is not specific for any disease process, but a positive result will indicate a need for further investigation with a colonoscopy, proctosigmoidoscopy, or a lower gastrointestinal x-ray that uses barium to visualize the digestive tract. Most commonly this test is ordered as a screen for asymptomatic patients, but it may also be used when there is anemia present with no identifiable cause or when the patient exhibits symptoms of other disorders that may result in a positive screen.

According to the Centers for Disease Control and Prevention (CDC), colorectal cancer is the second leading cancer killer in the United States. Early stages of this disease are usually asymptomatic; therefore, colorectal cancer is often overlooked until it has progressed to a point at which treatment options are limited. The CDC and the American Cancer Society recommend that all adults who are 50 to 75 years of age have a yearly fecal occult blood screening test performed. Those past the age of 75 should discuss the necessity of further testing with their physician. Earlier (before the age of 50) or more frequent screening tests may be necessary if a patient has a family history of colorectal cancer or if the patient has inflammatory bowel disease. For patients who are covered by Medicare, yearly fecal occult blood screening is a service that is covered for payment.

> **Test Your Knowledge 21-12**
>
> Why does the American Cancer Society recommend a yearly fecal occult blood screening?   (Outcome 21-9)

There are two types of fecal occult blood screening kits available. The **guaiac method**, usually referred to as the **FOBT** (for fecal occult blood test), uses a cardboard specimen holder containing a special guaiac paper inside. This paper is used for application of the specimen and the developer. If there is blood present in the stool, it oxidizes the guaiac, and when the developer (hydrogen peroxide solution) is added, the surrounding test paper turns blue where blood is present (Fig. 21-4). The guaiac reacts with heme present in the blood cells. This method has been available for many years, and is considered reliable if the patient follows the dietary restrictions and collection procedures as instructed. The guaiac method is not as sensitive or specific as the newer methods, but it is inexpensive, so many facilities still use it for their screening. Hemoccult (manufactured by Beckman Coulter) is most commonly used. Seracult (manufactured by Propper) is another screening kit that is available. To perform the collection process properly using guaiac-based kits, keep the following key points in mind:

1. Seven days prior to and during the collection, all NSAIDs (such as naproxen or ibuprofen) must be discontinued. One adult aspirin per day is allowed. Tylenol is also allowed.

2. Three days before and then during the collection, all vitamin C supplements must be discontinued, as well as citrus fruits or juices. For some test kits, turnips, broccoli, melons, radishes, and fresh fruit should also be discontinued. During this time, ingestion of red meat (beef, lamb, or liver) must be discontinued as well. Anticoagulant use may also cause false-positive test results, but patients must consult their healthcare provider before discontinuing these drugs.

3. The stool specimens should be collected from three consecutive bowel movements, preferably on three consecutive days. Follow directions provided concerning the volume of stool to apply, and to which side of the slide to apply it.

4.
> **Test Your Knowledge 21-13**
>
> Which of these substances should be avoided for 7 days prior to and then during the collection period for a FOBT?
>   a. Red meat
>   b. Caffeine
>   c. Sodium
>   d. NSAIDs
>
> (Outcome 21-10)

5.
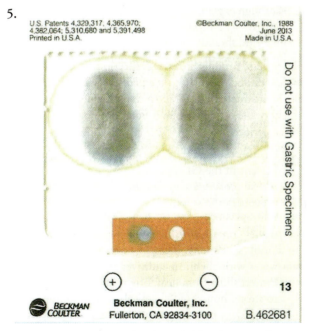

Figure 21-4 Positive fecal occult blood test result using guaiac method. Note the blue area around the specimens, which indicates a positive result and the presence of occult blood in the stool. In addition, there is a positive result on the control area of the slide. *Courtesy of Beckman Coulter.*

The other fecal occult blood testing method, the **iFOB,** which stands for immunochemical fecal occult blood, uses an immunochemical test to detect the presence of globin, part of the hemoglobin molecule. This test reacts only with human blood, and is more sensitive and specific than is the guaiac testing method. The iFOB has been shown to detect a positive result with less blood present in the stool, and to have fewer false-positives due to interfering substances. There are fewer dietary restrictions associated with this testing method; therefore, patient compliance may increase. The iFOB test may be available as a kit containing individual testing cartridges or as slides similar to the other type of fecal occult blood tests. It is still recommended that the sample be collected over three consecutive bowel movements over three days, as polyps and lesions in the GI tract may bleed intermittently, and this method of collection increases the opportunity to detect bleeding if present. Hemoccult ICT (manufactured by Beckman Coulter) is one example of this immunochemical testing method. Other manufacturers, such as Quidel, also produce a CLIA-waived rapid test that provides a qualitative result for the presence of fecal occult blood. The immunochemical tests for occult blood are much more expensive than are the guaiac tests, and are not commonly found in the physician office laboratory.

Regardless of the type of test used, the desired result is a negative one, indicating that no measurable occult blood is present in the stool. However, a positive result does not necessarily indicate colorectal cancer, or even a precancerous condition. The fecal occult blood test procedure is to be used as a screening tool only, and further testing is always necessary to identify the cause of any positive results. The test results for the FOBT and the iFOB are reported as a positive or negative result, indicating the presence or absence of occult blood in the specimen.

Procedure 21-3: Fecal Occult Blood Testing Using Guaiac Method

TASK

Provide patient instruction for the collection of the sample necessary and perform a test to detect the presence of fecal occult blood using the Hemoccult Sensa test cards and developer.

CONDITIONS

- Gloves
- Laboratory coat
- Hemoccult Sensa test cards
- Hemoccult Sensa developer
- Stool specimens
- Biohazardous waste container

CAAHEP/ABHES STANDARDS

 CAAHEP Standards

III.P. Psychomotor Skills, III. Applied Microbiology/ Infection Control, #2. Practice Standard Precautions

 ABHES Standards

- Apply principles of aseptic techniques and infection control.
- Use standard precautions
- Instruct patients in the collection of a fecal specimen

Procedure	Rationale
1. Greet and then identify patient using at least two unique identifiers.	All patients must be identified properly before collecting samples or performing laboratory testing.
2. Verify test ordered, and explain the specimen collection requirements to the patient.	All laboratory test orders should be verified by checking the chart and/or requisition form more than once. A thorough explanation of the collection procedure for the patient will ensure more cooperation. Written literature should also be provided so that the patient knows how to prepare appropriately and collect the specimens correctly. Preparation and collection instructions include the following: • Collect and apply samples from bowel movements from three different days to the slide. This increases the opportunity to detect blood that may be intermittently present from polyps or cancer present in the GI system. • Do not collect a sample if frank (obvious) blood is present in the stool. • For best results, collect the sample before the stool makes contact with the water present in the toilet. Stool specimens that are retrieved from toilet water with chemical additives are unacceptable. • Protect slides from heat, bright lights, and exposure to strong household chemicals such as ammonia. • For 7 days before and during the stool collection period, avoid NSAIDs such as aspirin and ibuprofen. One adult aspirin per day is acceptable. • For 3 days before and during the stool collection period, avoid vitamin C in excess of 250 mg/day and red meats. • Eat a well-balanced diet.

Procedure	Rationale
3. Provide the patient with a set of three slides, an applicator, collection tissues, and written instructions for collection. Let the patient know how and when to bring the specimens back to the laboratory. Make certain that the slides are correctly identified with the patient's name and account number.	Slides must be returned for testing within 14 days of collection. It is important that the date of each collection is recorded on the outside front of the slide. To apply the specimen to the slide, follow these steps: 1. Open the front of the slide. Using the applicator provided, place a small amount of stool specimen as a thin smear covering box A. Using the same applicator, choose a different part of the stool specimen and take another small amount to smear on box B. 2. Dispose of the applicator and close the front of the slide. 3. Patients must not open the back of the slide. This is for laboratory use only.
4. When the slides arrive back at the laboratory, wash hands and apply gloves before touching the slides.	Hands should always be washed between patients and before starting any procedures. Gloves are appropriate personal protective equipment (PPE) for this procedure.
5. Assemble the developer, and verify that all reagents are within the posted expiration dates.	The developer should be stored at room temperature and must be used before the expiration date.
6. Verify the patient identification on the cards.	Always verify that the correct specimen is in hand before completing the testing process.
7. Open the back of the slide. Place two drops of Hemoccult developer directly over the specimens in box A and box B. Results are to be read at 60 seconds after application of the developer. Any blue on or at the edges of the slide is considered to be a positive result for the presence of occult blood.	Guaiac occult blood test results should not be read by those who have color blindness, as they may not recognize the development of the blue color with a positive result.
8. Make a note of the result at 60 seconds.	The result must not be read before allowing 60 seconds for development or after 60 seconds has elapsed.
9. Before the results are considered to be valid, the quality control area of the slide must be developed.	Apply one drop of developer between the positive and negative designation of the QC testing area. Read the results at 10 seconds. • The positive area will turn blue, and no blue will develop in the negative area. • If results are not as expected when performing quality control, the patient results cannot be reported.
10. Repeat the testing process and quality control assessment on the other slides.	The procedure is the same for each slide.

Continued

Procedure 21-3: Fecal Occult Blood Testing Using Guaiac Method—cont'd

Procedure	Rationale
11. Dispose of the slide in the biohazardous disposal container.	Biohazardous specimens must be disposed of properly.
12. Put away developer, remove gloves, wash hands, and record specimen results.	Hands must always be washed after removing gloves.

Date	
8/19/2014:	Hemoccult slides tested; negative X3
11:50 a.m.	Connie Lieseke, CMA (AAMA)

Procedure 21-4: Fecal Occult Blood Testing Using iFOB Quickvue Method

TASK

Perform a fecal occult blood test using the Quickvue immunoassay method.

CONDITIONS

- Gloves
- Laboratory coat
- Hand sanitization supplies
- Specimen pouch containing
  - QuickVue collection tube (covered with identification label) contained in absorbent sleeve
  - Collection paper with adhesive
  - Patient instructions
  - Return mailer
- QuickVue test cassette
- Absorbent laboratory wipes or gauze pads
- Timer
- Quality control material (if necessary)
- Biohazardous waste container

CAAHEP/ABHES STANDARDS

 CAAHEP Standards

III.P. Psychomotor Skills, III. Applied Microbiology/Infection Control, #2. Practice Standard Precautions

 ABHES Standards

- Apply principles of aseptic techniques and infection control.
- Use standard precautions.
- Instruct patients in the collection of a fecal specimen.

Procedure	Rationale
1. Greet and then identify patient using at least two unique identifiers.	All patients must be identified properly before collecting samples or performing laboratory testing.
2. Verify the test ordered, and explain the collection procedure to the patient. Enter the patient identification information on the collection tube label.	All laboratory test orders should be verified by checking the chart and/or requisition form more than once. The collection process for this procedure is very specific, and must be followed carefully. Patient instructions include the following: • During the collection process, do not allow the fecal specimen to contact the toilet water. The specimen must also be protected from urine.

Procedure	Rationale
	• When ready to begin the collection, attach the collection paper to the toilet seat by removing the tape cover from the ends of the collection paper and attaching the adhesive material to the toilet seat across the back of the toilet. Attach the paper in such a way that it sags in the middle of the toilet. • Defecate on the collection paper. Do not remove the fecal specimen or the collection paper from the toilet seat at this point. • Unscrew the sampler from the collection tube. • Pierce the fecal specimen (while still on the collection paper) with the grooved end of the sampler device at least five times in different areas of the specimen. • Insert the sampler into the collection tube and close the cap securely. • Shake the tube to mix the buffer provided in the tube with the sample just added to the tube. • Flush the remaining collection paper and the fecal sample down the toilet.
3. Explain to the patient how to return the specimen to the laboratory for testing.	The specimens may be mailed using the provided mailer, or they may be delivered back to the laboratory. Specimens may be kept at room temperature for up to 8 days after collection.
4. When the specimen is returned to the laboratory, verify that the identification is appropriate and that the patient followed the correct collection procedure.	The specimen is invalid if the collection procedure is not followed.
5. Sanitize hands and apply gloves.	Hands should always be washed between patients and before starting any procedures. Gloves are appropriate personal protective equipment (PPE) for this procedure.
6. Assemble necessary equipment, and verify that all reagents are within the posted expiration dates.	The only additional equipment for this test would be the timer and the test cassette.
7. Remove the test cassette from the foil wrapper and place it on a level surface.	The test cassette should not be removed until right before use.
8. Remove the absorbent sleeve from the specimen pouch, and remove the collection tube from the absorbent sleeve.	The absorbent sleeve is provided in case of specimen leakage during transport.
9. Shake the collection tube well to mix the sample and the buffer solution.	The specimen and buffer must be well mixed for valid test results.

Continued

Procedure 21-4: Fecal Occult Blood Testing Using iFOB Quickvue Method—cont'd

Procedure	Rationale

10. Prior to performance of test, verify whether a quality control (QC) specimen needs to be tested, and if so, complete that test *before* the patient's test is performed.	External QC material should be tested following laboratory protocol and manufacturer's recommendations. Examples of when QC should be used to verify the test results include the following:
	  a. With a new shipment of the testing materials
	  b. Whenever a new lot number of reagents or QC is put into use
	  c. New operator; someone who is being trained on the procedure
	  d. Problems with storage, instrument, reagents, etc.
	  e. To ensure that storage conditions are fine, QC should be performed at least once monthly

11. Hold the collection tube upright and remove the light blue cap at the top of the tube.	It is important to hold the tube upright for this step.
12. Completely cover the exposed tip of the collection tube with the absorbent pad.	It is important to completely cover the exposed tip to avoid potential exposure to the specimen during the next step.
13. Without twisting, quickly snap off the tip of the collection container.	The tip will not snap off if a twisting motion is used.
14. Turn the collection tube upside down into a vertical position. Dispense six drops into the well of the testing cassette.	The tube should be held vertically to dispense the correct size of drop into the well.
15. Read the results in 5 to 10 minutes.	Some positive results will be evident at 5 minutes, whereas others may take up to 10 minutes to develop as a positive. Negative results should be reported within 10 minutes. Do not read the results after 10 minutes. Results are interpreted as follows: • Maroon lines will appear at the C and T area of the test cassette when the result is positive for the presence of occult blood. • Negative results will only exhibit a line at the C area. • If a line appears only at the T area of the test cassette or if no lines appear, the test results are invalid.
16. Dispose of the testing cassette and sample tube in the biohazardous disposal container.	These should all be disposed of as biohazardous materials because of the potential for the presence of blood or other biological hazards in the specimen.

Procedure	Rationale
17. Disinfect the work area.	The work area should always be disinfected after potential exposure to biological substances.
18. Remove gloves and sanitize hands.	Hands must always be sanitized after removing gloves.
19. Document the test results in patient chart and/or log sheet.	All results must be documented in the patient's chart.

Date	
8/17/2014:	IFOB test negative for occult blood ⁓⁓⁓⁓⁓⁓⁓⁓⁓⁓⁓⁓⁓⁓⁓⁓
12:50 p.m.	⁓⁓⁓⁓⁓⁓⁓⁓⁓⁓⁓⁓⁓⁓⁓⁓⁓⁓⁓ *Connie Lieseke, CMA (AAMA)*

SUMMARY

The comprehensive chemical analysis of urine is a frequently performed procedure as part of a routine urinalysis. Chemical analyses may also be limited to a few analytes, testing for the presence of substances such as glucose, ketones, and microalbumin. Urine reagent test strips contain pads that change color in the presence of various chemicals present in the urine specimen. The amount of color change is observed and recorded, either manually or automatically using an instrument. These color changes provide qualitative or semiquantitative results for the chemical analytes on the strip. Valuable information for the diagnosis and management of various renal diseases and other body system dysfunctions may be obtained by performing chemical urine testing. Fecal occult blood testing is performed as a screening test for the presence of colorectal cancer, allowing for early identification and treatment of that disease.

TIME TO REVIEW

1. What is the difference between glucosuria and glycosuria?   Outcome 21-1

2. Jaundice may include :   Outcome 21-1
   a. Yellow sclera of the eye
   b. Red, bloody urine
   c. Light-colored feces
   d. Pus in the urine

3. The sulfosalicylic acid precipitation test is used to detect which of these in the urine?   Outcome 21-8
   a. Glucose
   b. Ketones
   c. Bilirubin
   d. Protein

4. True or False: A positive blood test on a urine specimen is always indicative of intact red blood cells in the urine.   Outcome 21-2

5. The presence of ketones in the urine specimen is indicative of: Outcome 21-2
   a. High blood sugar
   b. Bile obstruction
   c. Increased fat metabolism
   d. Urinary tract infection

6. A positive nitrite result in the urine specimen may be indicative of: Outcome 21-2
   a. Hematuria
   b. White blood cells in the urine specimen
   c. Elevated specific gravity results
   d. Bacteria in the specimen

7. True or False: A urine specimen with a pH of 4.0 is considered to be outside of the reference range.   Outcome 21-3

8. True or False: Medication that causes the urine to appear bright orange is likely to cause interference on a urine chemistry test.   Outcome 21-4

9. Which of the following may   Outcome 21-4
   cause test interference on the urine chemistry tests?

   a. Vitamin C ingestion
   b. Dairy products
   c. Cold medication
   d. Excessive caffeine intake

10. List three safety precautions   Outcome 21-5
    applicable to urine chemistry testing procedures.

11. True or False: A positive fecal   Outcome 21-9
    occult blood test is always indicative of colorectal
    cancer.

Case Study 21-1: Exceptions to the rule?

Sally Steiner is at the physician's office because symptoms that may be indicative of a urinary tract infection. She has been urinating frequently and experiences pain when voiding. When the medical assistant in the laboratory performs the chemical analysis on her urine specimen, the nitrite test is negative.

1. Does this result eliminate the possibility that there may be bacteria present in the urine specimen? Why or why not?

RESOURCES AND SUGGESTED READINGS

Clinical and Laboratory Standards Institute, Urinalysis: Approved Guideline, ed. 3. CLSI document G16-A3. Wayne, PA, 2009
   Approved laboratory standards for collecting, processing, and testing urinalysis samples

"Galactosemia"
   The U.S. Library of Medicine, Genetic Home Reference, explains how galactosemia is passed genetically and the effect that it may have on the body http://ghr.nlm.nih.gov/condition=galactosemia

"Urinalysis, a Comprehensive Review"
   In-depth article from the American Association of Family Practitioners about the causes of urinalysis results, as well as information about false-positives and false-negatives http://www.aafp.org/afp/2005/0315/p1153.html

Chapter 22

Microscopic Examination of Urine

Constance L. Lieseke, CMA (AAMA), MLT, PBT(ASCP)

Learning Outcomes
After reading this chapter, the successful student will be able to:

22-1 Define the key terms.

22-2 Explain why urine microscopic examination procedures are performed.

22-3 List the various formed elements identified in urine specimens.

22-4 Describe the clinical significance of the formed elements in a urine specimen.

22-5 Contrast the standard methods used to prepare a urine specimen for microscopic analysis.

22-6 Describe how to focus the urine sediment specimen appropriately on the microscope for viewing.

22-7 Summarize the procedures for reporting formed elements in urine specimens.

22-8 Describe how a medical assistant may be involved in the performance of a urine microscopic analysis.

22-9 Detail what type of quality assurance and quality control procedures are necessary to perform with urine microscopic analysis.

22-10 Prepare a urine specimen for microscopic analysis.

CAAHEP/ABHES STANDARDS

 CAAHEP 2008 Standards

I.P.I.14. Perform Urinalysis
III.P.III.2. Practice Standard Precautions

 ABHES Standards

- Medical Office Clinical Procedures: b. Apply principles of aseptic techniques and infection control, i. Use standard precautions
- Perform Urinalysis

KEY TERMS

Artifacts	Hematuria	Reflexive
Casts	Mucus	Sediment
Crystals	Provider performed microscopy (PPM)	Spermatozoa
Epithelial cell		Supernatant
Fungus	Pyuria	

The final step in a complete urinalysis is the microscopic examination of the urine sediment. This procedure is performed to visualize and identify the formed elements that may be present. These microscopic structures may enter the urine while it is in the kidneys or as the urine passes through the lower urinary tract. The microscopic examination can detect infection, trauma, or damage to the urinary system, or provide information used to monitor certain disease states. In addition, some metabolic disorders may be detected because of the presence of pathological crystals in the urine specimen. Because the presence of the formed elements is not always clinically significant when they are present in small amounts, the microscopic examination provides quantitative information about the elements present in addition to the identification of the structures.

REASONS FOR PERFORMING URINE MICROSCOPIC EXAMINATIONS

The Clinical and Laboratory Standards Institute recommends the performance of a urine microscopic examination whenever the chemical or physical testing is abnormal on the urine specimen. Because of this recommendation, some laboratories always perform urine microscopic examinations when the chemical analysis or physical examination of the urine specimen is abnormal. This is known as **reflexive** testing. The decision for adding a urine microscopic examination may also be based on the appearance of the specimen; for example, if the specimen appears cloudy or bloody, then a microscopic examination may be added. In addition, the urine microscopic examination may be ordered by a healthcare practitioner to screen for a disease process or to monitor the progress of treatment. For example, the practitioner may need quantitative information about the amount of bacteria present in a sample in order to prescribe appropriate medication, or it may be necessary to determine if certain types of crystals are present in the specimen for a definitive diagnosis.

> **Test Your Knowledge 22-1**
>
> Provide one reason that a urine microscopic examination may be performed.   (Outcome 22-2)

COMMON FORMED ELEMENTS IN THE URINE AND THEIR CLINICAL SIGNIFICANCE

The formed elements that may be present in a urine specimen include epithelial cells, mucus, blood cells, spermatozoa, artifacts, casts, crystals, and various microorganisms. These structures are identified and the approximate amount present in the urine sediment is estimated and reported. Some of the structures are identified using the low-power objective on the microscope (10X), whereas others require the high-power objective (40X) for visualization.

Many normal urine specimens contain a few formed elements. It is important to appropriately report the quantity observed, because the presence of very small amounts of some structures may have clinical significance. The reference ranges and clinical significance of each formed element vary, as explained in the following sections.

Epithelial Cells

A common cell identified in the urine specimen is an **epithelial cell.** These cells are constantly added to the urine as they are shed from the lining of the urinary tract. There are three types of epithelial cells that may be present, and they are named according to the area where they originate within the urinary tract:

- *Squamous epithelial cells:* These are the most common epithelial cells present in the urine. Their presence is not considered to be clinically significant, as the cells naturally slough off from the lining of the lower urinary tract in both males and females, and from the vagina in females. Squamous epithelial cells are large, flat, and irregular in shape, with a large nucleus and abundant cytoplasm. Their shape may be described as having a "fried egg" appearance. Squamous epithelial cells are often the first formed element that is visible when focusing the microscope. They are reported using the low-power objective as rare, few, moderate, or many per low-power field. Usually there are at least a few squamous epithelial cells present in any urine sediment (Fig. 22-1).
- *Transitional epithelial cells:* These cells originate from the structures of the kidneys and the ureters, bladder, and upper urethra in males. They line the urinary tract in these locations, and their presence in small numbers in the urine is not considered abnormal. However, if the number of transitional epithelial cells is elevated, it may be indicative of a pathological condition such as a malignancy. Transitional epithelial cells may also appear in increased numbers after urinary catheterization or other invasive urological procedures. These cells are identified using the high-power objective and reported as rare, few, moderate, or many per high-power field.

A normal urine sample should not exhibit more than the rare transitional epithelial cell.

- *Renal tubular epithelial cells:* As the name implies, the renal tubular epithelial cells come from the renal tubules in the kidneys. The size and shape of the renal tubular epithelial cells differ, depending on the area of the tubules from which they originate. They are smaller than the other epithelial cells, and their appearance can vary from round to columnar. The presence of renal tubular epithelial cells in the urine specimen is clinically significant, as it may indicate conditions in which damage is occurring to the renal tubules. Examples include glomerulonephritis, viral infections, chronic or acute kidney disease, and other disease states that cause necrosis of the kidney tubules. Renal tubular epithelial cells are identified using the high-power objective, and reported as a number per high-power field. The presence of renal tubular epithelial cells in the urine sediment is always considered to be an abnormal result.

> **Test Your Knowledge 22-2**
>
> Is the presence of epithelial cells in a urine specimen always clinically significant? (Outcome 22-4)

Mucus

The presence of **mucus** in the urine specimen is very common. Mucus appears as thread-like strands made of protein. Figure 22-2 shows an example of mucus. The mucous membranes that line the lower urinary tract and the renal epithelial cells normally produce mucus. The strands may be difficult to visualize when the microscopic light source is at its brightest; it is often necessary to reduce light intensity to see mucus clearly. Mucus is not indicative of a pathological condition in the body, and has no clinical significance. Large amounts of mucus in the specimen may produce a positive protein result on the chemical urine analysis. Mucus is identified using the low-power objective, and is reported as rare, few, moderate, or many per low-power field. Normal urine specimens may include a moderate amount of mucus.

Blood Cells

Red blood cells and white blood cells are often identified as part of the urine microscopic examination. Their clinical significance varies with the number present and the type of blood cell visualized.

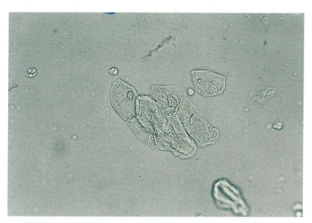

Figure 22-1 Squamous epithelial cells in urine sediment. *From Strasinger, SK, and Di Lorenzo, MS: Urinalysis and Body Fluids, ed. 5. FA Davis, Philadelphia, 2008, with permission.*

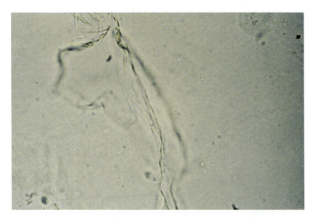

Figure 22-2   Threads of mucus; note the stringy appearance. *From Strasinger, SK, and Di Lorenzo, MS: Urinalysis and Body Fluids, ed. 5. FA Davis, Philadelphia, 2008, with permission.*

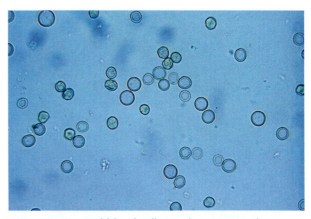

Figure 22-3   Red blood cells (erythrocytes) as they appear in urine sediment. *From Strasinger, SK, and Di Lorenzo, MS: Urinalysis and Body Fluids, ed. 5. FA Davis, Philadelphia, 2008, with permission.*

- *Red blood cells:* It is not uncommon to see one or two red blood cells when examining urine sediment with a high-power magnification. When the number of red blood cells is elevated, it is indicative of damage to the glomeruli of the kidney or trauma to the vessels surrounding the urinary tract. The presence of red blood cells in the urine is a called **hematuria.** The number of red blood cells present in the specimen is relative to the severity of the damage to the glomerulus or the vessels. Red blood cells may also be present in the urine specimen after strenuous exercise.

    Red blood cells may be difficult to identify when viewed in the urine specimen. They are colorless, smooth, and have no nucleus. Red blood cells appear as round biconcave disks that are difficult to distinguish from air bubbles, budding yeast, oil droplets, or artifacts in the specimen. The addition of stain to the specimen may aid in the identification and counting of the red blood cells. Figure 22-3 shows how red blood cells appear in the urine. Red blood cells are identified using the high-power objective, and are reported as the number seen per high-power field.

- **White blood cells:** A few white blood cells may be evident in a normal clean-catch midstream urine specimen when viewed under the microscope. Elevated numbers of white blood cells in the urine is called **pyuria,** which indicates infection or inflammation of the urinary tract. Prostatitis, pyelonephritis, and cystitis may cause elevated white blood cell counts in the urine specimen. Pyuria may also be present when there are tumors in the urinary tract, and other systemic inflammatory conditions.

It is easier to identify white blood cells in the urine specimen than it is to identify red blood cells. The white blood cells are larger, have a granular appearance, and contain a nucleus (Fig. 22-4). Most of those present in the urine specimen are neutrophils, although eosinophils or mononuclear cells may be elevated in certain situations. White blood cells are identified using the high-power objective and reported as the number visualized per high-power field.

Spermatozoa

Occasionally, **spermatozoa** may be present in urine specimens from both males and females after sexual intercourse. The spermatozoa will be identified by their distinctive shape, as they have an oval head that is

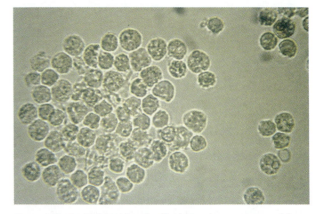

Figure 22-4   White blood cells. Note the presence of the nucleus and the cytoplasmic granules. *From Strasinger, SK, and Di Lorenzo, MS: Urinalysis and Body Fluids, ed. 5. FA Davis, Philadelphia, 2008, with permission.*

Occasionally the urine microscopic report for a female patient may include the presence of *clue cells.* This term is used to describe vaginal epithelial cells that are coated with the *Gardnerella vaginalis* bacterium. The clue cells are similar in appearance to the squamous epithelial cells, except that the clue cell borders are ill defined or completely obliterated with a coating of bacteria. The presence of these cells in the urine specimen may be indicative of an infection known as bacterial vaginosis, and they must be noted if viewed in the urine specimen.

There are numerous types of bacteria present as normal flora in the vagina at all times. Bacterial vaginosis is the result of an overgrowth of *G. vaginalis* when the balance of normal flora is disrupted. The use of broad-spectrum antibiotics may destroy healthy bacteria and allow the *G. vaginalis* to increase in number. Douching, retained tampons, use of intrauterine devices for contraception, and use of products that contain nonoxynol-9 may also cause the bacterial balance to shift in the vaginal tissues.

Bacterial vaginosis is the cause of 60% of vulvovaginal infections. It is important to diagnose and treat this condition promptly because it has been linked to an increased risk of pelvic inflammatory disease (PID). Pelvic inflammatory disease is a serious condition that may lead to infertility as well as being a component of many other disease processes.

somewhat teardrop shaped, and a long tail. Urine is toxic to spermatozoa, so it is unusual for these cells to exhibit the same amount of motility as they would in a semen specimen. The clinical significance of spermatozoa in a urine specimen is limited to situations of male infertility and retrograde ejaculation in which the sperm is released into the bladder instead of into the urethra. The presence of spermatozoa should be reported in any situation, whether or not the clinical significance is clear. Elevated amounts of spermatozoa in the urine specimen may cause the urine dipstick to test positive for protein. The presence of spermatozoa is noted with the rest of the microscopic examination results, but the manner in which is it reported is laboratory specific.

Test Your Knowledge 22-3

Is it possible to see spermatozoa in the urine of a female patient?

(Outcome 22-3)

Artifacts

Artifacts are contaminants that are visualized in the urine specimen. These may include fecal material, toilet paper, air bubbles, starch or powder, and clothing fibers. Artifacts are not usually reported as part of the urine microscopic examination, because they are not clinically significant. These structures are difficult to identify and may be confused with other formed elements in the urine specimen because of similarities in their shape and size.

Casts

The kidney tubules normally secrete a substance called the Tamm-Horsfall protein. This protein is not clinically significant unless certain conditions exist within the tubules that allow the Tamm-Horsfall protein to "gel" and form a protein-based mold of the tubule. Reduced urine flow, increased amounts of dissolved substances in the glomerular filtrate, and acidic urine conditions contribute to the formation of these **casts.** The casts assume the shape of the tubule or collecting duct in which they were formed. Any structures or substances that were present within the tubule or collecting duct when the cast was formed are trapped within the cast. These trapped substances may include bacteria, cells, or diffuse granules. Eventually, the protein making up the cast breaks away from the lumen of the tubules and flushes out with the urine. These casts can then be identified in the urine sediment when viewed under the microscope.

Casts are cylindrical because of the shape of the structure in which they were originally formed in the nephron tubules. They are classified using the names of the trapped substances within the protein structures. To visualize casts, the intensity of the light source on the microscope must be decreased, and the urine must be examined with the low-power objective. The presence of a few hyaline casts in a urine specimen is not considered abnormal, but the presence of any other type of cast may indicate damage to the kidney tubules. Some common types of casts identified in the urine sediment include the following:

- *Hyaline casts:* Clear, colorless, transparent. Hyaline casts may be difficult to see and to differentiate from threads of mucus. Figure 22-5 shows a hyaline cast. Strenuous exercise, heat exposure, or dehydration may cause an increased number of hyaline casts. Elevated numbers of hyaline casts may also be indicative of pyelonephritis, glomerulonephritis, or chronic renal disease. It is normal to see a few hyaline casts when

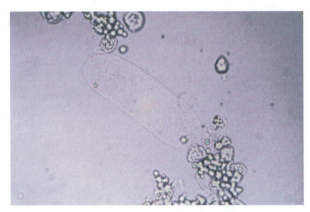

Figure 22-5 Hyaline cast. These casts are "hollow" and have no structures filling their core. *From Strasinger, SK, and Di Lorenzo, MS: Urinalysis and Body Fluids, ed. 5. FA Davis, Philadelphia, 2008, with permission.*

examining the urine under low magnification. Hyaline casts are reported as the number visualized per low-power field.

- *Granular casts:* Granular casts contain fine or coarse granules. These granules are disintegrated structures that were trapped in the renal tubule at the time that the cast was formed. Granular casts may be present in the urine sediment with stress or strenuous exercise, but they may also be evident with glomerulonephritis or pyelonephritis. Granular casts are identified using the low-power objective and reported as the number visualized per low-power field.
- *Cellular casts:* Cellular casts contain renal epithelial cells, red blood cells, or white blood cells. Renal epithelial cell casts are indicative of damage to the renal tubules and are not present in a normal urine specimen. Red blood cell casts may be seen after strenuous exercise, but their presence may also be indicative of bleeding within the nephron structure as in the case of glomerulonephritis. The red blood cell casts have a distinct orange-red color. White blood cell casts are present when there is inflammation or infection within the nephron. There may also be bacteria present in a white blood cell cast. Pyelonephritis is often characterized by the presence of white blood cell casts in the urine sediment. Cellular casts are identified using the low-power objective and are reported as the number visualized per low-power field.
- *Waxy casts:* Waxy casts appear smooth with an irregular outline. They are very refractive when examined with decreased light under low-power magnification. There are no trapped substances within the cast, but

the outline is easier to see than that of a hyaline cast. Waxy casts are indicative of an extreme decrease in the urine flow through the tubules that accompanies renal failure, and are not present in a normal urine specimen. They are identified using the low-power objective and reported as the number visualized per low-power field.

Crystals

The presence of **crystals** in normal urine sediment is common. Although many types of crystals are considered normal, it is important to report them when identified because their presence in increased numbers may be clinically significant. Crystals are formed from the dissolved substances (especially salts) in the urine. The precipitation of these dissolved substances into crystals is affected by the pH of the urine, as well as reduced temperature and increased specific gravity. Urine that has been at room temperature or refrigerated for a period of time will often contain abundant crystals in the urine sediment. In addition, highly concentrated urine (urine with a high specific gravity) with many dissolved substances will crystallize readily. The pH of the urine specimen plays a valuable role when attempting to identify crystals under the microscope, as certain types of crystals are evident in acidic urine, whereas others are present in alkaline urine. Various crystals can be seen in Figure 22-6.

Normal crystals may be present in acidic or alkaline urine specimens. These include the following:

- Amorphous (without a distinct shape) urates are present in acidic urine. The refrigeration of the specimen significantly contributes to the formation of amorphous urates in the specimen. The urine sediment may appear pink, and the amorphous crystals will appear as yellow-brown diffuse granules throughout the specimen when viewed under the microscope. Amorphous urate crystals may return to solution with the application of heat or addition of sodium hydroxide to the specimen.
- Uric acid crystals are evident in acidic urine, and appear with numerous shapes and a yellow-brown color. They may be present in increased numbers with leukemia when the patient is receiving chemotherapy, and occasionally in patients with gout.
- Calcium oxalate crystals are occasionally found in acidic urine or, more commonly, in urine with a neutral pH. They are seldom found in alkaline urine. These crystals appear as "envelopes" and are very refractive when viewed under the microscope.

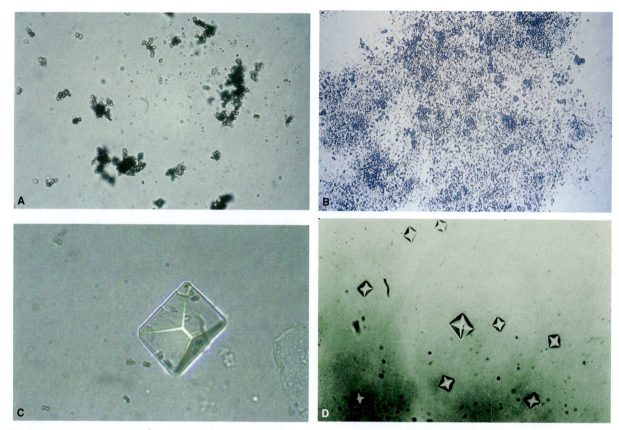

Figure 22-6   Various crystals. A. Amorphous urates. B. Amorphous phosphates. C. Triple phosphate crystals. D. Calcium oxalate crystals. *From Strasinger, SK, and Di Lorenzo, MS: Urinalysis and Body Fluids, ed. 5. FA Davis, Philadelphia, 2008, with permission.*

- Amorphous phosphates are present in alkaline urine. This crystallization is especially evident after refrigeration of the specimen. The amorphous phosphate crystals appear as diffuse granular particles that may obscure the other structures present in the sediment when viewed under the microscope. The urine specimen may take on a white color if amorphous phosphates are present. Amorphous phosphates dissolve with the addition of 10% acetic acid.
- Triple phosphate crystals are present in neutral or alkaline urine. They are colorless, and very refractive when viewed under the microscope. They are often described as a "coffin lid," shaped like a six-sided prism. Their presence is not clinically significant.

The presence of other crystals considered abnormal in the urine sediment may be indicative of metabolic diseases. Use of certain drugs (such as sulfonamides or ampicillin) may also result in crystal formation. Urine specimens with alkaline or neutral pH values rarely contain abnormal crystals. Fortunately, the abnormal urine crystals all have very characteristic shapes that are easily recognizable. Crystals that are considered abnormal include the following:

- Cystine crystals are present in patients with cystinuria, a metabolic disorder in which individuals are not able to reabsorb cystine in the renal tubules as a normal individual would. Cystine crystals are hexagonal.
- Cholesterol crystals are not usually visualized unless the urine specimen has been refrigerated. When they are present, they appear as flat rectangles with notches out of the corners of the structure. Their presence indicates a disorder that includes lipiduria (the presence of lipids in the urine), such as nephrotic syndrome.
- Tyrosine, leucine, and bilirubin crystals may be present in the urine of patients with liver disorders. Tyrosine needles look like clumps of needles, whereas leucine crystals look like yellow-brown, oily spheres. Bilirubin crystals are also described as lumps of needle structures, but they are yellow (like the color of bilirubin).

- Sulfonamide crystals have historically been present in urine sediment in patients undergoing sulfa drug treatment. However, the newer sulfonamide drugs are designed to be more soluble, which means that these crystals are rarely present now. If there are sulfonamide crystals present in the urine specimen, it may mean that the patient is not adequately hydrated. These crystals appear as bundles of needles or designs that resemble sheaves of wheat.
- Ampicillin crystals may also be present in urine when patients receive very large doses of the medication without adequate hydration. They also appear as colorless bundles of needles.
- Hippuric acid is increased in the urine when xylene and toluene are metabolized. Xylene and toluene are common industrial chemicals. Hippuric acid crystals may be an indication of increased exposure to these chemicals, as in workplace exposure or in those who abuse chemicals, such as sniffing glue products.

Microorganisms

When viewed with a compound microscope, various microorganisms may be visualized in the urine sediment. These include bacteria, fungi, and parasites. Smaller microorganisms such as viruses are not visible in the urine sediment with this type of magnification.

- *Bacteria:* It is not uncommon to see a few bacteria in urine specimens that are collected using the clean-catch midstream method. (See Fig. 22-7.) The presence of bacteria is usually the result of external contamination, especially in women. These bacterial contaminants multiply quickly after the urine is collected, and may cause the nitrite on the reagent stick to test positive if the urine is allowed to sit for more than an hour. When present in elevated numbers, the presence of bacteria will cause the urine pH to become more alkaline. (A pH above 8 may indicate the presence of excess bacterial contamination.) Bacteria must be visualized by using the high-power microscope objective because of their small size. The methods of reporting bacteria may vary among labs. Most commonly, bacteria is reported as few, moderate, or many, but a quantitative system of 1+, 2+, or 3+ may be used. Urinary tract infections may be caused by bacilli or cocci. When bacteria are present in the urine specimen in high numbers and white blood cells are evident, the urinalysis is generally followed up with a culture for positive identification of the bacteria and an antibiotic sensitivity.
- *Fungi: Candida albicans* is the most common type of fungi (yeast) present in urine. Yeast is commonly

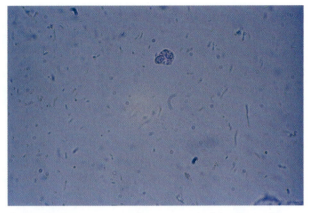

Figure 22-7   Bacteria as they appear in the urine sediment. *From Strasinger, SK, and Di Lorenzo, MS: Urinalysis and Body Fluids, ed. 5. FA Davis, Philadelphia, 2008, with permission.*

present in the urine of diabetic patients or those who are immunocompromised. Women who have the vaginal infection *candidiasis* may also have yeast present in their urine specimen. Yeast may be difficult to differentiate microscopically from red blood cells, as their size and shape are similar. Advanced yeast infections may present with yeast that is "budding" from stocks or branches as it multiplies and matures. The presence of yeast is reported in the same way that the presence of bacteria is reported.

- *Parasites:* The most common parasite present in the urine specimen is *Trichomonas vaginalis*. This is a sexually transmitted pathogenic microorganism that causes vaginal inflammation in females. Infection in males is often asymptomatic. *T. vaginalis* is often motile when viewed under the microscope in the urine sediment, and it may be recognized by the flagella that provides its movement. The motility of the organism is necessary for positive identification of the parasite. The presence of *T. vaginalis* is determined using the high-power objective and is reported as rare, few, moderate, or many per high-power field.

Test Your Knowledge 22-4

Which of the following microorganisms is not visualized in a urine sediment specimen using a compound microscope?

  a. Viruses
  b. Bacteria
  c. Fungi
  d. Parasites   (Outcome 22-4)

METHODS USED FOR URINE MICROSCOPIC EXAMINATION

The urine microscopic examination is the part of the routine urinalysis that is the least standardized from one laboratory to another. Each site may vary in the way that the specimen is prepared, in how much urine is used for preparation of the sediment, or by the way that the specimen is visualized during the examination. All procedures include the centrifugation of a specified volume of urine, separation of the **supernatant** (the fluid from the top of the specimen) from the **sediment** (the formed elements that have been compacted to the bottom of the tube), and examination of the urine sediment under a microscope. The formed elements are then examined using the low-power and/or high-power outcomes, and the results are reported.

The results of the microscopic examination may be affected by several factors. The age of the specimen and the conditions under which the specimen was stored can affect the integrity of the structures to be visualized. The volume of specimen centrifuged, the time of centrifugation, and the force of the centrifugation will determine the amount of sediment produced for the microscopic examination. The results may also be affected by the amount of supernatant discarded and the amount of sediment added to the slide for examination. The manner in which the results are reported may also differ according to laboratory protocol. Because of these variables, the Clinical and Laboratory Standards Institute has recommended that the process for preparing and performing urine microscopic examinations be standardized with use of commercial systems that minimize the variables in the process.

The KOVA system (manufactured by Hycor Biomedical, Inc.) is an example of a commercial urinalysis microscopic kit that uses a special pipette to standardize the amount of sediment prepared, has specific instructions concerning the rotations per minute and length of centrifugation to be used, and contains a special slide well used for examination of the sediment that dictates the amount of sediment used for the examination. The KOVA system also includes a stain that enhances the contrast of the formed elements to assist with identification. Procedure 22-1 details the use of the KOVA method for a microscopic examination. There are other commercial systems available, including the Urisystem manufactured by ThermoFisher Scientific and the Count-10 system manufactured by V-Tech, Incorporated.

Test Your Knowledge 22-5

Why might the KOVA system be used to prepare a urine microscopic specimen for examination?

(Outcome 22-5)

Regardless of the system used to process the urine and set up the microscopic examination, it is imperative that a fresh or properly stored urine specimen is used. If the urine specimen is allowed to remain at room temperature for an extended period of time (more than an hour), it may affect the results of the urine microscopic examination, in addition to the chemical analysis of the specimen. The formed elements present in the specimen will disintegrate and become distorted in specimens that are stored at room temperature for an extended period. The red blood cells, white blood cells, and hyaline casts are most affected. Specimens that are not analyzed within an hour may also exhibit an increase in bacterial growth, accompanied by an increase in pH.

Urine that is refrigerated prior to the performance of a microscopic examination will need to reach room temperature before the procedure is performed. If the urine is still very cold at the time of the examination, the precipitation of crystals will be visualized when viewed under the microscope. The presence of amorphous phosphates and amorphous urates in the refrigerated urine may obscure other clinically significant structures present in the specimen.

Medical assistants are often involved in the preparation of the urine sediment for the microscopic examination. In addition, the medical assistant may be asked to place the slide on the microscope stage and focus it appropriately so that the health-care provider (or another qualified laboratory professional) may perform the examination. To accomplish this, it is important that the medical assistant learn how to focus the microscope so that the formed elements are visible. Procedure 22-2 outlines the important concepts necessary to accomplish this task.

REPORTING URINE MICROSCOPIC RESULTS

As the various formed elements have been presented in this chapter, the reference ranges have been presented as well. It is important to remember that many normal urine specimens will include very few formed elements. If there are structures present in the urine sediment, it is important to report them in a way that is easy to interpret. The exact ranges and terminology used for

Procedure 22-1: Preparation of Urine Sediment for Microscopic Examination

TASK

Prepare a slide for urine microscopic examination using the KOVA system. Complete all steps within 15 minutes.

CONDITIONS

- Hand sanitization supplies
- Gloves
- Laboratory coat
- Face Shield
- Conical tube
- Freshly voided urine specimen
- KOVA System supplies, including tube cap, KOVA pipette, slide, and stain
- Centrifuge
- Test tube rack
- Microscope
- Biohazardous disposal container

CAAHEP/ABHES STANDARDS

 CAAHEP Standards

I.P.I.14. Perform Urinalysis   **III,P.III.2.** Practice Standard Precautions

 ABHES Standards

- Medical Office Clinical Procedures: b. Apply principles of aseptic techniques and infection control, i. Use standard precautions
- Perform Urinalysis

Procedure	Rationale
1. Sanitize hands, allow them to dry, and apply gloves.	Gloves protect the hands from exposure to potential bloodborne pathogens. Gloves should always be applied in the presence of the patient.
2. Gather necessary supplies. Urine must be at room temperature prior to use.	All supplies must be within reach so that the process can be completed in a timely manner. The urine must be at room temperature to avoid excess crystallization of the specimen.
3. Apply face shield and mix urine well by gently rotating the specimen cup or inverting the cup if necessary. Pour 12 mL of the specimen into the KOVA conical tube.	The application of the face shield protects the eyes and mucous membranes from potential splash and aerosol of the specimen. The urine must be well mixed for the results to be accurate, and the KOVA system instructions require 12 mL of urine to be added to the tube.
4. Apply the supplied cap to the tube, and centrifuge the specimen at 1,500 revolutions per minute for 5 minutes.	Centrifugation is necessary for the solid substances in the specimen to settle to the bottom of the tube so that they can be separated from the liquid at the top of the tube. The protective face shield can be removed at this time until the specimen is taken from the centrifuge, at which point it should be put on again.
5. When the centrifuge has come to a complete stop, remove the conical tube carefully.	Take care not to disturb the sediment in the bottom of the tube when handling the specimen.
6. Remove the cap and carefully insert the "petter" pipette included with the system into the urine specimen. Make sure the hook at the top of the pipette is settled into place over the edge of the conical tube.	The KOVA pipette is designed with a special hook device at the top of the apparatus. When the "petter" pipette is inserted correctly into the specimen, the hook will be firmly seated over the side of the conical tube.

Procedure	Rationale
7. With the pipette in place, carefully pour off the supernatant by inverting the tube over the sink to allow the liquid to pour out of the tube.	The KOVA pipette is specially designed with a bulb at the bottom of the pipette that holds the urine sediment in place as the supernatant is poured out of the tube. Approximately 1 mL of sediment is left in the bottom of the tube.

Courtesy of Fisher HealthCare, Inc.

Procedure	Rationale
8. Remove the pipette from the tube, but do not discard it at this time. Insert one drop of KOVA stain into the conical urine tube.	Only one drop of stain should be added so that the sediment is not diluted.
9. Reinsert the pipette into the tube and mix the stain with the sediment by application of gentle pressure on the bulb at the top of the pipette. Squeeze and release the bulb until the specimen is uniformly mixed.	The stain and the sediment must be thoroughly mixed, but excessive formation of air bubbles should be avoided.

Continued

Procedure 22-1: Preparation of Urine Sediment for Microscopic Examination—cont'd

Procedure	Rationale
10. Use the pipette to add a drop of the stained sediment to the KOVA slide. The slide is created with an opening at the top where the sediment can be added. The slide must not be overfilled or underfilled. At this point in the procedure, the protective face shield can be removed. Discard the pipette into the biohazardous disposal container.	If the slide is overfilled or underfilled, the results of the microscopic examination may be erroneous. When filling the slide, avoid the formation of air bubbles as much as possible. 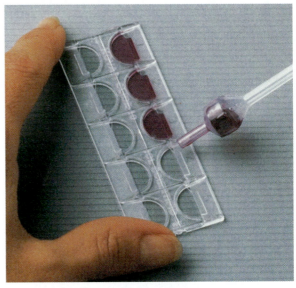 Courtesy of Fisher HealthCare, Inc.
11. Allow the specimen in the slide to settle for at least 1 minute before proceeding to the microscopic examination.	Focusing on the specimen too soon will make it difficult to identify or quantitate the formed elements correctly.
12. Complete the procedure necessary to focus the slide under the microscope.	The medical assistant may be involved in the focusing of the specimen, although he or she will not be performing the actual microscopic examination.

Procedure 22-2: Focusing the Urine Sediment Under the Microscope

TASK

Focus the urine sediment under the microscope to prepare it for identification and quantitation of formed elements. The process should be completed in less than 5 minutes.

CONDITIONS

- Hand sanitization supplies
- Gloves
- Laboratory coat
- KOVA slide with stained sediment added
- Biohazardous disposal container

CAAHEP/ABHES STANDARDS

 CAAHEP Standards

I.P.I.14. Perform Urinalysis   **III,P.III.2.** Practice Standard Precautions

 ABHES Standards

- Medical Office Clinical Procedures: b. Apply principles of aseptic techniques and infection control, i. Use standard precautions
- Perform Urinalysis

Procedure	Rationale
1. Sanitize hands, allow them to dry, and apply gloves.	Gloves protect the hands from exposure to potential bloodborne pathogens. Gloves should always be applied in the presence of the patient.
2. Move the mechanical stage all the way down, away from the microscope outcomes. Place the filled KOVA slide on the mechanical stage of the microscope. Use the clips on the stage to stabilize the slide.	The stage is moved away from the outcomes so that there is room to place the slide on the stage. All microscopic specimens are placed on the stage for examination. The clips allow the slides to be moved as needed for examination.
3. Move the 10X outcome into place for viewing. Minimize the light by using the adjustment knob at the base of the microscope and/or by closing the aperture opening where the light comes through to the slide.	Reduction of the light using the low-power outcome allows for better focus on the formed elements in the specimen.
4. Use the coarse adjustment knob to bring the stage as close as possible to the outcomes.	This will bring the slide into approximate focus when viewed through the eyepieces.
5. Look through the eyepieces, and use the coarse and fine adjustment knobs as needed to bring the specimen into focus. If necessary, move the slide across the stage to find a formed element to use as reference while focusing. Squamous epithelial cells are often present and easily identifiable.	Some specimens have very few formed elements; therefore, it may be necessary to scan several fields before a point of reference may be identified.
6. Inform the health-care practitioner or technologist that the slide is ready to be viewed. The microscopic examination should be completed within 5 minutes of the initial focus so that the specimen does not become dried out on the slide.	If the specimen dries out, it could lead to erroneous results because the concentration of formed elements on the slide can change with evaporation, and the appearance of the elements may change.
7. When the procedure is completed, discard the slide in the biohazardous disposal container, discard the tube with the rest of the stained sediment in the biohazardous waste container, disinfect the work site and microscope as needed, and remove gloves. Sanitize hands.	It is important to disinfect work areas and appropriately dispose of all laboratory specimens for infection control.

reporting may vary among laboratories. The differences in reporting methods may be the result of the system used for the examination (for instance, the commercial systems may have a grid that is used for counting and reporting the elements), or the differences may be the result of laboratory preference. Certain structures are reported as the number present per low-power field, whereas others report the number per high-power field. In addition, some of the formed elements are quantitatively reported as rare, few, moderate, and many, whereas others are reported using real numbers, such as 0 to 5, 5 to 10, and so on. Table 22-1 lists common formed elements and the units used for reporting.

> **Test Your Knowledge 22-6**
>
> True or False: All normal urine specimens contain a high number of formed elements.   (Outcome 22-7)

ROLE OF THE MEDICAL ASSISTANT IN MICROSCOPIC URINE PROCEDURES

The examination of urine sediment is not a CLIA-waived procedure. Medical assistants who perform this procedure in a physician office or other laboratory setting must possess the appropriate training and education to perform this moderately complex procedure. Urine microscopy examination may also be performed by the health-care provider in a physician office laboratory, as long as that laboratory has been registered appropriately with the Centers for Medicare & Medicaid Services as a site that is performing **provider performed microscopy**

(PPM). As part of the PPM process, the medical assistant will centrifuge the urine sample with added stain if necessary, place the sediment on the slide, and focus the specimen to prepare for the provider's microscopic examination. The medical assistant may also perform routine maintenance on the microscope.

> **Test Your Knowledge 22-7**
>
> List one duty that a medical assistant might perform in reference to the urine microscopic examination.
> (Outcome 22-8)

QUALITY CONTROL AND QUALITY ASSURANCE PROCEDURES FOR URINE MICROSCOPIC EXAMINATIONS

Quality assurance is a broad term used to describe the policies and procedures that ensure quality laboratory processes and patient care. For urine microscopic examinations, these parameters include the following components of the preanalytical phase of laboratory testing:

- Providing appropriate patient instructions for the collection of the specimen
- Ensuring adequate specimen volume
- Storing specimens correctly
- Using clean supplies
- Calibrating the centrifuge used to spin the specimen
- Separating the urine supernatant correctly
- Setting up the urine sediment correctly on the slide with the appropriate volume
- Focusing the specimen correctly in preparation for examination by a qualified laboratory professional

TABLE 22-1	
Common formed elements and method of reporting	
Common Formed Elements	**Units Used for Reporting**
Squamous epithelial cells	Rare, few, moderate, or many report per low-power field (lpf)
Mucus	Not reported by all laboratories; if reported, use rare, few, moderate, or many per low-power field (lpf)
Red blood cells	Average number visualized after counting 10 high-power fields (hpf). Reported as # per hpf
White blood cells	Average number visualized after counting 10 high-power fields. Reported as # per hpf
Spermatozoa	May or may not be reported according to laboratory protocol
Casts	Average number visualized after counting 10 low-power fields (lpf). Reported as # per lpf
Crystals	Reporting methods vary; usually rare, few, moderate, or many per high-power field
Bacteria	Rare, few, moderate, or many per high-power field
Yeast	Rare, few, moderate, or many per high-power field

Quality control refers more specifically to policies and procedures directly relating to the testing process. For urine microscopy, most medical assistants will not directly perform the microscopic quality control procedures because they are not qualified to perform examination of urine sediment under the microscope. However, it is important for medical assistants to know that they are still part of the quality control process. The medical assistant needs to verify that all reagents (such as stains) to be used are not expired. The instructions for use of commercial systems must be followed carefully to achieve desired results. Appropriate maintenance of the microscope is also part of quality control, because it is used directly in the testing process.

Medical assistants who have been properly trained to perform the urine microscopic examination may be responsible for quality control procedures that verify their ability to identify and quantitate the formed elements in the urine specimen correctly. These quality control procedures may include examination of commercially prepared specimens that contain known quantities of various formed elements. The laboratory will also participate in proficiency testing procedures in which results from standardized specimens are compared to those of other laboratories across the country to test for competency.

SUMMARY

The microscopic examination of urine specimens provides valuable information to health-care professionals. As the third part of a complete urinalysis, the knowledge gained from urine microscopy enhances the results obtained from the macroscopic and chemical examination of the specimen. The presence of formed elements in the urine such as blood cells, epithelial cells, crystals, and microorganisms provides valuable information to assist in a diagnosis of urinary tract infections, kidney disease or trauma, or metabolic disorders. The standardization of the specimen processing and microscopic examination procedure allows for more reliability in the results. To perform a urine microscopic examination, medical assistants would need appropriate education and training to meet the requirements for performance of a CLIA moderately complex procedure. However, medical assistants who have not received this additional training may still be responsible for preparing a specimen and focusing it under the microscope for reading by a qualified individual.

TIME TO REVIEW

1. The presence of white blood cells   Outcome 22-1
   in a urine specimen is called:
   a. Pyuria
   b. Hematuria
   c. Hemoglobinuria
   d. Cysturia

2. List two types of formed elements that   Outcome 22-3
   may be identified in a urine microscopic examination.

3. Which of the following may be   Outcome 22-4
   clinically significant if reported as part of a urine microscopic examination?
   a. The presence of a rare white blood cell
   b. Many bacteria
   c. The presence of a rare hyaline cast
   d. The presence of a rare squamous epithelial cell

4. Provide the name of one commercial   Outcome 22-5
   system used to prepare urine specimens for microscopic examinations.

5. When focusing the urine sediment   Outcome 22-6
   under the microscope, which microscope objective is used initially to bring the speciment into approximate focus?
   a. 10X
   b. 40X
   c. 100X
   d. None of the above

6. True or False: The presence of red   Outcome 22-7
   blood cells is reported as few, moderate, or many per lpf.

7. Which of the following represents   Outcome 22-8
   a typical task performed by a medical assistant in preparing for a urine microscopic examination?
   a. Counting the number of white blood cells present in 10 fields using the high-power objective
   b. Identifying the types of crystals present in the specimen
   c. Centrifuging the urine specimen
   d. Processing quality control specimens to verify competency with the procedure

8. True or False: Medical assistants are   Outcome 22-9
   not responsible for any quality control procedures pertaining to the urine microscopic examination.

9. How much supernatant is usually left   Outcome 22-10
   in the tube with the sediment when preparing the
   sediment to be placed on a slide for viewing?

   a. 5 mL
   b. 3 mL
   c. 0 mL
   d. 1 mL or less

Case Study 22-1: When is a specimen too cold?

Cassie Mason is a medical assistant working in a physician office laboratory at which urinalysis tests are performed. Cassie completed all the initial urinalysis test procedures before leaving for lunch. This included notation of the color and appearance of each specimen, as well as the chemical dipstick testing. She cleaned her work area, put all the specimens in the refrigerator, and left the results for the health-care practitioner to review before lunchtime.

When she returned from lunch an hour later, there was a note from the practitioner asking her to set up urine microscopic slides for two of the urine specimens for the practitioner to examine later that afternoon between appointments. About an hour later, Cassie removed the urine specimens from the refrigerator, centrifuged them, and immediately set up the slides and focused them on the microscope. Immediately thereafter, the practitioner came into the laboratory area and looked at the slide of the first specimen. After a cursory glance, she asked Cassie whether this specimen had been refrigerated. When Cassie acknowledged that it had, she told Cassie that she needed to pour another specimen, allow it to sit for at least a half an hour, then recentrifuge, and set up the slide again for viewing.

1. What did the practitioner see in the specimen that made her ask about the refrigeration?
2. How will it help to have the specimen sit at room temperature for a period of time before setting up another slide to be viewed?

Case Study 22-2: Normal results?

A patient drops off a urine specimen that was collected at home to the laboratory. The time of collection noted on the requisition form was several hours before the specimen was delivered to the laboratory. The medical assistant who is working in the laboratory performed a chemical analysis of the specimen, and notes that the pH of the specimen is 8, and that the nitrite result test produces a positive result.

1. In this scenario, what are the three details that provide a possible explanation for the test results obtained?
2. Should this specimen be used for a complete urinalysis?

RESOURCES AND SUGGESTED READING

University of Iowa Carver College of Medicine, practice tests for the Urine Microscopic Examination
  Presentation with questions and answers about the urine microscopic examination process http://www.medicine.uiowa.edu/cme/clia/modules.asp?testID=20
"Origin and composition of renal casts"
  Explains the origin and composition of the various types of renal casts http://www.agora.crosemont.qc.ca/urinesediments/doceng/doc_016.html

The typical urinalysis test consists of three components: physical examination, chemical examination, and microscopic examination. In many settings only the physical examination and chemical examination are routinely performed. A microscopic examination is only performed when the physical and/or chemical examination results suggest the presence of formed elements. Some situations in which a microscopic examination is typically indicated include the following:

- A sample that is cloudy or turbid
- A sample that is red in color
- A sample that has a large top layer of white or yellow foam
- A sample that has more than trace amounts of protein

It is important to correlate the results obtained in each of the urinalysis components performed. For example, one would expect to detect red blood cells on the dipstick test of a sample noted as being red during physical examination.

Case in Point

Recall Johnny, whom we met at the beginning of this section. He is an active 3-year-old who loves to play in the garage. He was rushed to his doctor's office after drinking antifreeze.

Examination of his urinalysis physical examination results reveals that both the color and clarity of Johnny's sample are abnormal. The fact that his urine is cloudy suggests that formed elements are present and indicate that a microscopic examination should be performed. The most important chemical examination result in this case is protein. Any amount more than a trace is considered abnormal and indicates the need to perform a microscopic examination.

These results are most likely the result of Johnny's ingestion of antifreeze, which is toxic to the kidneys. The kidneys typically respond to such substances by ceasing to produce urine. This stagnate state provides a perfect environment for the development of formed elements known as casts. Casts are cigar-shaped structures that contain a core matrix of a protein known as Tamm-Horsfall. Although this is a different protein from that which the corresponding dipstick test is designed to detect, presence of abnormal amounts of protein suggest that casts may be present. The best next course of action in this case is to perform a microscopic examination on Johnny's urine looking for formed elements, particularly casts.

On the Horizon

Advances in our understanding of how the body's immune system works have exploded in recent years. From this work, important discoveries have emerged. One such example is the fact that we now know that diabetes mellitus is associated with the immune system! No one would have even suspected this just a few short years ago. As a result of discoveries such as this, immunology has truly become a laboratory discipline within itself. Likewise, laboratory testing in this area, also known as immunology, has improved and expanded. In fact, there is much crossover of laboratory disciplines associated with immunology tests. Some laboratories have a section dedicated to performing immunology tests. In other settings, immunologic testing is performed throughout the laboratory.

Relevance for the Medical Assistant (Health-Care Provider)

As with so many other aspects of laboratory testing, medical assistants and other health-care support personnel often participate in immunologic testing by being involved in corresponding sample collection and processing. Furthermore, medical assistants often perform select CLIA-waived immunologic tests along with appropriate quality control. Medical assistants are also responsible for completing the documentation associated with this testing.

Case in Point

Four-year-old P.J. presented to the pediatrician's office where you work accompanied by his very worried father. In your initial conversation with P.J.'s father you learn that little P.J. had been battling a fever and sore throat for more than a week and was not showing any signs of improvement. Upon examination of the patient, the physician noted that the child had numerous yellow "spots" on the tonsillar area of his throat. "No wonder this little guy is so uncomfortable," you thought to yourself. The doctor ordered a strep screen test and requested that you perform the test. You obtain the following results: Rapid strip screen—Negative.

Questions for Consideration:

- What is the specimen type of choice for strep screen testing?
- What is the proper collection protocol for this specimen?
- What is the strep screen test designed to detect?
- What accounts for the negative strep screen results obtained?
- What could be done at this juncture to help determine the microbiological agent responsible for PJ's infection?

Section VI
Immunology

Chapter 23: Immunology provides the reader with a basic understanding of the immune system. Immunologic principles as they relate to blood typing and hemolytic disease of the newborn are covered. An introduction and overview of common immunology and serology test methods are presented.

Chapter 24: Immunologic-Based Rapid Testing includes a description of the common rapid tests that are routinely performed, including strep screen, infectious mononucleosis testing, pregnancy testing, *Helicobacter pylori* testing, and testing for influenzas A and B and HIV. The nature of each condition associated with these tests is examined. Appropriate follow-up testing is briefly discussed when indicated. Proper technique, normal test reference range, quality control, sources of error and interference, and test interpretation are described.

Chapter 23

Immunology

Constance L. Lieseke, CMA (AAMA), MLT, PBT(ASCP)

Learning Outcomes

After reading this chapter, the successful student will be able to:

23-1 Define the key terms.

23-2 Explain how serology and immunology are related to immunity.

23-3 Describe the mechanical barriers used by the immune system.

23-4 Explain how the internal defenses at the site of an invasion by foreign substances function.

23-5 Summarize how acquired immunity is activated in the body.

23-6 Distinguish what happens when the immune process malfunctions.

23-7 Examine how vaccinations activate the immune system.

23-8 Demonstrate understanding of the basic ABO and Rh blood typing systems and the role they play in hemolytic disease of the newborn.

23-9 Describe various immunology testing methods and common serology tests performed in hospital and reference laboratories.

23-10 Explain why some serology tests might be performed in physician offices rather than in reference laboratories.

23-11 Explain the clinical significance of the common CLIA-waived serology tests performed in physician offices.

CAAHEP/ABHES STANDARDS

 CAAHEP Standards

I.C.5. Describe the normal function of each body system
I.C.6: Identify common pathology related to each body system
III.C.10: Identify disease processes that are indications for CLIA-waived tests

 ABHES Standards

- Identify and apply the knowledge of all body systems; their structure and functions; and their common diseases, symptoms, and etiologies

KEY TERMS

Agglutination	Globulin	Macrophage
Allergy	Hemolytic disease of the newborn (HDN)	Mucous membranes
Antibody		Natural killer (NK) cells
Antibody-mediated immunity	Histamine	Normal flora
Antigen	Immunity	Pathogens
Autoimmune disease	Immunoglobulins	Phagocytes
B cells	Immunology	Phagocytosis
Cell-mediated immunity	Infection	Pus
Chemotaxis	Inflammation	RhoGam
Cilia	Interferons	RIA
Complement	In vitro	Serology
ELISA or EIA testing	In vivo	T cells
Erythroblastosis fetalis	Lateral flow immunoassay	Vaccine
Gammaglobulins	Lysozyme	

IMMUNITY AND IMMUNOLOGY

Our bodies are constantly under attack by an army of microorganisms, toxins, allergens and other substances that are recognized as foreign or "nonself." Luckily, our defenses are usually able to protect us from this ongoing attack. The recognition and destruction of these foreign substances by our bodies are known as **immunity**, and the study of this process is called **immunology**.

Immunity includes numerous protective mechanisms within our bodies. In order for these systems to function properly, we must be able to detect what is "self" and what is "nonself." When a foreign (or nonself) invader is

detected, the immune process is activated. A foreign substance capable of initiating an immune response is called an **antigen.** The antigen may be a microorganism (such as bacteria or viruses), an allergen (such as pollen or dander), a foreign body (such as a sliver), or even a cancerous cell from within the body.

Antibodies are substances that the body produces in response to certain antigens. The antibody is designed to attach to, or bond with, the specific antigen targeted. Antibodies are made of a type of protein called **globulin,** and because they are part of the immune process, they are known as **immunoglobulins.** The job of immunoglobulins is complex, and includes attachment to and destruction of the invader, as well as remembering the unique identity of the antigen so that if this invader comes into the body again, the body is ready to attack and destroy much faster than it was at the first exposure. Antibodies seek out and irreversibly bind to their specific antigen, rendering it ineffective.

A great deal of research has been performed on the immune responses of our bodies. We are now able to test for specific antibodies and antigens in the laboratory, using blood and other body fluids. This area of the laboratory may be known as the Immunology Department, but more commonly it is referred to as the Serology Department. **Serology** is the study of antigen and antibody reactions in serum, and may include methods such as radioactive laboratory testing, agglutination reactions, or simplistic tests such as those used to detect pregnancy.

Test Your Knowledge 23-1

How are antigens and antibodies related to immunity?

(Outcome 23-2)

Test Your Knowledge 23-2

Which department in the laboratory provides testing methods to monitor the immune system?

(Outcome 23-2)

THE IMMUNE PROCESS

If you've ever watched a movie about the Revolutionary War or Civil War, it is difficult to see the soldiers march forward on the battlefield in straight lines again and again to meet their enemies. Eventually, with a great deal of effort and substantial losses, this method of combat might affect the outcome of the encounter. On the other hand, the battles won with a minimal number of casualties were those that employed *multiple* strategies, or lines of defense.

We wage a similar battle in our bodies every day. The sheer number of foreign substances we encounter is overwhelming. We need more than one line of defense to defeat the invaders with minimal harm to ourselves. A healthy immune system makes use of three basic defense mechanisms (Fig. 23-1). These include mechanical and chemical barriers, internal defenses at the site of the invasion, and acquired or adaptive immunity created by the body in response to a specific antigen. The first two lines of defense are nonspecific, and function in a similar manner with any invader they encounter. These nonspecific mechanisms are protecting us all from birth or very soon afterward. The third defensive mechanism, however, is very specific and is something that we develop throughout our lives.

The First Line of Defense: Nonspecific Mechanical and Chemical Barriers

The first line of defense used by our immune system includes mechanical barriers, chemicals, organisms that are always present in our bodies, and protective reflexes. The goal of these mechanisms is to keep the invaders out of our bodies or prevent them from surviving long enough to cause any further harm.

Intact skin and the **mucous membranes** of our bodies are extremely important because they form a physical or mechanical barrier to many pathogens and other types of invaders. Their secretions also play an important role, by adjusting the pH to deter growth of most pathogens, and by trapping other invaders in a sticky environment where they can be destroyed or immobilized. The **cilia**

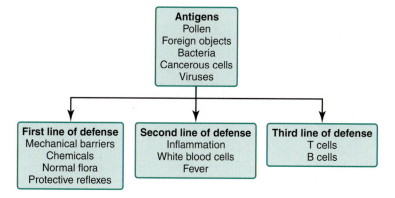

Figure 23-1   Flow chart showing the different kinds of immune responses and their triggers.

lining the mucous membranes constantly work to sweep out any trapped substances. Reflexes, such as sneezing or coughing, then move these potential **pathogens** out of the body. The acidic environment in our stomach and the enzymes in saliva also assist with this first line of defense. Earwax protects our ears, perspiration helps to flush away unwanted bacteria, and an enzyme in tears called **lysozyme** destroys many potential invaders.

In addition to the protective mechanisms already mentioned, our bodies are populated naturally by numerous types of bacteria. Although this might seem to be a bad thing, it is actually quite beneficial to our immune system. The presence of this **normal flora** creates a competitive environment in which most invading bacteria cannot survive. We have normal flora throughout our bodies, including in and on our skin, in our mouths, and in our intestinal tract.

Test Your Knowledge 23-3

How does a break in the skin trigger the first line of defense to respond?   (Outcome 23-3)

Test Your Knowledge 23-4

Are sneezes a good thing? Why or why not?
                                                         (Outcome 23-3)

The Second Line of Defense: Internal Nonspecific Response

If a foreign substance makes its way past the first line of immune defenses, it will be confronted with a wave of new defense mechanisms within the body. These are all part of the internal nonspecific response, also known as the second line of defense. Included in this arsenal are phagocytosis, inflammation, fever, and natural killer cells. This second line of defense is also known as natural or innate immune response.

When cells are injured, they release a chemical into the bloodstream that signals the second line of defense to activate. This signaling is called **chemotaxis,** and it attracts certain types of white blood cells to the scene of the invasion to act as **phagocytes.** The white blood cells (neutrophils and monocytes) are specially programmed to ingest and destroy the invaders. This process is called **phagocytosis.**

When a foreign substance has entered the body, we often observe the surrounding area become red, hot, and swollen. The internal process that causes this appearance is called **inflammation,** and if it is caused by a pathogen, it may be known as **infection.** Inflammation occurs as a result of injury to or irritation of a cell. When the cells become irritated or injured, they release **histamine.** The histamine causes the blood vessels in the area to dilate, or become larger. The blood flow increases to the irritated area, and this causes the heat and redness we see and feel. Histamine also causes the blood vessel walls to become "leaky," so more fluid leaks out of the bloodstream into the surrounding injured area, causing swelling. Pain is evident because the surrounding nerve receptors are stimulated by all the activity.

As the blood supply is increased, more phagocytes are brought to the area. While doing their job, these cells create a lot of debris. The built-up dead phagocytes, fluid, pathogens, and injured blood cells that accumulate are what we recognize as **pus.**

The next symptom we often note in a pathogenic invasion is fever, which occurs because the phagocytes that respond to the scene of the injury release a chemical that signals the brain to increase the body's temperature. The elevation in temperature helps the second line of defense by decreasing the ability of many pathogens to survive, as well as stimulating even more phagocytosis.

As if all the other activity weren't enough, protective proteins also assist at the scene of the invasion. There are two groups of protective proteins, known as **interferons** and **complement** proteins. Interferons are secreted by cells that have been infected by viruses, and they help other cells resist the spread and replication of the virus. Complement proteins are able to destroy bacteria by covering the surface of the bacterial cells and punching holes in the cell membrane, causing the bacteria to die.

The last component of the second line of defense is the **natural killer (NK) cells,** which are a special type of lymphocyte that responds to the invasion. NK cells can attack and destroy human cells that have been infected by pathogens. In addition, natural killer cells may be beneficial by destroying certain cancer cells before they can spread.

The Third Line of Defense: Acquired or Adaptive Immunity

Acquired or adaptive immunity is a defense mechanism that requires the body to "think" about the invaders. It involves three characteristics that are not present in the first or second line of defense. Recognition of an antigen as nonself must first occur, after which the antigen (invader) is identified very specifically. Then the body forms a memory of that antigen, so it will be immediately recognized in case of subsequent exposure. Usually this entire process requires 1 to 2 weeks after the first exposure to a specific antigen.

T cells and **B cells** are specifically programmed lymphocytes. They are both part of this third level of the immune process, but they each perform different functions when exposed to an antigen. T cells are involved in cell-mediated immunity, and B cells are involved in **antibody-mediated immunity,** also known as humoral immunity.

Cell-mediated immunity begins at the site of the invasion (Fig. 23-2). The T cells become "activated" toward a specific antigen when it is presented by a **macrophage.** (A macrophage is a type of phagocyte that leaves the bloodstream and goes into the tissues.) Once activated, this T cell creates four identical copies of itself, which all have specific functions:

- Killer T cells are produced to kill the antigens.
- Helper T cells are designed to stimulate other T cells and help the B cells.

- Suppressor T cells (also known as regulatory T cells) are created to inhibit the activity of the T and B cells when enough have been produced.
- Memory T cells are responsible for remembering the antigen for future encounters, which allows the cell-mediated immunity to occur faster with the next exposure.

Most of the lymphocytes in our circulation are T cells. Although no antibodies are produced by the T cells, they play an important role in many contact sensitivity reactions, as well as viral infections, fungal infections, and destruction of malignant cells.

Antibody-mediated immunity uses the lymphocytic B cells (Fig. 23-3). As with the cell-mediated immunity, the antigen must first be exposed, or introduced, to the B cell by presentation from the macrophage. The helper T cells release a chemical to assist with this recognition process. Once activated, the B cell produces two replicas of itself, which have their own duties:

- Plasma cells are created that secrete antibodies that are specific for a particular antigen. These antibodies

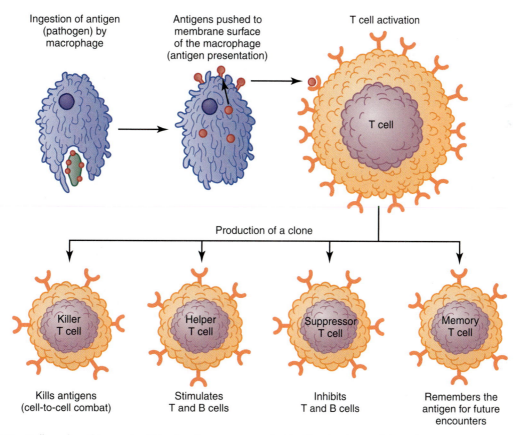

Figure 23-2 Cell-mediated immunity. This drawing represents the T-cell activation and the subsequent steps, creating four subsets of T cells.

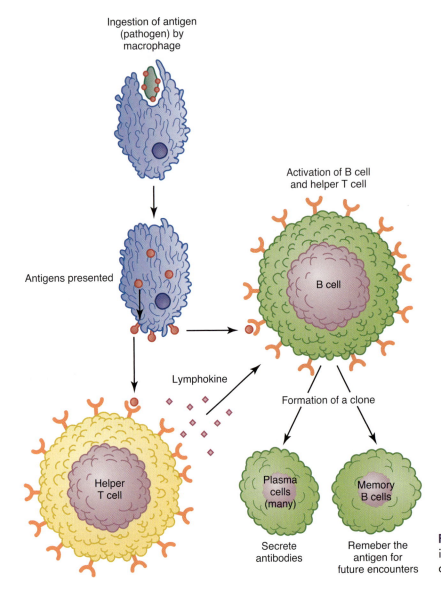

Ingestion of antigen
(pathogen) by
macrophage

Antigens presented

Activation of B cell
and helper T cell

B cell

Lymphokine

Formation of a clone

Helper
T cell

Plasma
cells
(many)

Memory
B cells

Secrete
antibodies

Remeber the
antigen for
future encounters

Figure 23-3   Antibody-mediated immunity. B-cell activation leads to antibody creation by plasma cells.

work like a lock and key and cannot be interchanged with other antigens. The antibodies bind to the antigens, blocking their ability to affect the cells of the body.

- Memory B cells form a "picture" of the antigen and remember it for future encounters.

Test Your Knowledge 23-5

True or False: Antigen exposure always triggers all three lines of defense.   (Outcome 23-4)

Test Your Knowledge 23-6

Which line of defense is "unique" toward a specific antigen?   (Outcome 23-4)

HOW IMMUNITY IS ACQUIRED

There are essentially four ways we can acquire immunity:

- *Natural active immunity acquired from an infection with a pathogen:* This causes the body to produce a memory of the antigen and protects the body on subsequent exposures. For instance, natural active immunity is produced when a person is infected with chicken pox. Once the person recovers, he or she is now immune to this pathogen. This is a long-term type of immunity.

- *Artificial active immunity acquired from a* **vaccine:** The typical antibody response of our body after exposure to an antigen is usually too slow to protect us from the initial infection. However, with subsequent exposures, the protection is so fast that we never become ill. Vaccines do this artificially. They contain an antigen that causes the body to develop antibodies as if it were being exposed for the first time. The vaccine may be a killed or weakened pathogen (known as *attenuated)* or it may just be part of a pathogen. Vaccines are available for many diseases, such as hepatitis A and B, measles, and mumps. The protection is long term with this type of immunity.
- *Natural passive immunity, such as the antibodies a mother passes on to an infant through the placenta or through breast milk:* This is a temporary type of immunity and fades as the child grows.
- *Artificial passive immunity:* This usually occurs with the injection of **gammaglobulins** (artificial antibodies). This immunity is short acting, and protects the individual in an emergency situation. For example, a family member has been diagnosed with hepatitis A, but the rest of the family is unvaccinated for that disease. The other family members are then injected with an "artificial antibody" (gammaglobulin) so that they will be protected until the infected individual recovers from the hepatitis A infection.

Test Your Knowledge 23-7

What does it mean when we say that we are "immune" to a certain disease?   (Outcome 23-5)

Test Your Knowledge 23-8

How do vaccines "fool" our immune systems? Which line of defense do they target?   (Outcome 23-5)

FAILURE OF OUR IMMUNE SYSTEMS

Unfortunately, our immune systems don't always work as they should. Sometimes our body's ability to recognize self and nonself is not fully developed, or is somehow dysfunctional. In this case, our body may attack its own cells, causing damage. This is the theory behind many

POINT OF INTEREST 23-1
Vaccines

Vaccines are used to prevent disease by introducing an antigen into the body to induce an immune response. After the vaccine is processed by the body, antibodies are created against that specific antigen. When the patient is exposed again to the disease-causing virus or bacteria, the body immediately produces large amounts of antibody that prevent the disease from developing.

The vaccine antigen may be attenuated, meaning that the antigen it is killed or weakened. Vaccines may also include parts of bacteria or virus particles that are capable of stimulating an immune response but not capable of causing disease. In addition, an inactivated toxin produced by the bacteria (called a toxoid) may be used. The tetanus and diphtheria vaccinations are toxoid vaccines.

forms of **autoimmune diseases,** such as rheumatoid arthritis. Also, as we age, our immune systems don't seem to detect the malignant or damaged cells in our bodies and destroy them as they should. This allows the cells to reproduce and cause cancer at a higher rate as we age.

In the case of an **allergy,** our immune system becomes hypersensitive after the initial exposure to an antigen. With subsequent exposures to that antigen, the immune response causes inflammation and organ dysfunction. Allergies may range from those with annoying symptoms (such as hay fever) to those that are truly life threatening, such as reactions to insect stings and certain medications. Table 23-1 provides examples of diseases associated with the immune system.

BLOOD TYPES

Blood types also involve antigens and antibodies, but in a different way. The antigens that determine blood types are on the surface of all red blood cells. Blood typing also involves natural and acquired antibodies in the plasma. There are several situations that might warrant a test for blood type, including transfusions, testing to prevent hemolytic disease of the newborn, and for investigative or forensic reasons. There are hundreds of different antigens present on the red blood cells of our bodies, all capable of causing transfusion complications. Fortunately, most serious complications from transfusions are due to the ABO and Rh blood groups, so much of our testing is focused on those groups.

TABLE 23-1

Common immune system disorders

Classification	Examples of Specific Disorders
Hypersensitivity (allergy)	Anaphylactic reactions, dermatitis or eczema, rhinitis, asthma
Autoimmune disorders	Systemic lupus erythematosus, type 1 diabetes, Graves' disease, celiac disease, myasthenia gravis, rheumatoid arthritis, systemic sclerosis
Malignancies of immune cells	Lymphocytic leukemias, lymphoma, multiple myeloma
Congenital immune disorders	Thymic hypoplasia, agammaglobulinemia
Secondary or acquired immunodeficiency	AIDS, transplant anti-rejection medication use, systemic infections, side effect of radiation treatment, overuse of antibiotics

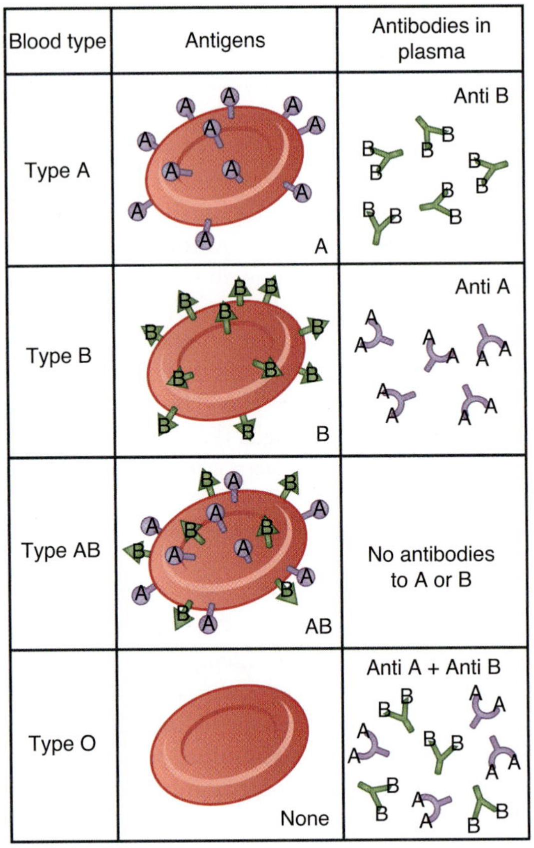

The ABO blood types include A, B, AB, and O, and they represent the antigens present (or absent) on the red blood cells of an individual. If people have a blood type of A, this means they have the A antigens on their cells. If B antigens are present, they are blood type B, and if both are present, the blood type is known as AB. Type O may be thought of as type "zero," as it means neither A or B antigens are present (Fig. 23-4).

The ABO blood typing system is unique, because in the plasma of each person there are natural antibodies to the antigens that are *not* present on their red blood cells. This means a person with a type A blood type has anti-B naturally in his or her plasma, and the plasma of a person with type B blood will contain antibodies to the A antigen. An individual who is type AB has neither anti-A nor anti-B in the plasma, and type O individuals naturally possess both anti-A and anti-B in their plasma. These plasma antibodies are created within the first few months of life as an immune response to dietary antigens and exposure to various environmental factors.

When patients receive blood transfusions, they generally receive a blood product known as packed red blood cells rather than whole blood. To prepare packed red blood cells, the unit of donor blood is centrifuged so that the plasma is separated from the cells, and most of the plasma and the white blood cells are separated from the red blood cells. Removal of the plasma avoids an overload of fluid for the patients needing multiple units to increase their red blood cell and hemoglobin concentration. The absence of white blood cells in the blood product helps to reduce the potential for an immune response.

Figure 23-4 Various blood type antigens and antibodies.

It is critical to consider the natural antibodies present in the plasma if a transfusion is needed. Ideally, a person should only be transfused with his or her own blood type. In an emergency situation, a person may be given a different type, but there are only a few alternatives that are safe. If a type B person received type A blood, the natural anti-A antibodies would cause the cells to clump (agglutinate), and eventually hemolyze (rupture). The by-products of this reaction could also clog the capillaries in the kidneys and cause renal failure. Blood type O is known as the universal donor, because there are no ABO antigens on the cells. When type O packed red blood cells are transfused to a patient with any other blood type, they are not rejected by the recipient and the natural anti-A and anti-B that was present in the plasma of the donor are not present in the packed cells to damage the recipient's blood cells. Type AB is known as the universal recipient, because there are no ABO antibodies in the plasma to damage any blood type that is transfused to these recipients. About 40% of the population is type A, 11% is type B, 45% is type O, and 4% is type AB (Table 23-2).

TABLE 23-2	
Percentage of various blood types in the U.S. population	
Blood Type	**Percentage of U.S. Population**
A	40%
B	11%
AB	4%
O	45%

Another very important red blood cell antigen is the Rh or D antigen. It was discovered in 1939 with work on rhesus monkeys, hence the designation Rh. Approximately 85% of the population has the D antigen on their cells, and they are known as Rh positive. Those who don't have the Rh (D) antigen on their cells are known as Rh negative.

Unlike the ABO blood types, Rh-negative individuals do not have naturally occurring Rh antibodies in their plasma. However, they can be sensitized to this foreign Rh antigen if exposed. This exposure may occur with a transfusion error, or it may occur with pregnancy and delivery. There is usually no problem evident with the first Rh exposure because the antibody production takes too much time. However, the antigenic response is *very* swift and strong with subsequent exposures to Rh-positive blood.

ERYTHROBLASTOSIS FETALIS

Erythroblastosis fetalis is a severe hemolytic anemia that affects Rh-positive newborns and occasionally other newborns with ABO incompatibility. This condition may also be known as **hemolytic disease of the newborn (HDN).** The Rh status of the blood cells is only an issue when the baby is Rh positive and the mother is Rh negative. During a first pregnancy, this incompatibility does not usually cause harm to the baby, as the mother's response to the Rh antigen does not happen quickly enough for the antibodies to attack the baby's red blood cells. However, during the first pregnancy, and especially during delivery of the baby and the placenta, there is an exchange of fetal blood with the mother, and the mother will become sensitized, which means that she will develop antibodies to the Rh antigens on the baby's red blood cells. If she becomes pregnant again with an Rh-positive baby, her antibodies to the Rh antigens will destroy the baby's red blood cells and the baby may be born with severe

POINT OF INTEREST 23-2
Kidney transplants for patients with incompatible blood types

Many potential kidney donors are rejected because their blood type is not compatible with that of the patients needing a kidney. There is now a process that allows patients to receive a kidney from a donor with an incompatible blood type.

The natural antibodies present in the plasma of the recipient of a kidney with an incompatible blood type usually cause the kidney to be destroyed. The process for ABO-incompatible kidney transplantation includes a procedure called plasmapheresis. The patient has a unit of blood removed from his or her body, and a portion of the liquid plasma is then removed. After each of the plasmapheresis procedures, the patient will receive replacement antibodies that are necessary to fight off other infections. The procedure may need to be repeated numerous times, until the level of ABO antibody detected in the blood is low enough to be considered safe for the transfusion.

Kidney transplant rejection rates for this procedure are not much different from the rate for patients who receive kidneys of the same ABO blood type. The patient will have more plasmapheresis and artificial antibody treatments after the transplant, depending on the individual needs of the patient. In addition, the recipient may also require a splenectomy, because the spleen is the organ in which the ABO antibodies are produced.

anemia, jaundice, and an enlarged spleen and liver, which may be fatal for the newborn.

An injection of **RhoGam** (anti-Rh gammaglobulin) during the pregnancy and shortly after delivery should be given to all Rh-negative mothers. This will keep the mother from becoming sensitized to the Rh antigen so she does not create the anti-Rh antibodies. When she becomes pregnant again with an Rh-positive baby, her body will react as if this were her first exposure, and the Rh incompatibility will not be a problem.

Test Your Knowledge 23-9

What antigens are present on the blood cells of an individual with a blood type of AB positive?

(Outcome 23-8)

IMMUNOLOGY TESTING METHODS

Various immunology testing methods are available for use in the medical office as well as hospital and reference laboratories. They can be performed **in vivo** (inside a living organism) as in allergy or tuberculosis testing; an antigen is placed under the skin, and the patient is monitored for a visible reaction. More often, they are performed **in vitro** (within a laboratory testing environment), where we commonly refer to them as serology tests.

Serology tests must be specific to the antigen or antibody being tested, and they must also be sensitive enough to detect even a small amount of the substance in the specimen. Many medications or other concurrent disease states can interfere with the specificity of a certain test, and sometimes can cause false-positive or false-negative results. The sensitivity of a testing method can be affected by high or low temperatures during shipping or storage, and also by minor errors that occur during the testing procedures. Package inserts should be examined carefully for specimen requirements, interfering substances, storage and handling directions, and testing procedures before performing any sort of serology testing.

All immunology tests are performed to determine the presence of a particular antibody or antigen. The specimen tested may be blood, serum, urine, oral fluids, or other body tissues. Various testing methods are used, including the following:

- Enzyme-linked immunosorbent assay tests (**ELISA or EIA**) tests usually involve a testing surface that is coated with an antibody or antigen bound to an enzyme. After the specimen is added, if the matching antibody or antigen is present, a color change will occur that can be read either by the testing personnel directly or by using an instrument to measure the amount of color change.
- An adaptation of the EIA principle, **lateral flow immunoassay** is used in many CLIA-waived tests. The specimen must be absorbed and must "flow" across the testing surface to reach the area imbedded with the antigen or antibody. If the test is positive, the antigen/antibody complex will cause a color change to occur in the testing area. These tests are read directly

by the testing personnel, and have a built-in quality control area as well.
- Radioimmunoassays (**RIAs**) use a radioactively labeled protein as the indicator of a positive result. The antigen/antibody complex formed in a specimen that is positive will combine with the radioactive protein rather than an enzyme as in the EIA method. The final result is obtained from the amount of radioactivity present in the sample at the end of the testing process. These assays are complicated, and are performed only by qualified personnel in hospital or reference laboratories.
- Agglutination is the formation of large insoluble aggregates (clumps) of cells that form when an antigen/antibody complex is present. Agglutination may use red blood cells and antibodies, as in the case of ABO and Rh blood typing, or it may use latex beads, as do some of the mononucleosis testing procedures. This reaction is read by the testing personnel directly, as the complex is visible to the naked eye.

COMMON SEROLOGY TESTS PERFORMED IN REFERENCE OR HOSPITAL LABORATORIES

Serology tests may share common methodology, but the complexity of the testing process can vary greatly. The tests mentioned below are usually performed only in reference or hospital settings, as they require additional training and/or credentials for the person performing the test.

- Testing for *ABO/Rh* major blood antigen groups uses agglutination techniques. Screening is also performed for other common red blood cell antigens, and compatibility tests are performed on the donor blood when a transfusion workup is necessary.
- *The antistreptolysin O (ASO)* test is used to detect antistreptolysin O antibodies, which are present in a patient with prior recent infection by group A streptococcus. The identification of those with prior infection is important, as group A streptococcus infection can lead to other complications such as glomerulonephritis, rheumatic fever, and bacterial endocarditis. The ASO antibody may be present for several months after the initial infection.
- *Cold agglutinins* are antibodies present with certain types of infections, pneumonias, cancers, or inflammatory autoimmune disorders. These antibodies can cause the red blood cells of the body to "clump" together when exposed to cold temperatures. This leads to hemolytic anemia and other complications.

- *The C-reactive protein (CRP)* test verifies the presence of that protein, which is present in the blood with acute systemic inflammation. It may be used as part of the diagnosis for a specific condition related to inflammation, or to monitor the effectiveness of treatment.
- *Hepatitis testing* determines which form of viral hepatitis (A through E) an individual has, and it may also provide more information about where an individual is in the disease process.
- Although a *pregnancy test* can be performed at home or in a physician office laboratory as a CLIA-waived test, it is sometimes necessary to use the more sensitive methods that are available in a larger laboratory. These methods can sometimes detect pregnancy sooner than can the CLIA-waived tests, and they can also quantitate the amount of human chorionic gonadotropin (HCG) present in the specimen. This quantitative analysis can be vital in the case of a suspected ectopic pregnancy, or in the diagnosis and treatment of testicular cancer, in which the hormone is also present in the bloodstream in male patients.
- Rheumatoid arthritis is a crippling and progressive autoimmune disease that affects the joints of the body. Those afflicted will have the *rheumatoid factor* present in their blood, which is a unique antibody used for diagnosis.
- *The most common tests used to detect syphilis* are the rapid plasma reagin (RPR) test and the venereal disease research laboratory (VDRL) test. The tests detect the presence of the microorganism *Treponema pallidum,* the causative agent of syphilis.

Test Your Knowledge 23-11

What do all serology tests have in common?

(Outcome 23-9)

Test Your Knowledge 23-12

True or False: The same disease may be detected by more than one serology test. (Outcome 23-9)

CLIA-WAIVED TESTS COMMONLY PERFORMED IN THE PHYSICIAN OFFICE LABORATORY

Tests performed in a physician office laboratory are very important for appropriate diagnosis and treatment of various diseases, as the results are available quickly within the same office where the patient is being examined. This section covers these tests, as well as their testing procedures, in more detail (Table 23-3).

- *Mononucleosis:* Mononucleosis is caused by the Epstein-Barr virus. The test performed for diagnosis identifies the presence of the heterophile antibody produced with this infection,.
- *Pregnancy:* Pregnancy tests determine the presence or absence of human chorionic gonadotropin (HCG) in urine or serum. CLIA-waived tests are qualitative in nature, with a positive or negative result.
- *Helicobacter pylori:* H. pylori is the bacterium responsible for many gastric and duodenal ulcers and gastritis. The test can be performed on serum and other body tissues.

TABLE 23-3

Commonly performed CLIA–waived immunology tests

Disease/Condition	Causative Agent	Test Performed	Required Specimen
Mononucleosis	Epstein-Barr virus	Mononucleosis screen or heterophile test	Blood
Pregnancy	Human chorionic gonadotropin (HCG)	Pregnancy (HCG) test	Serum or urine
H. pylori	Helicobacter pylori bacteria	H. pylori test	Blood or tissue sample
HIV	Human immunodeficiency virus	HIV test	Blood, oral fluids
Flu	Influenza virus	Influenza test	Nasal or nasopharyngeal swabs
Bladder cancer	Bladder tumor–associated antigen	BTA test	Urine
Strep throat	Group A streptococcus bacteria	Strep screen	Throat swab

- *HIV:* The human immunodeficiency virus screening test checks for the presence of the antibodies produced with HIV infection. This is designed to be a *screening* test only, and more definitive testing would then be performed on positive samples before the patient would be deemed HIV positive. Various body fluids can be tested for the presence of HIV.
- *Influenza:* The influenza test is performed during the winter months to detect the presence of influenza A or B, which causes a very serious respiratory infection.
- **Bladder tumor–associated antigen:** The screening test for bladder cancer uses a urine specimen.
- *Group A streptococcus infection:* The screening test for active infection with group A streptococcus uses a throat swab. The result is available in minutes after collection, allowing for much faster treatment than was previously available when only a throat culture was used.

Test Your Knowledge 23-13

Why might it be beneficial to perform simple serology tests in the physician office instead of a reference or hospital laboratory?   (Outcome 23-10)

Test Your Knowledge 23-14

What is the causative agent of mononucleosis?
(Outcome 23-11)

SUMMARY

Our immune systems are complex and protect us in various ways. We have three basic mechanisms that interact to provide this protection. They include various natural barriers, cellular and chemical responses to invaders, and antibody formation. We use vaccinations to protect us by activating our immune systems, and we also have naturally occurring antibodies to ABO blood types that are unlike our own. Blood type antibodies may be protective, but they can also cause serious health issues and must be considered during pregnancy to protect the unborn child.

Laboratory testing for immunity is known as serology. Various tests are performed in the physician office laboratory, as well as in hospital and reference laboratories. These tests may be qualitative or quantitative in nature, and are invaluable to aid in appropriate diagnosis of numerous disease states.

TIME TO REVIEW

1. A substance released in response to antigenic exposure that causes blood vessels to dilate is a(n):   Outcome 23-1

   a. Lymphocyte
   b. Histamine
   c. Interferon
   d. Chemotaxis

2. A(n) _____ is anything that our body recognizes as nonself.   Outcome 23-1

3. How are antigens and antibodies related to serology testing?   Outcome 23-2

4. What role does our stomach play in protecting us from antigens?   Outcome 23-3

   a. Inflammation destroys the pathogens
   b. The pH of the stomach acid helps to destroy microorganisms that may make their way into our bodies
   c. Antibodies are produced here to destroy the invaders; white blood cells engulf the antigens
   d. The stomach does not play a role in immunity

5. What is phagocytosis?   Outcome 23-1

   a. The process by which white blood cells engulf and destroy pathogens
   b. The process that occurs when a noncompatible blood type is given to a patient
   c. A term used to describe the first line of immunity
   d. The production of antibodies

6. True or False: Immunity provided by the mother at birth is lifelong for many diseases.   Outcome 23-5

7. True or False: Acquired immunity occurs only as a consequence of vaccinations.   Outcome 23-6

8. What is used in vaccinations to activate our immune systems?   Outcome 23-6

   a. Immunoglobulin
   b. Killed (attenuated) viruses or parts of viruses
   c. Normal flora
   d. B cells

9. Antibodies to blood type antigens A or B: Outcome 23-8

   a. Occur after exposure to another blood type
   b. Are naturally occurring and do not require exposure to develop

c. Do not exist in the bloodstream

d. Are harmless

10. True or False: Serology tests use a variety of testing methods.   Outcome 23-9

11. Which of the following are acronyms for tests used to detect syphilis infection?   Outcome 23-9

    a. VDRL and RPR

    b. HCG and IgG

    c. HET and RPR

    d. CRP and VDRL

12. Doctor Johnson is about to prescribe a medication to treat acne for Carly Lucas. This medication is not advised for those who are pregnant. Which CLIA-waived test might the physician order to be sure this drug is safe for Carly to take?   Outcome 23-9

    a. RPR

    b. *H. pylori*

    c. HCG

    d. Mononucleosis

13. True or False: All serology tests performed in physician office laboratories require blood samples as the speciment type.   Outcome 23-11

RESOURCES AND SUGGESTED READINGS

"How Your Immune System Works"
    Another explanation for how the immune system works http://www.health.howstuffworks.com/immune-system16.htm

"Overcoming Sensitivity Limitations of Lateral-Flow Immunoassays With a Novel Labeling Technique"
    Information about various medical devices and testing methods http://www.devicelink.com/ivdt/archive/06/05/010.html

"Quidel Rapid Diagnostic Products"
    Links to the Quidel point-of-care test kits, including CLIA–waived tests http://www.quidel.com/products/product_list.php?cat=1&by=brand&group=1

"Tests Waived by the FDA From January 2000 to Present"
    List of all CLIA–waived tests; updated regularly http://www.accessdata.fda.gov/scripts/cdrh/cfdocs/cfClia/testswaived.cfm

"What Does It Mean to Be Rh Negative?"
    Further information about Rh-negative immunity issues and the use of RhoGam. This site has information for patients and health-care professionals. http://www.rhogam.com/Patient/WhatRhNegativeMeans/Pages/default.aspx

---

Case Study 23-1: Could this be right?

Dr. Johnson has just handed his medical assistant a requisition form for a blood draw for Mr. Daniels, a 22-year-old male. The physician has ordered a β HCG test. The medical assistant is surprised, because she has only seen HCG tests ordered for females in the past. She is sure there is an error, and asks Mr. Daniels to wait a few minutes until she can confirm the order with the physician.

1. Is this test an appropriate one for a 22-year-old male? If so, why might the physician have ordered the test?

Chapter 24

Immunological Based Rapid Testing

Constance L. Lieseke, CMA (AAMA), MLT, PBT(ASCP)

CHAPTER OUTLINE

Immunology Methods and Procedures
Rapid Testing
    Advantages of Rapid Testing
    Common Procedural Elements of Rapid Testing
    CLIA–Waived Regulations and Their Application to
    Immunology -Based Rapid Testing
Common CLIA–Waived Rapid Tests and Their
Clinical Significance
    Group A Streptococcal Screening
    Mononucleosis Testing

Pregnancy Testing
Helicobacter pylori Testing
Influenzas A and B
HIV Testing
Summary
Time to Review
Case Study
Resources and Suggested Readings

Learning Outcomes

After reading this chapter, the successful student will be able to:

24-1 Define the key terms.

24-2 Analyze the advantages of rapid immunology testing.

24-3 Restate the common aspects of various rapid testing procedures.

24-4 Describe potential follow-up testing procedures that may be necessary based on rapid testing results.

24-5 Differentiate the clinical significance of strep screens, mononucleosis testing, rapid urine pregnancy tests, *Helicobacter pylori* testing, BTA tests, influenzas A and B, and HIV testing.

24-7 Perform CLIA-waived rapid testing procedures for a strep screen, a urine pregnancy test, and a test for mononucleosis.

CAAHEP/ABHES STANDARDS

 CAAHEP Standards

I.P.I.15. Perform immunology testing
III.P.III.2. Practice Standard Precautions
III.P.III.3. Select appropriate barrier/personal protective equipment (PPE) for potentially infectious situations
III.P.III.8. Perform CLIA-waived microbiology testing
I.C.I.6. Identify common pathology related to each body system
III.C.III.10. Identify disease processes that are indications for CLIA-waived tests

 ABHES Standards

• Perform selected CLIA-waived tests that assist with diagnosis and treatment, #6: Kit Testing, a. Pregnancy, b. Quick Strep
• Dispose of Biohazard Materials

KEY TERMS

Agglutination	Immunology	Sensitivity
Chromatographic	Lateral flow immunoassay	Serology
Colorimetric	Mononucleosis	Specificity
Epstein-Barr virus (EBV)	Qualitative	Streptococcal pharyngitis
Helicobacter pylori (H. pylori)	Quantitative	
Heterophile antibody	Quantitative HCG	
Human chorionic gonadotropin (HCG)	Rapid flow immunoassay	

Introduced in Chapter 23, **immunology** is defined as the study of the components of the immune system and their function. This includes numerous areas of specialty, such as autoimmune disorders, infectious disease, blood banking, and even tissue typing and organ transplantation. **Serology** describes the area of the laboratory where antigen-antibody reactions are studied. Serology implies that serum is used for the testing method, but immunology (or serology) testing performed today does not just use serum; urine, tissues, whole blood, and other body fluids may also be used. Immunology or immunoassay testing is performed to detect or identify antibodies or antigens in a specimen. The testing process may be **qualitative**, employing a positive or negative result, or **quantitative**, employing a numerical result, including varied levels of test complexity. Diseases such as mononucleosis, influenza, and hepatitis may be diagnosed using immunology tests.

Test Your Knowledge 24-1

How are immunology and serology similar?

(Outcome 24-1)

IMMUNOLOGY METHODS AND PROCEDURES

The majority of the common immunology tests are performed to detect the presence of a specific antigen or antibody in the specimen. The patient's specimen is mixed with the commercial solution that contains the antigen or antibody for that specific disease or condition. If the appropriate counterpart (antigen or antibody) is present in the specimen, a reaction will occur. In CLIA-waived immunology testing methods, a color change is evident when this reaction takes place. The CLIA-waived kits use an absorbent membrane that is treated with a chemical additive. Once the specimen and additional reagents are added to the membrane, a color change will occur, indicating whether the test is positive or negative. Testing methods that include a color change may be called **chromatographic** or **colorimetric** assays.

When choosing a certain test method, laboratories must consider whether the test method demonstrates **specificity** and **sensitivity** for the desired substance. The specificity of a certain method describes the ability to detect only the substance that is being tested for in the specimen. Testing methods that are not very specific will have an increased amount of false-positive test results because substances other than the one desired will also be detected by this method. The sensitivity of a testing method is related to the minimum concentration of the desired substance that will be detected. Ideally, laboratory testing methods will demonstrate a positive result when a very small amount of the substance is present in the specimen so that this presence is not overlooked.

Test Your Knowledge 24-2

If a test reacts positively with the presence of several different antigens, is this described as a lack of specificity or a lack of sensitivity? (Outcome 24-1)

Bladder tumor–associated antigen

Bladder tumor antigens (BTA) are produced by bladder tumor cells and shed into the urine of those individuals with bladder cancer. There are two CLIA-waived rapid tests that are designed to detect the presence of this antigen in the urine. This test has not been approved as a screening test for bladder cancer because of its low specificity. The BTA test may be positive in the presence of other disorders of the renal system, such as renal stones, nephritis, renal cancer, urinary tract infections, or recent trauma to the bladder or urinary tract. The CLIA-waived rapid screening test is used for monitoring residual or recurring bladder cancer after treatment. Positive results are often followed up with urine cytology, cystoscopy, and examination of biopsy samples.

RAPID TESTING

Rapid testing describes immunology and other laboratory tests that have results available in a very short time. Usually a rapid test can be completed and read within 30 minutes. For rapid immunology testing, the most common rapid testing methods used are **rapid flow immunoassay** procedures and **agglutination** tests. Rapid flow immunoassay procedures are testing methods in which the specimen and any additional reagents must be absorbed and "flow" across the testing surface before they can interact with the antigen or antibody present to display a result. This type of testing may also be known as **lateral flow immunoassay** procedures. These testing methods are usually chromatographic, which means that their results are evident as a color change on the surface of the testing area.

When agglutination testing is performed, the sample and reagents are mixed on a flat surface designed to allow full view of the mixture. The antibodies and antigens present in the specimen will aggregate (agglutinate) if they both are present. Agglutination is visible as clumps on the testing surface.

Test Your Knowledge 24-3
Provide two similarities present in most rapid testing procedures.   (Outcome 24-3)

Advantages of Rapid Testing

Many physician office laboratories perform rapid testing so that the health-care provider can obtain as much diagnostic information as possible in a short period of time. This can be especially advantageous when the testing is performed before the patient leaves the office. Testing in the physician office laboratory allows the health-care provider to prescribe medication or other treatment immediately without an additional office visit or phone call. Immediate results can save time and money for the patient, and often lead to better compliance with follow-up care.

Large laboratories may also choose to perform rapid testing rather than automated analysis for certain assays. In some situations, these rapid tests are the most cost-effective way to perform a specific assay. For tests that are not performed often, rapid testing kits may also be used to minimize potential waste of outdated reagents and controls. The CLIA-waived tests may be performed by employees with minimal training, allowing the laboratory professionals to perform tests of higher complexity. Rapid testing allows for the results to be available sooner than they might be if the tests were batched (tested together in large groups) and only performed at certain intervals as they often are in reference or hospital laboratories.

Test Your Knowledge 24-4
List two advantages of rapid testing procedures.   (Outcome 24-2)

Common Procedural Elements of Rapid Testing

Rapid testing methods differ by manufacturer and by test. However, there are similarities that are present no matter what type of test or which manufacturer is involved. These include the following:

- Relatively few reagents
- Small sample volume
- Detailed package inserts with images to use for result interpretation
- Qualitative results interpreted as positive or negative
- Lateral flow immunoassay tests have internal validation indicators that change color to indicate whether the device is working and the sample and reagents were added appropriately
- Testing methods that are timed for completion and usually take 10 minutes or less to complete

- Kits that include all supplies needed for the test, with the exception of personal protective equipment
- Positive and negative controls included with each kit

CLIA–Waived Regulations and Their Application to Immunology-Based Rapid Testing

Many rapid tests are CLIA-waived procedures. The U.S. Food and Drug Administration (FDA) has classified these as simplistic assays with minimal steps and easy-to-interpret test results. However, those rapid methods that require additional specimen preparation or multiple steps in the testing process may be categorized as moderately complex by CLIA standards. For instance, agglutination tests are relatively simple to perform, but reading the results requires subjective interpretation that places agglutination tests in the CLIA moderately complex category. Some rapid lateral flow immunoassay tests may be CLIA waived if whole blood is used for the testing process, but regarded as moderately complex if plasma or serum is used because of the additional steps required to process the specimen for the procedure. If the laboratory where the testing is performed is authorized to perform only CLIA-waived procedures, it is important to verify whether the testing method is appropriate for the qualifications of the personnel performing the test in the facility before it is used. The vendor should be able to verify whether the test is CLIA waived or of higher complexity, and often the CLIA-waived tests are labeled as such in bold letters to avoid confusion.

The instructions provided by the manufacturer must be closely followed for all CLIA-waived testing procedures, as well as those of moderate complexity. These instructions will specify the temperature at which the testing kit should be stored; the conditions for appropriate specimen collection, preparation, and storage; and the frequency at which quality control samples should be tested, in addition to the step-by-step testing procedure instructions. The package insert will also provide necessary information to interpret the test results correctly.

COMMON CLIA–WAIVED RAPID TESTS AND THEIR CLINICAL SIGNIFICANCE

Common immunology-based CLIA-waived rapid tests include strep screens, pregnancy tests, tests for the infectious mononucleosis, and tests for *Helicobacter pylori*.

CLIA-waived rapid tests for influenzas A and B and HIV are also available.

Group A Streptococcal Screening

Group A streptococcal infection is a common cause of **streptococcal pharyngitis,** more commonly known as strep throat. Common symptoms of group A strep throat infection include sore throat, fever, white or yellow deposits on the tonsillar area of the throat, swollen glands at the front of the neck, and an absence of cough. It is important to identify patients with streptococcal infections and treat them appropriately with antibiotics so that a more serious secondary disease does not develop. If a patient with pharyngitis has a negative group A strep screen but exhibits additional symptoms, the health-care provider may order a culture specimen to be set up to verify whether group A strep is present. Group A strep infection may cause inflammation of the joints, formation of scar tissue on the heart as a complication of endocarditis, or a dangerous kidney condition called glomerulonephritis.

> **Test Your Knowledge 24-5**
> What is a possible complication of untreated streptococcal infection?   (Outcome 24-5)

A group A strep screen is an uncomplicated test that can be completed in less than 10 minutes. A sterile throat swab (provided in the kit) is used to collect a specimen from the tonsillar area and back of the throat. Following the instructions included in the package insert, single drops of the kit reagents are added to the swab, after which the reaction is timed for the appropriate interval, usually 5 minutes. The specimen/reagent mixture will travel across the reaction area of the kit, and a positive result will be evident within the time frame indicated in the manufacturer's insert. The result must be read at the specified time after the addition of the reagent to the sample to be valid.

Mononucleosis Testing

Mononucleosis is an infectious disease caused by the **Epstein-Barr virus,** primarily infecting children and adolescents. It is spread through saliva, and is also called the "kissing" disease. Infectious mononucleosis is

Procedure 24-1: Perform a CLIA–Waived Rapid Strep Screening Procedure

Rapid strep screens are the most common CLIA-waived test performed in physician offices. They may also be performed in hospital or reference laboratories. In addition to patient samples, rapid strep screens may also be used by the microbiology departments in some settings to verify the identity of the growth on a culture specimen.

TASK

Perform a rapid strep screen on an appropriate specimen taken from the throat of a patient.

CONDITIONS

- Hand sanitization equipment
- Gloves
- Rayon collection swab inoculated with throat specimen
- Laboratory coat
- CLIA-waived rapid strep kit
- External quality control materials (if required by manufacturer's recommendations or laboratory policy)
- Timer or watch
- Control log sheet
- Test log sheet
- Manufacturer's insert with reference material for reading results
- Biohazardous waste container

CAAHEP/ABHES STANDARDS

 CAAHEP Standards

I.P.I. Anatomy and Physiology, #15 Perform immunology testing **III.P.III.** Applied Microbiology/Infection Control, #2 Practice Standard Precautions, #3 Select appropriate barrier/personal protective equipment (PPE) for potentially infectious situations, #8 Perform CLIA-waived microbiology testing

 ABHES Standards

- Perform selected CLIA-waived tests that assist with diagnosis and treatment, #6: Kit Testing, b. Quick Strep
- Dispose of Biohazard Materials

Procedure	Rationale
1. Verify the test ordered on the requisition form and the identification information on the specimen label.	The test and identification on the specimen label should be verified every time to avoid erroneous results.
2. Gather necessary supplies. Verify the expiration date on the kit and the required frequency for the quality control materials. Refer to the manufacturer's insert, if necessary, to verify the quality control (QC) frequency recommended for the kit.	Expired kits may not be used. The manufacturer's insert will provide minimum frequency for external quality control testing, as well as information about any internal quality control testing. Each laboratory may establish a unique schedule for QC testing; however, it may not be less frequent than that recommended by the manufacturer.
3. Wash hands (if they are visibly soiled) or apply hand sanitizer. Allow hands to dry completely.	Clean hands stop the spread of infection. Hands should be completely dry before attempting to apply gloves, or it will be difficult to put the gloves on the wet hands.

Continued

Procedure 24-1: Perform a CLIA–Waived Rapid Strep Screening Procedure—cont'd

Procedure	Rationale
4. If necessary, perform external quality control testing on the test kit. Log the results. Verify whether the kit is performing correctly before proceeding.	CLIA-waived kits usually come with external quality control testing materials. For those that do not include these materials, they may be purchased separately. Before patient testing may continue, it is important to verify that the positive and negative controls are testing in a valid range. If the controls are out of range, no patient testing can be performed until the problem has been identified and solved.
5. Perform the strep screen test as recommended by the manufacturer.	Test procedures will vary. Some kits use a test tube and dipstick, whereas others use a reagent well that is part of a test cassette. It is imperative that the instructions for the procedure are followed carefully. The number of drops and the timing of the different procedures are very important for accurate results.
6. Read the test result at the appropriate time. Test results are invalid after the time has elapsed, so they must be read immediately. Use the reference material included with the manufacturer's insert to interpret the results correctly. Record the results on the test log sheet and/or in a computer-based reporting system.	The result must be read at the appropriate time for the test to be valid. Reading results too soon or too long after the time interval has elapsed will result in erroneous results. The manufacturer's inserts will provide a chart to be used for reference when interpreting the color development changes for the kit.
7. Dispose of the throat swab and all testing materials in the biohazard disposal container.	All supplies should be disposed of properly for infection control reasons.
8. Remove gloves and wash hands.	Hands must always be washed after gloves are removed.
9. Record the results in the patient's chart, if available.	All results need to be charted immediately for the health-care provider to take appropriate action.

Date	
2/20/2014:	Rapid strep screen performed. Results negative
2:00 p.m.	Connie Lieseke, CMA(AAMA)

most common in those between the ages of 15 and 25. Fatigue, weakness, sore throat, headache, fever, and swollen lymph nodes are common symptoms of this infection. Sometimes the mononucleosis test may be ordered as a **heterophile antibody** test, because of the type of antibody produced by the body when infected with the Epstein-Barr virus. The antigen-antibody tests used to diagnose infectious mononucleosis use erythrocytes from sheep, horse, or cattle cells to interact with the heterophile antibodies.

The CLIA-waived mononucleosis tests demonstrate a positive result when the heterophile antibodies are present rather than reacting specifically with the Epstein-Barr virus. This means that false-positive results are not

Respiratory syncytial virus (RSV) is a virus that affects the respiratory system. In most cases, an infected individual will recover from this virus within 2 weeks of infection. However, some populations are severely ill with RSV infection. Some infants, young children, and older adults (over the age of 60) may be at risk for serious infection. In the United States, RSV is the most common cause of the inflammation of the small airways in the lung (also known as viral bronchiolitis) and pneumonia in infants younger than 1 year of age. Recent studies have also linked an increase in cases of severe respiratory illness in the older population to RSV infection.

There are rapid tests available for identification of RSV infection in respiratory specimens. Viral cultures are also commonly performed. RSV is especially sensitive to changes in temperature in the laboratory, which means that it may be expressed as a false-negative result if the specimen is not handled correctly. Older children and adults may need a blood test performed, as they historically have low viral levels present in the respiratory specimens.

uncommon. Patients with lupus or lymphoma may also have heterophile antibodies present in their specimen, even though they do not have infectious mononucleosis. The CLIA-waived tests may result in a false-negative result for young children because they often do not create heterophile antibodies even when infected with the Epstein-Barr virus.

Because the symptoms of infectious mononucleosis are very similar to those of streptococcal pharyngitis, the health-care provider may order a throat swab collection for a group A strep screen to be collected at the same time that the sample is obtained for the mononucleosis test. Procedure 24-2 explains the testing process for a CLIA-waived mononucleosis test.

Pregnancy Testing

CLIA-waived tests for pregnancy are designed to react in the presence of **human chorionic gonadotropin (HCG),** a hormone that is found in urine or blood during pregnancy. The developing placenta secretes HCG, and most rapid test kits can detect the presence in the urine or blood just a few days after conception. CLIA-waived HCG tests provide a qualitative positive or negative result. Procedure 24-3 explains how to perform a CLIA-waived pregnancy test in more detail.

Procedure 24-2: CLIA–Waived Mononucleosis Testing Using an OSOM Mononucleosis Testing Kit

Infectious mononucleosis is diagnosed using laboratory data and clinical symptoms of sore throat, fever, and swollen lymph glands. A positive laboratory test indicates the presence of heterophile antibodies, which are present with the Epstein-Barr virus infection in most patients with acute infectious mononucleosis.

TASK

Perform mononucleosis testing using the CLIA-waived OSOM mononucleosis testing kit, manufactured by Genzyme.

CONDITIONS

- Hand sanitization supplies
- Gloves

- Completed patient requisition form and patient chart
- Appropriate venipuncture supplies if a venous blood sample is to be used. EDTA or heparinized blood samples are acceptable.
- Supplies included in the test kit
  - Test stick
  - Test tube
  - Diluent
  - Positive and negative control material
  - Workstation
  - Capillary tubes and bulb for capillary blood samples
- Timer or watch
- Biohazardous disposal container
- Biohazardous sharps container

Continued

Procedure 24-2: CLIA–Waived Mononucleosis Testing Using an OSOM Mononucleosis Testing Kit—cont'd

Note: This test may be performed using a capillary blood sample or a sample obtained through venipuncture. Be certain to have the necessary supplies available for the method used for sample collection, as well as a biohazardous sharps disposal container and gloves. Either EDTA or heparin is an appropriate additive for venous samples for the OSOM mononucleosis test.

CAAHEP/ABHES STANDARDS

 CAAHEP Standards

I.P.I. Anatomy and Physiology, #15 Perform immunology testing **III.P.III.** Applied Microbiology/Infection Control, #2 Practice Standard Precautions, #3 Select appropriate barrier/personal protective equipment (PPE) for potentially infectious situations

 ABHES Standards

• Perform selected CLIA-waived tests that assist with diagnosis and treatment, #4 Immunology, #6 Kit Testing
• Dispose of Biohazardous Materials

Procedure	Rationale
1. Verify test ordered on requisition. Greet and then identify patient.	The requisition form should always be examined to be certain which test is ordered, and the patient identity must always be verified before proceeding.
2. Sanitize hands, allow them to dry, and apply gloves.	Gloves protect the hands from exposure to potential bloodborne pathogens. Gloves should always be applied in the presence of the patient.
3. Gather necessary supplies.	Supplies must be within reach before staring the process so that the timing of the testing is accurate.

Courtesy of Genzyme Corporation.

Procedure	Rationale
4. Verify whether quality control (QC) testing needs to be performed on the kit. If so, perform QC testing and verify validity of results before proceeding with patient testing.	The frequency of the QC testing is based on the manufacturer's and individual laboratory recommendations. Minimum recommendations from the Genzyme Corporation are that the positive and negative QC should be run with each new lot number and each new untrained operator. If the quality control results are not within the established range, patient testing cannot be performed until the problem has been solved.
5. Determine the method to be used for specimen collection. Collect the sample using appropriate techniques.	Capillary or venous whole blood may be used for this testing procedure.
a. If a capillary sample is to be tested, use the capillary tube and bulb supplied with the test kit. Follow appropriate procedures to fill the provided capillary tube with blood.	The capillary sample is the most common method of testing used in the physician office laboratory.
b. Blood obtained through venipuncture is acceptable, as long as it is collected into a tube containing EDTA or heparin.	Always follow appropriate venipuncture collection procedures.
6. Add the sample to the test tube.	For capillary samples, use the bulb provided to add the entire contents of the capillary tube to the test tube. If a venous sample is to be tested, add one drop to the test tube, using the transfer pipettes included in the test kit. Samples must be at room temperature at the time of testing.
7. Add one drop of diluent to the bottom of the test tube. Mix the diluent with the sample by gently moving the tube from side to side.	Slowly add the diluent so that it goes to the bottom of the test tube.
8. Remove a test stick from the container, and immediately recap the container.	The test sticks must not be exposed to moisture. The container must not be left uncapped for an extended period of time.
9. Place the absorbent (testing) end of the test strip into the sample/diluent mixture in the bottom of the tube and leave the strip in place.	One end of the test strip is absorbent, and the other end is designed to be handled during the testing procedure.
10. Set a timer (or note the time on a watch) for 5 minutes.	The test result is to be read at 5 minutes. Positive results may be read earlier, as long as the red control line is present.

Continued

Procedure 24-2: CLIA–Waived Mononucleosis Testing Using an OSOM Mononucleosis Testing Kit—cont'd

Procedure	Rationale
11. At 5 minutes, observe the test stick for the test results. a. If a blue line and the red control line are present, the test result is interpreted as a positive. b. If the red control line is present, but no blue line is evident, the test is interpreted as a negative result. c. If there is no red control line or if the background in the testing area is not clear (white), the test is considered to be invalid, and must be repeated.	It is important to pay close attention to the test stick to interpret the results appropriately. The red control line must always be visible for the test to be valid. Results are not to be reported as invalid. This is an indication that the test must be repeated with careful attention to the procedure. Quality control material should also be used to verify the performance of the test kit.
12. Make note of the test result.	It is not appropriate to chart the result while still wearing gloves that may be potentially contaminated.
13. Discard the pipette or capillary tube, testing strip, and test tube in the biohazardous disposal container.	Because blood was used in the testing procedure, all contaminated material must be disposed of as biohazardous substances.
14. Sanitize the work area and put away supplies.	The testing kit may be stored at room temperature. Follow laboratory protocol for storage of any unused specimens.
15. Remove gloves and sanitize hands.	Hands must always be sanitized after removing gloves.
16. Document the test results in the patient's chart.	All results must be documented in the patient's chart.

Date	
04/18/2013:	*Mono test performed from capillary puncture. Results negative*
11:33 a.m.	*Connie Lieseke, CMA (AAMA)*

In some situations, the HCG level in the blood or urine is not elevated enough to be detected by the rapid test procedure. This may be the case very early in pregnancy when the placenta has not had an opportunity to secrete enough of the hormone for the test to be positive. When a woman has an ectopic pregnancy, the hormone levels may never be elevated enough to produce a positive rapid test. In this situation, the healthcare provider may order a **quantitative HCG test,** which provides a number representing the level of hormone present in the blood. If the quantitative HCG result does not increase over time, the pregnancy is usually not viable. In a normal pregnancy, the HCG levels should continue to increase until approximately 3 months of gestation, at which time they will start to decline through the rest of the pregnancy.

Helicobacter pylori Testing

In 1982, it was discovered that most duodenal ulcers and many gastric ulcers were caused by a previously unknown bacteria, **Helicobacter pylori**. Until then, it was believed that ulcers were caused by stress, lifestyle, and food choices. Medications that reduced the production of stomach acid were often used to heal these ulcers, but recurrence was common once the treatment ended. In 1982, pathologist Robin Warren discovered that at least 50% of the biopsies examined from ulcer patients exhibited small, curved bacteria in the area of inflammation. Together with his partner, Barry Marshall, Warren provided evidence that these ulcers were caused by the bacteria he had observed and that the ulcers could be eradicated (without recurrence) with antibiotics and medication to reduce the acidity of the stomach. The bacteria cause inflammation and weaken the stomach lining, allowing stomach acids and bacteria to penetrate the layers and cause a hole or ulcer.

There are now numerous CLIA-waived rapid tests available to detect the presence of *H. pylori*. This bacterium is unique, as it has been isolated only from humans. It is thought that the transmission usually

---

Procedure 24-3: CLIA–Waived Urine HCG Testing Using the Beckman Coulter Icon 25 Testing Kit

Human chorionic gonadotropin (HCG) is secreted by the placenta shortly after implantation of a fertilized ovum. It may be detected in the urine specimen 7 to 10 days after conception, which may be as early as the first day of a missed menstrual period.

TASK

Perform urine HCG testing using the Beckman Coulter Icon 25 testing kit, and record the results appropriately. Complete all steps within 10 minutes.

CONDITIONS

- Hand sanitization supplies
- Gloves
- Completed patient requisition form and patient chart
- Supplies contained in test kit
- Test devices
- Disposable transfer pipettes
- Commercial quality control material
- Timer or watch
- Urine specimen collected in clean container
- Biohazardous disposal container
- Biohazardous sharps container

Note: The HCG test kit may be used for urine testing or serum testing. The test is only CLIA–waived when performed using urine samples.

CAAHEP/ABHES STANDARDS

 CAAHEP Standards

I.P.I. Anatomy and Physiology, #15 Perform immunology testing   **III.P.III.** Applied Microbiology/Infection Control, #2 Practice Standard Precautions   I#3 Select appropriate barrier/personal protective equipment (PPE) for potentially infectious situations

 ABHES Standards

- Perform selected CLIA-waived tests that assist with diagnosis and treatment, #6 Kit Testing, a. Pregnancy
- Dispose of Biohazardous Materials

Procedure	Rationale
1. Verify test ordered on requisition. Greet and then identify patient if present for collection.	The requisition form should always be examined to be certain which test is ordered, and the patient identity must always be verified before proceeding.
2. Sanitize hands, allow them to dry, and apply gloves.	Gloves protect the hands from exposure to potential bloodborne pathogens. Gloves should always be applied in the presence of the patient.

Procedure 24-3: CLIA–Waived Urine HCG Testing Using the Beckman Coulter Icon 25 Testing Kit—cont'd

Procedure	Rationale
3. Gather necessary supplies. Supplies and samples must be at room temperature for valid test results.	Supplies must be within reach before staring the process so that the timing of the testing is accurate. Courtesy of Beckman Coulter.
4. Verify whether quality control (QC) testing needs to be performed. If so, perform QC testing and verify validity of results before proceeding with patient testing.	The frequency of the QC testing is based on the manufacturer's and individual laboratory recommendations. The package insert for this testing procedure does not specify a minimum frequency for quality control testing.
5. Examine the urine specimen. If it appears cloudy, centrifuge the specimen before testing.	Excessive particulate matter needs to be removed from the specimen through centrifugation to ensure valid test results. The specimen should be collected in a clean container.
6. Remove the test device from the wrapper just prior to use.	The test device should not be exposed to room air (and potential exposure to moisture) for an extended period before use, as this may lead to an invalid test result.
7. Place the test device on a flat stable surface. Place three drops of urine in the sample well (marked with an S) using the supplied transfer pipette.	Avoid formation of air bubbles in the specimen during application.
8. Set the timer (or note the time on a watch) to 3 minutes.	The sample results are not valid before 3 minutes have elapsed.

Procedure	Rationale
9. At 3 minutes, observe the reaction area for the presence of red lines.	The test results need to be read precisely at 3 minutes. A delay in reading the results may allow for slight color development to occur, which may be erroneously interpreted as a positive result. Courtesy of Beckman Coulter.
a. A red line in the Control area in addition to the Test area is to be interpreted as a positive result.	To be a valid test, there must always be a red line in the Control area at three minutes.
b. A red line in the Control area without the presence of a red line in the Test area is to be interpreted as a negative result.	Look carefully at the Test area before reporting a result.
c. If there is no red line in the Control area, the result is not valid, and the test must be repeated.	Invalid tests are not to be reported as such; this is an indication that the test must be repeated with particular attention to procedural details. Quality control material should also be used to verify the performance of the test kit.
10. Make note of the test result.	It is not yet appropriate to chart the result, as the operator is still wearing gloves that may be potentially contaminated.
11. Discard the testing device and transfer pipette into the biohazardous trash.	The testing supplies were exposed to urine.
12. Put away the test kit, and store the specimen according to laboratory protocol.	The test kit may be stored at room temperature.
13. Sanitize the work area.	The work area must always be sanitized before proceeding to other tasks.
14. Remove gloves and sanitize hands.	Hands must always be sanitized after removing gloves.
15. Document the test results in the patient's chart.	All results must be documented in the patient's chart.

Date	
04/23/2013:	Urine HCG test performed. Results positive. Physician notified.
1:15 p.m.	Connie Lieseke, CMA (AAMA)

occurs early in life and that the microorganism is probably passed directly from one person to another. The most common specimen used for *H. pylori* testing is whole blood, but there are also CLIA-waived kits available for testing gastric biopsy specimens. Serum, plasma, and stool specimens may also be tested.

> ### Test Your Knowledge 24-6
>
> True or False: The presence of *Helicobacter pylori* in the stomach is linked to an infection of the lungs with the same bacteria.   (Outcome 24-5)

Influenzas A and B

The Centers for Disease Control and Prevention (CDC) estimates that every year 5% to 20% of the U.S. population comes down with the seasonal flu. More than 200,000 people are hospitalized with complications of this infection, and it leads to at least 36,000 deaths each year. Influenza flu viruses cause the flu. There are three types of human flu viruses, but only A and B are of clinical significance. Symptoms of the flu include fever, body aches, dry cough, headache, and sore throat. The duration of the symptoms may vary, but for many individuals the recovery time is a week or more. Human influenza C causes mild upper respiratory symptoms and is not vaccinated against. Yearly vaccination is recommended for the majority of the population against influenzas A and B.

Laboratory testing for identification and treatment of the flu virus is not always necessary. Many times the health-care professional will diagnose the patient with seasonal flu based on a clinical examination, and prescribe rest and symptomatic treatment. However, in situations in which the patient has other complicating factors (such as asthma, heart disease, or low immunity) it may be necessary to verify whether the patient is infected with influenza A or influenza B so that antiviral medications may be administered. Laboratory testing may also be indicated if the patient is living in a controlled, confined environment (such as a long-term care facility) so that the spread of the virus can be controlled with isolation of the patient and administration of antiviral medication.

Influenza cultures will provide detailed, specific information about the virus if it is present, but a culture result will usually take 3 to 10 days to be finalized, during which time the patient may be spreading the virus to others. Rapid CLIA-waived tests are a better option for the initial influenza screening, as the results are usually available within 15 minutes after collection. Examples of CLIA-waived tests include Quick Vue and BinaxNOW.

Many times the symptoms of the seasonal flu may mimic those of bacterial infections. Identification of the flu virus through rapid testing methods will also eliminate the use of unneeded antibiotics when bacterial infection is not present. All CLIA-waived testing methods, as well as the rapid tests that have been categorized as moderately complex use nasopharyngeal swabs for influenzas A and B. Nasal swabs, nasal rinses, or nasal aspirates may also be acceptable for some testing methods. Ideally, the specimen will be collected 3 to 4 days after infection is suspected. A viral culture may be indicated when an unexpected negative result is encountered, especially in situations in which the prevalence of the virus in the community is high. Blood testing may also be performed, using a method called reverse transcription polymerase chain reaction. This method is very sensitive and specific to the virus, and may allow for differentiation of variant strains present in the population.

> ### Test Your Knowledge 24-7
>
> When may a viral culture be indicated after a rapid influenza test is performed?   (Outcome 24-4)

HIV Testing

Approximately one individual out of every five infected with HIV is unaware of his or her positive status, according to the CDC. It is also estimated that there are approximately 40,000 new individuals infected by HIV annually in the United States. Historically, many of the individuals tested did not return to the health-care provider to receive their HIV results, so they were not treated appropriately, and continued to potentially spread the disease.

In 2004, the FDA approved several rapid testing kits to be used for HIV testing. This development was significant because it facilitated access to early diagnosis and treatment. The patient is now able to visit a health-care provider for pretest counseling and have the test run while waiting for the results. Before leaving the office, the patient will be provided with a result (although positive results are considered to be preliminary). The patient is also given information about appropriate interpretation of their HIV status and instructions before they leave. Only patients with a preliminary positive HIV screening test are required to return for their confirmatory results.

Test Your Knowledge 24-8

What is an advantage of rapid HIV testing?

(Outcome 24-4)

There are currently four CLIA-waived test procedures available for HIV testing:

1. OraQuick ADVANCED HIV-1/2 Antibody Test, by Orasure Technologies
2. Uni-Gold Recombigen HIV Test, by Trinity BioTech
3. Clearview HIV 1/2 Stat-Pak, by Inverness Professional Diagnostics
4. Clearview Complete HIV 1/2, also by Inverness Professional Diagnostics

All four are CLIA waived for whole blood testing from capillary or venous samples. Several may also be moderately complex if serum or plasma is used for the test procedure. The OraQuick and Clearview methods are capable of detecting two strains of HIV. HIV-1 is the most common strain worldwide, but an additional strain (HIV-2) has been identified, especially in West Africa. It is important to remember that any presumptive positive HIV rapid test result must be confirmed with a western blotting test or a immunofluorescent assay before the patient is considered HIV positive.

The newest CLIA-waived testing procedure for HIV (OraQuick) uses a sample of oral mucosal transudate rather than blood. Oral mucosal transudate is the fluid from the gums and cheek tissue. This method can benefit those patients who are reluctant to have their blood drawn for the test. The sample is obtained by handing the patient a special collection "paddle" and having him or her place it for a few seconds between the cheek and gum, after which it is rubbed over the gum area in the mouth. The end of the paddle that contains the specimen is then placed in a tube that contains the reagent for the test. If HIV antibodies are present in the sample, the reaction indicator on the paddle will demonstrate a positive result after 20 minutes. If the CLIA-waived rapid test is positive, another oral fluid specimen or a blood specimen must be collected for the confirmatory test. Negative test results are interpreted as a negative result for current HIV infection.

Although some of the processes involved in the rapid HIV testing procedures may vary, because a positive HIV test result is clinically significant, all rapid HIV testing procedures include specific federal requirements:

1. All patients must receive an information sheet (included with the testing kit) that explains HIV/AIDS, the testing process, and what the results mean, and provides information about the confirmation of positive results. Patients also sign a consent form before testing.
2. Quality control (QC) testing (positive and negative control samples) must be performed as directed. This includes QC testing whenever a new operator uses the test kit (prior to testing patient samples), whenever a new lot goes into use, and whenever a new shipment is received (even if it is the same lot number). Quality control testing must also be performed if the storage temperature drops below 35°F or rises above 80°F, or if the testing environment drops below 59°F or rises above 99°F. Each laboratory will also specify additional testing intervals for quality control.

SUMMARY

Immunologic-based rapid testing methods are commonly used as diagnostic tools for various diseases. The tests will identify the presence of antigens or antibodies present in whole blood or other body fluids. Many of the rapid testing procedures are CLIA-waived lateral flow immunoassays that indicate a positive result through a color change on the result area of the kit. Some of the rapid tests are used for confirmative diagnostic information so that the patient can be treated appropriately as soon as possible, whereas others may be used as an initial screening test or to follow up after disease treatment. Additional testing procedures are sometimes warranted once the rapid testing procedures are complete. The manufacturer's insert for the CLIA-waived rapid tests must always be followed closely to avoid erroneous results or invalid tests.

TIME TO REVIEW

1. If a test result is reported as positive   Outcome 24-1
   or negative, the test is _____.
   a. Qualitative
   b. Quantitative

2. How do rapid testing methods save   Outcome 24-2
   money for patients?
   a. Fewer office visits
   b. Inexpensive testing methods
   c. Less expensive antibiotics
   d. a and b

3. If a rapid test for HIV is positive,   Outcome 24-4
   what is the required follow-up testing procedure?
   a. HIV culture
   b. AIDS test
   c. Immunofluorescent assay or western blot test
   d. Neutrophil blood count

4. True or False: A negative urine   Outcome 24-5
   HCG test always means that the patient is not
   pregnant.

5. When performing a group   Outcome 24-6
   A strep screen, where should the sample be collected
   from the patient?
   a. Tonsillar area and the back of the throat
   b. Tonsillar area and the tongue
   c. Gum line
   d. Nasopharynx

6. How is an infection of   Outcome 24-5
   Helicobacter pylori treated?
   a. Surgical correction
   b. Antiseptic suppositories
   c. Antibiotics and acid reducing medications
   d. None of the above

7. Which of these may be an order   Outcome 24-5
   for a mononucleosis test?
   a. BTA
   b. Influenza A
   c. Heterophile
   d. GAS

Case Study 24-1: CLIA-waived testing procedures

James works as a "float" medical assistant at Briarcreek Medical Center. Today he has been assigned to work in the laboratory area at the busy obstetric/gynecology office of Dr. Stanton. The first patient of the day has a requisition with an FSH and a LH ordered, which both require serum for processing. James draws two tiger top tubes, thanks the patient, and cleans up his work area. Right after the patient leaves, Dr. Stanton tells James that he would also like a STAT pregnancy test to be performed on this patient.

1. Is it possible for James to perform a STAT HCG test on the specimen that he has in the laboratory?
2. What may keep James from performing the test?

RESOURCES AND SUGGESTED READINGS

"Tests Granted Waived Status under CLIA" https://www.cms.gov/CLIA/downloads/waivetbl.pdf

"Helicobacter pylori Fact Sheet for Health Care Providers" Information about *Helicobacter pylori* infection and treatment http://www.cdc.gov/ulcer/files/hpfacts.PDF

"Getting Tested"
San Francisco AIDS Foundation, "HIV Testing" http://www.sfaf.org/aids101/hiv_testing.html#urine

"Evaluation of Rapid Influenza Diagnostic Tests for Detection of Novel Influenza A (H1N1) Virus—United States, 2009" CDC Morbidity and Mortality Weekly Report, August 8, 2009 http://www.cdc.gov/mmwr/preview/mmwrhtml/mm5830a2.htm

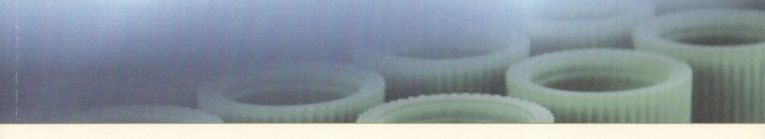

As this section clearly points out, immunology is an important aspect of laboratory testing that spans all of the other laboratory disciplines. Immunologic connections are often associated with advances, new discoveries, and findings in the field of medicine. Perhaps the most important concept in immunology testing is antigen-antibody complexes, that is, when antibodies targeted against specific antigens find them and bind together. Visualization of these complexes, as seen in the laboratory, is known as agglutination.

Case in Point

It was noted in the case of little P.J. that his strep screen test was negative, meanng that no agglutination was seen. Most strep screen tests are designed to detect group A streptococci antigens when present. A negative test indicates that the antigens being sought were not present. Because throat infections of this type may be caused by other bacterial or viral agents, the best step to take at this juncture is to submit a new, fresh specimen to the laboratory for microbial culture. Note that, in this case, if the strep screen was submitted to a clinical laboratory, it would likely be performed either in the microbiology area, because the test is looking for a microbiological agent or in a section dedicated to immunologic testing. The location of such tests being performed depends on the organization of the laboratory. Rapid tests such as the strep screen have revolutionized laboratory testing in terms of time and resources. In the case of strep screen results, what used to take 48 hours or more to complete is now available in about 10 minutes. Furthermore, because some of the rapid tests have been deemed CLIA-waived , trained medical assistants and other primary health-care providers can perform these tests in a physician office setting.

Reference Ranges

Reference Ranges for Glucose Testing Results

Fasting plasma glucose	70–100 mg/dL
2-hr PP glucose	Less than 140 mg/dL
Glycosylated hemoglobin (HbA1c)	
Nondiabetic	5%
Diabetes, well controlled	2.5%–6%
Diabetes, well controlled	>8%

From the American Diabetes Association.

Reference Ranges of Common Chemical Analytes (listed alphabetically)

Alanine aminotransferase (ALT)	10–35 U/L
Albumin (Alb)	3.5–5 g/dL
Alkaline phosphatase (ALP)	42–136 U/L
Amylase	30–70 U/L
Aspartate aminotransferase (AST)	0–35 U/L
Bilirubin, total (TBili)	0.3–1 mg/dL
Blood urea nitrogen (BUN)	10–20 mg/dL
Brain natriuretic peptide (BNP)	0–100 ng/L
Calcium (Ca)	8.2–10.5 mg/dL
Carbon dioxide (CO_2)	22–30 mEq/L
Chloride (Cl)	96–106 mEq/L
Cholesterol, total (Chol)	Less than 200 mg/dL
Creatine kinase (CK), aka Creatine Phosphokinase (CPK)	55–170 U/L
Creatinine (Creat)	0.6–1.2 mg/dL
Erythropoietin	5–35 IU/L
Ferritin, adult	10–150 ng/mL
High-density lipoprotein (HDL)	Greater than 50 mg/dL
Iron, serum adult	35–165 mcg/dL
Lactate dehydrogenase (LD, LDH)	100–190 U/L

Reference Ranges of Common Chemical Analytes (listed alphabetically)—cont'd

Low-density lipoprotein (LDL)	Less than 100 mg/dL
Magnesium	1.6–2.2 mg/dL
Myoglobin	Less than 90 µg/L
Potassium (K)	3.5–5.0 mEq/L
Phosphorus, adult	2.5–4.5 mEq/dL
Phosphorus, child	4.5–6.5 mg/dL
Sodium (Na)	136–145 mEq/L
Thyroid-stimulating hormone (TSH)	0.4–4.2 µU/mL
Thyroxine (T4)	4.5–11.2 µg/dL
Triglyceride (Trig)	Less than 150 mg/dL
Triiodothyronine (T3)	75–220 ng/dL

Reference Ranges for Urine Tests

Appearance and color	Clear; straw to yellow in color
pH	4.6–8.0
Protein	2–8 mg/dL (negative to trace)
Specific gravity	1.005–1.030
Leukocyte esterase	Negative
Nitrite	Negative
Glucose	Negative
Ketones	Negative
Leukocytes	Negative
Blood	Negative
Urobilinogen	0.1–1.0 mg/dL
White blood cells	3–4/hpf
White blood cell casts	Negative
Red blood cells	1–2/hpf
Red blood cell casts	Negative
Crystals	Few/negative

Reference Ranges for Hematology

Red blood cell, male	$4.6–6.2 \times 10^6$ cells/μL
Red blood cell, female	$4.2–5.9 \times 10^6$ cells/μL
Hemoglobin, male	13–18 g/dL
Hemoglobin, female	12–16 g/dL
Hematocrit, male	45%–52%
Hematocrit, female	37%–48%
White blood cell count	4,300–10,800 cells/mm³
Neutrophils	54%–65%
Lymphocytes	25%–40%
Monocytes	2%–8%
Eosinophils	1%–4%
Basophils	0%–1%
Platelets	150,000–450,000/mm³
Reticulocyte count, adult	0.5%–1.5% of all RBCs
Reticulocyte count, child	0.5%–2.0% of all RBCs
Erythrocyte sedimentation rate	
Adults: males younger than 50 years	<15 mm/hr
Adults: males older than 50 years	<20 mm/hr
Adults: females younger than 50 years	<20 mm/hr
Adults: females older than 50 years	<30 mm/hr
Children: 6 months–12 years	3–13 mm/hr

Reference Ranges for Coagulation

Fibrinogen	150–400 mg/dL
D-dimers	<250 ng/mL
Prothrombin time	11–13 sec
Activated partial thromboplastin time	25–31 sec
Bleeding time (Ivy method)	1–9 min

Appendix B
Test Your Knowledge Answers

Chapter 1

1-1. Reference laboratories have the most tests available. (Outcome 1-2)

1-2. The microbiology department would test the patient specimen to identify the microorganisms present in the wound. (Outcome 1-3)

1-3. b. The test is being performed to see if the patient is developing diabetes so that the disease can be treated early, or prevented if possible. (Outcome 1-4)

1-4. False. Medical assistants may work in specimen processing or as laboratory assistants performing a variety of duties in microbiology, histology, and the like. They may also work as phlebotomists if that laboratory provides this service. Medical assistants may also perform CLIA-waived or moderate-complexity tests with appropriate training. (Outcome 1-5)

1-5. Yes, as long as the training is appropriate and they have been designated as CLIA-waived or moderate-complexity tests. (Outcome 1-5)

1-6. There are various correct answers to this question. One reason is so that the results can be delivered or transmitted to the correct health-care provider upon completion. Another reason may involve reimbursement. Insurance companies require the name of the ordering practitioner for successful payment. (Outcome 1-6)

1-7. The ABN allows patients who have Medicare as their primary insurance to make an informed decision about whether they want to have laboratory tests performed that may not be reimbursed. The form offers an opportunity for the patient to refuse the test, or to accept the fee and have the test performed anyway. (Outcome 1-7)

1-8. To verify specimen requirements, tube stopper colors to be drawn, or any special handling procedures necessary for the test ordered. (Outcome 1-8)

1-9. They both contain important patient information, as well as the name of the ordering practitioner. They are both critical parts of the process, and both must be used for quality patient care. (Outcome 1-9)

1-10. The three phases of laboratory testing include the pre-analytical phase, the analytical phase, and the post-analytical phase. (Outcome 1-10)

1-11. The preanalytical phase. This error occurred prior to the performance or reporting of the test results, so it is included with the preanalytical phase of testing. (Outcome 1-11)

Chapter 2

2-1. Yes, a physician assistant may serve as a laboratory director in a physician office laboratory. (Outcome 2-2)

2-2. Yes, this is a role often assumed by a medical technologist. (Outcome 2-3)

2-3. A phlebotomist (in most states) is not required to have specific credentials gained by a national examination or formal education. A phlebotomist is required to have a high school education (or the equivalent) and documented training in phlebotomy. (Outcome 2-4)

2-4. No, they are not limited to drawing blood. They can perform a variety of duties, as long as there is documented training for these expanded duties. (Outcome 2-5)

2-5. CLIA '88 was designed to ensure reliable, accurate, and timely laboratory results. (Outcome 2-6)

2-6. The minimum level of education is as follows:
   a. High school graduate (or the equivalent)
   b. Same, but additional documented training (on the job is sufficient)
   c. At least an associate degree in a laboratory-based curriculum. (Outcome 2-7)

2-7. Assignment of complexity levels takes into account the difficulty of the actual test performance (how many steps involved, etc.) as well as the clinical significance of the test results. (If the test was reported incorrectly, what impact would it have on the patient and his or her treatment?) (Outcome 2-7)

2-8. A clinical laboratory scientist with four years of education could perform any level of testing as designated by CLIA. (Outcome 2-8)

2-9. The U.S. Food and Drug Administration assigns the categories to the laboratory tests. (Outcome 2-9)

Chapter 3

3-1. Viruses, fungi, and parasites are examples of other types of microorganisms. (Outcome 3-2)

3-2. No. (Outcome 3-3)

3-3. They appear different under the microscope. Staphylococci appear in clusters, and diplococci appear in pairs. (Outcome 3-4)

3-4. Bacilli appear as ovals or rod-shaped organisms. (Outcome 3-4)

3-5. Viruses have a different cellular makeup than bacteria; bacteria have cell walls and membranes, and contain various structures that allow them to survive and reproduce. Viruses have genetic material contained in a protein capsule, and depend on the cells of other living organisms to reproduce. Viruses are much smaller than bacteria. Antibiotics work to destroy bacteria, but not on viruses. (Outcome 3-5)

3-6. No, it is just medically aseptic, with most of the bacteria destroyed, with a special emphasis on pathogens. (Outcome 3-6)

3-7. By washing their hands. (Outcome 3-7)

3-8. She has broken the chain at the point of a susceptible host; she is no longer able to be affected by hepatitis A. (Outcome 3-7)

3-9. Everyone is considered infectious. (Outcome 3-8)

3-10. Hand washing. (Outcome 3-8)

3-11. Alcohol-based hand rubs. (Outcome 3-9)

3-12. Before eating or drinking, after removing gloves, between patients, when visibly contaminated. (Outcome 3-10)

3-13. So that the health-care worker doesn't contaminate his or her hands again by touching the dirty handles. (Outcome 3-10)

3-14. She touched the phone with her gloved hand; her gloves may be contaminated with pathogens and should be removed before she touches the phone or puts her hand near her face. (Outcome 3-9)

3-15. A laboratory coat and gloves. (Outcome 3-9)

3-16. Employees. (Outcome 3-11)

3-17. The laboratory assistant may look at the label on the container; it is required to contain the manufacturer's information. (Outcome 3-13)

3-18. There are nine required components. (Outcome 3-12)

3-19. The NFPA labels provide information about flammability, reactivity, health hazards, and other specific hazards for the chemical. They are color coded and have numeric symbols to indicate the severity of the hazard. (Outcome 3-14)

3-20. The letters are assigned to the fire extinguishers to indicate what type of fire they should be used to extinguish. (Outcome 3-14)

3-21. Other potentially infectious materials include semen, vaginal secretions, cerebrospinal fluid, pericardial fluid, pleural fluid, etc. (Outcome 3-16)

3-22. **False.** It was designed to protect health-care employees. (Outcome 3-15)

3-23. Determination of the employee risk of exposure, education, and implementation of appropriate use of personal protective equipment and other means to reduce the potential exposure of the employees; hepatitis B vaccination; postexposure evaluation procedures; and ongoing communication of hazards. (Outcome 3-17)

3-24. No; this is why it is so important to find out how to use the one that is in place at your worksite. (Outcome 3-18)

3-25. No; much of the waste generated in a laboratory is routine office waste, such as paper. (Outcome 3-19)

3-26. No. Hepatitis, or inflammation of the liver, can be caused by a variety of disease states. Viral hepatitis still has several forms; hepatitis A in particular is not a bloodborne pathogen. (Outcome 3-20)

3-27. They are both bloodborne pathogens, they are both caused by viruses, and they both have long-lasting effects on the body that may be or are fatal. (Outcome 3-20)

3-28. She should immediately rinse them out with water. (Outcome 3-21)

3-29. **True.** (Outcome 3-21)

Chapter 4

4-1. Both include documentation, both affect the quality of the test results, both involve employees, both involve written procedures, and both may involve external quality controls. (Outcome 4-2)

4-2. Incorrect laboratory results may result in improper treatment for the patient. Patients may not receive the necessary treatment, or they may be treated incorrectly based on the inaccurate results, leading to serious consequences. (Outcome 4-3)

4-3. No, they do not. They may provide information about whether the instrument is operating correctly, but they do not let you know whether a test is valid. (Outcome 4-4)

4-4. **d, a,** and **c.** (Outcome 4-4)

4-5. Cindy is following the procedure as she was taught; this means that the manufacturer's instructions may have changed since she was trained. Additional explanations may include the use of blood for a kit for which urine is the required specimen, or using an expired kit or one that has been stored incorrectly. This scenario stresses the need to follow the package insert instructions. (Outcome 4-6)

4-6. Without a date, there is really no reason to document the result, as it is not evident when the test was performed and which patient results were dependent on that result as verification that the testing device or instrument was working correctly. (Outcome 4-7)

4-7. No, it is not used to document qualitative results, only quantitative. It would not be possible to use this sort of chart to document positive and negative answers, as it is designed to show an acceptable range of results for a specific test. (Outcome 4-7)

4-8. A calibration sample has a known value, not a known range of acceptable values. Once the calibration specimen is tested, the instrument is adjusted until it reads precisely the known value. A quality control specimen has a known range of values, and it is designed to show that the machine is within calibration. (Outcome 4-8)

4-9. It is not required for all laboratories. Those that perform only CLIA-waived tests are not required to perform proficiency testing, although some sort of outside verification of performance is recommended. (Outcome 4-8)

4-10. The most important step that a medical assistant can take is to follow the manufacturer's instructions specifically. (Outcome 4-8)

Chapter 5

5-1. Enforcement: Laws are enforced by governmental agencies, and those who are noncompliant may be punished financially or even imprisoned. Ethics are not enforced or punished in the same way.

Creation: Laws are created by government agencies; ethics are either created personally by the individual based on morals and values or they are created by a professional organization. (Outcome 5-2)

5-2. b. Implied consent. (Outcome 5-3)

5-3. Yes, she has the right to get a copy of her medical record, although she might have to wait for it to be copied. No, it is not all right for her to take the entire original record from the office. (Outcome 5-4 and Outcome 5-5)

5-4. No; assault means the threat of injury, not the actual injury. (Outcome 5-1)

5-5. An intentional tort means that a wrong was committed by one person against another person intentionally, or on purpose. An unintentional tort is a case of accidental wrongdoing. (Outcome 5-6)

5-6. A medical assistant is certainly liable, and it is possible for him or her to be sued for malpractice. (Outcome 5-7)

5-7. No, the scope of practice may change state to state, depending on the laws for a particular state. (Outcome 5-8)

5-8. No, it also includes the portability of health insurance, and the method in which health-care information is transmitted for reimbursement, as well as standardization of health-care information. (Outcome 5-9)

5-9. Several standards are presented in the AAMA code of ethics, including respecting patients, keeping confidential information confidential unless it is required by law, upholding high principles of the profession, being a life-long learner, and being involved in the community. (Outcome 5-10)

5-10. This is most definitely an example of risk management, as appropriate documentation is very important to avoid potential legal issues. (Outcome 5-11)

Chapter 6

6-1. d. Compound microscope. (Outcome 6-2)

6-2. The stage is the surface where the slide is placed for observation/examination. (Outcome 6-3)

6-3. The condenser concentrates the light from the light source. (Outcome 6-3)

6-4. False; this outcome should be cleaned last. (Outcome 6-4)

6-5. c. Lens paper. (Outcome 6-4)

6-6. The coarse adjustment knob should be used first. (Outcome 6-5)

6-7. No, the stage should not be moved once the specimen is in focus with a lower magnification when changing from one outcome to another. (Outcome 6-5)

6-8. b. Electron microscope. (Outcome 6-2)

6-9. Generally, medical assistants do not perform microscopic examinations in which they are identifying different formed elements in a specimen. However, with appropriate training, a medical assistant may be able to perform a normal manual differential count, and also to perform urine microscopic examinations. (Outcome 6-6)

6-10. Answers may vary, but they may include cleaning the centrifuge, using a tachometer to monitor the rpms, checking the centrifuge for any cracks or discolorations, and checking the electrical system for wear. All these procedures would, of course, be documented. (Outcome 6-7)

6-11. Whenever the centrifuge is used, a container of similar size with the same volume of liquid must be placed across from the specimen before turning on the centrifuge. (Outcome 6-7)

6-12. Temperatures should be monitored at least daily. In situations in which the temperature control is critical (as in blood bank facilities), the temperatures must be monitored continuously. In these critical situations, an alarm system is also in place to verify that the temperature stays within the established range for that storage unit. (Outcome 6-8)

6-13. Answers may vary, but could include the following:
- On-site testing allows for a definitive diagnosis to be established as well as a plan of treatment while the patient is still in the office.
- CLIA-waived tests performed in the office may be less expensive.
- Patients are often more compliant because the tests can be performed in the office during an office visit. (Outcome 6-10)

6-14. This method of measurement uses an electrical current. When the specimen is passed through an aperture that runs between the two electrodes for the current, the number, size, and other characteristics of the cells in the specimen can be measured. The amount of disruption (or impedance) to the electrical current provides the information needed for the measurement. (Outcome 6-11)

6-15. d. Whole blood. (Outcome 6-13)

6-16. Yes, the results are visible on the screen of the instrument, and often the instrument is capable of printing the results at the time of the test as well. (Outcome 6-13)

6-17. The Cholestech LDX is a common CLIA-waived instrument used for cholesterol testing in the physician office laboratory. (Outcome 6-14)

6-18. No, it is not measured from intact red blood cells. The cells must be broken (or lysed) before the hemoglobin test can be performed. (Outcome 6-15)

6-19. No, the glucometer is an instrument used to test glucose levels in the blood, which is a type of chemistry test, not a hematology test. (Outcome 6-14)

6-20. d. Meniscus. (Outcome 6-17)

Chapter 7

7-1. Demographic information, documentation of test ordered, ICD-9 codes, last dose of medication if a drug level is ordered, type of fluid to be tested, wound source, date of testing, name of ordering physician. (Outcome 7-2)

7-2. Both types of panels are designed to assist the healthcare provider with an easier diagnosis by grouping tests that complement one another in a panel. (Outcome 7-3)

7-3. This is not an acceptable order, because standing orders cannot be extended for more than a year. (Outcome 7-4)

7-4. No repeat collections needed, quicker opportunity for diagnosis, faster treatment. (Outcome 7-5)

7-5. No, it should not because there is no way of verifying if it is the armband that belongs to the patient who is in the bed. (Outcome 7-6)

7-6. The medical assistant should ask him if he has had coffee in the past 12 hours before she begins the blood draw. (Outcome 7-8)

7-7. The reference ranges for most laboratory tests are dependent on many factors, including the collection method. Reference ranges for arterial blood are different from those of venous specimens, which are different from capillary specimens. In addition, the reimbursement for the collection may be different for the various types of blood specimen collections. (Outcome 7-10)

7-8. Initials or identification of the person who has collected the specimen, date and time of collection, patient name, and unique identifier (such as patient ID or birth date). (Outcome 7-12)

7-9. The specimen has a special label placed over the top of the container that is tamper evident. Also, the chain of custody form provides documentation of all those who had access to the specimen. The specimen should be kept in a locked area with limited access when it is not in the possession of a laboratory employee. (Outcome 7-13)

Chapter 8

8-1. The heart, arteries, veins, and capillaries. (Outcome 8-1)

8-2. Arteries have a pulse, veins do not. Arteries carry bright red blood that has just been oxygenated, whereas the blood in veins is darker. Veins have valves to help the blood to move in one direction; arteries have blood pulsing through and do not need the valves. Upon palpation, they feel different—the arteries are a bit stiffer; veins are spongier. (Outcome 8-3)

8-3. No. Capillaries are much smaller; they are microscopic in size. (Outcome 8-4)

8-4. The antecubital area. (Outcome 8-5)

8-5. No. They are also performed on the heel when drawing an infant. (Outcome 8-6)

8-6. Not always; there are times when there is no other choice, so certain precautions have to be taken before drawing the blood near a site at which an IV is running. (Outcome 8-7)

8-7. The edema can add additional fluid to the sample, causing erroneous results. There is an increased chance of infection, and the blood draw may be very difficult. (Outcome 8-7)

8-8. Needle, tubes, sharps biohazardous disposal container, gauze, alcohol pads, tube holder or syringe, gloves. (Outcome 8-8)

8-9. No. The ones used for the evacuated tube system have two ends that are sharp; syringe needles have only one end that is sharp, and they screw onto the syringe. Butterfly systems have needles that are much shorter and attach to a long piece of tubing. (Outcome 8-8)

8-10. Because they have the air removed from the tube to create a vacuum and allow the blood to enter without any additional "pulling" action. (Outcome 8-8)

8-11. The stoppers are color coded to indicate the type (or absence of) additives. (Outcome 8-10)

8-12. To avoid potential crossover contamination from one type of tube to another. This contamination may cause erroneous results. (Outcome 8-11)

8-13. Because the reference ranges are different for each type of blood specimen. The capillary specimens generally have more fluid contamination so the results may be much different. (Outcome 8-13)

8-14. No, it is not. The capillary samples don't have the potential contamination issues from each tube that the venipuncture procedures have, so the order of draw is based more on the tubes that might clot accidentally if they are left unattended too long. (Outcome 8-11)

8-15. Proper patient identification procedure is the most important aspect. (Outcome 8-14)

8-16. The specimens must be drawn into a tube that does not contain anticoagulant. After the draw is complete, the sample must sit for at least half an hour undisturbed at room temperature to allow for a clot to form. After a clot has formed, the sample can be centrifuged for at least 10 minutes so that complete separation can occur. Finally, the serum may be separated using various techniques. (Outcome 8-17)

8-17. Serum does not contain clotting factors, as they are used up in the blood clot. Plasma does contain the clotting factors. Serum is taken from a tube that does not contain anticoagulant. Plasma is taken from a tube that contains anticoagulant. (Outcome 8-18)

8-18. False. Tests that require whole blood must be thoroughly mixed prior to testing. (Outcome 8-17)

8-19. d. All of the above. (Outcome 8-19)

8-20. False. The angle at which the needle is inserted for venipuncture plays a significant role in the success of the procedure and avoidance of the negative outcome. (Outcome 8-20)

Chapter 9

9-1. Diagnosis of urinary tract infections, chemical analysis. (Outcome 9-2)

9-2. Labeling procedures, documentation of medication, documentation of collection times for specimen, communication to the patient for collection procedures. (Outcome 9-2)

9-3. To avoid external contaminants which may lead to a misdiagnosis and incorrect patient treatment. (Outcome 9-2)

9-4. The urine specimen container should be labeled before it is given to the patient. (Outcome 9-6)

9-5. A straight or intermittent catheterization procedure is used to collect a urine specimen for culture, if needed. (Outcome 9-3)

9-6. The patient should be told not to urinate directly into the container. (Outcome 9-7)

9-7. The first morning void specimen is collected immediately after waking up. The 24-hour urine specimen is collected over 24 hours. (Outcome 9-3)

9-8. Because it is not possible to control the urination times of an infant, the device has to be ready to collect the specimen whenever it is generated. (Outcome 9-3)

9-9. Because microscopic pathogens may be present, and OSHA recommends that gloves are worn whenever there is a potential for exposure to body fluids. (Outcome 9-4)

9-10. The bacterial count. (Outcome 9-5)

Chapter 10

10-1. Pathogen. (Outcome 10-1)

10-2. Specimen source, patient name, name or ID for collector, date, and time of collection. (Outcome 10-2)

10-3. Ideally, the sample should be collected before the antibiotic therapy has been initiated. (Outcome 10-2)

10-4. It may differ in the form that it takes (liquid versus solid), the container it is provided in, and by how selective it may be for specific types of samples. (Outcome 10-3)

10-5. Bacterial samples will grow more quickly than the other types listed. (Outcome 10-4)

10-6. No, this will contaminate the specimen with organisms that were not present in the area of specimen collection. (Outcome 10-2)

10-7. They both use swabs for their collection, and they are both collected from the same area at the back of the throat. Also, the PPE used for both types of collection is the same. (Outcome 10-5)

10-8. No, it is best to collect two swabs, as one is used for the strep screen and one is used for the culture. If one swab is collected and the culture is set up before the strep screen is performed, there is a chance that the strep screen could produce a false negative because of an insufficient sample volume. If the strep screen is performed first, the culture cannot be set up from the swab afterward, as there are chemicals added to the swab that would affect the bacterial growth. (Outcome 10-5)

10-9. No, they are not. Ideally, for both types of collections, the medical assistant will touch areas that appear most inflamed, and if there are any white pustules, those will be areas to target as well. (Outcome 10-5)

10-10. Many of the pathogens present in the sputum of infected patients are spread by droplets while the patient is coughing or sneezing. Collection of the sputum specimen in the waiting area could potentially expose all those who are present and even those who follow, as the droplets may land on surfaces that they touch. Sputum specimens should be collected in a private area; it is recommended that the patients collect them in the privacy of their home. (Outcome 10-6)

10-11. a. Specimens taken from indwelling catheters. (Outcome 10-7)

10-12. The bottles include different nutrition sources and additives. One bottle is designed to encourage the growth of aerobic microorganisms, whereas the other is designed for anaerobic microorganism growth. (Outcome 10-8)

10-13. b. Two times (Outcome 10-8)

10-14. The CSF tubes must be marked according to their order of collection. This allows the laboratory to process them appropriately when performing chemistry, hematology, and microbiology testing procedures. (Outcome 10-9)

10-15. c. Swabs (Outcome 10-10)

10-16. False. It is definitely advisable to wash a wound before collecting a culture specimen, so that any extraneous (transient) microorganisms are washed away from the area. (Outcome 10-11)

10-17. It is important because stool specimens include a great deal of normal flora. The media used for this type of specimen encourages the growth of the pathogenic microorganisms that are present in the GI tract, while discouraging the growth of the normal flora to avoid overgrowth. This is more important for stool specimens than it is for any other type of specimen because the normal flora occurs in such high numbers. (Outcome 10-12)

10-18. It reduces the discomfort of using a dry swab in the eye; these patients usually are already in pain from the eye infection. (Outcome 10-13)

10-19. a. Otitis externa. This is often linked to swimming or introduction of liquid to the ear canal, as can occur in bathing or showering. (Outcome 10-14)

10-20. No, fungal infections can occur in any area of the body. (Outcome 10-15)

10-21. KOH preps and wet mounts are similar in that they are used for examination of microorganisms in their living state, without preservative or staining. Ideally, the movement of the organisms can be evaluated, as well as the morphology. They are also similar in that both methods may be used to examine samples taken from the same areas of the body. KOH preps are different from wet mounts because the KOH prep is designed specifically to clear away all elements from the sample that are not fungal in nature; the wet mount allows for examination of everything in the specimen. (Outcome 10-16)

10-22. a. The O&P collection procedures include containers with preservative solution, but the stool culture samples procedures do not. (Outcome 10-17)

10-23. To collect the sample for detection of pinworms or their ova, clear adhesive tape is pressed against the rectum to pull out the worms or eggs. The adhesive tape is then placed on the slide to be examined under the microscope. (Outcome 10-18)

10-24. The two different types of stains allow for bacteria to be differentiated with the staining procedure. By using two different colors of stains, it is possible to identify bacteria as gram positive (those that absorb the purple stain in their cell walls) or gram negative (those that absorb the pink counterstain in their cell walls). If only one stain were used, it would not allow a chance to examine the bacteria that did not absorb the initial stain, as they would be colorless. (Outcome 10-19)

10-25. d. All of the above. (Outcome 10-20)

10-26. Antibiotic discs are used to apply different types of antibiotics to the bacteria so that the microbiologist can determine which antibiotic may be most effective to treat the infection. The antibiotics that do not allow the bacteria to grow close to their borders are more effective in treating that specific bacteria than are those antibiotics that allow the growth to continue right up to their borders. (Outcome 10-21)

10-27. C&S means "culture and sensitivity." This is a procedure in which the specimen is cultured and the infection-causing pathogen is identified Then an antibiotic sensitivity is performed to determine which medication is most effective for use. A C&S is not performed for viral or fungal cultures, as antibiotics are not used to treat these infections. (Outcome 10-22)

Chapter 11

11-1. Erythrocytes, leukocytes, and thrombocytes (red cells, white cells, platelets) make up the formed elements in blood. (Outcome 11-3)

11-2. Hematopoiesis is the process of the production of blood cells. (Outcome 11-2)

11-3. *Pluripotent* means "having the ability to differentiate into several types of specialized cells." (Outcome 11-2)

11-4. No, the nucleus is expelled from the red blood cell before it enters the general circulation. Mature red blood cells do not include a nucleus. (Outcome 11-3)

11-5. There may be an increase in the number of reticulocytes following blood loss. (Outcome 11-4)

11-6. The neutrophil is the white blood cell that first fights bacterial infection; therefore, the numbers increase as the cells are employed. (Outcome 11-5)

11-7. The eosinophil count may increase in an allergic reaction. It is a granulocytic white blood cell with a bilobed nucleus and bright red-orange granules in the cytoplasm. (Outcome 11-5)

11-8. The lymphocyte has forms that make antibodies and are active in cell-mediated immunity. (Outcome 11-5)

11-9. Platelets stick together to form the platelet plug to fill the break in the vessel, release serotonin to help the vessel contract, and start the chemical reactions of coagulation to increase the stability of the platelet plug. (Outcome 11-7)

11-10. Three CLIA-waived procedures are hemoglobin, hematocrit, and erythrocyte sedimentation rate testing. (Outcome 11-8)

Chapter 12

12-1. The CBC (complete blood count) tests are the hemoglobin, hematocrit, red blood cell count, white blood cell count, and the differential. The erythrocyte indices and a platelet count are often included. (Outcome 12-2)

12-2. The normal range is 4.2 to 6.2 million red blood cells per cubic millimeter of blood. (Outcome 12-3)

12-3. The white blood cell count is increased in bacterial infection and in leukemia. (Outcome 12-4)

12-4. The red blood cell indices describe the size of red blood cells and the amount of hemoglobin that they contain. (Outcome 12-6)

12-5. The appearance of the white blood cell nuclei and the cytoplasm is used for differentiation. In addition, the colors added by the polychromatic stain aid in the identification process. The nuclei, cytoplasm, and granules all absorb different colors. (Outcome 12-7)

12-6. From greatest in number to least, they are neutrophils, lymphocytes, monocytes, eosinophils, and basophils. (Remember—Never let monkeys eat bananas.) (Outcome 12-7)

12-7. The normal red blood cell is circular, with a pale center. (Outcome 12-9)

12-8. A pale red blood cell that has a decreased amount hemoglobin is hypochromic. (Outcome 12-9)

12-9. *Poikilocytosis* is the word used to describe a variety in the shapes of red blood cells on the blood smear. (Outcome 12-9)

Chapter 13

13-1. Hemoglobin is made up of one molecule of globin and four molecules of heme. (Outcome 13-2)

13-2. Oxygen delivery to the tissues of the body. (Outcome 13-2)

13-3. Answers may vary, but examples of abnormal hemoglobin strains are Hb S, Hb C, Hb D, Hb G, Hb J, and Hb M. (Outcome 13-3)

13-4. No, the cells must be lysed first. (Outcome 13-4)

13-5. Errors may include overfilling or underfilling the tube, sealing inadequately with the clay on the end of the tube, using an incorrect speed for the centrifuge, allowing the specimen to sit for too long before reading the result, contaminating with interstitial fluid, and using an incorrect reading technique. (Outcome 13-5)

13-6. The hematocrit is the amount of space occupied by red blood cells in a sample of whole blood. It is reported as a percentage. (Outcome 13-5)

13-7. The centrifuge is used to create the three layers in performing the hematocrit. (Outcome 13-5)

13-8. Anemia is the disorder in which there is low oxygen-carrying capacity of blood. (Outcome 13-9)

13-9. The physician could order a hemoglobin and/or hematocrit. The red blood cell count and indices could also give additional information for anemia. (Outcome 13-8)

13-10. Iron deficiency, pernicious, aplastic, and sickle cell anemias are examples. (Outcome 13-10)

Chapter 14

14-1. The sedimentation rate is a laboratory test where the settling of red blood cells is observed. (Outcome 14-1)

14-2. Rouleaux formation is the stacking of red blood cells on top of one another, as in a stack of coins. It occurs when the red cells are no longer repelled from one another. (Outcome 14-1)

14-3. Increased fibrinogen and certain globulin levels in the plasma decrease the negative charge on the red blood cells, and they are not as repelled from each other and will stack more easily into the rouleaux formation. (Outcome 14-2)

14-4. There is less surface area to the volume of the stacked cells so the stack will settle faster in the plasma than single red blood cells. (Outcome 14-3)

14-5. For those younger than 50 years of age, the normal value for men is less than 15 and the normal value for women is less than 20 mm/hr. (Outcome 14-4)

14-6. The inflammatory process causes the shift in proteins that will lead to an increased ESR. (Outcome 14-5)

14-7. The Sediplast Westergren erythrocyte sedimentation system and the Wintrobe ESR system. (Outcome 14-6)

14-8. Any two of the following procedure errors will affect the value of the ESR: using a clotted sample could cause erroneous results; using an EDTA tube that is not well mixed; using a sample that is at refrigerated temperature; leaving air spaces in the column that is filled with the aliquot of blood; not keeping the column vertical during the hour of the procedure; placing the column in direct sunlight or in an area where there is vibration or movement. Also, reading the test at less than 60 minutes would cause an erroneous result. (Outcome 14-7)

Chapter 15

15-1. It may be done to screen for possible coagulation disorders or to monitor medication use. (Outcome 15-2)

15-2. No; there are other factors that are involved in addition to the platelets. (Outcome 15-3)

15-3. The constriction of blood vessels in the immediate and surrounding area is the body's first response to vessel injury. (Outcome 15-3)

15-4. This term refers to a series of events that seal off vessel injury and secondary coagulation steps that follow the formation of the initial platelet plug. (Outcome 15-3)

15-5. A thrombus is a blood clot that is stationary; an embolus is a part of a blood clot or a whole blood clot that has left the point of formation and has traveled through the body. (Outcome 15-4)

15-6. DIC and DVT are similar because they both involve formation of blood clots. DVT is a deep vein thrombosis that is contained in a particular vessel, whereas DIC is intravascular coagulation that is spread throughout the body. (Outcome 15-5)

15-7. Thrombocytopenia is different because it is a disorder specific to the number of platelets; all the other disorders discussed are in reference to other aspects of the clotting process. (Outcome 15-5)

15-8. No, the INR is used when monitoring a patient who is taking warfarin or Coumadin, not for initial screening. It may be reported as part of the initial screening, but the health-care provider will not use the INR to make a decision on potential coagulation defects without the prothrombin time result as well. (Outcome 15-6)

15-9. c. Heparin. (Outcome 15-8)

15-10. The patient may exhibit slow or inadequate blood clotting with blood vessel injury, resulting in excessive bruising and/or bleeding. (Outcome 15-11)

15-11. The answers may vary, but should include the following: results are not reproducible; aspirin has a profound effect; other medications and health conditions may affect the result to a high degree; and the bleeding time result does not seem to correlate well to the true risk of bleeding in surgical situations. (Outcome 15-10)

15-12. **False.** It is imperative that these tubes are filled to the point at which the vacuum is exhausted. (Outcome 15-13)

Chapter 16

16-1. Qualitative tests provide a result that indicates whether the specimen is positive or negative for a specific substance. Quantitative tests provide an actual number that indicates the amount of a substance that is present in the specimen. (Outcome 16-1)

16-2. a. Serum. (Outcome 16-2)

16-3. Glucose testing may be performed in a physician office laboratory to screen for the presence of diabetes mellitus or gestational diabetes, or to monitor the progress of a patient who is being treated for these conditions. (Outcome 16-4)

16-4. **b.** LDL. (Outcome 16-5)

16-5. **d.** Cadmium. (Outcome 16-6)

16-6. Panels allow the health-care provider to have access to a variety of test results, which can often aid in a differential diagnosis.

If the provider orders only one test at a time, the patient may need to return to the office several times to have specimens collected, which would be cumbersome and time consuming.

Some panels also allow the health-care provider to evaluate more than one organ system at once, which can help to establish a diagnosis.

Panels may be less expensive in some situations. (Outcome 16-8)

16-7. **True.** This is the most common reason that these tests are ordered. (Outcome 16-7)

16-8. When damage to the heart muscle occurs, the specific cardiac enzymes become elevated at different rates. To determine whether a myocardial infarction occurred, it is essential to collect a series of specimens to see if the enzymes have become elevated. (Outcome 16-10)

16-9. **a, b,** and **c.** (Outcome 16-11)

16-10. **a.** Lipemia. (Outcome 16-13)

Chapter 17

17-1. Glycogen is the storage form of glucose in the body; it is produced when there is excess glucose present in the bloodstream and stored in the liver and the adipose tissues. (Outcome 17-1)

17-2. **a.** Formation of glycogen. (Outcome 17-3)

17-3. Answers may vary and might include the following: Type 1 and type 2 diabetes both exhibit elevated levels of blood glucose. They both may exhibit similar symptoms. Both type 1 and type 2 diabetes are diagnosed using blood glucose levels, in addition to physical examination and medical history. Both types of diabetes are caused by problems with insulin in the body: a decrease in the amount of glucose, or cellular resistance to glucose. (Outcome 17-4)

17-4. Diabetic neuropathy, damage to the optic nerve, cardiovascular damage, irreversible kidney damage, poor healing. (Outcome 17-6)

17-5. Gestational diabetes is more like type 2 diabetes because in both there is adequate insulin present,

but the cells develop a resistance to the action of the insulin. In type 1 diabetes, the patient does not have enough insulin produced. (Outcome 17-5)

17-6. Untreated gestational diabetes may lead to macrosomia (an excessively large fetus). (Outcome 17-7)

17-7. **c.** A glucose level drawn at any time of the day without any previous preparation. (Outcome 17-8)

17-8. **True.** A laboratory postprandial test involves the ingestion of a glucose drink. A postprandial blood glucose test done at home is performed a certain amount of time after a meal. (Outcome 17-9)

17-9. The blood is drawn a minimum of four times if the test is completed entirely. This includes a fasting, 1-hour, 2-hour, and 3-hour draw. (Outcome 17-10)

17-10. **c.** 3 months. (Outcome 17-11)

17-11. The plasma glucose will be higher than the whole blood glucose. (Outcome 17-12)

17-12. Medical assistants may assist with this process in many ways. These include helping the patients understand how their plasma glucose and whole blood levels will be different from one another, showing the patients how to use their blood testing equipment properly, helping patients find an instrument that works well for them, explaining how to document blood glucose levels properly, and assisting with proper use and disposal of lancets. MAs may also assist patients with reimbursement for diabetes testing supplies by researching the policies of their insurance. (Outcome 17-13)

Chapter 18

18-1. Ingested cholesterol comes from animal products (like meat), dairy products, and processed foods. (Outcome 18-2)

18-2. LDL and VLDL. (Outcome 18-3)

18-3. Yes, it is desirable to have high HDL levels and low LDL levels, respectively. (Outcome 18-4)

18-4. No, this result is not within the desirable range. The reference range (or desirable range) is less than 200 mg/dL. (Outcome 18-4)

18-5. Elevated LDL levels are considered a health risk because they directly contribute to plaque buildup by depositing cholesterol on the lining of the blood vessels. (Outcome 18-5)

18-6. **a.** Consumption of excess calories. (Outcome 18-6)

18-7. **b.** Excess fat particles. (Outcome 18-7)

18-8. **False.** Electrolytes exhibit a positive or negative charge when dissolved in water. (Outcome 18-1)

18-9. The electrolyte most commonly associated with arrhythmia is potassium. (Outcome 18-13)

18-10. c. Nitrogen. (Outcome 18-14)

Chapter 19

19-1. The physical examination of the urine specimen includes observations of the urine that can be seen with the naked eye; the microscopic procedures require the use of a microscope for magnification and are generally performed on urine sediment. (Outcome 19-7)

19-2. The function of the urinary system is the filtration of blood, excretion of waste, and the regulation of the body's fluid and acid-base balance. (Outcome 19-2)

19-3. c. Located on either side of the vertebral column with one slightly lower than the other. (Outcome 19-3)

19-4. Because urine is formed in the nephron. (Outcome 19-3)

19-5. Reabsorption and secretion. (Outcome 19-4)

19-6. No, ureters are only involved in the transportation of urine, not in the actual formation of urine. (Outcome 19-4)

19-7. False. Urinalysis testing is performed for a variety of reasons, including screening of asymptomatic individuals. (Outcome 19-6)

19-8. The physical examination procedures include observation of color, clarity, and sometimes the odor of the urine. (Outcome 19-7)

19-9. c. Chemical analysis. (Outcome 19-7)

19-10. d, a, and **b.** (Outcome 19-9)

Chapter 20

20-1. Urochrome is the pigment that gives urine its characteristic yellow color. (Outcome 20-1)

20-2. The bright orange color present in the urine is not clinically significant; it is merely a result of the medication she was given, probably pyridium, which is prescribed to those with recurrent urinary tract infections. (Outcome 20-2)

20-3. Using some sort of print or object behind the urine specimen allows the person performing the test to assess the transparency of the urine with more accuracy; it gives a point of reference. (Outcome 20-3)

20-4. b. Decreased. (Outcome 20-4)

20-5. No, there are other causes for strong odors in addition to a urinary tract infection. (Outcome 20-4)

20-6. False. A high specific gravity means that the specimen has a lot of dissolved substances; this does not necessarily mean that the urine is cloudy. High levels of large molecules such as glucose and protein do not make the urine cloudy. (Outcome 20-5)

20-7. No, this is not correct. Urine specific gravity must always be reported with three spaces to the right of the decimal point, the first of which is a zero, for example, 1.025. (Outcome 20-7)

20-8. Refractometers take only a drop of urine, they are relatively inexpensive, and they may be portable. (Outcome 20-6)

20-9. No, partly hazy is not a valid description of the clarity of the urine specimen. (Outcome 20-8)

Chapter 21

21-1. False. The reference range for many of the analytes is actually a negative result; this means that they are not normally present in the specimen. (Outcome 21-3)

21-2. Bile obstruction or liver dysfunction. (Outcome 21-2)

21-3. a. Intact red blood cells. (Outcome 21-3)

21-4. No. If the diabetic has too much glucose in the bloodstream at any given time, the urine may be positive for glucose. However, if the blood glucose level is under control (through diet, exercise, medication, or insulin use), then the urine may be negative for glucose. The values can fluctuate quite a bit throughout the day. (Outcome 21-2)

21-5. False. The leukocyte esterase result will not always be positive when white blood cells are present in the urine specimen, because not all white blood cells contain this enzyme. However, the only ones that do not secrete this enzyme are the lymphocytes, and they are not usually the type of white blood cell present in an infection. (Outcome 21-3)

21-6. b. Fever. (Outcome 21-3)

21-7. The strips can be exposed to moisture by leaving the lid off the container they are kept in or removing the desiccant packaged with the strips. They can also be exposed to direct light, excessive heat, or volatile liquids. They can be used past their expiration date or when discolored. (Outcome 21-4)

21-8. b. Allowing the reagent strip to remain in the urine for 60 seconds before removing the strip. (Outcome 21-4)

21-9. The most common route of exposure is through mucous membrane exposure by splashing or aerosol exposure. (Outcome 21-5)

21-10. True. Some only test for one or two analytes (e.g., glucose and ketones), and some do or do not provide an opportunity for specific gravity testing even if they are the more comprehensive strips. (Outcome 21-6)

21-11. Less opportunity for operator error, less time intensive for the person performing the test, and opportunities for multiple testing procedures to occur at once are all advantages of automated urine chemistry testing. (Outcome 21-6)

21-12. Because the FOBT is a means of detecting early, asymptomatic colorectal cancer. (Outcome 21-9)

21-13. **d.** NSAIDs. (Outcome 21-10)

Chapter 22

22-1. It may be added as a reflexive test when the chemical tests are abnormal. The urine microscopic may also be performed when ordered by the practitioner; this may occur if the practitioner suspects the presence of certain formed elements in the urine specimen, such as crystals or casts. (Outcome 22-2)

22-2. No, the presence of squamous epithelial cells is not considered clinically significant. (Outcome 22-4)

22-3. **b** Yes, spermatozoa may be present in the urine of females if they have recently been involved in sexual intercourse. (Outcome 22-3)

22-4. **a.** Viruses. (Outcome 22-4)

22-5. The KOVA system allows for a standardized amount of sediment to be visualized, and it also adds a stain to the sediment before it is placed on the slide for visualization. The stain will allow for more contrast with structures that appear similar, which will aid with identification. (Outcome 22-5)

22-6. **False.** Many normal urine specimens have very few formed elements present in the urine sediment. (Outcome 22-4)

22-7. A medical assistant may be responsible for providing instructions to the patient for specimen collection; accepting and logging in the specimen; pouring off some of the sample into a tube to be centrifuged; centrifuging the urine specimen; processing the centrifuged specimen to place the sediment on a slide; adding stain to the sediment for visualization; focusing the microscope for visualization of the formed elements on the slide. (Outcome 22-8)

Chapter 23

23-1. Antigens stimulate an immune response in our bodies, and antibodies may be produced in response to protect us. (Outcome 23-2)

23-2. It is usually tested in the serology area of the laboratory. (Outcome 23-2)

23-3. The injured cells release a chemical that signals for the internal nonspecific responses to begin. These include histamine production and white blood cell migration. (Outcome 23-3)

23-4. They are good for our immune system. They often occur in response to a foreign object in our nasal passages, and they can expel this before it causes a problem for our body. (Outcome 23-3)

23-5. No. If the first or second line of defense destroys the foreign invader, the subsequent level is never involved in the process. (Outcome 23-4)

23-6. The third line of defense is the one that is very specific toward each antigen. This includes antibody production. (Outcome 23-4)

23-7. It means that we have been exposed (either naturally or artificially) to that disease before, and our body has produced antibodies that will react immediately to protect us in subsequent exposures. (Outcome 23-5)

23-8. Vaccines "fool" our immune system into producing antibodies to a specific antigen without ever becoming ill with that disease. They target the third line of defense. (Outcome 23-5)

23-9. A antigens and B antigens. (Outcome 23-8)

23-10. Yes, she will probably be receiving a RhoGam injection to keep her body from forming anti-Rh that might cause harm to this fetus or those in the future. (Outcome 23-8)

23-11. They involve antigen/antibody reactions as part of the testing procedure. (Outcome 23-9)

23-12. Yes. An example may be the tests for syphilis VDRL and RPR. (Outcome 23-9)

23-13. The results are available quickly so that the physician can take immediate action. They are also usually less expensive than other methods may be for the patient. (Outcome 23-10)

23-14. The Epstein Barr virus. (Outcome 23-11)

Chapter 24

24-1. Immunology is the study of the immune system, including the antigens and antibodies involved in the process. Serology is the study specifically of the antigens and antibodies; therefore, it is part of immunology. They are similar because they both include the study of the reactions of antigens and antibodies. (Outcome 24-1)

24-2. The test is demonstrating a lack of specificity. (Outcome 24-1)

24-3. Most are immunoassays in which the reagents and the sample are mixed and move across the testing surface to produce a chromatographic result indicating a positive or a negative. They are also similar because they usually take less than 15 minutes to obtain a result. (Outcome 24-3)

24-4. Answers may vary, but should include the following: The rapid tests allow for faster treatment and better patient compliance because the patients are in the facility when the diagnosis is made and treatment is prescribed; the tests are usually cost effective, especially so for tests that are seldom performed; the results are ready in a short period of time. (Outcome 24-2)

24-5. Complications include glomerulonephritis, inflammation of the joints, and endocarditis. (Outcome 24-5)

24-6. No, it is not present elsewhere. (Outcome 24-5)

24-7. When there is an unexpected negative result with a high prevalence of influenza in the population. (Outcome 24-4)

24-8. The patient doesn't need to return for results, so it allows the health-care provider to provide education and counseling to the patient at the same time that the test specimen is collected. This helps to control the spread of the disease by those at high risk who are unaware of their HIV-positive status. (Outcome 24-4)

Tube Guide for BD Vacutainer Venous Blood Collection

BD Vacutainer® Venous Blood Collection
Tube Guide

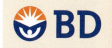

Helping all people live healthy lives

For the full array of BD Vacutainer® Blood Collection Tubes, visit www.bd.com/vacutainer.
Many are available in a variety of sizes and draw volumes (for pediatric applications).
Refer to our website for full descriptions.

BD Vacutainer® Tubes with BD Hemogard™ Closure	BD Vacutainer® Tubes with Conventional Stopper	Additive	Inversions at Blood Collection*	Laboratory Use
Gold	Red/Gray	• Clot activator and gel for serum separation	5	For serum determinations in chemistry. May be used for routine blood donor screening and diagnostic testing of serum for infectious disease.** Tube inversions ensure mixing of clot activator with blood. Blood clotting time: 30 minutes.
Light Green	Green/Gray	• Lithium heparin and gel for plasma separation	8	For plasma determinations in chemistry. Tube inversions ensure mixing of anticoagulant (heparin) with blood to prevent clotting.
Red	Red	• Silicone coated (glass) • Clot activator, Silicone coated (plastic)	0 5	For serum determinations in chemistry. May be used for routine blood donor screening and diagnostic testing of serum for infectious disease.**Tube inversions ensure mixing of clot activator with blood. Blood clotting time: 60 minutes.
Orange		• Thrombin-based clot activator with gel for serum separation	5 to 6	For stat serum determinations in chemistry. Tube inversions ensure mixing of clot activator with blood. Blood clotting time: 5 minutes.
Orange		• Thrombin-based clot activator	8	For stat serum determinations in chemistry. Tube inversions ensure mixing of clot activator with blood. Blood clotting time: 5 minutes.
Royal Blue		• Clot activator (plastic serum) • K_2EDTA (plastic)	8 8	For trace-element, toxicology, and nutritional-chemistry determinations. Special stopper formulation provides low levels of trace elements (see package insert). Tube inversions ensure mixing of either clot activator or anticoagulant (EDTA) with blood.
Green	Green	• Sodium heparin • Lithium heparin	8 8	For plasma determinations in chemistry. Tube inversions ensure mixing of anticoagulant (heparin) with blood to prevent clotting.
Gray	Gray	• Potassium oxalate/sodium fluoride • Sodium fluoride/Na_2 EDTA • Sodium fluoride (serum tube)	8 8 8	For glucose determinations. Oxalate and EDTA anticoagulants will give plasma samples. Sodium fluoride is the antiglycolytic agent. Tube inversions ensure proper mixing of additive with blood.
Tan		• K_2EDTA (plastic)	8	For lead determinations. This tube is certified to contain less than .01 µg/mL(ppm) lead. Tube inversions prevent clotting.

BD Vacutainer® Tubes with BD Hemogard™ Closure	BD Vacutainer® Tubes with Conventional Stopper	Additive	Inversions at Blood Collection*	Laboratory Use
	Yellow	• Sodium polyanethol sulfonate (SPS) • Acid citrate dextrose additives (ACD): **Solution A -** 22.0 g/L trisodium citrate, 8.0 g/L citric acid, 24.5 g/L dextrose **Solution B -** 13.2 g/L trisodium citrate, 4.8 g/L citric acid, 14.7 g/L dextrose	8 8 8	SPS for blood culture specimen collections in microbiology. ACD for use in blood bank studies, HLA phenotyping, and DNA and paternity testing. Tube inversions ensure mixing of anticoagulant with blood to prevent clotting.
Lavender	Lavender	• Liquid K₃EDTA (glass) • Spray-coated K₂EDTA (plastic)	8 8	K₂EDTA and K₃EDTA for whole blood hematology determinations. K₂EDTA may be used for routine immunohematology testing, and blood donor screening.*** Tube inversions ensure mixing of anticoagulant (EDTA) with blood to prevent clotting.
White		• K₂EDTA and gel for plasma separation	8	For use in molecular diagnostic test methods (such as, but not limited to, polymerase chain reaction [PCR] and/or branched DNA [bDNA] amplification techniques.) Tube inversions ensure mixing of anticoagulant (EDTA) with blood to prevent clotting.
Pink	Pink	• Spray-coated K₂EDTA (plastic)	8	For whole blood hematology determinations. May be used for routine immunohematology testing and blood donor screening.*** Designed with special cross-match label for patient information required by the AABB. Tube inversions prevent clotting.
Light Blue Clear	Light Blue	• Buffered sodium citrate 0.105 M (≈3.2%) glass 0.109 M (3.2%) plastic • Citrate, theophylline, adenosine, dipyridamole (CTAD)	3-4 3-4	For coagulation determinations. CTAD for selected platelet function assays and routine coagulation determination. Tube inversions ensure mixing of anticoagulant (citrate) to prevent clotting.
Clear	New Red/ Light Gray	• None (plastic)	0	For use as a discard tube or secondary specimen tube.

Note: BD Vacutainer® Tubes for pediatric and partial draw applications can be found on our website.

BD Diagnostics
Preanalytical Systems
1 Becton Drive
Franklin Lakes, NJ 07417 USA

BD Global Technical Services: 1.800.631.0174
BD Customer Service: 1.888.237.2762
www.bd.com/vacutainer

* Invert gently, do not shake
** The performance characteristics of these tubes have not been established for infectious disease testing in general; therefore, users must validate the use of these tubes for their specific assay-instrument/reagent system combinations and specimen storage conditions.
*** The performance characteristics of these tubes have not been established for immunohematology testing in general; therefore, users must validate the use of these tubes for their specific assay-instrument/reagent system combinations and specimen storage conditions.

Printed in USA   07/10   VS5229-13

1 or 2 hours postprandial (1 hr pp or 2 hr pp) – A specimen drawn 1 or 2 hours after a meal.

24-hour urine collection – A urine specimen collected over a 24-hour period to be used for chemical analysis.

Accuracy – A statistical term representing how close a laboratory result is to the true value.

Acidosis – An increase in the acidity of the blood and body tissues (decrease in pH) because of a buildup of acids in the blood.

Activated partial thromboplastin time (aPTT or PTT) – A test used to measure the time required for a fibrin clot to form after the activation factor, calcium, and a phospholipid mix have been added to the plasma. The results are recorded in seconds.

Advance Beneficiary Notice of Noncoverage (ABN) – A form that must be filled out for Medicare patients when the laboratory test ordered is not likely to be reimbursed.

Aerobes – Bacteria that require oxygen to grow and reproduce.

Aerobic – An organism that requires oxygen to survive and replicate.

Afferent arteriole – The arteriole that transports blood toward the center of the glomerulus of the kidney.

Afibrinogenemia – A condition in which a patient lacks fibrinogen in the bloodstream.

Agar – A solid, jelly-like culture medium usually provided in Petri dishes or tubes.

Agglutination – The clumping of particles (living or nonliving) in fluid. This is often a visible reaction that may be viewed under the microscope.

Aggregate – To come together or cluster in a mass.

Agranular – A classification used to describe white blood cells that do not have granules in their cytoplasm.

AIDS – Acquired immune deficiency syndrome.

Albumin – A plasma protein that functions as a carrier molecule for transporting various chemicals throughout the body. Albumin also functions to prevent plasma from leaking out of the capillaries. Patients with poor glycemic control may have albumin present in their urine, indicating damage to the kidneys.

Aliquot – A small portion of the whole specimen.

Alkalosis – An increase in blood alkalinity resulting from an increased number of alkaline substances or a decrease in the number of acidic substances. The pH will be elevated from the normal range in a state of alkalosis.

Allergy – An immune response to a foreign antigen that results in a hypersensitivity to that antigen. The immune response includes inflammation and dysfunction of body organs or systems.

Ambulatory – Able to walk or transport oneself; not confined to bed.

Ambulatory care – Care provided to patients who are able to ambulate (walk) into the premises. Generally refers to physician offices, urgent care facilities, emergency rooms, and the like.

Amorphous phosphates – A granular diffuse precipitate in alkaline urine that is made up of crystallized calcium and phosphate.

Amorphous urates – A granular diffuse precipitate in acidic urine that is made up of crystallized uric acid.

Anaerobes – Bacteria that do not need oxygen for growth and reproduction.

Anaerobic – An organism that does not need oxygen to survive and replicate. The growth of this type of organism is often actually inhibited by the presence of oxygen in its environment.

Analysis – Assists with differential diagnosis of congestive heart failure or respiratory disease.

Analyte – A chemical substance that is being tested or analyzed.

Anemia – A reduction in the oxygen-carrying capacity of the blood.

Anion – An ion that carries a negative charge. Electrolytes are ions when dissolved in water, and those with a negative charge (such as chloride and bicarbonate) are anions.

Anisocytosis – Condition in which there is inequality in the size of red blood cells.

Antecubital area – The area of the arm that is directly in front of the elbow. This is the preferred area for venipuncture procedures.

Anterior – Directional term meaning "to the front."

Antibiotic sensitivity testing – Performed to determine how effective antimicrobial therapy is against a certain type of bacteria.

Antibody – A protein substance developed in response to antigenic exposure.

Antibody-mediated immunity – A term used to describe an immune response using antibodies; the third line of defense.

Anticoagulants – Substances added to keep blood from coagulating or clotting.

Antigen – A substance that the body detects as "foreign" or "nonself." This may initiate the formation of antibodies.

Antiphospholipid syndrome – A disorder with increased systemic thrombi formation, in which patients have high levels of antibodies against phospholipids in their system.

Anuria – The absence of urine production.

Aperture – An opening or hole through which a controlled amount of a substance, liquid, or light is admitted.

Aplastic anemia – Anemia caused by deficient red cell production in the bone marrow.

Apolipoproteins – Proteins that combine with and transport cholesterol in the bloodstream.

Arm – Part of a microscope that connects the base of the microscope to the tube where the optical lenses are attached.

Arteries – Blood vessels that carry blood away from the heart.

Arterioles – Small arteries that lead into a capillary at its distal end.

Artifacts – Contaminating substances in the urine specimen that have no clinical significance.

Asepsis – A term that means that a surface is without pathogenic microorganisms.

Aseptic – Free of pathogens.

Assault – A term used to describe a threat to inflict injury, with the apparent means to accomplish the threat.

Asymptomatic – Without symptoms or obvious outward signs of disease.

Atherosclerosis – Sclerosis or hardening of the arteries because of the buildup of a waxy, sticky coating on the inside of the vessel walls.

Atrial fibrillation – A disorder in which there is ineffective ejection of blood into the atria. Those with atrial fibrillation have a rapid and irregular heartbeat.

Autoantibodies – An antibody that is produced by the body against the cells of the same body. Autoantibodies are thought to be the cause of the destruction of the insulin-producing islets of Langerhans, leading to type 1 diabetes.

Autoimmune disease – A disease in which the body does not recognize the antigens on the surface of its own cells; it sees these cells as nonself.

Autoimmune response – The response the body when it no longer recognizes all the cells of the body as "self" and begins to damage these cells.

B cells – A type of lymphocyte that remembers an antigen after exposure to it.

Bacilli – Bacteria that are oval or rod shaped when viewed under the microscope.

Bacteria – Single-cell microorganisms that possess a cell wall in addition to the cell membrane that human cells possess.

Balanced – The practice of placing a tube of equal size and similar volume across from the specimen to be processed in the centrifuge. This allows the centrifuge to operate with symmetry, and not be "pulled" to one side or the other as it spins.

Band cell – An immature, unsegmented neutrophil.

Base – The bottom of a microscope that sits on the bench top.

Basic metabolic panel (BMP) – A group of eight tests that have been approved by the CMS for overall health screening and/or for monitoring certain disease states.

Basilic vein – A vein in the antecubital area that is on the inner side (medial) running over the top of the brachial artery. This vein is the last choice of the major veins in this area for venipuncture procedures.

Basophil – A granulocytic white blood cell essential to the nonspecific immune response in inflammation.

Battery – Touching another without his or her consent.

Beaker – A glass container that may be used in the laboratory to hold, mix, or heat chemicals. Beakers usually have a cylinder shape and a flat bottom.

Bence Jones protein – An immunoglobulin (protein) that is present in the renal tubules and excreted in the urine of patients having multiple myeloma.

Bevel – The slanted area of the needle that creates a sharp point at the tip.

Bilirubin – A product produced from the degradation of hemoglobin; it is yellow or orange in color.

Bilobed – Having two lobes or sections.

Binocular – A term used to describe a microscope that has two oculars so that both eyes can be used at once to view the specimen.

Biohazard symbol – Symbol used to mark bags or containers that hold items that are biohazardous in nature.

Biohazardous waste – Liquid or semiliquid blood or other potentially infectious materials. This includes contaminated items that would release blood (or OPIM) in a liquid or semiliquid state if compressed. It also includes items that are caked with dried blood (or OPIM) that are capable of releasing these substances while being handled. This classification also includes pathological or microbiological waste that contains blood or other potentially infectious materials. (See also Regulated waste.)

Bladder – The urinary bladder is a muscular "sac" that holds urine until it is expelled from the body.

Blast – Immature stage in cellular development.

Blood urea nitrogen (BUN) – A by-product of protein metabolism that should be cleared from the blood by the kidneys. Elevated amounts in the blood are indicative of renal dysfunction.

Bloodborne pathogens (BBPs) – Pathogenic microorganisms present in human blood that are transmitted by direct contact to blood or mucous membranes of another person.

Bloodborne Pathogens Standard (1910.1030) – A regulation created by the Occupational Safety and Health Administration to educate and protect health-care workers from occupational exposure to blood or other potentially infectious materials. Originally created in 1988; there have been several addendums since that time.

Body mass index (BMI) – A statistical calculation comparing the weight and height of a person. This calculation is used to estimate whether a patient may be overweight or underweight according to his or her weight.

Bowman's capsule – A portion of the renal tubules that collects the initial urinary filtrate when it is forced from the glomerulus.

Brain natriuretic peptide (BNP) – Enzyme secreted by the muscular walls of the ventricles.

Broth – A liquid culture medium.

Buffer – Compound that reacts with strong acids or bases to minimize pH changes in the body.

Butterfly system – A system used for venipuncture that includes a short needle attached to a length of tubing. The tubing is then attached to a syringe or directly to an evacuated tube for blood withdrawal.

C&S – Culture and sensitivity; includes the growth and identification of the bacterial microorganisms present in a specimen as well as the determination of the antibiotics best suited for treatment of the infection.

Calibration – Standardization of an instrument by comparison of the results produced against those of a known value, and appropriate adjustment of the instrument as needed to achieve optimal results.

Calibration verification – The verification of the success of a calibration process by analyzing quality control samples.

Calyx – A cup-like drainage vessel that collects urine as it is formed in the renal pyramids and transports the urine to the renal pelvis to be expelled from the kidneys.

Candle jar – A setup using a jar and a candle that encourages growth of bacteria that prefer less oxygen in their environment. A candle is placed in the jar with the culture plates and then lit. The jar is closed tightly, and the candle uses up the oxygen in the jar, after which it goes out.

Capillaries – The smallest blood vessels. Capillaries are microscopic in size and connect the arterial and venous systems.

Capillary action – A surface tension that attracts liquid to fill a capillary tube or elevates liquid when touched by a solid.

Capillary puncture – A method of blood collection during which an incision is made in through the skin, which passes through the epidermis into the dermal layer.

Capillary tubes – Small, hollow plastic or glass tubes used to perform microhematocrit testing.

Carbohydrate – An organic molecule that is used as an energy source by the body. Carbohydrates are broken down during digestion to provide glucose, which is easily used by the cells of the body.

Carcinogenic – Anything capable of causing cancer.

Cardiovascular – Pertaining to the heart, arteries, veins, and/or capillaries.

Carriers – Someone who is infected (or carrying) a pathogen in the body without symptoms. Sometimes these individuals may have already undergone the complete disease process but keep the causative agent in the blood, and sometimes they have never been symptomatic.

Casts – Protein "shells" formed in the glomerular tubules. Casts may be filled with white cells, red cells, granules, or other substances. All but hyaline casts may be clinically significant.

Cations – An ion that carries a positive charge. Electrolytes are ions when dissolved in water, and those with a positive charge (such as potassium and sodium) are cations.

CD4 cell – A type of lymphocyte (a white blood cell) that is attacked by HIV.

Cell mediated – A term used to describe all the activities of the T cells during the specific immune response to an antigen.

Centers for Disease Control and Prevention (CDC) – The premier public health agency in the United States. The CDC is part of the Department of Health and Human Services, and it protects the public health through research and implementation of recommendations for education, vaccination, infection control, and proper treatment of disease.

Centers for Medicare & Medicaid Services (CMS) – The organization responsible for enforcement of the CLIA regulations. Its members perform site visits and collect the fees associated with the registration process.

Centrifugal force – An outward force caused by the rotation of an object. The centrifugal force causes the specimen that is being centrifuged to separate into layers based on their relative weight or density.

Centrifuge – An instrument that spins specimens at a high speed to force the contents outward and separate the components as needed.

Cephalic vein – A vein in the antecubital area that is on the outer (lateral) side of this area when the arm is placed in the appropriate position for a venipuncture.

Cerebrospinal fluid (CSF) samples – Used to help diagnose various diseases of the central nervous system.

Chain of Custody – A form used to document all those who have possession of or process a legal specimen through all the steps of collection, testing, and disposal.

Chemotaxis – The process that signals more white blood cells to come to the scene of an invasion by a foreign substance.

Cholesterol – A soft, waxy lipid that is found in various parts of the human body, including the bloodstream.

Chromatographic – Analysis of substances on the basis of color changes that occur during the testing process.

Cilia – Slim, thread-like projections on the inner surface of mucous membranes that sweep away foreign objects such as pollen and dust.

Cirrhosis – A chronic liver disease characterized by scarring and ineffective function.

Clarity – The clearness of appearance. A term used to describe urine transparency.

Clean-catch midstream urine specimen – A procedure to be followed for urine specimen collection in which the potential for contamination with microorganisms from outside the urinary tract is minimized.

CLIA '88 – Clinical Laboratory Improvement Amendment of 1988.

CLIA-waived – Laboratory tests that have been determined by the FDA to fit this category. These tests are very simple to perform, need very little interpretation, and result in minimal clinical significance if they are performed or interpreted incorrectly.

Clinical chemistry – The quantitative or qualitative measurement of clinical compounds in the fluid portions of the body. This includes analysis of blood, urine, CSF, and other fluid specimens from the body.

Clinical significance – Meaningful results or actions affecting the clinical outcome or treatment of a patient.

Clot activators – Substances (such as silicone) that accelerate or aid in the clotting process within an evacuated tube.

Clotting cascade – The clotting process in which each step is dependent on the step prior until the clot has been formed.

Clotting factor – Enzymes and chemicals that interact in the clotting cascade to form a clot.

Coarse adjustment knob – The knob used on a microscope to bring an object into approximate focus.

Cocci – Round bacteria, which can then be classified further by their appearance when examined microscopically.

COLA – An independent company that accredits laboratories.

Colonies – Clusters of microorganisms visible on a culture.

Colorimetric – Analysis of the amount of a substance present in a sample, based on the amount of light absorbed by the substance. True colorimetric analysis often uses an instrument called a colorimeter to read the results. Colorimetric may sometimes be used synonymously with chromatographic.

Competency assessment – A process used to verify whether an employee is performing a testing procedure properly.

Competency testing – See Competency assessment.

Complement – A protein that assists in the second line of defense by destroying pathogens and sending signals to stimulate phagocytosis and inflammation.

Complete blood count (CBC) – A hematology test that includes hemoglobin concentration, hematocrit, red blood cell count, red blood cell indices, white blood cell count, leukocyte differential, and a platelet count.

Complexity – Level of intricacy, difficulty, or complication.

Compound microscope – A microscope that has two means of magnification that are "compounded" or multiplied for a higher level of magnification.

Comprehensive metabolic panel (CMP) – A group of 14 tests ordered together to provide a comprehensive analysis of overall patient health. This panel has been approved for reimbursement by the CMS.

Condenser – A lens on many microscopes that concentrates the light as it comes through an aperture.

Conjugated bilirubin – Bilirubin that has been changed by the liver to be water soluble. Conjugated bilirubin is also known as direct bilirubin.

Contagious – Anything that is capable of being transmitted from one person to another.

Contaminated sharps – Sharps (needles or other sharp objects such as lancets or glassware) that have been contaminated with blood or other potentially infectious materials. Essentially, any contaminated object that can penetrate the skin.

Contraindications – Any reason that a procedure would be inadvisable or inappropriate.

Coumadin – An anticoagulant medication used to prevent or treat blood clots. Coumadin is taken orally, and monitored with the PT/INR test.

Cover slip – A thin piece of glass or plastic that is placed on top of a liquid specimen when viewed under the microscope.

Creatine kinase (CK) – A by-product of muscle metabolism. May also be known as CPK.

Creatinine – A by-product of muscle metabolism that is cleared from the blood by the kidneys. Elevated levels of creatinine in the blood may be indicative of renal dysfunction.

Credentialed – Formal recognition of competence achieved by an examination. ASCP provides credentialing opportunities to laboratory professionals.

Critical results – Results that are very far outside the expected reference range for a specific test and indicate a critical or crisis condition for the patient. These results are considered to be something that must be acted on immediately by notifying the health-care provider who ordered the test. The critical result ranges are established by the practice (in the case of a physician office laboratory) or the pathologist in a larger laboratory.

Crystals – The precipitation of dissolved substances in the urine. Some of these may be clinically significant.

Culture – The growth of microorganisms in special medium that contains chemicals and/or nutrition to encourage and support their growth.

Current procedural terminology (CPT) codes – These codes are developed and monitored by the American Medical Association and are assigned to individual procedures to be used for reimbursement.

Cyanmethemoglobin – A colored compound used to measure hemoglobin. Hemoglobin is converted to this form so that the color change can be measured and quantitated.

Cylinder – A slim, round glass container used to measure liquids in the laboratory setting.

D-dimer – A breakdown product when clots are dissolved in the bloodstream. D-dimers are specifically formed when fibrin is broken down. It is is used as a diagnostic tool for different types of thrombosis.

Deep vein thrombosis (DVT) – Blood clots formed in the deep veins of the extremities, especially the legs.

Diabetes – A general term used to describe a group of diseases that demonstrate excessive urination. This is most commonly used to describe diabetes mellitus, which is diabetes with hyperglycemia.

Diabetes insipidus – Diabetes characterized by excessive urination resulting from the inability of the kidneys to concentrate urine.

Diabetes mellitus – Diabetes that includes high levels of blood glucose. Diabetes mellitus is caused either by a failure of the pancreas to produce insulin (type 1 diabetes) or by the resistance of the cells of the body to the presence of insulin (type 2 diabetes).

Diabetic ketoacidosis – A condition in which the blood pH is acidic, caused by an accumulation of ketones from an extended state of high blood glucose.

Diabetic neuropathy – Nerve damage caused by vascular and metabolic changes in those with diabetes mellitus. This may cause numbness, tingling, or pain, especially in the extremities. The loss of sensation in the feet may lead to serious damage.

Diapedesis – The movement of white blood cells out of small arterioles, venules, and capillaries as part of the inflammatory process.

Differential – A procedure whereby a blood sample is stained and WBCs are identified and counted by type.

Diluent – A liquid (such as water or saline) used to dilute another ingredient.

Diplococci – Round bacteria that appear in pairs when viewed under the microscope.

Disclosure – Sharing of the patient's information.

Disinfection – The application of a substance to materials and surfaces to destroy pathogens.

Disk-diffusion method – A procedure in which antibody-impregnated disks are used to test for antibiotic sensitivity on an agar plate.

Dissecting microscope – A microscope used to achieve a low level of magnification of three-dimensional objects, often those that are untreated and/or unstained.

Disseminated intravascular coagulation (DIC) – A disorder in which the coagulation process is stimulated throughout the body instead of in a localized area.

Distal convoluted tubule – A section of the renal tubule that is surrounded by capillaries in the nephron. The distal convoluted tubule is a twisted tubule that is distal to the Bowman's capsule.

Distal urethra – The part of the urethra that is closest to the outside of the body, or furthest from the bladder.

Diurnal variation – The change seen in a urinary or blood chemical at different times during a 24-hour day.

Documentation – Recording of pertinent information. This may be documentation of patient results, quality control results, or maintenance procedures, in a chart or on maintenance charts or logs.

Duress – The use of threats to accomplish a goal.

Dysfibrinogenemia – Any abnormality in the structure or function of the fibrinogen present in the bloodstream.

Ectoparasites – Parasites evident on the outside of their host.

Edema – A condition in which body tissues contain an excessive amount of fluid. An edema an be localized or systemic, and can result from many disease processes.

Efferent arteriole – The arteriole that transports blood away from the center of the glomerulus. The efferent arteriole is smaller in diameter than the afferent arteriole.

Efficacy – The capacity for producing a desired result or effect; a measurement of how effective a mechanism is toward reaching a desired goal.

Electrical impedance – A process for counting blood cells that depends on their resistance to the flow of an electrical current.

Electrolyte – A substance that is capable of conducting electricity when dissolved in water. In the human body, common electrolytes include sodium, potassium, and chloride.

Electron microscope – A specialized microscope that uses electrons to create a visual image with great detail.

Electronic quality control devices – Devices that are used to verify the accuracy of an instrument. These electronic devices should produce results that are within a narrow range every time they are tested on the instrument.

Emancipated – Not constrained or restricted; in the case of emancipated minors, this is a legal procedure that releases a child from the control of the parents, and releases any responsibility that the parents may have for the child.

Embolus – A mass of undissolved material traveling in the bloodstream. An embolus may be a blood clot that has broken away from its point of origin, or other foreign material such as a cluster of bacteria.

Endogenous cholesterol – Cholesterol that is created by the liver for use in the body.

Endoparasites – Parasitic infection within the host.

Endothelial cell lining – Flat epithelial cells that line the interior of the blood vessels.

Engineering controls – Devices that are used to limit or eliminate the potential for exposure to bloodborne pathogens in the workplace.

Enuresis – Inability to control the flow of urine.

Enzyme-linked immunosorbent assay (ELISA) testing – Also called EIA testing, ELISA testing is a common method of identifying the presence or absence of antibodies and/or antigens in a serum or plasma specimen.

Eosinophil – Granulocytic white blood cells with a lobed nucleus and cytoplasmic granules that stain red/orange with Wright's stain. Eosinophils contribute to the destruction of parasites and to allergic reactions by releasing chemical mediators.

Epidemiology – The study of the spread of disease.

Epithelial cells – Cells from the epithelial lining of the urinary tract. These may be squamous, renal tubular epithelial cells, or transitional epithelial cells. They are classified according to their point of origin.

Epstein-Barr virus (EBV) – The virus that causes infectious mononucleosis.

Erythroblastosis fetalis – A severe hemolytic disease of the newborn characterized by anemia and jaundice.

Erythrocyte – Mature red blood cell.

Erythrocyte sedimentation rate (ESR) – A nonspecific laboratory test of the speed at which erythrocytes settle out of anticoagulated blood.

Erythroid – Pertaining to erythrocytes.

Erythropoiesis – The process that results in the formation of red blood cells.

Erythropoietin – A protein made by the kidneys that stimulates the proliferation of red blood cells.

Ethics – Moral standards and behavioral codes that dictate the behavior of an individual.

Etiology – The cause of a disease.

Eustachian tube – A flexible hollow tube that extends from the middle ear to the nasopharynx.

Evacuated tube system – A system used to draw blood that involves the use of a multipoint needle, a needle holder, and an evacuated tube.

Exogenous cholesterol – Cholesterol that is introduced to the body through ingestion of meat and dairy.

Exposure control plan – A plan that must be created by employers to educate and help protect employees from bloodborne pathogen exposure. This plan includes education, vaccination, safety procedures, and follow-up in case of exposure.

Expressed consent – Consent for a behavior that is expressed fully and personally by the patient; it may be an oral or written expression.

External quality control specimens – Quality control specimens that are purchased from an outside source, or those that are included in a test kit, but are separate from the testing system. These are usually liquid controls.

Extracellular – Outside the cells. Used to describe substances outside the cells of the body, in the plasma or interstitial fluid.

Extrinsic pathway – Part of the blood-clotting cascade that includes chemicals that are secreted into the bloodstream in response to vessel injury.

Exudate – A fluid that is released from the human body. Exudates are classified according to the solid substances present in the drainage, or the level of protein present.

Eyepiece – The part of the microscope for viewing.

Fasting – A period of at least 12 hours during which a patient forgoes food or drink (other than water). Generally done in preparation for a blood specimen to be drawn.

Fasting blood sugar (FBS) – The glucose level performed in a laboratory on a fasting blood specimen.

Fasting plasma glucose (FPG) – The level of glucose tested in the plasma (liquid portion of the blood) after a patient has fasted for at least 8 hours.

Fasting urine specimen – Urine collected during the second morning void. This urine will indicate the state of the body after a prolonged fast.

Fecal occult blood testing (FOBT) – Testing that identifies the presence of occult (hidden) blood in the stool. This test screens for the early stages of colorectal cancer, as well as additional sources of bleeding.

Fecal occult blood – Blood, which cannot be seen, that is present in the feces of an individual.

Fecal-oral route – A method of transmitting infective microorganisms. The pathogen is shed in the feces of the infected individual and then transferred to the skin. It is then spread to food, water, inanimate objects, or other people.

Fibrates – A class of medication used to treat elevated triglyceride levels. Fibrates may also decrease the LDL levels, but to a lesser extent.

Fibrin degradation products (FDPs) – Substances present in the bloodstream when clot dissolution occurs in the body. Fibrin degradation products include the by-products of fibrinogen as well as fibrin that may be involved in the blood clots.

Fibrinogen – A protein that is created in the liver and is present in blood plasma. Fibrinogen is converted into fibrin by the action of ionized calcium.

Fibrinolysis – The breakdown of fibrin in blood clots, allowing them to dissolve. Fibrinolysis occurs spontaneously in the body, and can also be accomplished by use of medications.

Fibrinolytic drugs – Also called clot busters.

Filtration – The process of removing large particles from a solution by allowing the liquid to pass through a semipermeable membrane.

Fine-adjustment knob – The focusing knob used on the microscope to provide fine, detailed focus at higher levels of magnification.

First morning void – A urine specimen collected right after waking from sleep. This specimen usually is more concentrated, and is the recommended collection method for some tests.

Flanges – Flared edges at the bottom of the evacuated tube holder that allow for leverage when inserting or removing a tube.

Flask – A glass container used to mix or store chemicals. Flasks are generally smaller at the top than they are at the bottom.

Fomites – A substance or surface that adheres to and transmits infectious microorganisms.

Formed elements (blood) – The cellular components of blood: erythrocytes, leukocytes, thrombocytes.

Formed elements (urine) – Substances in the urine specimen that may be viewed microscopically, such as cells, bacteria, and fungal elements.

Fraud – A dishonest or deceitful act that is performed with the intent to hide the truth.

Fungal elements – Fungus microorganisms present in the urine specimen. The most common are yeast.

Fungi – A type of microorganism that causes disease in humans. This type of infection is called a mycotic infection. Examples of fungal infections in humans are yeast infections, athlete's foot, and thrush.

Gammaglobulin (also known as immune globulin) – A fluid that contains active antibodies against a particular antigen that may be given to offer short-term, immediate protection to the recipient.

Gauge – A term used to describe the diameter of the hollow interior portion of a needle. Gauge number is inversely related to the size of the needle.

Gestational diabetes – Hyperglycemia detected during pregnancy in women who did not have diabetes before becoming pregnant.

Glass slides – A piece of finely ground glass that is uniform in shape. Specimens are applied to the glass slide to be viewed under the microscope. Some specimens require staining or some sort of treatment before viewing, whereas others are viewed as they appear naturally.

Globulin – One of the group of plasma proteins that controls colloidal osmotic pressure (oncotic pressure) within the capillaries, participates in the immune response, and binds with substances to transport them in blood.

Glomerular filtration – The filtration process that occurs in the glomerulus. Because the afferent arteriole is much larger in diameter than the efferent arteriole, pressure builds up in the glomerulus, forcing filtrate and small molecules from the capillary bed while retaining large molecules in the bloodstream.

Glomerulus – A group of twisted capillaries encircled by the Bowman's capsule in the nephron of the kidney. The hydrostatic pressure in the glomerulus forces out the initial filtrate from the blood, which eventually becomes urine.

Glucagon – A hormone created by the islets of Langerhans in the pancreas that offsets the effects of insulin on the cells of the body.

Glucose – A type of sugar in the bloodstream that results from digestion of carbohydrates. Glucose is the most commonly used energy source in the body.

Glucose challenge – A process in which a patient is given a glucose drink that contains 50 g of glucose to ingest. The blood is drawn for a glucose test 1 hour after the glucose drink has been ingested.

Glucose tolerance test – A test that screens for diabetes (or occasionally hypoglycemia), which involves serial blood draws following ingestion of a drink containing glucose. Sometimes known as an oral glucose tolerance test, or OGTT.

Glucose tolerance urine specimen – A specimen collected as part of a glucose tolerance test. These are tested specifically for the presence of glucose and sometimes for ketones.

Glucosuria – The presence of glucose in the urine.

Glycated hemoglobin – Hemoglobin that is irreversibly changed with the addition of glucose to the molecule. This occurs when there have been elevated blood glucose levels for an extended period of time.

Glycemic control – A term used to describe the balance or control of blood glucose levels. Good glycemic control means that the patient does not have extremely high or low levels of blood glucose.

Glycogen – A storage form of glucose when there are excessive amounts present in the bloodstream. Glycogen is stored in the liver and some of the cells of the body, to be used for energy when glucose levels are low.

Glycogenolysis – The breakdown of glycogen to allow for the release of glucose when needed. This often occurs during periods of fasting, or when there is an elevated need for energy, such as during exercise.

Glycolysis – The first steps of the use of glucose by the cells of the body; a series of reactions that convert glucose to pyruvic acid and energy.

Glycosuria – The presence of sugar in the urine. This may be glucose, pentose, galactose, or fructose. Further testing is necessary to identify the type of sugar present in the specimen.

Glycosylated hemoglobin (HbgA1c) – Hemoglobin that has been changed by the addition of glucose molecules to the protein. The measurement of the percentage of glycosylated hemoglobin in the blood provides an indication of the glucose levels present in the bloodstream over the past 3 months. A subtype of hemoglobin (Hb A) is glycated when the blood glucose is elevated for an extended period of time, as in the case of uncontrolled diabetes mellitus.

Graduated cylinder – A cylinder that is marked in different quantities for measuring liquids.

Gram stain – A staining method that allows the classification of bacteria dependent on the color of the stain that they absorb. Gram-positive bacteria retain the crystal violet dye used in the process, and appear purple. Gram-negative bacteria do not keep the crystal violet dye in their cell membranes, and instead absorb the color from the safranin counterstain. They appear pink when viewed under the microscope.

Granular – A classification used to describe white blood cells that contain granules in their cytoplasm.

Granulocyte – White blood cells that have names ending in –phil (neutrophil, eosinophil, and basophil) and have distinct granules visible in their cytoplasm.

Granulocyte-macrophage colony-stimulating factor (GM-CSF) – A glycoprotein that stimulates the production and functional activity of neutrophils, monocytes, and macrophages.

Guaiac – A type of tree resin used for fecal occult blood testing. Guaiac interacts with the heme in the hemoglobin molecule present in red blood cells. If there is blood present, the interaction makes the guaiac paper turn blue when hydrogen peroxide developer solution is added.

Hanging drop slide – A slide with a depression in the center. This allows a drop of fluid containing the specimen to be suspended from a cover slip over the depression for observation microscopically.

Hazard communication standard – A document created to educate and protect employees from the chemicals in use at their workplace.

Hb A – The normal adult hemoglobin, composed of two alpha and two beta chains.

Hb A1c; HgbA1c – See Glycosylated hemoglobin (HgbA1c).

Health Information Portability and Accountability Act (HIPAA) – A federal law that affects the security, standardization, and confidentiality of health-care information. It also affects the rights of those who have insurance coverage when they change jobs.

Health care–associated infection – An infection contracted by an individual at a health-care facility. Refers specifically to an infection that the individual did not come into contact with in any other way.

Helicobacter pylori (H. pylori) – A type of bacterium that causes gastric and duodenal ulcers.

Hematocrit (Hct) – The volume of erythrocytes packed by centrifugation in a given volume of blood.

Hematology – The study of blood and blood-forming tissues.

Hematoma – A mass of blood caused by damage to a blood vessel.

Hematopoiesis – Production and development of blood cells, normally in the bone marrow.

Hematuria – The presence of blood in a urine specimen.

Hemoconcentration – A condition resulting from a tourniquet that is too tight or is left on too long, causing a relative increase in the cells in the antecubital area and possibly resulting in erroneous test results.

Hemocytometer – A counting chamber for determining the number of cells in a stated volume of blood.

Hemoglobin – The protein in red blood cells that carries oxygen.

Hemoglobin (Hgb) – The iron-containing pigment of red blood cells that carries oxygen from the lungs to the tissues.

Hemoglobin and hematocrit (H&H) – Hemoglobin and hematocrit testing is often ordered together as H&H.

Hemoglobin electrophoresis – The movement of hemoglobin on a medium as a result of changes in electrical potential, used to determine type of hemoglobin present.

Hemoglobinopathies – Any one of a group of genetic diseases caused by or associated with the presence of one or several forms of abnormal hemoglobin in the blood.

Hemoglobinuria – Hemoglobin in the urine.

Hemolysis – The destruction (lysis) of the red blood cell membrane with the release of the fluid contents. A visible reddish tint becomes evident in the plasma if there is marked hemolysis in the specimen.

Hemolytic disease of the newborn (HDN) – A neonatal disease, usually the result of an Rh incompatibility in which the antibodies of the mother cross the placenta and "attack" the neonate. May cause neonatal anemia, jaundice, edema, and enlargement of the liver and spleen.

Hemolytic uremic syndrome – An abnormal reaction to infection with the *E. coli* strain O157:H7. The *E. coli* bacteria secrete a toxin that causes an inflammatory process, resulting in blood clot formation in the capillary vessels of the body. As the red blood cells of the body pass through these clogged capillaries, it causes them to become damaged, which consequently causes damage to the kidneys as they attempt to process these damaged cells. The patient must be treated for the anemia and renal failure immediately.

Hemophilia – Blood-clotting disorders in which the patients have deficiencies of specific clotting factors.

Hemostasis – A stoppage of bleeding or of circulation.

Heparin – A naturally occurring anticoagulant in the human body. Heparin is also provided as a fast-acting anticoagulant, administered via IV or subcutaneously.

Hepatic function panel – A group of tests that are ordered together to monitor liver function.

Hepatitis – Inflammation of the liver. Hepatitis may be caused by a viral infection or other disease state that causes the liver to be inflamed.

Hepatitis A virus (HAV) – A type of virus that causes inflammation of the liver in infected patients. Hepatitis A is transferred via the fecal-oral route, and usually does not cause permanent liver damage. Vaccinations are available for this disease.

Hepatitis B virus (HBV) – A type of virus that causes inflammation of the liver in infected patients. Hepatitis B is bloodborne, and is transferred through sexual contact, contaminated needles, mucous membrane exposure, or other direct blood-to-blood contact. Hepatitis B infection may lead to permanent liver damage. Hepatitis B is the most common bloodborne pathogen to be transmitted to health-care workers. There are vaccinations available for this disease.

Hepatitis C virus (HCV) – A bloodborne virus that causes inflammation of the liver. Hepatitis C infection usually leads to permanent liver damage, and is often asymptomatic until the liver damage has become quite advanced. There is no vaccination available for this disease.

Hepatitis D – A type of virus that causes liver inflammation. This is considered a genetic mutation or variant of the hepatitis B virus, as it is present only in those who are already infected with hepatitis B. There is no vaccination for this disease.

Heterophile antibody – A nonspecific type of antibody that is present in those with infectious mononucleosis. Heterophile antibodies are also present in other inflammatory situations.

Heterozygous – A genetic term in which the two genes for one characteristic are not the same.

High complexity – Laboratory tests that have been determined by the FDA to be complex enough so that the procedures can be performed only by highly trained laboratory professionals.

High-density lipoprotein (HDL) – A lipid subgroup; this is known as the "good" cholesterol because it helps to reduce the plaque buildup on the interior of the blood vessels.

Hilum – The indented (concave) portion of the kidney.

Histamine – A substance produced by the body in response to antigenic exposure that causes dilation of the blood vessels, increased secretion of acid in the stomach, smooth muscle constriction, mucus production, tissue swelling, and itching (during allergic reactions).

Histogram – A graph of the distribution of cell sizes made during cell counting on an automated analyzer.

Homeostasis – The internal balance of the body that is necessary for good health. Homeostasis includes minor adjusting to outside stimuli.

Homozygous – A genetic term in which the two genes for one characteristic are the same.

Hospital laboratories – Laboratories that are usually housed within a hospital and provide services primarily to patients of that institution. Hospital laboratories may be owned by the hospital or contracted to provide their services.

Human chorionic gonadotropin (HCG) – A hormone that is secreted by the trophoblasts of a fertilized ovum early in pregnancy. This hormone maintains the corpeus luteum so that it will secrete estrogen and progesterone. The presence of HCG in blood and urine is indicative of pregnancy.

Human immunodeficiency virus (HIV) – This is a retrovirus that invades the CD4 cells of humans and causes the failure of their immune systems. Infection leads to the eventual development of AIDS. It is a bloodborne pathogen, and may be transmitted through sexual contact, mucous membrane exposure, or parenteral exposure.

Hyperchromic – Pertaining to excess hemoglobin concentration in the erythrocyte.

Hyperglycemia – Blood glucose levels elevated above acceptable reference ranges.

Hyperkalemia – Elevated levels of potassium in the blood plasma.

Hyperlipidemia – Excessive levels of lipid in the bloodstream.

Hypernatremia – Elevated levels of sodium in the blood plasma.

Hyperthyroidism – A condition in which the thyroid gland is overactive.

Hypochromic – A condition of the blood in which the erythrocytes have a reduced hemoglobin content and appear pale in color.

Hypofibrinogenemia – Low levels of circulating fibrinogen in the bloodstream.

Hypoglycemia – Decreased blood glucose levels below acceptable reference ranges.

Hypokalemia – Decreased levels of potassium in the blood plasma.

Hyponatremia – Decreased levels of sodium in the blood plasma.

Hypothyroidism – A condition in which the thyroid gland is underactive.

Icteric – A term used to describe the serum or plasma of a patient with hepatic dysfunction. An icteric specimen has a yellowish green color.

iFOB – An acronym used to describe an immunochemical method of testing for fecal occult blood. It uses an antigen-antibody interaction with the globin portion of the hemoglobin molecule and is an alternative testing procedure to the guaiac method for the presence of fecal occult blood.

Immunity – Protection from diseases.

Immunoglobulins – Plasma proteins that play a role in protection from disease. These may occur on the surface of the lymphocytes, or may be secreted in response to antigenic exposure.

Immunology – The study of the components of the immune system and their function.

Impaired fasting glucose (IFG) – A term used to describe prediabetics who exhibit elevated fasting plasma glucose levels.

Impaired glucose tolerance (IGT) – A term used to describe prediabetics who exhibit elevated glucose levels after drinking a glucose solution.

Implied consent – Consent for a procedure that is implied by the actions of the individual.

International Classification of Diseases, 9th ed. (ICD-9) – Codes assigned by the CDC to symptoms or disease states. These codes must be included for reimbursement for laboratory procedures.

In vitro – Latin for "in glass," referring to testing done outside of the body.

In vivo – Latin for "in the living body," referring to something occurring inside the body, such as antigen-antibody reactions within a living subject.

Incubators – A device by which the temperature, and sometimes humidity, of the environment can be controlled. Incubators are often used to help bacterial specimens grow for testing or to assist with the completion of a testing procedure.

Indwelling catheter – A plastic tube that is allowed to remain in the urinary bladder for a period of time to facilitate drainage of urine as it is formed.

Infection – A disease state caused by pathogenic microorganisms, including bacteria, viruses, parasites, or fungi. Infections may be localized or may spread throughout the body. Symptoms often include pain, fever, redness and swelling, and loss of function.

Infection control – Policies and procedures to help minimize the spread of infection and to analyze data in relation to infection within a health-care facility.

Infectious – A term used to describe a subject who is capable of transmitting disease to others. The transmission may occur directly or indirectly.

Inflammation – A immunological defensive mechanism of the body, including increased blood flow, tissue swelling, increased white blood cell presence, and release of chemical toxins.

Informed consent – Approval that is obtained in writing after the patient has been informed about the specifics of the proposed procedure, the risks of the procedure, alternative treatments, and information about what may happen if the patient decides against the procedure.

Inoculation – Addition of a specimen to a culture medium for growth.

Insulin – A hormone produced by the islets of Langerhans of the pancreas. Insulin is necessary for the cells of the body to absorb glucose to be utilized as energy.

Insulin dependent – Diabetes that requires injections of insulin to control blood glucose levels. Patients with type 1 diabetes are usually insulin dependent.

Insulin resistance – A condition in which cells have a diminished ability to interact appropriately with insulin.

Intentional tort – A wrongful act that is committed by one person against another person deliberately.

Interferons – A group of proteins produced in the body having antiviral properties.

Interleukin – A hematopoietic growth factor affecting growth and differentiation of lymphocytes.

Intermittent (straight) catheter – A catheter (hollow, plastic tube) placed directly into the bladder to facilitate drainage. The catheter is removed as soon as the bladder has drained.

Internal quality control – Quality control that is built into the testing kit, provided by the manufacturer.

International normalized ratio (INR) – A mathematical calculation used to standardize treatment based on prothrombin time (PT) results. PT results may vary, depending on lot numbers of reagents and different instruments used for testing. The INR is a calculation that takes these variables into account and provides a tool for monitoring those patients on anticoagulant therapy. Most patients on anticoagulant therapy should have an INR between 2.0 and 3.0.

Interstitial – Between the cells.

Interstitial fluid – The fluid between cells.

Intracellular – Within the cells.

Intravascular lysis – The destruction of red blood cells within the vessels of the body.

Intrinsic factor – A glycoprotein secreted by the parietal cells of the gastric mucosa, necessary for the absorption of vitamin B_{12}.

Intrinsic pathway – Part of the blood-clotting cascade that uses chemicals that are normally present in the bloodstream.

Ions – An atom or group of atoms that has lost or gained electrons so that it possesses an electrical charge. Electrolytes are substances that become ions when dissolved in water.

Iris diaphragm – A device with a variable diameter that controls the amount of light that is used to view a specimen through a microscope.

Iron-deficiency anemia – Anemia resulting from a greater demand on stored iron than can be supplied.

Ischemia – An insufficient supply of blood to an organ or body part. This term is often used to describe a lack of blood flow to areas of the heart when the patient has atherosclerosis, causing partial blockage of the vessels.

Islets of Langerhans – Specialized groups of pancreatic cells that produce insulin and glucagon. Insulin and glucagon are necessary for controlling the levels of blood glucose in the body.

Jaundice – A yellow staining of body tissues and the fluids of the body as a result of excess bilirubin in the bloodstream in patients with hepatic dysfunction.

Ketones – A chemical that is elevated in the bloodstream with increased fat metabolism. This is usually associated with dysfunctional carbohydrate utilization, as in the case of diabetes mellitus.

Ketonuria – The presence of ketones in the urine.

Kidneys – Organs that create urine.

Kirby-Bauer method – A method used to test specific bacteria for antibiotic sensitivity, utilizing antibody-impregnated disks on special agar plates.

KOH (potassium hydroxide) – A solution used for examination of a sample under the microscope which is performed immediately after collection to search for the presence of fungi.

Labile – Describes a substance or sample that is not fixed, and is easily changeable. These types of specimens generally must be tested immediately to provide accurate results.

Laboratory – Any site where specimens may be collected, processed, or tested.

Laboratory directory – A reference document in which specimen requirements and other useful information might be found. It includes all the tests offered by a particular laboratory.

Laboratory report – A document used to transmit laboratory results and reference ranges.

Laboratory requisition – A form used to order laboratory tests.

Laboratory thermometer – A thermometer used to measure temperatures in a controlled environment, such as a refrigerator, freezer, or incubator.

Lateral flow immunoassay – A test used to determine the presence of an antigen or antibody in a specimen. In this type of test, the sample moves laterally across the testing surface, resulting in a color change if the antibody and/or antigen is present in the specimen. This testing method is used in many CLIA-waived tests.

Laws – Regulations established by a governmental authority that are enforced and punishable for noncompliance.

Leukemia – A class of hematological malignancies in which immortal clones of immature blood cells multiply at the expense of normal blood cells.

Leukocyte – White blood cell.

Leukocyte esterase – An enzyme secreted by granulated white blood cells and monocytes.

Leukocytosis – Abnormal increase in white blood cell (leukocyte) count.

Leukopenia – Abnormal decrease in white blood cell (leukocyte) count.

Liability – Legally responsible for an action.

Libel – A false statement in print.

Light source – The origin of light or illumination for a specimen to be viewed on a microscope. For most compound microscopes, this is a light bulb located in the base of the unit.

Lipemia – The presence of excessive lipids in the blood. This term is used to describe the "milky" appearance of the plasma or serum in specimens with elevated lipid content.

Lipid – A term used to describe fats in the body. Cholesterol and triglycerides are types of lipid molecules.

Lipoproteins – Simple proteins bound to lipids or fats in the bloodstream. Lipoproteins are the method by which cholesterol travels in the bloodstream; they are further differentiated as HDL, LDL. or VLDL.

Lobulated – Having lobes or sections.

Loop of Henle – The middle portion of the renal tubules where exchanges occur as part of the formation of urine from the renal filtrate.

Low-density lipoprotein (LDL) – A subclass of cholesterol present in the body; this is known as the "bad" cholesterol because it contributes to plaque buildup on the blood vessel walls.

Lumbar puncture – A procedure used to obtain samples of cerebrospinal fluid for examination and testing.

Lumen – The term used to describe the interior hollow portion of the needle. This term may be used to describe the inside of any hollow object, such as a vein or artery.

Lymphocyte – A white blood cell responsible for much of the body's immune protection.

Lymphoid – Pertaining to lymphocytes.

Lysed – The action of cell destruction (lysis) by chemical or mechanical methods, releasing the contents of the cells.

Lysozyme – An enzyme found in various cells and body fluids that damages bacterial cell walls.

Lytes – See Electrolytes.

Macrocyte – Cells larger than normal size.

Macrocytic – Abnormally large erythrocytes exceeding 10 μ in diameter.

Macrophage – Cells that are capable of phagocytosis.

Macroscopic – A description of a structure that is large enough to be seen or examined without magnification.

Macrosomia – An abnormally large baby. An infant who has a birth weight above the 90th percentile of the standardized growth curve exhibits macrosomia. This may be caused by gestational diabetes in the mother.

Malabsorption – Inadequate or incomplete absorption of nutrients from the digestive tract.

Malfeasance – Performance of a wrong and unlawful act.

Malpractice – The negligence of a professional person.

Mastectomy – The removal of breast tissue.

Material Safety Data Sheets (MSDS) – A descriptive sheet required by law to accompany chemicals upon delivery. These sheets contain essential safety information about the chemical, as well as contact information for the manufacturer.

Mean – The mathematical average of a set of results.

Mean corpuscular hemoglobin (MCH) – The average weight of hemoglobin in red blood cells in a sample.

Mean corpuscular hemoglobin concentration (MCHC) – The average weight of hemoglobin in a given volume of packed blood cells.

Mean corpuscular volume (MCV) – The average volume of a red blood cell in a sample.

Media – Plural of *medium;* a term used to describe the substance that supports growth of microorganisms.

Median cubital vein – The middle vein of the antecubital area; this is the first vein of choice for venipuncture procedures.

Medical asepsis – A state of cleanliness and disinfection that has reduced the number of microorganisms and pathogens to a significant degree.

Megakaryocyte – A large bone marrow cell with large or multiple nuclei from which platelets are derived.

Meniscus – A curve in the surface of a liquid in a cylinder caused by surface tension between molecules.

Metabolic syndrome – The presence of four interrelated risk factors for atherosclerosis: insulin resistance (hyperglycemia), hypertension, hyperlipidemia, and obesity.

Methicillin-resistant *Staphylococcus aureus* (MRSA) – *Staphylococcus aureus* organisms that show resistance to the methicillin family of antibiotics. This strain is a growing concern to the health-care profession.

MIC – See Minimum inhibitory concentration.

Microalbumin – Small amounts of albumin.

Microalbuminuria – Small amounts of albumin in the urine. This may be an indication of poor blood glucose control and kidney damage because of high glucose levels.

Microcollection containers – Small blood collection containers designed to be used for small amounts of blood. Often used for capillary draws, or situations in which the venipuncture is very difficult.

Microcytes – A small erythrocyte with a diameter of less than 5 μ.

Microcytic – Small erythrocytes less than 5 μ in diameter.

Micrometer (micron, μ) – One millionth of a meter, or 10^{-6}.

Microorganisms – Living organisms that are too small to be seen without the aid of a microscope.

Microscopic – A description of a structure that cannot be seen or examined without the use of magnification.

Micturition – Urination or the voiding of urine.

Minimum inhibitory concentration (MIC) – A term used to describe the lowest concentration of an antibiotic that will inhibit bacterial growth. This term is used to describe a procedure using a plate of wells that have specific antibiotics at known concentrations.

Misfeasance – Performance of a lawful act in an improper manner.

Moderate complexity – Laboratory tests that have been determined by the FDA to be moderately complex in nature. These tests require more quality control procedures, proficiency testing, and comprehensive documented personnel training than the CLIA-waived tests.

Monocular – A term used to describe a microscope that has only one ocular for viewing.

Monocyte – A mononuclear phagocytic white blood cell derived from myeloid stem cells.

Mononucleosis – An infectious disease caused by the Epstein-Barr virus.

Morphology – Description of the structure and form; term used to describe the shape of cells in a complete blood count.

Motility – Spontaneous movement; a term often used when describing microorganisms viewed in their natural state without preservation or staining.

MRSA – Acronym for methicillin-resistant *Staphylococcus aureus*. (See also Methicillin-resistant *Staphylococcus aureus*.)

Mucous membranes – Membranes lining body cavities that open to the outside of the body.

Mucus – A viscous fluid secreted by the epithelial cells.

Multiple myeloma – A malignant condition in which the bone marrow is overcome by nonfunctional cancer cells.

Multisample needle – A needle used with the evacuated tube system having a point at both ends.

Mycoses – Fungal infections.

Mycotic – A term used to describe fungal infections.

Myeloid – Pertaining to the precursor cell for granulocytes, monocytes, erythrocytes, and megakaryocytes.

Myocardial infarction – A blockage of the coronary blood vessels, resulting in damage to and death of the heart muscle.

Myoglobin – A protein that stores and uses oxygen in cardiac and skeletal muscle tissue. The blood myoglobin concentration will become elevated with damage to the heart or the skeletal muscle of the body.

Myoglobinuria – The presence of myoglobin in the urine.

Nasopharyngeal collection technique – A sample taken from the portion of the pharynx just above the soft palate. This specimen is obtained by insertion of a collection swab through the nasal cavity to the back of the throat.

Nasopharynx – The portion of the pharynx located directly behind the nose, just above the soft palate.

National Fire Protection Association (NFPA) – A nonprofit organization established in 1896 whose mission is to use education, codes and standards, research, and training to reduce fire and other hazards. This organization is known worldwide for its fire-prevention efforts.

Natural killer cells – Large lymphocytes that bind to invading cells and inject toxins, causing cell lysis.

Negligence – Occurs when a professional does not act with reasonable care.

Nephrons – The functional unit of the kidney where urine is formed.

Neutrophil – A granulocytic white blood cell responsible for much of the body's protection against infection.

Niacin – A B vitamin used to treat elevated triglyceride and cholesterol levels.

Nitrite – Nitrites are important components of the blood because they dilate blood vessels, reduce blood pressure, and perform other functions.

Nocturia – Excessive or frequent urination at night.

Nonintact skin – Skin that is broken. This may be caused by a scratch or puncture, but it may also be caused by irritation, such as develops with use of gloves and frequent hand washing.

Nonfeasance – The failure to perform a necessary medical act.

Normal flora – Resident bacteria normally present in specific areas of the body. This bacterial presence is not pathogenic.

Normal ranges – A range of results that are expected for a specific test within a certain population. Also referred to as reference ranges.

Normochromic – A red blood cell with sufficient hemoglobin.

Normocytic – A red blood cell of normal size, which is of 6 to 8 μ.

Nosocomial infection – An infection contracted in a hospital or other inpatient care facility.

O&P – Ova and parasites.

Objective lenses – The lenses of the microscope that are closest to the specimen. Compound microscopes have various levels of magnification available by using different lenses.

Occlude – To close up or obstruct, such as when a blood vessel has been blocked by a clot or plaque buildup.

Occupational exposure – Exposure that occurs while performing duties in the workplace. Occupational exposure does not always mean that there was an error in the way a task was performed; some types of exposure are inherent to all careers. For laboratory and health-care personnel, occupational exposure to bloodborne pathogens is commonplace.

Occupational Safety and Health Administration (OSHA) – A governmental agency within the Department of Labor. OSHA's mission is to ensure the health and safety of all American workers.

Ocular lenses – The lens that is closest to the eyepiece. These lenses provide a low level of magnification that is not adjustable.

Oil immersion lens – The most powerful objective lens (usually 100X magnification) that is used with a drop of oil between the lens and the slide. This allows for the light to be focused fully on the specimen without an opportunity for scatter.

Oliguria – Diminished urinary output of less than 400 mL per day.

Oncologist – A physician who specializes in the field of tumors and/or cancer treatment.

Opportunistic pathogens – Infections that usually do not cause disease in a healthy individual. When the immune system of an individual is compromised, or when there is an imbalance of some sort present, a pathogen may take advantage of the situation and cause an opportunistic infection.

Oral glucose tolerance test (OGTT) – A screening test for diabetes mellitus in which the patient is given a standardized glucose solution to drink, then has blood glucose levels checked at hourly intervals to monitor the response to the ingestion.

Other potentially infectious materials (OPIMs) – This category includes semen, vaginal secretions, cerebrospinal fluid, synovial fluid, pleural fluid, pericardial fluid, peritoneal fluid, amniotic fluid, saliva during dental procedures, breast milk, and any body fluids that are visibly contaminated with blood.

Otitis – Inflammation of the ear.

Otitis externa – Inflammation or infection of the outer ear.

Otitis media – Inflammation or infection of the middle ear.

Ova and parasite (O&P) examination – An examination of a stool sample for the presence of parasitic microorganisms or their eggs (ova).

Ovalocyte – An elliptical red blood cell.

Packed cell volume – A synonym for the hematocrit, the volume of erythrocytes packed by centrifugation in a given volume of blood.

Palpation – Process of examination by the application of the hands or fingers; assessing an area of the body by use of touch.

Panels – Groups of laboratory tests that are ordered together. These are often organ or disease specific. Also known as profiles.

Panic results – See Critical results.

Parasites – Any organism that lives on or within another living organism, often at the expense of the host organism.

Parenteral exposure – Exposure that occurred with a piercing of the skin.

Partial thromboplastin time (PTT) – Measurement of the efficacy of the intrinsic coagulation pathway. This pathway includes the actions of clotting factors VIII, IX, XI, and XII. The PTT is measured in seconds.

Pathogen – A microorganism that is capable of causing disease.

Pathological thrombosis – Formation of thrombi unnecessarily or excessively, not only in response to vessel injury.

Patient identifiers – Personal information that may identify a patient seeking care including demographics, Social Security numbers, birth dates, and the like.

Peak collection – A blood specimen drawn at the time when a medication is at its highest level in the bloodstream.

Percutaneous – Through the skin.

Peritoneum – The membrane that lines the abdominal cavity.

Pernicious anemia – A chronic macrocytic anemia in which the stomach secretes insufficient intrinsic factor for B_{12} absorption.

Personal protective equipment (PPE) – Equipment that is worn as protection for the employee, including goggles, masks, respirators, laboratory coats, or face shields.

Petri dish – A small, round dish with a flat bottom and a lid. Agar is often contained in a Petri dish for culture procedures. Petri dishes may be made of glass or plastic.

Phagocytes – A cell that has the ability to ingest and destroy antigens.

Phagocytosis (phagocytic; phagocytize) – A three-stage process by which phagocytes (certain white blood cells) engulf and destroy microorganisms, antigenic substances, and cellular debris.

Phlebotomist – A person who draws blood from a vein, capillary, or artery.

Physician office laboratories (POL) – Laboratories that are located within a physician's office that perform testing on the specimens collected from the patients of that practice.

Physiology – The study of the function of the human body.

Pinworm – Infection caused by the parasite *Enterobius vermicularis,* which is the most common type of worm infection in the United States.

Pipette – A device used in the laboratory to transfer liquid from one place to another.

Pisse prophets – Nonmedical practitioners who used urine to diagnose and predict disease without scientific basis for the practice.

Plaque – Deposits of cholesterol within blood vessels.

Plasma – The liquid portion of blood within the body. This term is also used to describe the liquid portion of a specimen when it has been drawn into a tube containing anticoagulant.

Plasma separator tubes (PST) – Tubes containing a thixotropic separating gel to form a barrier between the blood cells and the liquid portion of the blood after centrifugation.

Plasmin – An enzyme involved in the breakdown of blood clots.

Platelet – Formed element in the blood that aids in blood clotting.

Platelet count – The quantity of platelets (thrombocytes) present in a blood sample. Adequate numbers are essential for effective coagulation.

Pluripotent – Having the ability to differentiate into several types of specialized cells, a quality that stem cells are said to have.

Poikilocytosis – Variations in the shape of red blood cells.

Point-of-care testing (POCT) – Testing that is performed at the bedside or chairside of a patient, with results available within minutes.

Polychromatic stain – A staining process consisting of both an alkaline stain and an acidic stain that allows for cells to stain a variety of colors.

Polycythemia – Having an excess of red blood cells.

Polydipsia – Excessive thirst.

Polymorphonuclear – Possessing a nucleus consisting of several parts or lobes connected by fine strands.

Polyphagia – Excessive hunger.

Polyuria – Excessive urine production.

Postexposure prophylaxis (PEP) – Protective measures taken immediately after exposure to a chemical or other type of hazard. This may include medication, but may also include other types of precautions taken "just in case" after a chemical or biohazardous exposure.

Postprandial – After eating.

Precision – A statistical term that is used to describe the reproducibility of the results for a test to each other.

Prediabetes – A condition in which a patient shows early evidence of impaired carbohydrate metabolism or impaired secretion of insulin.

Privacy Rule – An expansion of the original HIPAA mandate that applies to confidentiality of health information, and the rights of patients to control access to their own records.

Proficiency testing – A process in which the test results for a specific analyte are compared to those of other laboratories that use the same testing method to verify the accuracy of the test results.

Proficiency testing – A standardized, formal assessment of the quality of test results. These are commonly performed when the laboratory is sent a sample with a known value to see how competent its testing methods are when the specimen is tested.

Profiles – A group of tests often ordered together that test for a specific body system or a specific disease process. Also known as panels.

Prophylactic – A treatment that is used to prevent a disease process or prevent an unwanted outcome.

Prostatitis – Inflammation of the prostate.

Prostatitis specimen – A urine specimen collected to identify a bacterial infection of the prostate.

Prostatitis specimen collection process – A special procedure for collecting urine in which there are three specimens collected in close progression.

Protected health information (PHI) – All information about a patient included in his or her medical record.

Proteinuria – The presence of protein in the urine.

Prothrombin time (PT; protime) – A measurement (in seconds) of the time needed for blood to clot when thromboplastin and calcium are added to a plasma specimen. This test is used to evaluate those who are on oral anticoagulant therapy as well as to screen for potential clotting disorders.

Protime – See Prothrombin time.

Protoporphyrin – A substance included in the heme portion of the hemoglobin molecule. Necessary to make iron functional and available to attach to the oxygen.

Protozoa – Complex single-cell microorganisms, most of which are nonpathogenic.

Provider-performed microscopy (PPM) – Microscopy examinations performed by a health-care provider in the office. To perform these legally, the laboratory will need to be registered with CLIA as a facility that performs PPM.

Provider-performed microscopy procedures (PPMPs) – These are laboratory procedures that are performed by a midlevel provider or a physician using a microscope.

The examinations are performed on specimens that are unfixed and time sensitive, such as urine sediment microscopic examinations and wet mounts. There are specific quality control requirements that accompany this type of laboratory procedure, including maintenance on the microscope used for the examination.

Proximal convoluted tubule – The proximal part of the renal tubule where the renal filtrate first enters after it leaves the Bowman's capsule.

Plasma separator tubes (PSTs) – PSTs contain a thixotropic gel that separates the blood cells from the liquid when spun in a centrifuge.

Pus – The liquid product of inflammation, including dead cells, fluid, and pathogens.

Pyuria – The presence of white blood cells or "pus" in the urine specimen.

Qualitative – A term used to describe results which indicate whether or not a substance is present in a specimen, rather than the amount of the substance that is present. Qualitative tests provide a positive or negative result.

Qualitative result – A test that determines the presence or absence of a substance, having a yes/no or positive/negative result.

Quality assurance – All the processes used to assure quality in laboratory testing, including all phases of the laboratory experience: before, during, and after the test is performed.

Quality control (QC) – Practices used in the laboratory to ensure that the results for a given test are correct.

Quantitative HCG – A test that provides a numeric result for the presence of human chorionic gonadotropin (HCG) in serum. This test may be necessary if an ectopic pregnancy or fetal demise is suspected.

Quantitative result – A test that determines the amount of a specific substance in a sample. The result is expressed as a number or percentage.

Quantitative test – A test that provides a numeric result, indicating the level of the analyte present in the specimen.

Quantity not sufficient (QNS) specimen – A specimen that is not of sufficient quantity for testing.

RACE – An acronym used to remind employees of the order of action in the event of a fire. R: Rescue those who might be in danger; A: Alarm, activate the alarm system; C: Confine the fire as much as possible by closing doors and windows; E: Extinguish the fire if possible.

Radioimmunoassay (RIA) testing – A testing method in which the antigen or antibody in the specimen binds to a radioactive substance to be measured.

Random – Without plan or purpose or pattern. When used in connection with urine specimen collection, *random* refers to specimens collected at unspecified intervals.

Random collection – A specimen that can be drawn at any time of the day without limitations or special preparation.

Rapid flow immunoassay – A term that may be used interchangeably with lateral flow immunoassay. Rapid flow immunoassay also describes test methods in which the specimen/reagents do not flow laterally across the surface.

Reabsorption – The process by which water and other necessary substances are reabsorbed into the body through the capillaries that surround the renal tubules.

Reagent dipstick – A plastic strip that is imbedded with various reagent pads that test for chemicals in urine specimens.

Reagent strips – Strips of material (usually some type of plastic) that have been covered or treated with chemicals. These are designed to change color or produce certain substances as part of a chemical reaction. Reagent strips are designed to be used one time only, and may be used to detect the presence of a certain substance in a specimen or to measure the amount of a specific substance.

Red blood cell (RBC) – Formed element in the blood; primary function of red blood cells is to transport oxygen.

Red blood cell index – A calculated value that helps to classify RBCs in terms of size and hemoglobin concentration.

Reference laboratory – A reference laboratory is a private commercial laboratory that tests a high volume of specimens, and often performs highly specialized tests that are not available at a physician office laboratory or a hospital laboratory. The reference laboratory receives specimens from other laboratories, and hospital or physician office laboratories, not just from their general community. Specimens may be shipped from all over the country.

Reference ranges – The expected ranges for a specific population for an analyte. These ranges can vary by age, gender, or race. Ranges are established by each laboratory, based on testing method.

Reflexive testing – A policy in which follow-up tests are added automatically to a specimen when abnormal results are found with the initial testing ordered. This often applies to culture and urine specimens.

Reflexive – The automatic performance of additional laboratory testing in response to abnormal test results. For urine, the urine microscopic examination is often added on as a reflexive test for abnormal urine chemistry results.

Refractive index – A measurement of how much light is deflected from its normal path when it passes through a different media. The amount of deflection may be affected by the concentration of dissolved substances in the medium.

Refractometer – An instrument used to determine the specific gravity of a liquid.

Regulated waste – See Biohazardous waste.

Renal cortex – The outer layer of the kidney.

Renal medulla – The inner layer of the kidney.

Renal pelvis – A basin-shaped hollow structure that collects urine as it is formed before it exits the kidney through the ureters.

Renal tubule – The area of the nephron where reabsorption and secretion occur as urine is formed.

Reportable condition – A condition or disease that has been deemed a threat to the public.

Resident bacteria – Another term used to describe normal flora.

Resistant – A bacterial microorganism that is not affected by the properties of a specific antibiotic.

Reticulocyte – The last immature stage of red blood cells; when stained with a supravital stain, the darkly staining granules are fragments of the endoplasmic reticulum.

Reticulum – A mesh-like microscopic network in a cell.

Retroperitoneal – Behind the peritoneum.

Revolving nosepiece – The part of a microscope where the objectives attach. The revolving nosepiece can be turned as the different objectives are utilized.

RhoGam – A type of immune globulin used to protect neonates who have Rh-negative mothers.

Risk management – Ways of reducing potential risk to patients, employees, and employers.

Rotations per minute (rpm) – Used to measure the speed at which a centrifuge operates.

Rouleaux – A group of red blood cells that are stuck together, resembling a roll of coins.

Rugae – A fold or crease in the cells lining various areas of the body that allows for more stretching and flexibility of these areas.

Sanitization – To remove microorganisms from equipment or surfaces.

Scabies – An infection of the skin with a parasitic mite that causes intense itching.

Scope of practice – The various activities that a professional is qualified to perform. This may be based on education and/or experience and differs by profession.

Secretion – The final process in urine formation within the renal tubules. During secretion, substances are added to the urine filtrate from the capillaries that are wrapped around the renal tubules.

Sediment – Formed elements in the urine specimen that settle to the bottom of the urine specimen when spun in the centrifuge.

Semiquantitative – A type of testing procedure that provides an approximate amount of a substance.

Sensitive – A bacterial microorganism that is killed or kept from multiplying by the use of a specific antibiotic.

Sensitivity – The minimum concentration of the desired substance that will be detected.

Septicemia – Infection of the bloodstream by a pathogenic microorganism.

Sequela – A secondary complication or infection as a result of the primary infection.

Serially – A series at set intervals. This term is used to describe laboratory samples that are to be collected at specific intervals over a period of time.

Serology – The study of the antigen and antibody components in the liquid portion of the blood or other body fluids.

Serotonin – A chemical vasoconstrictor.

Serum – The liquid portion of the blood without the various clotting factors. Serum is taken from a blood specimen that has been allowed to clot before centrifugation.

Serum separator tubes (SST) – Tubes that contain a thixotropic separating gel that is designed to form a barrier between the blood cells and the liquid portion of the blood after it is centrifuged.

Sharp – Any object that has projections, corners, or edges that are capable of piercing the skin. If the object has come into contact with blood or other potentially infectious materials, it is a biohazardous sharp. These must be disposed of in a special, puncture-proof container.

Shift – A sudden change in quality control values. This may be a shift from one side of the mean to another, or a significant jump in values on the same side of the mean.

Short draw – When there has been a loss of vacuum in the evacuated tube, blood will not enter the tube, or it will fill incompletely. Often, this requires that the specimen be redrawn.

Sickle cell – Red blood cell changed to a crescent shape by low oxygen tension. These cells contain the abnormal hemoglobin, Hb S.

Sickle cell anemia – An inherited autosomal recessive trait in which the individual's red blood cells contain hemoglobin S.

Sickle cell trait – Condition of being heterozygous for Hb S in which each red blood cell has Hb A and Hb S; these cells become sickled under extremely low oxygen tension.

Slander – Untrue statements that are spoken about another person.

Slant – A tube with agar added and allowed to harden in a slanted form to allow for maximum surface area for bacterial growth.

Specific gravity – The weight of a substance as compared to an equal volume of distilled water. The specific gravity of urine provides an indication of the amount of dissolved substances present in the specimen.

Specificity – The ability to detect only the desired substance in the specimen.

Specimens – A piece or part of something that is designed to show the characteristics of the whole.

Spectrophotometer – A machine (or part of a machine) that is used to measure how much light of a certain wavelength has been absorbed by a specimen.

Spectrophotometrically – An estimation of coloring matter in a solution by wavelength of light.

Splenomegaly – An enlarged spleen.

Spermatozoa – A mature male sex cell.

Spherocyte – An erythrocyte that assumes a spheroid shape and has no central pallor.

Spirilla – Bacteria that have a spiral shape when viewed under the microscope.

Spores – A dormant bacterial form that is resistant to heat and moisture. Spores are the form that many bacteria assume when conditions are unfavorable, and this protective form allows them to survive until the conditions become more comfortable for growth and replication.

Sputum – Mucus that is expelled from the lungs and lower respiratory system with a deep cough.

Stage – The portion of a microscope where the glass slide is placed for viewing.

Standard of care – An acceptable level of performance for the employees within a profession.

Standard precautions – Guidelines developed by the CDC to assist with the spread of infectious disease in health-care facilities.

Standing orders – Orders for laboratory tests to be drawn at specific intervals over a period of time.

Staphylococci – Bacteria that are round and appear in grape-like clusters when viewed under a microscope.

STAT – Something that is to be accomplished immediately.

Statins – A classification of drugs used to treat patients with elevated lipid levels. Statins are especially effective for treatment of elevated LDL levels and triglycerides.

Statutes – Laws established by the legislative branch of a government entity.

Stem cells – Precursors of all blood cells that are present in the bone marrow.

Stereomicroscope – A microscope that allows a specimen to be viewed from two different angles to create a three-dimensional image. Also known as a dissecting microscope.

Sterilize – A process by which all microorganisms are destroyed on a surface.

Strep screens – CLIA-waived procedures often performed in a physician office laboratory. These tests employ a throat swab specimen and produce results within minutes. Strep screens test for group A streptococci, and allow for timely treatment of streptococcal throat infections.

Streptococcal pharyngitis – Inflammation and infection of the pharynx and tonsillar area caused by group A streptococcal bacteria.

Streptococci – Bacteria that appear round and in small "chains" when viewed under the microscope.

Stroke – A loss of neurological function that is caused by vessel injury or occlusion in the blood vessels of the brain. Also known as a cerebrovascular accident (CVA).

Sulfosalicylic acid precipitation test – A test that uses turbidity as a measure of the presence of protein in the urine.

Supernatant – The clear part of the urine specimen left at the top of the tube after the sediment has settled out to the bottom of the tube.

Suprapubic aspiration – A procedure used to remove urine from the bladder when traditional catheterization is not an option. Suprapubic aspiration uses a syringe and needle to aspirate urine directly from the bladder. The needle is inserted through the external abdominal wall.

Surgical asepsis – The destruction of all pathogenic organisms before they enter the body. This involves the use of sterile supplies for invasive procedures.

Susceptible – Having very little or no defense from infection by a specific microorganism.

Syringe system – A method of drawing blood that involves a syringe with a needle attached. This method is used when a patient has veins that may not be able to withstand the evacuated tube method, which applies a lot of reverse pressure all at once, which may collapse the vein.

T cells – Specialized lymphocytic white blood cells that are programmed in the thymus to serve as part of the immune response.

Tachometer – An instrument used to measure rotation speed.

Target cell – An erythrocyte that has a reduced hemoglobin concentration and appears with a little color around the edge of the cell and a dark central area.

Thalassemia – Inherited disorders in which abnormal hemoglobin is produced by either a defective production rate of the alpha or beta globin chains or a decreased synthesis of the beta chain.

Thrombin – An enzyme that converts fibrinogen to fibrin, which is necessary for definitive blood clot formation.

Thrombocytes – Platelets.

Thrombocythemia – Overproduction of platelets by the bone marrow.

Thrombocytopenia – An abnormal decrease in the number of platelets.

Thrombocytosis – An increase in the number of platelets.

Thrombopoietin – A growth factor that acts on the bone marrow to stimulate platelet production as well as the production of other cell lines.

Thrombosis – A blood clot formed in response to vascular injury, or pathological formation of a blood clot.

Thrombus – A blood clot that adheres to the wall of a vessel or organ.

Thyroid-stimulating hormone (TSH) – A hormone produced by the pituitary gland that stimulates the thyroid gland to produce thyroxine, thyrocalcitonin, and triiodothyronine.

Thyroxine (T4) – A hormone produced by the thyroid gland that affects the rate of metabolism of the cells throughout the body.

Tort – Wrongs that are committed that do not involve a contractual agreement.

Tourniquet – A stretchy, rubber-like band that is applied to the arm to facilitate the location of veins to be used for blood draws.

Transient bacteria – Bacteria that are not part of the normal flora of the body. These are the bacteria that are picked up on the hands and skin during daily activities and those that are washed off when washing the hands.

Transmissible – Something that is capable of being passed, or transmitted, to another.

Trends – A slow, steady incline or decline in the quality control values over time.

Trichomoniasis – Infection with a parasite that often lives in the vagina in women or urethra in men. This parasite causes discharge, itching, and burning, and may be transmitted through sexual intercourse.

Triiodothyronine (T3) – A hormone produced by the thyroid gland that affects the rate of metabolism of the cells throughout the body.

Troponin – A muscle protein that is found in skeletal and cardiac muscle, but not smooth muscle. An elevated cardiac troponin level is one of the first indicators of heart trauma.

Troubleshooting – Investigative processes employed when the quality control specimens are not within the expected ranges.

Trough collection – A specimen drawn at the time when a medication is at the lowest level in the bloodstream. This is usually drawn immediately before the next dose is due.

Type 1 diabetes – Diabetes that results from inadequate or absent insulin secretion. Extended periods of hyperglycemia result, and treatment involves insulin injections.

Type 2 diabetes – Diabetes that results from insulin resistance. Type 2 diabetes is usually successfully treated with lifestyle changes and oral medications.

Unintentional tort – A wrongful act that is accidentally committed by one person against another person.

Universal precautions – The concept that all blood products and other potentially infectious materials are to be treated as if they are infected with bloodborne pathogens.

Ureters – The tubes that carry urine from the kidney to the bladder. Most individuals have two ureters, one for each kidney.

Urethra – The tube that extends from the bladder to the outside of the body through which urine travels.

Urinalysis – Analysis of a urine specimen. The urinalysis usually includes a macroscopic examination of the specimen for color and clarity, measurement of the specific gravity of the specimen, testing for various chemicals, and may also include microscopic examination for suspended structures in the specimen.

Urinary frequency – An increase in the urge to urinate.

Urinary incontinence – Involuntary urination.

Urinary meatus – The external opening of the urethra.

Urine culture – The process by which a urine specimen is added to a medium containing nutrients that nurture the growth of pathogenic microorganisms.

Urine microscopic – The examination of urine sediment under the microscope for detection and quantification of structures suspended in the urine.

Urinometer – A type of hydrometer used to measure specific gravity of urine. A urinometer has a float that will fall to a depth measured at 1.000 when used with distilled water, but will not fall to this depth in urine specimens with an increase in dissolved substances.

Urobilinogen – A derivative of bilirubin; bilirubin is converted to urobilinogen by intestinal bacteria.

Urochrome – A pigment that gives urine its characteristic yellow color.

Uroscopy – The name originally used to describe the analysis of urine specimens. This name is no longer used routinely.

U.S. Department of Health and Human Services (HHS) – An agency that assumes the overall responsibility for laboratory quality assurance as designated in CLIA '88.

U.S. Food and Drug Administration (FDA) – The federal agency responsible for assigning the level of complexity for various laboratory tests.

Vaccine – A substance containing altered antigenic material used to stimulate an immune response to a particular pathogen and provide protection. Vaccines are usually injected.

Vacuum – A space that has all the air removed, creating a "vacuum" when it is opened (or pierced in the case of the vacuum tubes used for venipuncture).

Valid – A term used to describe a test result that can safely be reported. This usually refers to qualitative tests, in which there is an indicator on the testing device to show that the test result is valid. This is independent of whether the result is positive or negative.

Vasodilation – An enlargement of a vein due to the relaxation of the vessel walls.

Vasovagal syncope – Loss of consciousness, usually related to a stressful or upsetting event, such as a blood draw.

Vector – A carrier of pathogenic microorganisms. The vector is usually unaffected by the pathogen that it carries, but it is able to transmit it to a susceptible individual.

Veins – Blood vessels in the body that carry blood from the capillary beds back to the heart.

Venules – The smallest vessels in the venous system. Capillary vessels gradually enlarge and change in structure to become venules. Venules then become veins.

Virus – A microorganism that is too small to be seen without the aid of a microscope with advanced technology. Viruses consist of genetic material wrapped in a protein coating, and they use the genetic information of the host cell to reproduce themselves.

Viscous – Thick, sticky, or syrupy.

Very low-density lipoprotein (VLDL) – A subclass of cholesterol. Elevated VLDL levels are linked to an increased chance of plaque formation in the blood vessels.

von Willebrand's factor – A glycoprotein that is present in plasma. It carries clotting factor VIII, which is necessary for blood hemostasis. von Willebrand's factor also interacts with other processes in the clotting cascade.

Warfarin – An oral anticoagulant.

Water baths – A tank filled with water to be heated to a specific temperature. Test tubes are suspended in the heated water to speed up certain chemical reactions during testing procedures.

Westergren erythrocyte sedimentation rate (ESR) – A test performed in which the anticoagulated blood is mixed with a sodium citrate or saline solution prior to transfer into the pipette for testing.

Wet mount – A method used to observe living organisms microscopically without staining or preserving the specimen. This is especially useful when observing the movement (or motility) of microorganisms. A wet mount is essentially a suspension of the specimen placed on a slide for observation under the microscope.

White blood cell (WBC) – Formed element in the blood; the primary function of white blood cells is to provide immunity for the body.

Window period – The period of HIV infection when the infected individual does not test positive in typical laboratory tests, but is still capable of transmitting the disease. This period can last for several months after infection.

Winged infusion set – A butterfly setup. The winged infusion set consists of a needle (usually a half inch in length) attached to a piece of plastic tubing. The needle has plastic "wings" on both sides where the fingers grip the device while drawing blood.

Wintrobe erythrocyte sedimentation rate (ESR) – A method of performing the ESR in which the anticoagulated blood is placed directly into a short Wintrobe tube specifically designed to perform the ESR. The tube is graduated in millimeters for reading the results. The tubes are usually made of glass.

Wood's lamp – A lamp used for examination of the skin. The Wood's lamp uses ultraviolet light to detect organisms or areas of the body that fluoresce. Many mycotic infections produce fluorescence.

Work practice controls – Controls that alter the manner in which a task is performed to minimize the risk of exposure to bloodborne pathogens.

Zone of inhibition – The area around a specific antibiotic disk where the growth of the microorganism is absent. The organism on the culture plate is sensitive (susceptible) to the antibiotic that is on the disk.

INDEX

Note page numbers followed by an *f* indicate figures; page numbers followed by a *t* indicate tables.